Kimberly A. Sackheim
Editor

Pain Management and Palliative Care

A Comprehensive Guide

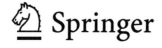 Springer

Editor
Kimberly A. Sackheim
Department of Rehabilitation Medicine
Interventional Pain Management
New York University
Langone Medical Center
New York, NY, USA

ISBN 978-1-4939-2461-5   ISBN 978-1-4939-2462-2   (eBook)
DOI 10.1007/978-1-4939-2462-2

Library of Congress Control Number: 2015933514

Springer New York Heidelberg Dordrecht London

Springer Science+Business Media LLC New York is part of Springer Science+Business Media (www.springer.com)

To my beautiful daughters. May you get everything you want in life. Always follow your dreams.

In loving memory of Anita.

Foreword

The 2011 Institute of Medicine (IOM) report—"Relieving Pain in America: A Blueprint for Transforming Prevention, Care, Education, and Research"—highlights a sobering statistic: Chronic pain affects approximately 100 million American adults, more than heart disease, cancer, and diabetes combined. Pain is a major reason for visits to healthcare professionals, and most people with chronic pain seek help outside the healthcare system whether or not they obtain medical care. Very few patients with pain ever see a physician with subspecialty training in pain management or palliative care. Most patients with chronic pain are older and have one or more chronic medical disorders. Numerous studies have linked pain with the use of multiple medications and other treatments, and many have demonstrated the association between pain and impaired work and role functioning, disturbed mood and sleep, stress on the family, and relatively poor quality of life. The combined pain-related cost of treatment and loss of workforce productivity may reach as much as $635 billion annually.

These observations underscore the reality that chronic pain is both a profound clinical issue and a public health challenge. From the public health perspective, the IOM has called for a strategy that embraces population-level changes that can raise consciousness among professionals and the public and improve pain assessment and management in the diverse systems that deliver health care. In so doing, government will certainly seek to apply those precepts that are at the heart of healthcare reform. These include a focus on quality, safety, and patient satisfaction and the elimination of disparities in access to care. They also focus on cost containment through incentives for attainable outcomes and, most important, a shift from a fee-for-service system to one that shares risk for managing populations in varied models. Hopefully, the public health imperative in unrelieved chronic pain can be simply incorporated within the broad changes now emerging in health care, and ultimately, the efforts made to improve the public health will favorably affect the clinical work necessary to help the individual with chronic pain.

From the clinical perspective, the observations highlighted in the IOM report support the view that pain is best understood as a serious illness in its own right. Although clinical management always should include a search for an underlying pathology that can explain the persistence of pain, neither the association between pain and chronic disease nor the hopeful fact that disease management can sometimes relieve pain diminishes the distinct importance of the pain phenomenon itself. Patients always deserve access to competent assessment and management of pain, even if there are likely to be effective treatments for its cause.

Those with pain commonly engage in self-management strategies, often with the input of those who promote and sell products and services that purport to help. If this reflects self-efficacy, it may be salutary; if indicative of impeded access to medical care, it is part of the problem in need of redress. Patients who do access medical care for pain may do so through primary care or specialty care, or in pain subspecialty practices. The array of potentially useful treatments available to providers in all these settings is impressive: dozens of drug therapies, interventions such as injections and implants, rehabilitative approaches, psychoeducational and behavioral techniques, neurostimulation approaches, and complementary and alternative therapies.

In accessing care for pain, patients rely on the knowledge, skills, and judgment of healthcare professionals. Many pain therapies, such as long-term administration of opioids or

NSAIDs, spinal injections or neural blockade, and implanted generators or pumps, may or may not benefit the individual and carry substantial risks over time, and patients must trust that the professionals they see are knowledgeable and competent as they navigate the complex arena of pain management.

The IOM emphasizes the need for an educated professional force. Education about pain is essential for physicians and nonphysicians and for generalists and specialists alike. There should be content about the complex biological and psychosocial aspects to pain, pain syndromes, and the best practices supporting the use of both self-help and therapeutic approaches to ameliorate pain and aid in adaptation to the pain that remains. Undergraduate and graduate programs should offer information about pain, and continuing education that is current and readily accessible is needed for primary care providers and specialists alike. Professionals need to understand the evidence base, and as research slowly expands what is known, educated clinicians can ensure that treatments based on the best available evidence and expert experience are undertaken with increasing safety and efficacy.

Clinical materials are essential tools in broadening access to education, and there is a never-ending need for materials in varied formats. There is great value in books, such as Sackheim's *Pain Management and Palliative Care*: *A Clinical Guide*, that offer clinically relevant information for a medical audience about an array of topics relevant in both generalist and specialist practice. This volume emphasizes common syndromes and treatments, with particular attention to pharmacotherapy and interventions. It is useful information for those who manage chronic pain and a piece of a broader foundation in pain assessment and management essential in addressing the public health and clinical imperatives of poorly controlled pain.

New York, NY, USA   Russell K. Portenoy, M.D.
                                                                          Director
                                           MJHS Institute for Innovation in Palliative Care
                                                                Chief Medical Officer
                                                        MJHS Hospice and Palliative Care
                                                               Professor of Neurology
                                                       Albert Einstein College of Medicine
                                                                     New York, NY

Preface

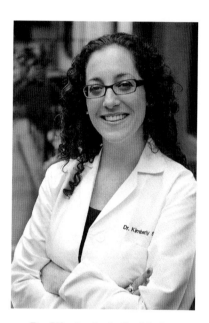

Dr. Kimberly A. Sackheim

This book is a comprehensive yet concise guide to interventional and medical pain management and palliative care. It can be used as an invaluable daily companion for physicians in all specialities as a quick reference and guide to the diagnosis and treatment of these patients and conditions. Whether being treated for an infection, fracture, or chronic medical condition, all patients experience pain which should be properly managed.

New York, NY, USA

Dr. Kimberly A. Sackheim

Contents

Part V Interventional Management for the Pain Patient

Contributors

Editor

Kimberly A. Sackheim Department of Rehabilitation Medicine, Interventional Pain Management, New York University Langone Medical Center, New York, NY, USA

Authors

Andrew Kamal Abdou, B.S. New York University—Rusk Institute for Rehabilitation Medicine, Physical Medicine & Rehabilitation, Ambulatory Care Center, New York, NY, USA

Kathy Aligene, M.D. Department of Rehabilitation Medicine, Mount Sinai School of Medicine, Physical Medicine and Rehabilitation, New York, NY, USA

Division of Pain Medicine, Department of Anesthesiology, Icahn School of Medicine at Mount Sinai, New York, NY, USA

Jared D. Anderson, M.D. Department of Anesthesiology/Pain Medicine, Baylor Scott & White Health/Texas A&M College of Medicine, College Station, TX, USA

Melinda Aquino, M.D. Department of Family and Social Medicine, Montefiore Medical Center, Albert Einstein College of Medicine, Bronx, NY, USA

Department of Anesthesiology, Montefiore Medical Center, Albert Einstein College of Medicine, Bronx, NY, USA

Sait Ashina, M.D. Department of Pain Medicine and Palliative Care, Beth Israel Medical Center, New York, NY, USA

Levan Atanelov, M.D., M.S. Department of Physical Medicine and Rehabilitation, Johns Hopkins Hospital, Baltimore, MD, USA

Shan Babeendran, D.O. Department of Rehabilitation Medicine, New York University Langone Medical Center, New York, NY, USA

Christopher J. Burnett, M.D., F.I.P.P. Department of Anesthesia and Perioperative Care, University of California San Francisco Medical Center, University of California San Francisco, Temple, TX, USA

Tim Canty, M.D. Comprehensive Spine and Pain Center, State University of New York Downstate Medical Center, New York, NY, USA

Tita Castor, M.D., F.A.C.P. Palliative Care Service, Elmhurst Hospital Center, Elmhurst, NY, USA

Geriatrics and Palliative Medicine, Icahn School of Medicine at Mount Sinai, New York, NY, USA

SriKrishna Chandran, M.D. Department of Physical Medicine and Rehabilitation, Johns Hopkins Hospital, Baltimore, MD, USA

Richard G. Chang, M.D., M.P.H. Department of Physiatry, Hospital for Special Surgery, New York, NY, USA

Halland Chen, M.D. Manhattan Pain Management & Rehabilitation, New York, NY, USA

Houman Danesh, M.D. Division of Pain Medicine, Department of Anesthesiology, Icahn School of Medicine at Mount Sinai, New York, NY, USA

Laurie Daste, M.D. Department of Anesthesiology, Ochsner Medical Center, New Orleans, LA, USA

Anjuli Desai, M.D. Interventional Pain Physician, Capitol Pain Institute, Austin, TX, USA

Jignyasa Desai, D.O. Interventional Pain Management Physician, Edgewater, NJ, USA

Sudhir Diwan, M.D., F.I.P.P., A.B.I.P.P. Manhattan Spine and Pain Medicine, SUNY Downstate Medical Center, Lenox Hill Hospital, New York, NY, USA

Adam C. Ehrlich, M.D., M.P.H. Department of Medicine, Section of Gastroenterology, Temple University Hospital, Philadelphia, PA, USA

Brandon Rock Esenther, M.D. Department of Anesthesiology, New York Presbyterian—Columbia, New York, NY, USA

Brian Richard Forzani, M.D. Department of Rehabilitation Medicine, New York University Langone Medical Center, New York, NY, USA

Michelle S. Gentile, M.D., Ph.D. Department of Radiation Oncology, Northwestern Memorial Hospital, Chicago, IL, USA

Clifford Gevirtz, M.D., M.P.H. LSU Health Sciences Center, New Orleans, LA, USA

Somnia Pain Management, New Rochelle, NY, USA

Joslyn Gober Nova Southeastern University College of Osteopathic Medicine, Fort Lauderdale, FL, USA

Karina Gritsenko, M.D. Department of Family and Social Medicine, Montefiore Medical Center, Albert Einstein College of Medicine, Bronx, NY, USA

Department of Anesthesiology, Montefiore Medical Center, Albert Einstein College of Medicine, Bronx, NY, USA

Joyce Ho, M.D. University of California Irvine, Physical Medicine and Rehabilitation, Irvine, CA, USA

Melanie Howell, D.O. Department of Rehabilitation Medicine, New York University Langone Medical Center, New York, NY, USA

Anthony Isenalumhe Jr., M.D. Pain Management/Anesthesiology, Stanford Medical Center, Mountain View, CA, USA

Robin Iversen, M.D. Rutgers New Jersey Medical School, The Valley Hospital, Ridgewood, NJ, USA

Alan David Kaye, M.D., Ph.D. Department of Anesthesiology, Interim LSU Hospital and Ochsner Kenner Hospital, New Orleans, LA, USA

Department of Pharmacology, Interim LSU Hospital and Ochsner Kenner Hospital, New Orleans, LA, USA

Yury Khelemsky, M.D., Division of Pain Medicine, Department of Anesthesiology, Icahn School of Medicine at Mount Sinai, New York, NY, USA

Surendra B. Kholla, M.D. Department of Urology, UCI Medical Center, Orange, CA, USA

Phong Kieu, M.D. Department of Orthopedics and Sports Medicine, John Peter Smith Hospital, Arlington, TX, USA

Lisa Kilcoyne, M.D. Department of Anesthesiology, Division of Pain Medicine, New York Presbyterian Hospital, Columbia University, New York, NY, USA

Jonathan S. Kirschner, M.D., R.M.S.K. Department of Physiatry, Hospital for Special Surgery, Assistant Professor of Clinical Rehabilitation Medicine, Weill Cornell Medical College, New York, NY, USA

Stephen Kishner, M.D. Department of Physical Medicine and Rehabilitation, Louisiana State University School of Medicine, New Orleans, New Orleans, LA, USA

Holly M. Koncicki, M.D., M.S. Department of Medicine, Division of Kidney Diseases and Hypertension, Hofstra North Shore-LIJ School of Medicine, Great Neck, NY, USA

Rodney R. Lange, M.D. Department of Anesthesiology/Pain Medicine, Baylor Scott & White Health/Texas A&M College of Medicine, Marble Falls, TX, USA

Angela Lee, M.D. Department of Anesthesiology, Columbia University Medical Center, New York Presbyterian Hospital, New York, NY, USA

Marc S. Lener, M.D. Department of Psychiatry, Icahn School of Medicine at Mount Sinai, New York, NY, USA

Alyssa Lettich, M.D. Intermountain Neurosciences Institute, Intermountain Medical Center, Murray, Utah, USA

Eric Leung, M.D. Department of Rehabilitation Medicine, Icahn School of Medicine at Mount Sinai, New York, NY, USA

Aleksandr Levchenko, D.O. Department of Rehabilitation Medicine, New York University Langone Medical Center, New York, NY, USA

Felix S. Linetsky, M.D. Department of Osteopathic Principles and Practice, Nova Southeastern University of Osteopathic Medicine, Clearwater, FL, USA

Jackson Liu, M.D. Department of Physical Medicine and Rehabilitation, New York University Langone Medical Center, Woodside, NY, USA

Benjamin P. Lowry, M.D. Department of Anesthesiology, Baylor Scott & White Health/Texas A&M College of Medicine, Temple, TX, USA

Rudy Malayil, M.D. Beth Israel Medical Center, New York, NY, USA

Anuj Malhotra, M.D. Division of Pain Medicine, Department of Anesthesiology, Icahn School of Medicine at Mount Sinai, New York, NY, USA

Leena Mathew, M.D. Division of Pain Medicine, Department of Anesthesiology, New York Presbyterian Hospital, Columbia University, New York, NY, USA

Staicy Mathew, M.D. Department of Orthopedics, Hospital for Joint Disease at NYULMC, New York, NY, USA

Russell K. McAllister, M.D. D.A.B.P.M. Department of Anesthesiology, Baylor Scott & White Health/Texas A&M College of Medicine, Temple, TX, USA

Niall G. Monaghan, M.D. Department of Rehabilitation Medicine, New York Presbyterian Hospital, New York, NY, USA

Geet Paul, M.D. Department of Rehabilitation Medicine, Mount Sinai Medical Center, New York, NY, USA

Tamer Refaat, M.D., Ph.D., M.S.C.I. Department of Radiation Oncology, Northwestern University, Chicago, IL, USA

Thomas A. Riolo, D.O. Department of Rehabilitation Medicine, New York University Langone Medical Center, New York, NY, USA

John-Ross Rizzo, M.D. Department of Rehabilitation Medicine, New York University Langone Medical Center, New York, NY, USA

Jeremy J. Robbins, D.O. Department of Anesthesiology, University of Missouri Health System, Columbia, MO, USA

Julia Sackheim, D.O. Department of Internal Medicine, Stony Brook University Hospital, Stony Brook, NY, USA

Adam M. Savage, M.D. Department of Anesthesiology—Pain Management, Scott & White Hospital, Temple, TX, USA

Yolanda Scott, M.D. Department of Rehabilitation Medicine, Icahn School of Medicine at Mount Sinai, New York, NY, USA

Sovrin M. Shah, M.D. Department of Urology, Female Pelvic Medicine and Reconstructive Surgery, Icahn School of Medicine at Mount Sinai Mount Sinai Beth Israel, New York, NY, USA

Jason W. Siefferman, M.D. Division of Pain Medicine, Department of Anesthesiology, New York University School of Medicine, New York, NY, USA
Manhattan Pain Medicine, New York, NY, USA

Earl L. Smith, M.D., Ph.D. Department of Rehabilitation Medicine, Emory Palliative Care Center, Emory University, Atlanta, Georgia, USA

Eli Soto, M.D., D.A.B.P.M., F.I.P.P. Anesthesia Pain Care Consultants, Tamarac, FL, USA

Ariel C. Soucie, D.P.T. Aureus Medical Group, Portsmouth, NH, USA

Amir Soumekh, M.D. Department of Medicine, Division of Gastroenterology and Hepatology, Weill Cornell Medical College, New York, NY, USA

David Spinner, D.O. Beth Israel Deaconess Medical Center, Harvard Medical School, Brookline, MA, USA

Danna Ogden, D.O. Department of Hospice and Palliative Medicine, Kaiser Permanente, Portland, OR, USA

Fani Thomson, D.O., D.A.B.I.P.P. Physical Examination, Valley Institute for Pain, Valley Hospital, Paramus, NJ, USA

Samir Tomajian, M.D. Gulfport Memorial Hospital, Gulfport, MS, USA

Juliet P. Tran, M.D., M.P.H. Department of Family Medicine, East Jefferson General Hospital, Metairie, LA, USA

Andrea M. Trescot, M.D. Pain and Headache Center, Wasilla, AK, USA

Kiran Vadada, M.D. Interventional Spine and Sports Medicine, Spine Center and Orthopedic Rehabilitation of Englewood, Englewood, NJ, USA

Christopher A.J. Webb, M.D. Department of Anesthesia and Perioperative Care, University of California San Francisco Medical Center, University of California San Francisco, San Francisco, CA, USA

Paul D. Weyker, M.D. Department of Anesthesia and Perioperative Care, University of California San Francisco Medical Center, University of California San Francisco, San Francisco, CA, USA

Matthias H. Wiederholz, M.D. Performance Spine and Sports Medicine, Lawrenceville, NJ, USA

Isaac Wu, M.D. Department of Anesthesiology, New York Presbyterian Hospital, Columbia University Medical Center, New York, NY, USA

James F. Wyss, M.D., P.T. Department of Rehabilitation Medicine, Hospital for Special Surgery, Weill Cornell Medical College, New York, NY, USA

Part I

Evaluation of the Pain Patient

Physiology of Pain

1

Eric Leung

Abbreviations

ACC	Anterior cingulate cortex
CNS	Central nervous system
CRPS	Complex regional pain syndrome
GABA	Gamma-aminobutyric acid
NDMA	N-Methyl-d-aspartate
PAG	Periaqueductal gray
RVM	Rostral ventromedial medulla
TRPV	Vanilloid receptor
VPL	Ventroposteriolateral
WDR	Wide dynamic range

Definitions

Pain: a conscious experience that is affected by the peripheral nervous system, central somatosensory processing, and psychosocial/emotional processes [1]

Nociception: the physiologic activation of neural pathway by stimuli (noxious, thermal, mechanical, or chemical) that are potential or currently damaging [2]

Afferent nerve: a sensory or receptor neuron; carries impulse from organ to CNS

Efferent nerve: a motor neuron; carries impulse away from CNS to muscle

Pathway of Pain (Fig. 1.1)

1. *Transduction*—peripheral (primary) afferent nerves convert noxious stimuli to a unique frequency of electrical impulses (action potentials) that travel down the nerve

E. Leung, M.D. (✉)
Department of Rehabilitation Medicine, Icahn School of Medicine at Mount Sinai, One Gustave L. Levy Place, Box 1240, New York, NY 10029, USA
e-mail: eric.leung@mountsinai.org

toward the dorsal horn of the spinal cord where it synapses with second-order neurons.

- Three types of peripheral afferent nerves; **Aß, Aδ**, and **C-fibers** (see Table 1.1).
- **C-fibers** can be further broken down into different fiber nociceptors, for example [3–5]
  - *Temperature-sensitive nociceptors*
    - C-mechanoheat, C-mechanocold, C-mechanoheatcold
  - *Mechanical-sensitive nociceptors*
    - C-mechanonociceptors, C-fiber low-threshold mechanoreceptors
  - *C-mechanoinsensitive*
    - Not excitable by physiologic heat or mechanical nociception
    - Thought to be activated by inflammation and involved in complex regional pain syndrome (CRPS) [6]
- Both large fiber (Aß) and small fiber (Aδ, C) neuropathies can produce pain
  - **Small fiber (Aδ, C) neuropathic pain** is associated with reduced sensation to both pinprick and temperature; autonomic symptoms (changes in local vasoregulation, dry skin, decreased sweating, discoloration of skin, impaired vasomotor control) [7]
  - **Large fiber (Aß) neuropathic pain** is associated with reduced proprioception, numbness, loss of muscle-stretch reflexes, and muscle weakness [7, 8]
- Noxious stimuli are converted to **action potentials**, a series of electrical impulses. This is mediated by ion channels:
  - *Sodium channels* are responsible for depolarization of the nerve. When current passively spreads, voltage gated sodium channels are opened causing an influx of sodium causing a change in voltage and allows for further propagation of the action potential. This mechanism can be blocked with sodium channel antagonists such as lidocaine [9].

K.A. Sackheim, *Pain Management and Palliative Care: A Comprehensive Guide*,
DOI 10.1007/978-1-4939-2462-2_1, © Springer Science+Business Media New York 2015

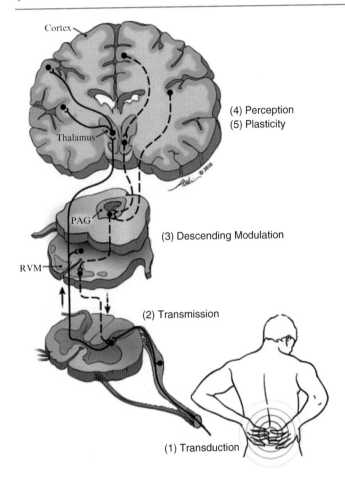

Fig. 1.1 Pathway of pain

- *Potassium channels* play a role in repolarization. The outflux of potassium ions correct the positive charge caused by the rapid influx of sodium. If blocked, there is a prolonged action potential. Continued blockage prevents repolarization and failure of the cell to generate another action potential.
- *Calcium channels* are essential for the release of neurotransmitters at nerve endings after synaptic depolarization. These can be blocked with calcium channel blockers such as gabapentin (Table 1.2).

2. *Transmission*—Aδ and C-fibers synapse at **Rexed laminae** [10, 11] (located at the dorsal horn of the spinal cord) to second-order neurons.
   - The dorsal horn is anatomical separated into layers called **lamina** [3]. The layers of lamina were first described by Rexed 1952 in his study of the spinal cord of a cat (Fig. 1.2).
     - Aß fibers terminate at lamina III–V
     - Aδ fibers terminate at lamina I, V
     - C-fibers terminate at the superficial lamina I, II

- **Two major types of second-order neurons**—spinal neurons that receive input from primary afferent fibers
  - *Wide dynamic range (WDR)*—receives input from both Aδ and C-fibers. Consistently active, but has increased responsiveness to painful stimuli.
  - *Nociceptive Specific*—receives input from C-fibers, normally inactive but responds to painful stimuli
- *Second-order neurons* receive both excitatory stimuli from the peripheral afferents and inhibitory stimuli from descending nerves and interneurons via neurotransmitters (see Table 1.2).
- *Second-order neurons* ascend rostrally toward the **supraspinal** structures
  - **Spinothalamic tract**: crosses the midline near the level of the cell body to the contralateral anterolateral spinal region and ascends rostrally to synapses at the *ventroposteriolateral (VPL) thalamus, ventroposteriormedial thalamus (VPM) thalamus* [1]. This is the primary perception pathway
  - **Spinoreticular tract**: synapses to the brainstem (periaqueductal *gray matter, hypothalamus, reticular system*) en route to the *intralaminar nucleus of the thalamus*. This tract ascends ipsalaterally and contralaterally. This controls the autonomic response to pain.
  - **Spinomesencephalic tract**: synapses to the midbrain tectum and periaqueductal gray where it integrates somatic sensation with visual and auditory information
- *Third-order neurons* distribute to the cerebral cortex to areas known as the "pain matrix."
  - The "pain matrix" consists of the **somatosensory cortex, insula cortex, anterior cingulate cortex (ACC)** [12]

3. *Modulation*—Pain is heavily modulated both centrally via descending pathways and peripherally via interneurons. The main mechanisms behind modulation are:
- Descending inhibition—The limbic system of the brain (responsible for emotions) project to the **periaqueductal gray (PAG)** and **rostral ventromedial medulla (RVM)** before descending down to synapse at the dorsal horn.
  - **PAG**—projects to RVM, then descends down to Rexed lamina where it releases serotonin and norepinephrine.
  - **Serotonin** plays an important role in antinociception; however, given the many subtypes of serotonin receptors has made it difficult to develop effective medication to target specific serotonin receptors in the dorsal horn. It is synthesized at the *nucleus raphe magnus*.

Table 1.1 Peripheral nerves

Speed (slowest) → (fastest)				
C-fiber	**B**	**Aδ**	**Aß**	**Aα**
Sensory afferent	Preganglionic sympathetic	Sensory afferent		Motor efferent
Thin, *un*myelinated	Thin, myelinated	Thin, myelinated	large, myelinated	large, myelinated
"Slow" pain burning, tingling, dull, achy	Autonomic function	"Fast" pain sharp, intense pain	Light touch, proprioception, pressure	Motor

Modified from [1, 3, 4]

Table 1.2 Neurochemistry of pain

Inhibitory	Excitatory
Gamma-aminobutyric acid glycine (GABA)	Substance P, K
Glycine	Neurokinin A
Serotonin	Glutamate
Dopamine	Aspartate
Norepinephrine	Calcitonin gene-related peptide
Endogenous opioids (*enkephalins, dynorphins, beta-endorphins*)	Cholecystokinin
Cannabinoids	
Somatostatin	

Adapted from [2–4]

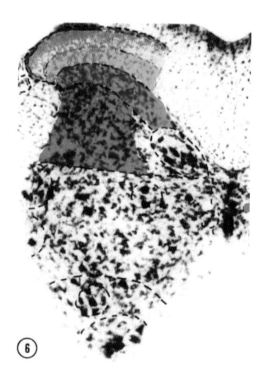

Fig. 1.2 Laminar organization of dorsal horn at the level of L1. *From top to bottom: red*—laminae I, *yellow*—laminae II, *green*—laminae III, *blue*—laminae IV, *pink*—laminae V. *Right center: orange*—laminae X [10, 11]

– **Norepinephrine** activates postsynaptic alpha 2-adrenergic receptors for modulation. It is synthesized at *locus coeruleus*.
• Local Modulation—Interneuron in the dorsal horn can also provide local modulation of pain transmission. The frequency of nociception or its persistence can elevate pain transmission.
– Excitation
▪ **Vanilloid receptor (TRPV)**—activated by inflammatory mediators (*bradykinin*) resulting in a lower threshold for excitation and increased proportion of nerves that respond to nociception [2].
▪ **NMDA receptors**—recruited only by an intense/prolong somatosensory stimulus that is sufficient to relieve the tonic Magnesium/Zinc cation blockade. Persistent activation leads to sensitization of dorsal horn neurons, decreased activation threshold, and prolong depolarization [2]. NMDA antagonist includes methadone and ketamine.
– Inhibition
▪ Mediated by interneurons that synapse at the dorsal horn. The neurotransmitters **GABA** and **glycine** are the best established (see Table 1.2).
• Endogenous opioids—*enkephalins, dynorphins, beta-endorphins.* Opioid receptors mainly found in laminae I, II of the dorsal horn, and PAG in the brain.
4. *Perception*—This is the subjective sensation of pain. It is the summation of the ascending signals from the peripheral nervous system, a psychosocial/emotional process, and central somatosensory processing.
• Facial emotions of others have been shown to change one's perception of pain [13].
5. *Neural plasticity*—Both the peripheral and central nervous system undergo changes in response to pain.
• *"Wind Up"*—Repeated activation of C-fiber nociceptors at 0.5–1 Hz can sensitize the peripheral afferent nerve and increase the duration of the excitatory response by dorsal horn neurons. WDR becomes increasingly excitable.

- Changes to "pain matrix"—In subjects with chronic pain (low back pain [14], fibromyalgia [15]), functional MRI and diffusion tensor imaging have shown the reorganization of the "pain matrix," as well as, changes in pattern of activation of the brain.

References

1. Cavanaugh DJ, Basbaum AI. Basic mechanisms and pathophysiology. In: Lynch ME, Craig KD, Peng PWH, editors. Clinical pain management: a practical guide. West Sussex: Wiley-Blackwell; 2010. p. 14–23.
2. Dougherty PM, Raja SN, Boyette-Davis J. Chapter 2—Neurochemistry of somatosensory and pain processing. Essentials of pain medicine. 3rd ed. Saint Louis: W.B. Saunders; 2011. p. 8–15.
3. Raja S. Anatomy and physiology of somatosensory and pain processing. In: Benzon H, Raja SN, Fishman SM, Liu S, Cohen SP, editors. Essentials of pain medicine. 3rd ed. Philadelphia: Elsevier/Saunders; 2011. p. 1–7.
4. Miller R. Miller's anesthesia: expert consult—online and print. 7th ed. Philadelphia: Churchill Livingstone; 2009.
5. Garcia-Anoveros J, Corey DP. The molecules of mechanosensation. Annu Rev Neurosci. 1997;20:567–94.
6. Maihofner C, Seifert F, Markovic K. Complex regional pain syndromes: new pathophysiological concepts and therapies. Eur J Neurol. 2010;17(5):649–60.
7. Mendell JR, Sahenk Z. Clinical practice. Painful sensory neuropathy. N Engl J Med. 2003;348(13):1243–55.
8. Tavee J. Small fiber neuropathy: a burning problem. Cleve Clin J Med. 2009;76(5):297–305.
9. Mao J, Chen LL. Systemic lidocaine for neuropathic pain relief. Pain. 2000;87(1):7–17.
10. Molander C, Xu Q, Grant G. The cytoarchitectonic organization of the spinal cord in the rat. I. The lower thoracic and lumbosacral cord. J Comp Neurol. 1984;230(1):133–41.
11. Rexed B. A cytoarchitectonic atlas of the spinal cord in the cat. J Comp Neurol. 1954;100(2):297–379.
12. Iannetti GD, Mouraux A. From the neuromatrix to the pain matrix (and back). Exp Brain Res. 2010;205(1):1–12.
13. Heckel A, Rothmayr C, Rosengarth K, Hajak G, Greenlee MW, Eichhammer P. Aversive faces activate pain responsive regions in the brain. Neuroreport. 2011;22(11):548–53.
14. Baliki MN, Chialvo DR, Geha PY, Levy RM, Harden RN, Parrish TB, et al. Chronic pain and the emotional brain: specific brain activity associated with spontaneous fluctuations of intensity of chronic back pain. J Neurosci. 2006;26(47):12165–73.
15. Jensen KB, Loitoile R, Kosek E, Petzke F, Carville S, Fransson P, et al. Patients with fibromyalgia display less functional connectivity in the brain's pain inhibitory network. Mol Pain. 2012;8:32.

Obtaining a Pain History

Andrew Kamal Abdou, John Ross Rizzo, and Jackson Liu

Abbreviations

ADL	Activities of daily living
COMM	Current Opioid Misuse Measure
DAST-10	Drug Abuse Screening Test
DN	*Douleur Neuropathique*
GED	General educational development
IADL	Instrumental activities of daily living
MMTP	Methadone Maintenance Treatment Program
ORT	Opioid Risk Tool
PMQ	Pain Medication Questionnaire
SISAP	Screening Instrument for Substance Abuse Potential
SOAPP	Screener and Opioid Assessment for Patients with Pain
VAS	Visual analog scale

Obtaining a Pain History

1. *Chief complaint*
   - Patient's self-reported symptoms or areas of pain leading them to seek care

A.K. Abdou, B.S.
New York University—Rusk Institute for Rehabilitation Medicine, Physical Medicine & Rehabilitation, 240 East 38th Street, NYU Ambulatory Care Center, Room # 1776, New York, NY 10016, USA
e-mail: Andrew.Abdou@nyumc.org

J.R. Rizzo, M.D. (✉)
New York University Langone Medical Center, Rehabilitation Medicine, 240 B 38th St., Office 1776, New York, NY 10016, USA
e-mail: Johnross.rizzo@nyumc.org

J. Liu, M.D.
New York University Langone Medical Center, Physical Medicine and Rehabilitation, 812 Queens Boulevard, Apt. 7i, Woodside, NY 11377, USA
e-mail: jackson.liu@nyumc.org

2. *History of present illness*
   - Approach to questioning
     - Build upon the chief complaint in a detailed and comprehensive manner through the use of open-ended questions (e.g. Tell me about your pain?)
     - How/when did it start? Were you doing a certain activity when pain started? Have you had this same issue previously?
     - Assess for new issues or changes in chronic conditions
     - Rule out acute medical issues that may require immediate referral for emergency care such as new or worsening neurological symptoms etc. bowel or bladder incontinence.
     - Obtain and review previous work up done to assess condition
     - Obtain most recent labs to assess other medical conditions that may effect your treatment
   - *Characterizing pain* [1]
     - *Location*: ex back vs. leg vs. both, neck vs. shoulder vs. arm/hand
     - *Radiation*: Where to? How far down extremity? What digits specifically?
     - *Intensity*: Severe enough to take medications or seeking other treatment options?
     - *Quality of pain*: Sharp, dull, electrical, shooting, etc.
     - *Frequency*: pain only at times or all day long?
     - *Temporal aspects*: Onset, duration, and changes since onset
     - Setting and time of day in which pain occurs
     - Characteristics of any breakthrough pain, how often
     - *Mitigating and exacerbating factors*: position change, bending forwards/backwards, sitting/walking, lifting, stairs, sneezing/coughing, etc.
     - *Associated symptomology*
       - Restriction of range of motion, stiffness, or swelling
       - Muscle aches, cramps, or spasms

- Weakness
- Sensory disturbances (e.g., dysesthesias, itching, numbness, tingling)
- Bowel or bladder changes
- Color or temperature changes in effected body part
- Changes in sweating, skin, hair, or nail growth
  - Mnemonics
    - **"SOCRATES"** (**S**—site, **O**—onset, **C**—character, **R**—radiation, **A**—associations, **T**—timing, **E**—exacerbating & relieving factors, **S**—severity)
    - **"OPQRST"** (**O**—onset, **P**—provocation, **Q**—quality, **R**—radiation, **S**—severity, **T**—time)
- Patient's thoughts and feelings about his/her pain
  - Subjective changes of pain throughout its development alongside corresponding objective pain scale values (see *Pain Scales* section)
- Subjective changes of pain throughout its development alongside corresponding objective pain scale values (see *Pain Scales* section)
- Previous treatments and effectiveness
  - *Pharmaceutical*
    - Obtain full details of previous use of topical, oral, intravenous, and pump therapy with dosage and frequency
      Know which medications and doses caused side effects and which were tolerated, did they help manage the pain and to what extent?
    - Previous pain physicians or other physicians who have written opiates or administered treatment—contact recent prescribers to confirm patient is no longer seeing them and to confirm compliance
      Ask if patient was ever discharged from a pain practice and why prior to making these calls, can help to establish trusting relationship if honest
    - History and reason of recent dose escalations
    - Any aberrant behavior (doctor shopping, multiple pharmacies, etc.)
      Check state database program prior to every visit to assure compliance
  - *Physical or occupational therapy*
    - How long was treatment? How often? Did this help?
    - Type of program e.g., specific to body part and exercises learned
    - Compliance with a home exercise program
    - Modalities
      Use of TENs with or without success? Relief/exacerbation with heat or ice?
  - Osteopathic *manipulations or chiropractic treatments*—helpful?
  - *Complementary and alternative therapies*
    - Herbs, acupuncture +/− moxibustion, cupping
    - Naturopathy or traditional Chinese medicine
    - Mind–body therapies, cognitive behavioral therapy, mediations, aromatherapy, expression or art-based therapies
    - Comprehensive interdisciplinary pain clinic enrollment
  - *Peripheral joint injections*
    - Injectable therapies may include anesthetics, anti-inflammatory medications, viscosupplementation, and platelet-rich plasma
    - Which were given? How many times? Did they help? For how long?
  - *Spinal Interventions*
    - Various procedures/injections which may include nerve blocks, spinal injections, intraspinal opioids, spinal cord stimulators, peripheral nerve stimulators, or implantable drug delivery systems
    - Which injections were done? Did they decrease pain? How much of a decrease and for how long?
  - *Surgeries to affected region*
    - Did this initially help? Is pain same as prior to surgery? What changes?
- Include pertinent positive or negative findings from other sections of the history

3. *Past medical history*
- General history of childhood and adult illnesses
  - History or cardiac, gastric, liver, or renal pathology that may interfere with medications or cause worsening of pathology
  - History of psychiatric illnesses
    - Prior hospitalizations
    - Suicidal or homicidal ideations or attempts
    - Review psychiatric medications for possible interactions
    - Contact treating psychiatrist or psychologist for complete history and permission to use opiates

4. *Past surgical history*
- Dates of all surgeries

5. *Social history*
- Provides a more detailed assessment of the patient which can reveal suspicions or inconsistencies in the

reported history as well as risk factors for substance abuse and addiction

- Educational Level (e.g., High School, GED, College)
- Home environment and living circumstances
- Patient's support system including family and friends
  - Ask patient if there are young children in their home and if/how medication is kept secure
- Substance use/abuse history (details below)
- Sexual history/history of abuse
- Criminal history
- Involvement in a problematic subculture or contact with high-risk individuals
- Past Substance abuse history
  - Higher risk of abusing/misusing opiates if history of previous abuse
  - Some physicians choose not to give opiates to patients with history of alcohol or illicit substance abuse
- Prior/current participation in a Methadone Maintenance Treatment Program (MMTP)
  - Determine compliance with this program
    - Ask how often methadone is administered
      Patients who have to pick this up daily are not as reliable
    - Ask how often urine toxicology is checked
    - Get contact information of the MMTP counselor
      Counselor can help you determine if patient is reliable enough to have added opiates for pain control
      Many physicians choose not to treat patients on MMTP with additional opiates

6. *Family history*
   - Any family history of substance or prescription drug use/misuse or abuse
   - Family history of alcoholism
   - Family history of psychiatric disorders
   - Serious medical issues in family
   - History of family abuse
   - Documents risk factors for aberrant behavior such as a family history of prescription drug or alcohol abuse

7. *Allergies*: specifically ask about medications used during injections such as anesthetics, steroid, shellfish, iodine, or contrast

8. *Medications*
   - General medications
     (i) Important for side effects, cross-reactivity, and metabolism
   - Pain-related medications
     (i) Ask patient to bring in bottles for pill counts and to assess information off the prescription bottle (pharmacy used, previous physician, date prescription filled, etc.)

(ii) Confirm all pain medications tried in past, if they helped and if any side effects

(iii) Opioid medication history
   - Inquire about the patient's current medication regimen used to control pain
     - Name of medications, dosage, and frequency
     - Patient satisfaction with current regimen
     - Associated side effects
     - How long have they been on these medications?
     - Name of prescribing physician
     - How long has this physician been prescribing these medications?
   - Obtain a list of pharmacies used to fill prescriptions
     - All pharmacies should be contacted on initial visit to verify compliance and assure no doctor shopping
     - Patients should be encouraged or mandated to use same pharmacy each month to fill controlled substances
   - Ask patient about prior care under other pain management physicians
     - Previous opioid prescribing physician(s) should be contacted on initial visit
     - Ask why the patient is seeking a new pain management physician
     - Ask patient about prior/recent discharge from a physician's care for noncompliance, abusive behavior, or any other reason
       - Be cautious when accepting patients who have been discharged previously for appropriate reasons
     - Ask patient when last prescription was received
       - How many pills remaining?
       - Do they have enough medication to last for at least 2 weeks or until next follow-up appointment after urine results are recorded?

9. *Functional evaluation*
   - Normal activity level prior to pain initiation
   - Current independence measures including bed mobility, transfers, mode of locomotion, and use of assistive devices
   - Activities of Daily Living (ADLs) and Instrumental Activities of Daily Living (IADLs) [1]
     - ADL—walking, bathing, dressing, toileting, brushing teeth, eating
     - IADL—cooking, driving, using the telephone or computer, shopping, keeping track of finances, managing medication

- Changes in function with pain onset
  - Attempt to document with objective measures e.g., number of blocks the patient is able to walk
  - Assess improvement or deterioration of function in temporal relation to use of medications or injections
10. *Review of systems*
- Assess for expected side effects of opiate use e.g., constipation, dry mouth
- Assess for signs and symptoms of opiate withdrawal/overuse
- Assess for reasons to avoid opioids or other medications such as dizziness, imbalance, and history of falls
11. *Confirming patient's history*
- Collateral information from other sources relating to the patient can provide useful information and help unveil potential inconsistencies in the history
  - Family member or caregiver with patient permission
  - Primary care physician or previous opiate-prescribing provider
    - Prescription and illicit drug history
    - History of noncompliance
    - Patient's reason for leaving the provider's office ex discharge
    - History of a urine toxicology test results
- Pharmacy
  - Use of multiple pharmacies by the patient
  - Names of all previously prescribed pain medications
  - *Names* and numbers of all previous providers—this can help recognize doctor
- Shopping
  - Last filled prescription to give rough estimate of remaining pill count
- Assess for signs and symptoms of aberrant behavior, dependence, abuse, addiction
  - Identify possible signs of drug-seeking behavior
  - *Are* they demanding certain medications only, not willing to try all options
  - Unusual appearance (e.g., untidiness, sleepy during history, not answering questions appropriately)
  - Unusual knowledge of controlled substances and/or gives medical history with textbook symptoms; or gives evasive or vague answers to questions regarding medical history
  - Reluctant or unwilling to provide reference information

- Imaging
  - Verify all imaging reports. Many patients seeking opioids have falsified reports. Confirm with imaging location that report is valid or examine imaging CD directly
12. *Supplemental assessment tools*
- Pain scales
  - (i) *Unidimensional*
    - Visual Analog Scale (VAS) [2, 3]
      - Measures a characteristic across a continuum of values
      - Horizontal line, 100 mm in length
      - The patient marks on the line the point that they feel represents their perception of their current state
      - Score is determined by measuring in millimeters from the left hand end of the line to the point that the patient marks
    - Numerical rating scale [3, 4]
      - The patient is asked, "What number would you give your pain right now?"
      - 0 = No pain
      - 1–3 = Mild pain (nagging, annoying, interfering little with ADLs)
      - 4–6 = Moderate pain (interferes significantly with ADLs)
      - 7–10 = Severe pain (disabling; unable to perform ADLs)
    - Verbal descriptor scale [3, 5]
      - Used more for articulate patients, who can use verbal terms to express the level of their pain
      - Six levels of intensity ranging from "no pain" to "the most intense pain imaginable"
      - Have patients place a check mark next to the phrase that best describes the current intensity of their pain
        Score the mark, "no pain" = 0 and "the most intense pain imaginable" = 6
    - Wong-Baker FACES pain rating scale [3, 6]
      - Explain to the person that each face is for a person who feels happy because he has no pain or sadness because he has some or a lot of pain
      - Ask the person to choose the face that best describes how he or she is feeling
      - Rating scale is recommended for patients aged 3 years and older (Fig. 2.1)

Fig. 2.1 Wong-Baker FACES pain scale. Hockenberry MJ, Wilson D: *Wong's essentials of pediatric nursing*, ed. 8, St. Louis, 2009, Mosby. Used with permission. Copyright Mosby

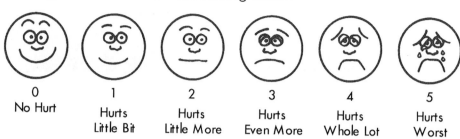

Wong-Baker FACES Pain Rating Scale

| 0 No Hurt | 1 Hurts Little Bit | 2 Hurts Little More | 3 Hurts Even More | 4 Hurts Whole Lot | 5 Hurts Worst |

  (ii) *Multidimensional* [7]
    – Brief pain inventory
    – McGill pain questionnaire
 (iii) *Neuropathic pain* [8]
    – Neuropathic pain scale
    – Leeds assessment of neuropathic symptoms and signs
    – DN (*Douleur Neuropathique*) [4]
    – Risk assessments for aberrant behaviors, misuse, dependence, abuse, and addiction [9]
      ▪ Screener and Opioid Assessment for Patients with Pain (SOAPP)
      ▪ Opioid Risk Tool (ORT)
      ▪ Pain Medication Questionnaire (PMQ)
      ▪ Current Opioid Misuse Measure (COMM)
      ▪ Drug Abuse Screening Test (DAST-10)
      ▪ Screening Instrument for Substance Abuse Potential (SISAP)

References

1. Bickley LS, Szilagyi PG. Bates' guide to physical examination and history taking. 11th ed. Philadelphia: Wolters Kluwer Health/Lippincott Williams & Wilkins; 2013.
2. Crichton N. Visual analogue scale (VAS). J Clin Nurs. 2001; 10:697–706.
3. Schofield P, Aveyard B. The management of pain in older people: a workbook. 1st ed. M & K Update: Keswick; 2007.
4. McCaffery M, Beebe A. Pain: clinical manual for nursing practice. 1st ed. St. Louis: Mosby; 1989.
5. Young DM, Mentes JC, Titler MG. Acute pain management protocol. J Gerontol Nurs. 1999;25(6):10–21.
6. Wong DL, Hockenberry MJ, Wilson D, Winkelstein ML. Wong's essentials of pediatric nursing. 7th ed. Elsevier Mosby: St. Louis; 2005.
7. Younger J, McCue R, Mackey S. Pain outcomes: a brief review of instruments and techniques. Curr Pain Headache Rep. 2009; 13(1):39–43.
8. Cruccu G, Truini A. Tools for assessing neuropathic pain. PLoS Med. 2009;6(4):e1000045.
9. Passik SD, Kirsh KL. Screening for opioid abuse potential. Int Assoc Study Pain. 2008;16(7):1–4.

Physical Examination: Approach to the Pain Patient

3

Jeremy J. Robbins, Fani J. Thomson, and Julia Sackheim

Abbreviations

AC	Acromioclavicular
ASIS	Anterior superior iliac spine
ATFL	Anterior talofibular ligament
DIP	Distal interphalangeal
DTR	Deep tendon reflex
EOMI	Extraocular muscles intact
FADIR	Flexion adduction internal rotation
MCP	Metacarpophalangeal
PERRLA	Pupils equal round reactive light
PIP	Proximal interphalangeal
PROM	Passive range of motion
PSIS	Posterior superior iliac spine
ROM	Range of motion
SI	Sacroiliac
SLR	Straight leg test
TMJ	Temporomandibular joint

Introduction

Physical examination is important as it helps to rule out serious pathology and can lead to a more focused treatment once etiology is established. Below is a basic approach to the physical examination for the pain management physician.

J.J. Robbins, D.O.
Department of Anesthesiology, University of Missouri Health System, One Hospital Drive, Columbia, MO 65212, USA
e-mail: robbinsjj@health.missouri.edu

F.J. Thomson, D.O., F.A.A.P.M.R., D.A.B.I.P.P. (✉)
Physical Examination, Valley Hospital, Valley Institute for Pain, Luckow Pavilion, 1 Valley Health Plaza, 3rd Floor, Paramus, NJ 07652, USA
e-mail: fanifab@aol.com

J. Sackheim, D.O.
Department of Internal Medicine, Stony Brook University Hospital, Stony Brook, NY, USA

Muscle Strength Scale [1] (the Same Scale Is Used for each Section of the Physical Examination)

- 0 = No contraction
- 1 = Visible muscle twitch but no movement of the joint
- 2 = Weak contraction insufficient to overcome gravity
- 3 = Weak contraction *able to overcome gravity*
- 4 = Contraction able to overcome some resistance but not full resistance
- 5 = Normal; able to overcome full resistance

Deep Tendon Reflex (DTR) Grading Scale [1]

- 0 = No observable reflex
- 1 = Trace reflex
- *2 = Normal reflex*
- 3 = Very brisk increased reflex
- 4 = Clonus

Head/Facial Exam

- *Inspection*:
  - Head/Face: Lesions/masses/swelling/bruising
  - Eyes: PERRLA, EOMI
  - TMJ: Swelling/erythema [2]
- *Palpation*:
  - Note any tenderness, tightness, restricted motion, or warmth [1]
  - Note areas of hyperalgesia, hypoalgesia, allodynia, and/or decreased sensation
  - TMJ: Place fingers just anterior to the ears and ask patient to open and close mouth, this will allow your fingertips to drop into joint space. Examine for swelling, tenderness, clicking, and snapping [2].
  - Palpate muscles of mastication:

Locate the masseters at the angle of the mandible, examine for local tenderness and possible reproduction of pain

Locate the temporal and pterygoid and examine them during clenching and relaxation [2], note any tenderness

- *Range of motion:*
  - TMJ: Have the patient open, close, protrude, retract, and perform lateral motion/deviation (moving side to side) with their jaw.

    Mouth should open wide enough to put three fingers between teeth.

    Jaw should protrude enough to allow the bottom teeth to be in front of the upper teeth [2].

Upper Extremity

Shoulder Exam

- *Inspection*: Examine for muscle atrophy, erythema, bruising, asymmetry of shoulder heights, deformity [3]
- *Palpation*:
  - *Bony landmarks and joints*: (Figs. 3.1)

    Sternoclavicular joint (medial), Acromioclavicular (AC) joint, Coracoid process of scapula (inferior and medial from AC joint) [2]
  - *Biceps tendon*: This can be located at the divot of the intertubercular groove at the anterior shoulder [2].

- *Bursas and rotator cuff muscles*: Passively extend the humerus in order to allow these structures to move anterior to the acromion [2].

  Subacromial bursa

  Subdeltoid bursa

  Supraspinatus (under acromion), Infraspinatus (posterior to supraspinatus), Teres Minor (posterior and inferior to supraspinatus) [2]

- *Range of motion (ROM)*: Perform passively and actively. ROM can be restricted in rotator cuff tears, capsulitis, sprains, tendonitis, bursitis, dislocations [2, 4]
  - Feel for Crepitus when evaluating ROM
  - *Decreased active ROM AND passive ROM is indicative of adhesive capsulitis. If active ROM is limited, but the examiner is able to perform full passive PROM on patient than this is not adhesive capsulitis*
  - Decreased abduction can indicate supraspinatus muscle pathology

Table 3.1 Range of motion of the shoulder

Action	Normal range
Flexion	180°
Extension	45°
Abduction	180°
Adduction	40°
External rotation	90°
Internal rotation	80°

- *Muscle strength testing*: Extension, Flexion, External rotation, Internal rotation, Abduction, and Adduction against resistance [2, 3, 5]

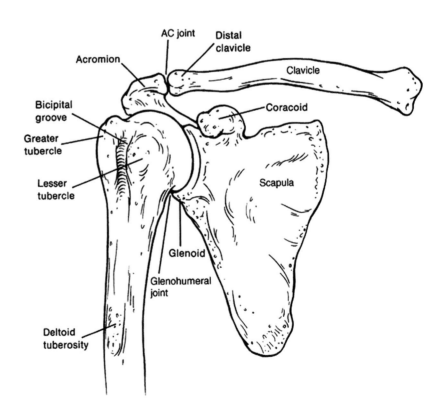

Fig. 3.1 Anterior view of the bony processes of the scapula. *With permission from: The Shoulder, by Wiesel, Brent B.; Carroll, Raymond M. Book: Essentials of Orthopedic Surgery Book DOI: 10.1007/978-1-4419-1389-0 Chapter: 8 Chapter DOI: 10.1007/978-1-4419-1389-0_8 Published: 2011-01-01. Springer*

- **Provocative maneuvers for stability**
  - *Anterior stability—Apprehension test*: Abduct and externally rotate the arm while putting pressure on the posterior humeral head. Pain or apprehension is positive for anterior instability or dislocation [3].
  - *Posterior stability—Jerk test*: Internally rotate the patient's arm and flex both the arm and forearm to 90°. While monitoring the shoulder joint, adduct the patient's elbow. A jerk is felt when the humeral head glides of the glenoid fossa [3].
  - *Inferior stability—Sulcus sign*: With patient's arm in a neutral position apply inferior traction at the patient's upper arm/shoulder (not forearm). A gapping between humerus and acromion is positive for inferior shoulder laxity [3].

Table 3.2 Provocative maneuvers for testing the shoulder

Diagnosis	Muscles being tested	Test	Method	Positive test
Impingement/ rotator cuff pathology	Supraspinatus, infraspinatus, teres minor, subscapularis	Neer's	While stabilizing the scapula from behind, internally rotate the patient's arm and passively flex the shoulder past 90°	Pain at the shoulder Fig. 3.2
Impingement/ rotator cuff pathology	Supraspinatus, infraspinatus, teres minor, subscapularis	Hawkins	Flex patient's shoulder to 90', flex elbow to 90' while forearm in neutral. This test can be done at varying degrees of internal rotation of the shoulder	Pain at the shoulder
Bicipital tendonitis		Speed's	Flex patient's shoulder to 90°, supinate the hand, extend elbow. Resist the patient's upward (flexion) motion of the shoulder by pushing downward on their forearm and palpating the intertubercular groove of the biceps tendon	Pain at the intertubercular groove overlying the biceps tendon *Weakness (may indicate superior labral tear)* Fig. 3.3
Bicipital tendonitis		Yergason's	Flex patient's elbow to 90° and fully pronate the forearm. Place your hand in the patients palm and ask them to resist you by having them move supinate the wrist and flex the elbow	"Snapping" or pain at intertubercular groove overlying the biceps tendon Fig. 3.4
Rotator cuff tear	Supraspinatus, Infraspinatus, Teres Minor, Subscapularis	Empty can	Flex the shoulder to 90° with the elbow fully extended and fully internally rotate the arm. Have the patient resist as you push downward on their arm	Weakness in resistance or patient "giveway" to resistance can indicate pathology with the supraspinatus muscle Fig. 3.5
Rotator cuff tear	Supraspinatus, Infraspinatus, Teres Minor, Subscapularis	Drop arm	Patient fully abducts arms to shoulder height with elbow extended and then slowly lowers them	Arm falls down abruptly instead of being slowly lowered down
Rotator cuff tear	Supraspinatus, Infraspinatus, Teres Minor, Subscapularis	Apley scratch	Patient touches the opposite scapula by abducting and external rotating arm and then adducting and internally rotating arm	Pain
AC joint arthritis		SCARF sign/cross arm adduction test	Flex shoulder to 90', adduct arm across the body	This will elicit pain in AC joint if there is arthritic joint
Labral tear		O'Brian's test	Forward flex shoulder to 90° with elbow extended. Apply downward resistance with arm fully internally rotated and then externally rotated	Pain in the internally rotated position that is then relieved in the externally rotated position

Elbow Examination

- *Inspection*: Examine for erythema, swelling, ecchymosis, and bony arthritic changes. Note carrying angle (the angle formed by the humerus and the forearm) 5–8° is normal [6].
- *Palpation*: 3.6
  - *Lateral/medial epicondyle*: Tenderness at or slightly distal to the medial or lateral epicondyles suggest epicondylitis.
  - *Olecranon*: Palpate for tenderness, bursa swelling [6].
- *Range of motion*: Perform passively and actively [4, 7]

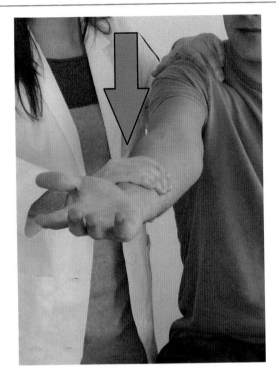

Fig. 3.2 Speed's test—Resist the patient's forward flexed and supinated hand

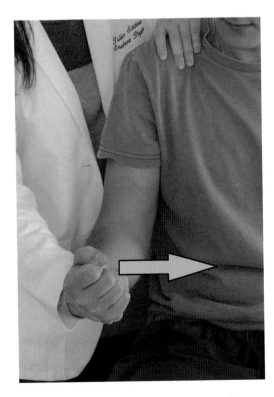

Fig. 3.3 Yergason's test—Have the patient supinate forearm against resistance with the elbow flexed 90°

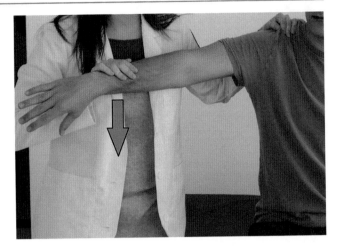

Fig. 3.4 Empty can—Patient pronates arm and abducts shoulder against resistance

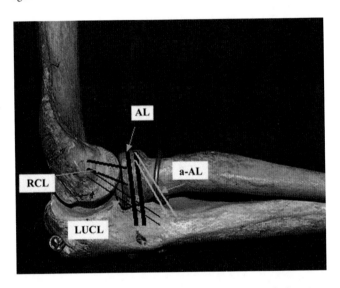

Fig. 3.5 Lateral view of the ligaments of the elbow: Anatomical preparation of the elbow joint with schematically presented ligaments on the lateral side of the joint (*AL* annular ligament; *a-AL* accessory annular ligament; *LUCL* lateral ulnar collateral ligament; *RCL* radial collateral ligament)

Table 3.3 Range of motion of the elbow

Action	Normal range
Flexion	150°
Extension	0–10°
Supination	80°
Pronation	80°

- *Muscle strength testing*: Flexion, extension, supination, pronation against resistance [4].
- *Provocative maneuvers*:
  - *Varus stress test*: Apply varus stress to the medial side of the elbow while the forearm is in pronated position. This will test for stability of the lateral collateral ligament [6].

- *Valgus stress test*: Apply valgus stress to the lateral side of the elbow while forearm is stabilized in a supinated position. This will test for stability of the ulnar collateral ligament.
- *Mills*: Pain at the lateral epicondylitis while passively extending the elbow, pronating the forearm and flexing the wrist. Indicates lateral epicondylitis.
- *Cozen's*: Pain with resisted wrist extension indicates lateral epicondylitis.
- Pain with resisted wrist flexion indicates medial epicondylitis [6].

Table 3.4 Muscle actions of the upper extremity

Muscles	Action
Biceps and brachioradialis	Flexion
Triceps	Extension
Pronator teres	Pronation
Supinator	Supination

Wrist Examination

- *Inspection*: Examine for bony arthritic changes/prominences, swelling of joints, atrophy over the thenar or hypothenar or intrinsic muscles [6].
- *Palpation*: Note any bony arthritic changes, swelling, tenderness at the following locations: Figs. 3.6 and 3.7
  - Distal radius and ulna bones, ulnar groove (medial elbow) [2]
  - Anatomical snuff box—pain here could indicate scaphoid pathology [2]
  - Carpal bones, metacarpals, and phalanges
  - MCP joints—tenderness could indicate arthritis [2]. Most commonly noted at the thumb
  - PIP and DIP [2]
  - Carpal tunnel, de Quervains tendons—abductor pollicis longus and the extensor pollicis brevis
  - Prominences at dorsal and palmar regions, which could be ganglion cysts [6]
- *Range of motion*: Actively and passively [4, 7]

Table 3.5 Range of motion of the wrist

Action	Normal range
Flexion	80°
Extension	70°
Abduction (ulnar deviation)	20°
Adduction (radial deviation)	35°

- *Muscle strength testing*: Flexion, extension, adduction, and abduction against resistance. Test hand grip strength, by asking patient to squeeze your first two fingers [2].
- *Sensory testing:*
  - Test all cervical dermatomes (see dermatome figure) and all upper extremity peripheral nerves

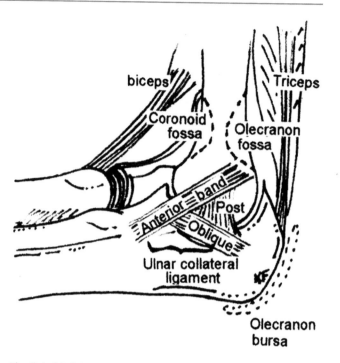

Fig. 3.6 Medial view of the elbow: Medial view of the elbow joint, demonstrating the orientation of the ulnar (medial) collateral ligament

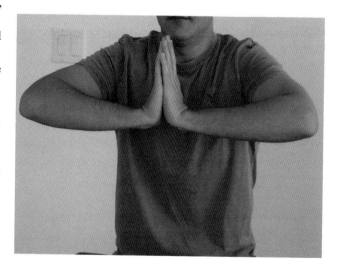

Fig. 3.7 Reverse phalens/prayer test: patient extends wrists against each other

- *Provocative maneuvers for de Quervain's Tenosynovitis*:
  - *Finkelstein's test*: Have the patient make a fist with the thumb inside the fingers and place the fist into ulnar deviation. If this elicits pain over the dorsal radial compartment of the wrist, this indicates de Quervain's tenosynovitis [6].
- *Provocative maneuvers for Carpal Tunnel Syndrome*:
  - *Tinel sign*: Tap over the carpal tunnel at the palmar wrist—paresthesias indicate positive entrapment of the median nerve [6]

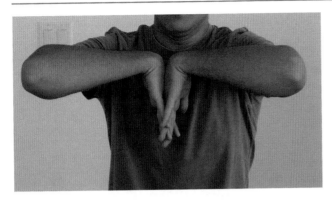

Fig. 3.8 Phalen's test: patient flexes wrists against each other

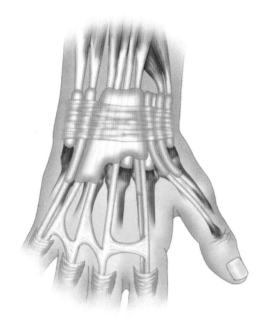

Fig. 3.9 Dorsal view of the ligaments and sheath of the hand

– *Phalen's maneuver*: Flex the patient's wrists to 90° and keep them in this position for 60 s. Numbness or tingling is indicative for Carpal Tunnel Syndrome [6] Fig. 3.8

– *Reverse Phalen's test*: Extend the patient's wrist to 90° against each other (palms against palms). Keep them there for 60 s. Numbness or tingling is indicative of Carpal Tunnel syndrome (Fig. 3.9) [11].

• *Provocative maneuvers for MCP Arthritis*:
  – MCP grinding: Extend the patient's finger and while holding the distal phalanx, apply compression along the axis of the finger, pain at the MCP joint indicates probable arthritis [8]

Lower Extremity

Hip Examination

• *Inspection*:
  – Observe the patients gait as they enter the room. Observe the width of the base, shift of the pelvis, and flexion of the knee [2].
    ▪ *Gait*
      Observe/Test for:
      • *Instability*: Patient looks prone to fall and/or grabs on to rails for assistance [3]
      • *Toe walking*: Difficulty could indicate weakness in plantar flexors (S1)
      • *Heel walking*: Difficulty could indicate weakness in dorsiflexors (L4, L5)
      • *Tandem gait*: Difficulty could indicate balance issues and/or weakness
      • *Wide-based gait*: Can indicate unsteadiness in numerous neurological disorders
      • *Favoring of extremity/antalgic gait*: May indicate pain of favored extremity [6]
      • ***Trendelenberg gait***: *Patient's contralateral hip will drop when standing on one foot due to weakness of the ipsilateral hip abductors (Gluteus medius and minimus). Can indicate superior gluteal nerve injury* [3].
  – With the patient supine, assess for leg length discrepancy [2]
  – Inspect for any bruising or muscle atrophy in the lower limb [2]
• *Palpation*:
  – Bony anatomy: Iliac crest, ASIS, PSIS, pubic symphysis, SI joint Fig. 3.9
  – Bursas: Psoas bursa (below the inguinal ligament), Trochanteric bursa (over greater trochanter), ischiogluteal bursa (over ischial tuberosity)
• *Range of motion*: Actively and passively

Table 3.6 Range of motion of the hip

Action	Normal range
Flexion	100°
Extension	30°
Abduction	40°
Adduction	20°
Internal rotation	45°
External rotation	45°

• *Muscle strength testing*: Against resistance. Flexion, extension, abduction, adduction, external rotation, internal rotation [4, 7, 9]

- *Provocative maneuvers SI joint pain*:
  - *FABER test*: (flexion abduction—external rotation)—while the patient is supine, place hip into flexion, abduction, and external rotation. Then apply downward pressure on the knee. If pain is elicited, the hip or SI joint may be affected [6].
  - *Gaenslen's test*: Patient is supine with thighs draped off of table. Maximally flex the hip on one side while extending the other hip joint simultaneously. Pain in either joint is a positive finding for SI joint dysfunction [3].
  - *Fortin's finger test*: Apply pressure with one finger over SI joint. If patient has reproducible pain, this is suggestive of SI joint pathology [6].
- *Provocative maneuvers hip joint pain*:
  - *FADIR test*: (Flexion Adduction Internal Rotation)—while the patient is supine, place hip into flexion, adduction, and internal rotation. Pain in the groin suggests hip osteoarthritis or pathology [6].
- *Provocative maneuvers for gluteus medius weakness*:
  - *Trendelenburg test*: Tests for gluteus medius weakness
    - Patient stands on one leg. If gluteus medius strength is normal, the contralateral iliac crest will not drop and thus the pelvis remains level.
    - A positive finding for gluteus medius weakness occurs when the contralateral iliac crest drops (i.e., a lower iliac crest on the right side indicates left gluteus medius weakness) [3].

Knee Examination

- *Inspection*: Observe gait and examine for valgus (knock knees) or varus (bowleg) deformities. Examine for quadriceps atrophy, hamstring or calf atrophy. Inspect for knee effusion [6].
- *Palpation*:
  - Medial and lateral epicondyles of femur and tibia and medial and lateral collateral ligaments
  - Patella
  - Suprapatellar pouch (along margins of patella), prepatellar bursa and anserine bursa (both on the posterior medial side) [2]
  - Palpate for knee effusion
  - Palpate the calves and Achilles tendon
- *Range of motion*: Passively and Actively. Test knee flexion, knee extension, internal rotation (sit and swing lower leg medially) and external rotation (sit and swing lower leg laterally) [2, 4, 7]

Table 3.7 Range of motion of the knee

Action	Normal range
Flexion	150°
Extension	0–10°

- Muscle strength testing: Test extension and flexion against resistance from your hand
- *Provocative maneuvers:*

Table 3.8 Provocative maneuvers for testing the knee

Structure	Provocative maneuver	Positive test
Patella	*Patellar apprehension sign*: With the patient supine, flex the patient's knee to 30°. Using both your thumbs on the medial edge of the patella, displace it laterally	Pain with displacement is a positive result of patella dislocation [3]
Patella	*Patellar grind test*: With the patient supine, place your hand on the patient's leg with the webbing between your thumb and index finger along the superior curvature of the patella. Have the patient contract the quadriceps	Pain upon contraction is positive for patellofemoral syndrome [3]. Figure 3.13
Meniscus/ligament	*Apley's test*: With patient prone and knee flexed 90°, stabilize the patient's thigh with your knee. Apply a superior distraction force while rotating the leg both internally and externally	Pain or restricted motion may indicate a ligament lesion. Conversely, repeating the test while applying compression may indicate a meniscus lesion [2]. Figure 3.14
MCL/LCL	*McMurray's Test*: With patient supine, flex both the thigh and knee to 90°. While stabilizing the medial and lateral aspects of the knee, externally rotate the leg and apply a valgus force while extending the knee	Pain or a click is a positive result for a MCL tear. Conversely, to test for a LCL tear, internally rotate the leg and apply a varus force [3]. Figures 3.15 and 3.16
MCL	*Valgus stress test*: With patient supine, drape the leg over the exam table, flex the knee to 30°, and slightly abduct the leg. Use one hand to stabilize the lateral aspect of the knee and then apply an abducting stress on the ankle	If the knee seems to open up on the medial side it is a positive finding for an MCL tear [3]
LCL	*Varus stress test*: With patient supine, drape the leg over the exam table, flex the knee to 30°, and slightly abduct the leg. While holding the ankle with one hand, place the other hand on the medial aspect of the knee and apply an adducting stress to the knee	If the knee seems to open up on the lateral side it is a positive finding for a LCL tear [3]

(continued)

Table 3.8 (continued)

Structure	Provocative maneuver	Positive test
ACL	*Anterior drawer test*: With patient supine, flex the hip to 45° and the knee 15°. Stabilize the leg by sitting on the foot. With your thumbs on the tibial plateau and fingers behind the tibia, apply anterior force	Excessive forward displacement is positive for ACL tear [3]. Figure 3.17
	Lachman test: Same as Anterior Drawer Test but the knee is only flexed 30°. Excessive forward displacement is positive for ACL tear [3]	
PCL	*Posterior Drawer Test*: With patient supine, flex the hip to 45° and the knee 15°. Stabilize the leg by sitting on the foot. With your thumbs on the tibial plateau and fingers behind the tibia, apply posterior force	Excessive posterior displacement is positive for PCL tear [3]. Figure 3.18
Illiotibial band	*Ober's sign*: Patient lies on unaffected side with that side of the hip flexed. While stabilizing the hip, flex the patient's leg to 90°. Proceed to abduct and extend the hip. Then lower/adduct the patient's leg	If the patient's leg will not adduct then it is a positive finding for iliotibial band tightness [3]
Knee effusion	*Bulge sign*: With knee extended, apply pressure above the knee and on the medial aspect of the knee in order for pushing fluid downward and laterally. Tap the knee behind the lateral margin to evaluate for fluid wave [2]	Fluid wave present

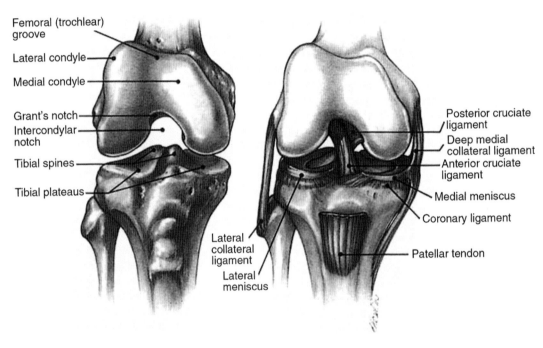

Fig. 3.10 The anterior and posterior views of the bony structures in the knee. *With Permission from*: *The Knee by Evans, Brian G.; Zawadsky, Mark W. Book*: *Essentials of Orthopedic Surgery Book DOI*: 10.1007/978-1-4419-1389-0 *Chapter*: *12 Chapter DOI*: 10.1007/978-1-4419-1389-0_12 *Published*: 2011-01-01

Ankle Examination

- *Inspection*: Examine for high arch (pes cavus), flat foot (pes planus), callus, nodules, deformities, swelling and increased pronation of the ankle while standing.
- *Palpation*:
  - With thumbs, palpate the anterior aspect of each ankle joint [2].
  - Palpate the heel, achilles tendon, calcaneal bursa, and length of plantar fascia

  - Palpate the lateral and medial malleolus
  - Palpate the metatarsophalangeal joints, by compressing the forefoot between thumb and fingers. Evaluate for pain, which could present in rheumatoid arthritis [2]
- *Range of motion*: Inversion and eversion, dorsiflexion (ankle extension) (point foot to the ceiling) and plantar flexion (ankle flexion) (point foot to the floor) [2]
  - Pain/limitation in dorsiflexion can be seen in Achilles tendonitis [4].

Table 3.9 Range of motion of the ankle

Action	Normal range
Plantar flexion	40°
Dorsiflexion	20°
Inversion	30°
Eversion	20°

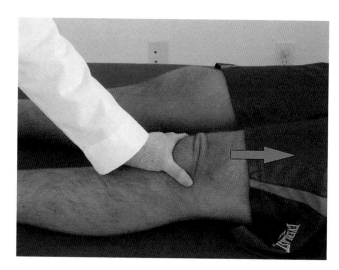

Fig. 3.11 Patellar grind—Grasp caudad to the kneecap and apply cephaled pressure

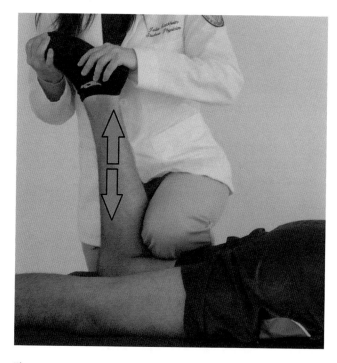

Fig. 3.12 Apley's distraction/compression—Applying pressure into the joint should illicit pain while tractioning the joint (distracting) should relieve pain

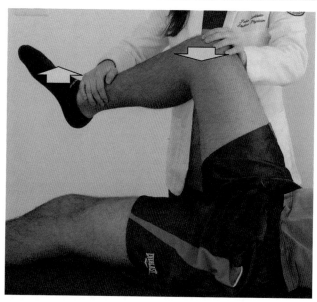

Fig. 3.13 McMurray's—Valgus stress being applied to test for an MCL tear

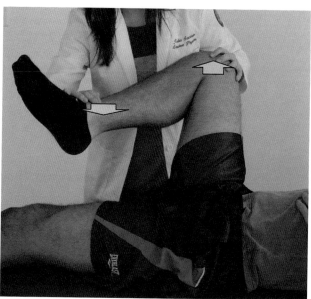

Fig. 3.14 McMurray's—Varus stress being applied to test for an LCL tear

- *Muscle strength testing*: Inversion, eversion, dorsiflexion, and plantar flexion against resistance
    - Extensor hallucis longus, anterior tibialis, peroneal longus and brevis, posterior tibialis [6]
- *Provocative maneuvers*:
    - *Anterior drawer test*: With the ankle in a relaxed position, grasp the distal end of the tibia with one hand. With the other hand grasp the heel and apply

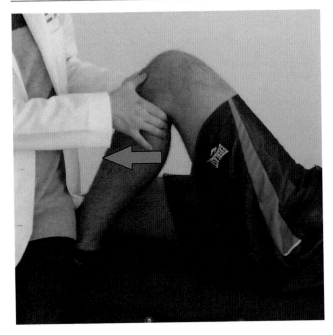

Fig. 3.15 Anterior drawer—Apply anterior force to assess any laxity

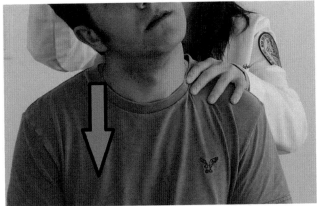

Fig. 3.17 Spurling's maneuver—Compress the cervical spine during side bending and extension with slight downward force to reproduce radicular pain

also be heard with squeezing the metatarsals while applying a superior/inferior translator motion [3].

- *Thompson test*: While patient is prone, squeeze their calf. If Achilles tendon is ruptured, the calf will not plantar flex as it should [10].

Spine

Cervical Spine Examination

- *Inspection* [6]:
  - *Posture*: Examine for increased kyphosis, scoliosis, asymmetry
  - Loss of lordosis
  - Rash
- *Palpation*:
  - Occipital protuberances [6]
  - Paraspinal muscles
  - Spinous processes, transverse processes
  - Facets joints (lie about 1 in. laterally to spinal process at each vertebral level) [2]
- *Range of motion*: Passively and actively
  - *Flexion*: Limited range or increased pain can indicate radiculopathy
  - *Extension*: Limited range or increased pain can indicate facet arthropathy
  - Torticollis (Sternocleidomastoid muscle spasm) can be seen with neck rotation and side-bending.

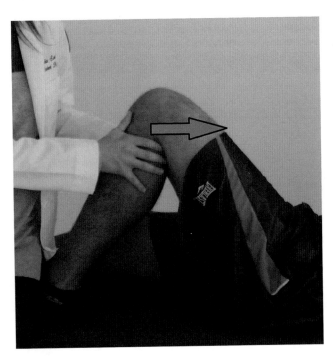

Fig. 3.16 Posterior drawer—Apply posterior force to assess any laxity

an anterior force. Excessive forward displacement is a positive finding for lateral ankle ligaments or ATFL [3].

- *Talar tilt test*: Stabilizing the distal tibia with one hand, invert the talus. Excessive inversion is a positive finding for a calcaneofibular ligament sprain or tear [3].
- *Morton's neuromas*: Squeeze in between the metatarsals to palpate any neuromas. "Mulder's click" can

Table 3.10 Range of motion of the cervical spine

Action	Normal range
Flexion	60°
Extension	50°
Rotation	80°
Sidebending	45°

- *Neurological testing*: Including muscle strength testing, reflexes, and sensation of all cervical dermatomes. See appropriate figures and tables.

- *Provocative maneuvers for cervical radiculopathy*:
  - *Spurling's maneuver*: Extend neck and sidebend head towards affected side while placing axial pressure

Table 3.11 Cervical dermatomes/muscles/reflexes

Nerve root	Innervated muscles	Action	Sensory	Reflex
C5	**Deltoid**, SITS, **biceps**	Shoulder abduction and External rotation	Upper lateral arm	Biceps (C5/6)
C6	Biceps, brachioradialis, supinator, **extensor carpi radialis longus**, scalene muscles	Elbow flexion and wrist extension	Lateral forearm to digits 1, 2	Brachioradialis (C5/6)
C7	**Triceps**, pronator teres, flexor carpi radialis	Elbow extension and wrist flexion	Middle of forearm into digit 3	Triceps
C8	Triceps, **flexor digitorum superficialis, flexor digitorum profundus**, flexor carpi ulnaris, abductor pollicis longus, extensor pollicis longus, opponens pollicis	Thumb extension and ulnar deviation Finger flexion	Medial forearm to digits 4, 5	None
T1	**intrinsic muscles of the hand**	Finger abduction	Upper medial arm and axilla	None

(applying pressure on the top of the head). Reproducible radicular arm pain is positive for a cervical radiculopathy Fig. 3.17 [1].

- *Bakody's sign*: Externally rotate and abduct the ipsilateral arm/shoulder above the patient's head. Relief of pain indicates a positive finding for cervical radiculopathy [3].
- *Valsalva maneuver*: Radicular pain is a positive result and can indicate presence of a space occupying lesion [3].
- *Manual neck distraction test*: Vertical upward traction is applied under the jaw and at the occiput. If pain is relieved

by this maneuver, this is indicative of cervical radiculopathy due to relief of the pressure on the nerves [1].

- *Upper motor neuron signs*:
  - *Hoffman reflex*: Flick the tip of middle fingernail. A positive result is thumb flexion which indicates spinal cord lesion/pathology in the neck region [3].
  - *Babinski reflex*: Tracing along the curvature of the sole, sweep the foot from heel to toe. A positive result is hallux extension, which indicates spinal cord lesion/pathology in the cervical region [3].

Table 3.12 Cervical spine pathology

Diagnosis	Pain distribution	Onset of pain	Levels typically affected	Flexion
Cervical spondylosis	Unilateral or bilateral	Gradual	C5-C7	May decrease pain (pain can increase with extension)
Cervical stenosis	Unilateral or bilateral	Gradual	Varies	May decrease pain
Cervical disk herniation	Unilateral more commonly	Sudden	C5-6	May increase pain

Thoracic Spine Examination

- *Inspection*: Observe for scoliosis, kyphosis, asymmetry
- *Palpation*:
  - Muscles: Paraspinals, rhomboids, supraspinatus, infraspinatus mucles
  - Bony Anatomy: Vertebral bodies, Spinous Processes, Facet joints, Ribs

- *Range of motion*: Passively and actively [11]
- *Sensation*: See Fig. 3.18

Table 3.13 Range of motion of the thoracic spine

Action	Normal range
Flexion	20–45°
Extension	25–45°
Sidebending	20–40°
Rotation	35–50°

The dermatomes: the segmental cutaneous supply of the skin

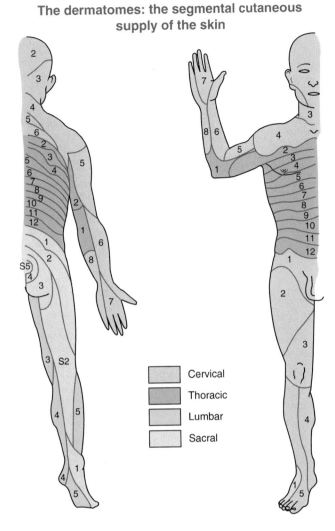

Cervical

Thoracic

Lumbar

Sacral

Fig. 3.18 Posterior and anterior dermatomes

Lumbar Spine Examination

- *Inspection*:
  - Posture: Loss/increased lordosis, scoliosis

- *Pain in certain positions*:
  - Sitting (indicative of disc pathology)
  - Standing
  - Bending forwards (indicative of disc pathology)
  - Bending backwards (indicative of facet diseas)
  - Frequent changes in position (which indicates increased severity of pain)
  - Use of assistive device (cane, rolling walker, etc.)
- *Palpation*:
  - Muscles: Parapspinals, gluteals, piriformis
  - Facet joints
  - Spinous processes
  - SI Joint
  - PSIS
  - Coccyx
  - Greater trochanteric bursa
  - Iliotibial band
  - Palpate for vertical step offs to check if one spinous process is more prominent than another, which could indicate spondylolisthesis [2]
- *Range of motion*: Other details under inspection
  - *Flexion*: Limited range or increased pain with this motion can indicate radiculopathy or disc pathology.
  - *Extension*: Limited range or increased pain with this motion can indicate facet arthropathy or spondylolisthesis Table 3.14 [3, 11].

Table 3.14 Range of motion of the lumbar spine

Action	Normal range
Flexion	90°
Extension	30°
Rotation	40°
Sidebending	30°

- *Muscle strength testing*: Hip flexors (L1-2) and extensors, knee extensors (L3–4) and flexors, ankle dorsiflexors (L4), Toe extensors (extensor hallucis longus) (L5) and ankle plantar flexors against resistance

Table 3.15 Lumbosacral dermatomes/muscles/reflexes

Nerve root	Innervated muscles	Action of muscle	Paresthesia	Reflex
L1	Iliopsoas, adductors	Hip flexion	Groin	None
L2	(Same as L1)	Hip flexion	Front of thigh	None
L3	Quadriceps	Knee extension	Inner knee, anterior lower leg	None
L4	Tibialis anterior	Foot dorsiflexion	Medial calf and ankle	Patellar reflex
L5	Extensor hallucis longus, gluteus medius and minimus	Toe extension	Lateral leg, toes 1–3	None
S1	Gastrocnemius, gluteus maximus	Ankle plantarflexion	Toes 4 and 5, lateral leg, plantar side of foot	Achilles reflex
		Ankle eversion		
		Hip extension		
		Knee flexion		

- *Sensation*: Refer to dermatome figure
- *Reflexes*:
  - L4: Patellar reflex
  - S1: Achilles reflex
- *Upper motor neuron signs*:
  - *Ankle clonus*: Rapidly dorsiflex the foot upward and hold. Several "beats" of the foot is positive for ankle clonus [3].
  - *Lower extremity spasticity*: Tightness of in muscles. Evaluate gait. Gait abnormalities greatly vary in each patient [3].
  - *Babinski sign*: Stroke lightly on plantar surface of the foot and look for great toe extension, which is a sign of spinal cord involvement [3].
- **Provocative maneuvers for lumbar radiculopathy**:
  - *Straight leg test (SLR)*: Patient lays supine, examiner elevates affected leg while keeping knee extended.
    + SLR is noted if patient has pain radiating down examined leg at 30–70° [3]
  - *Crossed straight leg raise*: Positive test can be elicited with lifting asymptomatic side and causing pain on symptomatic side [6].
  - *Slump test*: Patient sits on the side of the table and flexes forward (in a slumping position). Gently flex the cervical spine. Then extend the patient's knee. If no pain is reproduced, continue by dorsiflexing the patient's foot. A positive finding is reproducible pain, which indicates possible dura, spinal cord, or nerve root impingement [11].
  - *Seated straight leg raise*: Distraction technique to discern between amplification of pain. Extend patient's knee while talking. If patient does not extend back, no radicular pain is elicited [6]. Used to assess if patient is malingering.
  - *Reverse straight leg test*: While the patient is prone, lift the hip into extension with the knee straight. This test will be positive with upper lumbar nerve root involvement (*This is for upper lumbar radiculopathy as opposed to the other maneuvers which are for lower lumbar radiculopathy diagnosis*) [6].

Signs of Malingering

(a) **Waddell's Signs**:
  - *Distraction*: Repeat any positive tests while the patient is distracted. Malingering patients may not respond in pain while distracted.
  - *Overreaction*: Disproportionate noises or visual expressions of pain. Malingering patients may over-exaggerate pain to ensure they get their desired result.

- *Regional disturbances*: Affected regions not to follow dermatome/anatomical patterns. However, patients may have researched such features of the pain they are faking.
- *Simulation tests*: Pretend to perform a test that the patient thinks may elicit pain. Malingering patients will voice pain despite it being a test that does not cause any pain.
- *Tenderness*: Real pain is usually localized to one particular neuromuscular structure. Malingering patients may display one of the following:
  - *Superficial*: Skin is tender to light touch or pinch
  - *Nonanatomic*: Deep tenderness that is not localized to one structure [3]

Pelvic and Abdomen Examination (See More Details in Pelvic and Abdominal Pain Chapter)

- *Percuss*: Note any dull areas that could be due to an underlying mass or tympany due to excess gas.
- *Palpation*: Palpate lightly and deeply. Note any tenderness, tightness, restricted motion, rigidity, guarding, masses, or warmth. Palpate the liver borders.

References

1. UpToDate [Internet]. Lexi-comp online™. Hudson, OH. Evaluation of the patient with neck pain and cervical spine disorders. 2013. http://www.uptodate.com/contents/evaluation-of-the-patient-with-neck-pain-and-cervical-spine-disorders?source=search_result&search=neck+exam&selectedTitle=1~150#H30. Accessed 13 Feb 2013.
2. Bickley L, Szilagyi P. Bates' guide to physical examination and history taking. 10th ed. Philadelphia: Lippincott Williams & Wilkins; 2009.
3. Magee DJ. Orthopedic physical assessment. 4th ed. Edmonton: Saunders Elsevier; 1954.
4. Range of joint motion evaluation chart. http://www.dshs.wa.gov/pdf/ms/forms/13_585a.pdf. Accessed 4 Mar 2014.
5. Luke A. Shoulder physical examination. http://orthosurg.ucsf.edu/patient-care/divisions/sports-medicine/conditions/physical-examination-info/shoulder-physical-examination/. Accessed 4 Mar 2014.
6. Griffin L. Essentials of musculoskeletal care. 3rd ed. Rosemont: American Academy of Orthopaedic Surgeons; 2005.
7. Choi H, Sugar R, Fish D, Shatzer M, Krabak B. Physical medicine and rehabilitation pocketpedia. Philadelphia: Lippincott Williams & Wilkins; 2003.
8. http://ahn.mnsu.edu/athletictraining/spata/wristhandfingermodule/specialtests.html
9. Roach K, Miles T. Normal hip and knee active range of motion: the relationship to age. J Am Phys Ther Assoc. 1991;71(9):656–65. http://www.physther.net/content/71/9/656.full.pdf. Accessed 5 Mar 2014.
10. Cuccurullo S. Physical medicine and rehabilitation board. New York: Demos Medical; 2010.
11. Malanga GA. Musculoskeletal physical examination. 1st ed. Philadelphia: Elsevier Mosby; 2006.

Diagnostic Imaging

4

Paul Weyker, Christopher Webb, Isaac Wu,
and Leena Mathew

Abbreviations

AP	Anterioposterior
CPP	Chronic pelvic pain
CRPS	Complex regional pain syndrome
CT	Computed tomography
MRI	Magnetic resonance imaging
STIR	Short-tau inversion recovery
TVUS	Transvaginal ultrasound
US	Ultrasound

Introduction [1]

Diagnostic radiology traces its origins to 1895 when Wilhelm Roentgen produced the first X-ray image.

Different modes of diagnostic radiology include:
- Plain X-ray, computed radiography
- Computed axial tomography (CT)
- Magnetic resonance imaging (MRI)
- Ultrasound (US)
- Fluoroscopy

P. Weyker, M.D. • C. Webb, M.D.
Department of Anesthesia and Perioperative Care, University of California San Francisco Medical Center, University of California San Francisco, San Francisco, CA, USA

I. Wu, M.D.
Department of Anesthesiology, New York Presbyterian Hospital, Columbia University Medical Center, New York, NY, USA

L. Mathew, M.D. (✉)
Division of Pain Medicine/Department of Anesthesiology, New York Presbyterian Hospital, Columbia University, New York, NY, USA
e-mail: Lm370@columbia.edu

Two types of risk with radiation:
- Stochastic:
  - Affects probability of a condition
  - Severity will be dose independent
  - Examples are: fetal abnormalities, cancer and genetic effects
- Non-stochastic (deterministic):
  - Effect has known threshold radiation dose: erythema, cataracts

Plain X-Ray

- *Physics*
  - An X-ray beam is passed through the body onto a film cassette.
- *Contrast agents*:
  - Not generally used for plain X-rays
- *Indications*:
  - X-rays: used to detect bony lesions such as fractures or tumors
  - Spine flexion/extension films: used to evaluate for spondylolisthesis and dynamic instability
  - Joint pain: to look for arthritis, loose bodies, fractures
- *Contraindication*:
  - Pregnancy
- *Risks*:
  - Radiation exposure

Magnetic Resonance Imaging [1]

- *Physics*:
  - Uses very powerful static magnetic field and radiofrequency gradients that alters the alignment of protons
  - Energy given off by protons is detected and a computer is used to create an image.

K.A. Sackheim, *Pain Management and Palliative Care: A Comprehensive Guide*,
DOI 10.1007/978-1-4939-2462-2_4, © Springer Science+Business Media New York 2015

- Tissues are differentiated by differences in T1 and T2 relaxation times.

  T1 measures how quickly a tissue becomes magnetized and T2 measures of how quickly a tissue loses magnetization.

  T1-weighted scans are good at differentiating fat from water, with water appearing darker, and are good for providing anatomic detail.

  T2 images are useful for imaging edema and pathologic conditions, with fat appearing darker and water lighter.

- *Contrast agents*:
  - Gadolinium chelates are used as contrast agents to detect blood–brain barrier disruptions and to accentuate other pathology such *as infections and tumors*.

    Contrast is also recommended when imaging a patient who has undergone prior spine surgery.

- *Indications*:
  - MRI is superior to CT scans in detecting soft tissue lesions such as tumors and infection. MRIs are commonly used to evaluate muscular/tendon/ligament and vertebral disc pathology.
  - MRI can be safely used in pregnancy, if necessary, as it produces no ionizing radiation.
  - MR neurograms are used to evaluate the course peripheral nerves such as the sciatic nerve.
  - MR angiograms are used to evaluate vasculature.

- *Contraindications*:
  - Implants that are electrically, magnetically, or mechanically activated are generally contraindicated.

    Most spinal cord stimulators

    Intrathecal pumps

    Pacemakers

    Cochlear implants are variable

    Pacing wires

    Swan–Ganz catheters

    Ferromagnetic implants

    Any metal in body such as—bullets and shrapnel

    Note that generally titanium joint replacements are considered safe. With any of these implants it is recommended to check with the manufacturer to determine compatibility prior to ordering an MRI.

Computed Tomography (CT) [1]

- *Physics*:
  - CT is accomplished by rotating an X-ray tube 360° around a patient.
  - Detectors opposite the X-ray tubes collecting the X-ray beams
  - A computer reconstructs the cross-sectional images of the patient's body.

- *Contrast agents*:
  - Water-soluble molecules containing iodine atoms
  - Iodinated contrasts are ionic, high-osmolality or non-ionic, low-osmolality.
  - *Low osmolality agents associated are with a lower incidence of adverse reactions.*
  - Contrast is used to enhance density differences between normal tissue and lesions such as infections and tumors. It is also used to define vascular anatomy and patency.

- *Indications*:
  - CT scans are superior to MRI in detecting bony lesions and fractures.
  - CT scans without contrast are used to detect acute intracranial hemorrhage.
  - CT can be used safely in patients with implanted devices.

- *Contraindications*:
  - Relative contraindications:

    Pregnant women should avoid the ionizing radiation unless absolutely necessary for emergency care. If possible, US and MRI are preferred in this situation when absolutely required.

    Contrast use should be avoided unless absolutely necessary in patients with renal dysfunction or iodinated contrast allergy. Premedication can be given when needed to avoid allergic reaction.

Ultrasound [1]

- *Physics*:
  - A transducer emits a high frequency sound wave that is transmitted into tissues.
  - Sound waves are reflected where there are density changes between layers of tissues.
  - A receiver collects these reflected sound waves to create an image.

- *Indications*:
  - Used for diagnosis of musculoskeletal pathology, abdominal and pelvic pain syndromes
  - Use is gaining popularity among physicians for pain image-guided treatment/injection

    It is quickly becoming the imaging modality of choice for performing peripheral nerve blocks by many anesthesiologists.

    A few examples of injections that can be done with ultrasound guidance include stellate ganglion blocks, facet injections, sacroiliac joint injections, ilio-inguinal, and transversus abdominis plane blocks.

  - Safe in pregnancy

- *Contraindications*:
  - None

Imaging Recommendations for Specific Pain Conditions

Chronic Headache [2]

- New imaging is not required for history of chronic headache with no new features, as long as prior imaging was previously completed.
- MRI head/brain without and with contrast when history/ physical positive for new features (worst headache, change in headache, new headache, acute worsening of symptoms, seizures, advancing age, visual changes, mass effect, focal deficits, slurred speech)
- Please see more details in Chap. 16

New/Change Headache in Non-immunocompromised [2]

- *Sudden onset of severe or "worst headache of life" or headache associated with neurologic deficits*: head CT without contrast to rule of acute brain hemorrhage
- *If suspect stroke*: head CT without contrast and/or MRI without contrast, MRI may not show evidence of stroke initially, this may take time to show on MRI
- *Trauma*: head CT without contrast to rule out fracture

New Headache in Immune Compromised [2]

- *New onset headache in HIV/cancer/infections/ immunotherapy*: MRI brain with and without contrast to rule out infection

Temporal Arteritis [2]

- MRI brain without contrast with diffusion-weighted sequences

Nontraumatic Painful Myelopathy [3]

- MRI spine without contrast
- CT spine without contrast

Brachial Plexopathy [4]

- *Brachial plexus MRI*: depicts subtle changes in signal intensity of the nerves or enhancement and aid in refining the differential diagnosis.

- MRI sequences such as fat-saturated T2-weighted spin echo
- Short-tau inversion recovery (STIR)
- Gadolinium-enhanced T1-weighted spin-echo sequences: lumbosacral → MRI pelvis without and with contrast

Lumbar Spine [4–6]

- Suspected herniated disc or spinal stenosis
  - MRI lumbar spine without contrast
- Risk factors for cancer (advanced age/history of cancer/ presence of primary tumor)
  - Lumbosacral plain radiography AP and Lateral to rule out bony lesion
  - MRI lumbar spine with and without contrast if initial imaging is negative but high degree of suspicion remains
- Suspected instability (elderly, prior instrumentation, pain with flexion and extension, trauma, osteoporosis)
  - Plain X-rays with flexion and extension
- Neurologic deficits
  - MRI lumbar spine without contrast
- Risk factors for spinal infection (fever/sweats/chills/ increasing low back pain, spinal instrumentation/epidural or spinal interventions)
  - MRI lumbar spine with and without contrast
- Suspected vertebral compression fracture (elderly, patient on chronic steroids, multiple myeloma, cancer)
  - Lumbosacral plain radiography
- Risk factors for/signs of Cauda Equina syndrome (progressive or new onset sensory and motor deficit with or without bowel and bladder incontinence)
  - MRI lumbar spine without contrast
- Suspected ankylosing spondylitis
  - Lumbosacral plain radiography
  - Anterior–posterior pelvis plain radiography

Cervical Spine

- X-ray C-spine: AP, lateral, open mouth, oblique views
  - Open mouth view is to capture the odontoid for possible pathology
- MRI cervical spine without contrast: if X-rays are normal and neurologic signs/symptoms present

Facial Pain [7–10]

- *Trigeminal neuralgia and atypical facial pain*:
  - MRI face and brain with and without contrast: focus on trigeminal nerve

Complex Regional Pain Syndrome (CRPS) [11, 12]

- X-ray, MRI, or CT scan to rule out other differential diagnosis
- Triple phase bone scan: may be done to identify osteopenia but is not essential since CRPS is a clinical diagnosis

Abdominal/Pelvic Pain [13, 14]

- Chronic pelvic pain (CPP):
  - Transvaginal ultrasound (TVUS): modality of first choice
  - MRI of the abdomen or pelvis: if TVUS is equivocal or nondiagnostic
  - See Chap. 22 for more details

Joint Pain

- Plain X-ray
- MRI without contrast: if X-ray nondiagnostic or displays effusion [15]
- X-ray arthrography of hip, knee, and shoulder: using contrast, local anesthetic ± corticosteroid, if X-ray is non-diagnostic/equivocal
- MR arthrogram: detects tears in ligaments or labrum, cartilaginous defects, intra-articular bodies, surgical planning

References

1. Brant WE, Helms CA. Fundamentals of diagnostic radiology. 4th ed. Philadelphia: Wolters Kluwer/Lippincott Williams & Wilkins Health; 2012.
2. American College of Radiology. Headache. 1996 [updated 2009; cited 25 Nov 2012]. Available from: http://www.acr.org/~/media/ACR/Documents/AppCriteria/Diagnostic/Headache.pdf.
3. American College of Radiology. Myelopathy. 1996 [updated 2011; cited 25 Nov 2012]. Available from: http://www.acr.org/~/media/ACR/Documents/AppCriteria/Diagnostic/Myelopathy.pdf.
4. American College of Radiology. Low back pain. 1996 [updated 2011; cited 25 Nov 2012]. Available from: http://www.acr.org/~/media/ACR/Documents/AppCriteria/Diagnostic/LowBackPain.pdf.
5. Chou R, Qaseem A, Snow V, Casey D, Cross Jr JT, Shekelle P, et al. Diagnosis and treatment of low back pain: a joint clinical practice guideline from the American College of Physicians and the American Pain Society. Ann Intern Med. 2007;147(7):478–91. PubMed PMID: 17909209, Epub 2007/10/03.eng.
6. Chou R, Qaseem A, Owens DK, Shekelle P. Diagnostic imaging for low back pain: advice for high-value health care from the American College of Physicians. Ann Intern Med. 2011;154(3):181–9. PubMed PMID: 21282698, Epub 2011/02/02.eng.
7. American College of Radiology. Sinonasal disease. 2009 [updated 2012; cited 24 Nov 2012]. Available from: http://www.acr.org/~/media/ACR/Documents/AppCriteria/Diagnostic/SinonasalDisease.pdf.
8. Siccoli MM, Bassetti CL, Sandor PS. Facial pain: clinical differential diagnosis. Lancet Neurol. 2006;5(3):257–67. PubMed PMID: 16488381, Epub 2006/02/21.eng.
9. Ogutcen-Toller M, Uzun E, Incesu L. Clinical and magnetic resonance imaging evaluation of facial pain. Oral Surg Oral Med Oral Pathol Oral Radiol Endod. 2004;97(5):652–8. PubMed PMID: 15153880, Epub 2004/05/22.eng.
10. Martin DS, Awwad EE, Maves MD. Imaging facial pain of trigeminal origin. Am J Otolaryngol. 1995;16(2):132–7. PubMed PMID: 7793509, Epub 1995/03/01.eng.
11. Cappello ZJ, Kasdan ML, Louis DS. Meta-analysis of imaging techniques for the diagnosis of complex regional pain syndrome type I. J Hand Surg. 2012;37(2):288–96. PubMed PMID: 22177715, Epub 2011/12/20.eng.
12. Bailey J, Nelson S, Lewis J, McCabe CS. Imaging and clinical evidence of sensorimotor problems in CRPS: utilizing novel treatment approaches. J Neuroimmune Pharmacol. 2012;11. PubMed PMID: 23054370, Epub 2012/10/12.eng.
13. Cody Jr RF, Ascher SM. Diagnostic value of radiological tests in chronic pelvic pain. Baillieres Best Pract Res Clin Obstet Gynaecol. 2000;14(3):433–66. PubMed PMID: 10962636, Epub 2000/08/30.eng.
14. Cheong Y, Stones W. Investigations for chronic pelvic pain. Rev Gynaecol Pract. 2005;5:227–36.
15. American College of Radiology. Nontraumatic knee pain. 1995 [updated 2008; cited 25 Nov 2012]. Available from: http://www.acr.org/~/media/ACR/Documents/AppCriteria/Diagnostic/NontraumaticKneePain.pdf.

Painful Surgical Spine Referrals and Emergencies

5

Anthony Isenalumhe Jr.

Abbreviations

AAA	Abdominal aortic aneurysm
AIDS	Acquired immunodeficiency syndrome
AP	Anteroposterior
CSF	Cerebral spinal fluid
CT	Computed tomography
FEV	Forced expiratory volume
FVC	Forced vital capacity
IV	Intravenous
MRI	Magnetic resonance imaging
PFTs	Pulmonary function tests

Introduction

It is important to differentiate a pain complaint that does not require surgery from one that requires routine surgery and even more important to recognize a surgical emergency. Taking a comprehensive history, physical exam, and obtaining appropriate imaging can help to distinguish between these circumstances.

- Time of symptomatic onset and the mechanism of injury provide a sense of the acuity of the patient's condition as well as the extent of injury that may have been sustained.
  - Sudden onset of intense pain following an event is often indicative of significant tissue trauma (i.e., a fracture) or of rapidly progressive pathology (i.e., an epidural hematoma).
  - Insidious onset of pain, on the other hand, occurs mostly in situations where the surrounding tissue and the body at large have time to accommodate/compensate (i.e., tumor and osteoarthritis) [1, 2].

- Mechanism of injury provides the practitioner with an idea of the extent of possible tissue damage—motor vehicle accident versus impact with a bicycle [2, 3].
- *Red flags*—ominous signs and symptoms that may clue you into a specific diagnosis. These flags are discussed along with each diagnosis in this chapter.
- *When should a diagnostic test be ordered and how should it guide your decision?*
  - **X-ray**—delineates the bony anatomy, not as reliable as a CT scan
    To optimize benefit, it is important to get dynamic imaging—flexion, extension films, particularly when worried about dynamic pathology in a patient with positional pain. X-rays can help with the diagnosis of micro- fracture, misalignment, scoliosis, aberrant bone growth, and any calcified lesion that may be missed by non-X-ray imaging such as MRI.
  - **Computed tomography (CT)**—used to assess the degree of bony involvement, better resolution than X-ray, with thin cut cross-sectional areas of the body that can also be reconstructed to provide a 3-dimensional image. Greater risk of radiation. Can evaluate for herniated disc or spinal stenosis. Of note, metallic implant may generate artifacts. Used in patients with metal implants such as non-mri compatibles spinal cord stimulators, etc.
  - **MRI**—best modality currently for visualization of soft tissue structures such as nerve, muscles and discs. Safer method of imaging [3, 4].
  - **Ultrasound**—provides the benefit of real-time image. No risk of radiation. Safe for pregnancy. It also provides good delineation of tissue relationship, but its poor bone penetration, high operator dependence, and limited field of view at any given time makes it **not** the imaging modality of choice for spinal pathology. When utilized by a trained ultrasonographer, it is very effective for extraspinal examination (i.e., joints, peripheral nerves, bursas, ligaments, and such peripheral tissues that are not encased in bone).

A. Isenalumhe Jr., M.D. (✉)
Pain Management/Anesthesiology, Stanford Medical Center, 2275 Latham Street, Apt 52, Mountain View, CA 94040, USA
e-mail: isenalumhe@gmail.com

K.A. Sackheim, *Pain Management and Palliative Care: A Comprehensive Guide*, DOI 10.1007/978-1-4939-2462-2_5, © Springer Science+Business Media New York 2015

Consider non-spine-related causes of neck and back pain which may require surgical intervention or specialty evaluation.

Examples listed below (these do not represent complete differential diagnoses): [4–6]

- **Neck pain**:
  - Thoracic outlet syndrome
  - Esophagitis
  - Angina
  - Vascular dissection
- **Back pain**:
  - AAA
  - Aortic dissection
  - Retroperitoneal pathology (pancreatitis, renal pathology—i.e., stones)
  - Gallbladder disease
  - Retroperitoneal hematoma

Reasons For Spinal Surgical Referral

1. **Severe Scoliosis**—abnormal lateral curvature of the spine
   - Type is mostly defined by etiology: idiopathic (unknown cause—the most common), congenital (birth defect), neuromuscular (consequence of muscular disease such as cerebral palsy, polio, and muscular dystrophy), and osteopathic (bony abnormality) [6, 7].
   - Diagnosis of scoliosis can be made with *Adams forward bend test*—patient bends forward, feet together and knees straight, and the provider can evaluate the symmetry of either side of the spine and its curvature. If positive, an AP X-ray is indicated to examine the spine. From the X-ray a "Cobb's angle" can be measured.
     - *Cobb's angle*—a measurement used for evaluation of curves in scoliosis on an AP radiographic projection of the spine. Cobb's angle of 10° is minimum angulation to define scoliosis.
   - Surgery is indicated with Cobb's angle >45–50°, as an angle >50° progress even after skeletal maturity [7].
   - Scoliosis in the thoracic region progress more rapidly than other areas of the spine; therefore, surgery should be considered sooner.
   - Concerns with progression of scoliosis in the thoracic region are not for aesthetic reasons primarily but rather significant morbidity and mortality from compression of intrathoracic organs
     - *Respiratory*—causing loss of pulmonary function as well as predisposing the patient to pneumonia, even resulting in respiratory failure at larger curvatures (Cobb's angles >60° by 40–50 years of age). The associated decreased chest wall compliance and consequent progressive atelectasis increase the work of

breathing. The increased work of breathing progressively weakens respiratory muscles. Pulmonary function test can provide an easy and reliable means for evaluation and follow-up.

Patients with Cobb's angle ranging between 100° and 150° and poor PFTs with FVC ratio $\leq 65\%$, FEV1 ratio $\leq 65\%$, and PEF ratio $\leq 65\%$ are at significantly higher risk for postoperative pulmonary complications, and therefore poor surgical candidates [7, 8].

Key: postoperative pulmonary complications are thought to be associated with the surgical approach, preoperative PFTs (primarily FVC ratio $\leq 65\%$), and concomitant thoracoplasty [7–9].
- *Cardiac*—restrictive cardiomyopathy can occur with scoliosis as spinal rotation deform the thoracic cage, decreasing the chest wall compliance and accordingly compromises the ventilatory volume of lung and respiratory capacity. The poor ventilation and increased pulmonary resistance progressively increases the afterload of the right heart leading to cor pulmonale over time.

However, they do tolerate surgery well, but are at risk of decompensating in the perioperative period and accordingly, perioperative monitoring with transthoracic echocardiogram should be highly considered [9–11].

2. **Spondylolisthesis**—an anterior or posterior displacement of a vertebra in relation to the vertebra below [3, 6]
   - Etiologies—classified as congenital (dysplastic), spondylolytic (isthmic), degenerative, traumatic, pathologic, or iatrogenic
   - Percentage of slippage in comparison to the vertebra below determines the grade of spondylolisthesis
     - Grade 1—0–25 %
     - Grade 2—25–50 %
     - Grade 3—50–75 %
     - Grade 4—75–100 %
   - Grade 1 and 2 may present with pain in the lower back and buttock with tightness and spasm in the hamstrings. Treated mostly with conservative methods: exercise, back brace
   - Grade 3 and 4 may shift the intra-abdominal content presenting as a protruding abdomen, difficulty walking, and radiating pain indicative of nerve compression, as these high grades do cause narrowing of the neural foramina.

   Grades 3 or higher may require surgical intervention if conservative methods fail to relieve the symptoms.

3. **Spinal stenosis**—narrowing of the spinal canal with compression of the neural structures
   - Lumbar spine—most common region for spinal stenosis

- Spinal stenosis is the most common reason for lumbar spine surgery in adults >65 years of age.
- Lumbar spinal stenosis often presents with radicular leg pain or neurogenic claudication (progressive pain with walking or prolonged standing, which is relieved by sitting down or lumbar flexion).
- In comparing surgical vs. nonsurgical therapy for lumbar spinal stenosis, patient with imaging-confirmed spinal stenosis without spondylolisthesis and leg symptoms prolonged for at least 12 weeks did better with surgery compared to the nonsurgical group with relief of symptoms and improving function for at least 2 years [3, 6, 12].

4. **Disc herniation** [1, 2, 12]
   - Most patients do well with conservative treatment (i.e., physical therapy, medications, epidural injections), which provides symptomatic relief and obviates unnecessary surgery.
   - 50 % of patients with herniated discs recover in 1 month
   - 96 % recover by 6 months
     When should surgery be considered?
     - Severe weakness
     - Disabling pain, despite exhausted conservative efforts
     - Unremitting or severe neurological symptoms—e.g., loss of control of bowel or bladder
     - Persistent radicular pain with progressive weakness and numbness despite conservative treatment
     - Importantly, clear delineation of a surgically amenable disc herniation on imaging (MRI, CT scan, or myologram) that correlate to a likely site of nerve compression which explains the patient's dermatomal and myotomal presentation.

5. **Neoplasm**—spinal tumors include a wide range of abnormal growth of cells of various origins
   Type of cell/tissue from which they originate classifies spinal tumors [13].
   - *Intramedullary tumor*—tumors arising from within the spinal cord itself. Normally benign, however, based on their location, they can cause significant neural compromise as they grow.
     - Astrocytomas—originate from glial cells (the supporter cell of neurons of the central nervous system).
     - Ependymomas—originate from the epithelial-like cells that line the CSF-filled ventricles in the brain and the central canal of the spinal cord.
     - Hemangioblastomas—arise from the vascular system
   - *Intradural-extramedullary tumor*—as the name suggests, originates from the protective layers of the spinal cord but are outside the spinal cord.
     - Meningiomas—arise from the meninges

- Schwannomas and neurofibromas—arise from Schwann cell
- *Extradural tumors*—most common spinal tumors, also known as vertebral column tumors—include metastatic tumors and tumors that originate from surrounding bone and cartilage.
  - Common primary tumors that metastasize to the spine are lung, breast, prostate, and kidney.
    - Initial presentation of these tumors can be localized pain in the neck or back. However, progression of symptoms occurs as the tumor grows and is mostly the result of compression of neural tissue based on the location of occurrence—cervical, thoracic, lumbar, or sacral.
    - Depending on the severity and acuity of presentation, the patient may benefit from a regimen of steroids and/or localized radiation to decrease the associated inflammation and tumor size, respectively, allowing time for a schedule surgical intervention.
    - Emergent surgical intervention is necessary whenever there is progressive threat with neurological symptoms, which can occur with spinal tumors based on type (poorly defined, rapidly growing) or location (proximity to vital spinal tissue). This can present as progressive loss of sensory and motor function in the legs based on compression of the lumbrosacral nerve fibers, or arrhythmia based on local compression or infiltration of the cardiac accelerators (the upper thoracic neural fibers T1-T4). An understanding of spinal innervation is necessary for proper correlation of the presenting symptoms to the location of pathology [13].

6. **Spinal hemangiomas** [1, 2, 13]
   - Hemangiomas are benign tumors formed due to abnormal proliferation of blood vessels; such lesions can also form in the skin and other organs. The vertebrae and skull are the most common sites of formation in the skeletal system.
   - Most common location in the spine: Thoracic > Lumbar > Cervical; Commonly between 50 and 70 years of age; females twice likely to be affected than males.
   - Majority are asymptomatic, incidental finding on imaging—no treatment required
   - About 1 % are symptomatic: presenting as axial back pain or with neurological symptoms (sensory and/or motor deficit). Symptoms are either due to pathological/compression fractures (due to structural destabilization from the replacement of bony tissue with blood vessel intrinsic to hemangioma formation) or cord

compression (which can occur when the hemangioma lesions extend out of the vertebral body or bleed).
- Diagnosis: MRI with contrast is helpful in discerning tissue relationship; however, CT with contrast is a reasonable alternative.
- Surgical treatment if indicated:
  - *Nonemergent* (no cord compression)
    - Vertebroplasty/kyphoplasty
    - Radiation therapy
    - Emolization
  - *Emergent* (cord compression)
    - Intralesion alcohol injection
    - Embolization with subsequent surgical removal of tumor and bracing with bone grafts and metallic prosthesis

7. **Spinal cysts: ganglionic and synovial** [14, 15]
   - The difference between a ganglionic cyst and a synovial cyst is the existence of a synovial lining in a synovial cyst. Otherwise, both share the same clinical presentation, treatment, and prognosis.
   - *Epidemiology*: occur in patients primarily in the sixth decade of life; slightly higher incidence in females
   - *Symptoms*: based on the progressive mass effect of the cyst as it grow and is therefore based on location and the tissue being compressed (neural versus nonneural tissue, i.e., bony component of the spine). Most common symptoms: #1 Radiculopathy, #2 Neurogenic claudication
   - Most common location for a spinal cyst to occur is in the lumbar region, primarily L4-5, but it can affect multiple levels and can be bilateral.
   - The formation of spinal cysts is mostly associated with spinal instability i.e., facet joint arthropathy, and degenerative spondylolisthesis, and therefore a concomitant fusion procedure may be performed if a surgical approach is elected.
   - *Diagnosis*: MRI is the image of choice; a noncontrast MRI is sufficient as the variation of the different sequences (T1, T1, Stir) helps differentiate it from other possible pathologies and delineate the relationship of the adjacent tissue.
   - Spinal cyst are rarely emergencies but can be if they hemorrhage and bleed into the surrounding soft tissue or spinal canal causing acute compression of the spinal cord.
   - *Treatment*:
     - Conservative: oral analgesics, physical therapy
     - Interventions: needle aspiration, intra-articular or epidural steroid injection
     - Invasive: surgery
     - Regardless of which modality is chosen. Note that the cyst can recur.

8. **Spinal infections** [1, 2, 4]— primarily the result of vascular spread or direct introduction via instrumentation of the spinal column and its contents leading to:
   - *Meningitis or encephalitis*—present with headache, neck stiffness, loss of neurologic functions, or CSF finding
   - *Epidural abscess*—most commonly bacterial in origin but can be caused by a virus or fungus
   - *Osteomyelitis*
     - Patients susceptible to osteomyelitis include:
       - Elderly patients
       - Intravenous drug users
       - Immunocompromised individuals
   - *Pott's disease*—Tuberculosis of the spine; should be evaluated with a CT with contrast; also well visualized on an MRI
   - *Discitis*—inflammation of the vertebral disc space, usually associated with infection via hematologic spread
     - Most common location—Lumbar > Cervical > Thoracic spine
     - *Risk factors*: IV drug user and immunosuppressive states, i.e., AIDS and diabetes, may also occur after surgery involving the disc space
     - *Clinical presentation*: insidious onset of pain and localized tenderness of the affected spinal level. Pain is worse with movement. May be associated with fever; of note, neurological deficits may occur, primarily when the infection is at the cervical level.
     - X-ray (show narrow disc space, end plate irregularity, and calcification of the annulus); however, it may be normal—especially in the beginning.
     - MRI is the most sensitive and specific study with contrast (always better to use contrast to evaluate vascular lesions—infection, tumors, etc.).
     - Initial treatment is via parenteral antibiotics for 6–8 weeks. Surgical treatment may be needed if there are neurological deficits, or no response with antibiotic therapy.

   Treatment for each type of spinal infection is initially conservative and is based on the type of pathogen: bacterial, viral, fungal, parasitic, with treatment with antibiotics, antivirals, antifungals, supportive therapy (i.e., steroids), respectively.

   Surgery is required for:
   - Urgent for: debridement (drainage of abscess and removal of necrotic tissue) and infections that are intractable despite optimization of drug delivery (including intravenous and intrathecal)
   - Emergent for: decompression, when there is development of mass effect by an abscess with compression of neural tissue (brain, spinal cord, or nerves)

Conditions Requiring Emergent Surgical Intervention

Sudden severe or progressive nerve/cord compression (a concern also in unstable spinal fractures, ex. vertebral compression fracture, burst fractures, and "jumped facets", which are not discussed in this chapter as these are due to major trauma and present to the ER and not the out-patient clinic). Any evidence of spinal cord injury may require emergent surgical intervention as well.

Cauda Equina Syndrome [16, 17]

- A constellation of symptoms brought on by compression/damage of the cauda equina—nerve roots of L2-S5. Causes of cauda equina syndrome include central or centerolateral disk prolapse and other space-occupying lesions; infections such as meningitis; rare causes such as abdominal aortic dissection; and complications after surgery, spinal manipulation, or epidural injections.
- One of the following symptoms must be present for the diagnosis of Cauda equina syndrome:
  - Bladder and/or bowel dysfunction (check anal tone on exam)
  - Reduced sensation in the saddle area (check sensation including perianal region)
  - Sexual dysfunction with possible neurologic deficits in the lower extremities, which may include loss of motor, sensory, or reflex function.
  - *Treatment*: mostly involves urgent surgical decompression, primarily if the clinical signs and symptoms are sudden. As the innate pathology is a condition (tumor burden, disc protrusion, trauma, hemorrhage, etc.) causing mass effect on the lumbrosacral nerve root with threat to nerve survival. The chance of avoiding long-term neurological damage is dependent on time to decompression. Surgery is the fastest means of decompression. Other forms of decompression include radiation for tumor burden and steroids for associated inflammation.

Vascular/hematologic pathology [18, 19]

Epidural hematoma
- *Etiology*: rupture of the Batson vertebral venous plexus
- Can occur spontaneously or secondary to minor trauma—i.e., lumbar puncture or epidural anesthesia
- *Risk factors*: include spinal instrumentation, blood dyscrasia, and coagulopathy (please review the ASA guidelines for each anticoagulation therapy and recommended timing for spinal interventions).

- *Presentation*:
  - Neck, back, or abdominal pain, depending on the location of the hematoma; accordingly, there may be a radicular pain component into the extremities, chest, abdomen.
  - Difficulty with urinating and bowel movement
  - Numbness and/or weakness of extremities
- *Imaging*: MRI or CT with contrast is preferred
- *Treatment*:
  - No time to waste with onset of clinical signs of nerve compression:
  - Best outcomes are with surgical decompression ≤ 8 h
  - Poor outcome are when decompression does not occur in ≤ 48 h.

Infection [19, 20]

Epidural abscess—can occur via hematogenous spread, continuous spread from infected neighboring structures, or non-sterile instrumentation
- Most common organism is staphylococcus aureus
- *Risk factors*: Intravenous drug abuse, diabetes mellitus, existing infection, alcoholism, as well as other forms of immunosuppressive states, including AIDS
- *Clinical presentation*: similar to the presentation an epidural hematoma but presents days later; may be preceded by an epidural hematoma which creates a conducive environment for bacterial growth. Presentation for abscess includes fever and malaise.
- *Labs/imaging*: blood culture (not always positive); MRI or CT with contrast
- *Treatment*:
  - Decompression: when there is development of mass effect by an abscess with compression of neural tissue (brain, spinal cord, or nerves).

References

1. Chou R, Baisden J, Carragee EJ, Resnick DK, Shaffer WO, Loeser JD. Surgery for low back pain; a review of the evidence for an American Pain Society Clinical Practice Guideline. Spine (Phila Pa 1976). 2009;34(10):1094–109.
2. Henschke N, Maher CG, Refshauge KM, Herbert RD, Cumming RG, Bleasel J, York J, Das A, McAuley JH. Prevalence of and screening for serious spinal pathology in patients presenting to primary care settings with acute low back pain. Arthritis Rheum. 2009;60(10):3072–80.
3. Watters III WC, Baisden J, Gilbert TJ, Kreiner S, Resnick DK, Bono CM, Ghiselli G, Heggeness MH, Mazanec DJ, O'Neill C, Reitman CA, Shaffer WO, Summers JT, Toton JF, North American Spine Society. Degenerative lumbar spinal stenosis: an evidence-based clinical guideline for the diagnosis and treatment of degenerative lumbar spinal stenosis. Spine J. 2008;8(2):305–10. Epub 2007 Dec 21.

4. Wright M, Tidy C, Huins H. Spinal disc problems (including red flag signs). Patient.co.uk. 2012. http://www.patient.co.uk/doctor/spinal-disc-problems-including-red-flag-signs#ref-2

5. Douglass AB, Bope ET. Evaluation and treatment of posterior neck pain in family practice. J Am Board Fam Pract. 2004;17 Suppl:S13–22.

6. Gibson JN, Grant IC, Waddell G. The Cochrane review of surgery for lumbar disc prolapse and degenerative lumbar spondylosis. Spine (Phila Pa 1976). 1999;24(17):1820–32.

7. Maruyama T, Takeshita K. Surgical treatment of scoliosis: a review of techniques currently applied. Scoliosis. 2008;3:6.

8. Barois A. Respiratory problems in severe scoliosis. Bull Acad Natl Med. 1999;183(4):721–30.

9. Loa L, Weng X, Qiu G, Shen J. The role of preoperative pulmonary function test in the surgical treatment of extremely severe scoliosis. J Orthop Surg Res. 2013;8:32.

10. Primiano Jr FP, Nussbaum E, Hirschfeld SS, et al. Early echocardiographic and pulmonary function findings in idiopathic scoliosis. J Pediatr Orthop. 1983;3(4):475–81.

11. Liu L, Xiu P, Li Q, Song Y, Chen R, Zhou C. Prevalence of cardiac dysfunction and abnormalities in patients with adolescent idiopathic scoliosis requiring surgery. Orthopedics. 2010;33(12):882.

12. Hu SS, et al. Lumbar disc herniation section of disorders, diseases, and injuries of the spine. In: Skinner HB, editor. Current diagnosis and treatment in orthopedics. 4th ed. New York: McGraw-Hill; 2006. p. 246–9.

13. Thakur NA, Daniels AH, Schiller J, Valdes MA, Czerwein JK, Schiller A, Esmende S, Terek RM. Benign tumors of the spine. J Am Acad Orthop Surg. 2012;20:715–24.

14. Lyons MK, et al. Surgical evaluation and management of lumbar synovial cysts: the Mayo Clinic experience. J Neurosurg. 2000;93 (1 Suppl):53–7.

15. Khan MA, Girardi F. Spinal lumbar synovial cysts. Diagnosis and management challenge. Eur Spine J. 2006;15(8):1176–82.

16. Fraser S, Roberts L, Murphy E. Cauda equina syndrome: a literature review of its definition and clinical presentation. Arch Phys Med Rehabil. 2009;90(11):1964–8.

17. Arrigo RT, Kalanithi P, Boakye M. Is cauda equina syndrome being treated within the recommended time frame? Neurosurgery. 2012; 70(5):1324–5.

18. French KL, Daniels EW, Ahn UM, Ahn NU. Medicolegal cases for spinal epidural hematoma and spinal epidural abscess. Orthopedics. 2013;36(1):48–53.

19. Song KJ, Lee KB. The poor outcome of the delayed diagnosis of acute spontaneous spinal epidural hematoma: two cases report. J Korean Med Sci. 2005;20(2):331–4.

20. Chao D, Nanda A. Spinal epidural abscess: a diagnostic challenge. Am Fam Physician. 2002;65(7):1341–6. Review.

Urine Toxicology Screen

6

Joyce Ho

Abbreviations

AED	Antiepileptic drug
CLIA	Clinical Laboratory Improvement Amendments
EPPD	2-Ethylidene-1,5-Dimethyl-3,3-Diphenylpyr-rolidine
ER	Emergency Room
EtOH	Ethanol
GM	Gas chromatography
HPLC	High performance liquid chromatography
IA	Immunoassay
LC/MS/MS	Liquid chromatography tandem mass spectro-metry
LSD	Lysergic Acid Diethylamide
MDMA	3,4-Methylenedioxy-N-methylamphetamine
MDPV	Methylenedioxypyrovalerone
MMTP	Methadone Maintenance Treatment Program
MS	Mass spectrometry
PCP	Phencyclidine
POC	Point of care
RDS	Random drug screen
TCA	Tricyclic
THC	Tetrahydrocannabinol
UDS	Urine drug screen
UTOX	Urine toxicology

Reasons to Order Urine Toxicology Screen [1]

- Assure prescribed medications taken as directed, i.e., establish compliance
- Detect possible diversion of medications
- Detect the presence of non-prescribed drugs and/or illicit substances

J. Ho, M.D. (✉)
University of California Irvine, Physical Medicine and
Rehabilitation, 1 Medical Plaza Drive, Irvine, CA 92697, USA
e-mail: joyceh3@uci.edu

When to Order Urine Toxicology Screen [2]

- Prior to initiation of an opioid: Assess for the presence of illegal and possible prescribed/non-prescribed drugs
- Change of opioid prescriber: Assess for the presence of illegal drugs and currently prescribed opiate
- Suspect substance misuse/abuse
- Routine random testing

Appropriate Frequency

- No specific rule in terms of frequency of drug testing but risk stratification appears to be the best way to determine frequency
  - **Low risk**
    Randomly, approximately every 6 months
  - **Intermediate risk**
    3 to 4 times a year
  - **High risk**
    As often as once a month
- May be subject to state and local statutes and regulations
- *Documentation:* Reasoning behind the frequency of testing as well as the need for confirmatory testing is required, including evidence of risk assessment

Helpful History for Identifying Higher Risk Individuals

- Inconsistent history
- Comorbid psychiatric disorder such as depression, anxiety, bipolar disorder, and/or personality disorder
- Current or history of alcohol or psychoactive drug use
- Past inconsistent drug screen
- History of substance abuse (including EtOH, and or illicit drugs, dependence/addiction including history of enrollment in treatment program such as MMTP) [3]

K.A. Sackheim, *Pain Management and Palliative Care: A Comprehensive Guide,*
DOI 10.1007/978-1-4939-2462-2_6, © Springer Science+Business Media New York 2015

- Patient or family considers patient to be addicted
- Patient's care previously terminated by a provider
- Patient changes providers frequently
- Unstable and/or dysfunctional social situations
- Decreased functioning
- History of buying medications "on the street"
- History of sharing medications with a friend or family member or taking their medications

Physical Examination for Identifying Higher Risk Individuals

- Observed intoxication (walking "funny," slurred speech, drowsy, EtOH breath)
- Strange affect (liable emotion, not reactive, disinterested, agitated)
- Needle track marks
- *Drug-seeking behaviors*
  - Focusing (excessively) on opiate issues
  - Self-increasing dosage/frequency
  - Persistently asking the prescriber to escalate dosage/frequency
  - Frequently requesting early refills
  - Reporting lost/spilled/stolen medications/prescriptions
  - Showing up unscheduled
  - Failing to keep regular appointments or persistent late arrivals
  - Failing to improve in function or decrease in pain
  - Going to other providers including ER for more medications
  - Using medications for symptoms other than pain (insomnia, anxiety, depression)
  - Failing to bring in unused medications upon request for pill counting
  - Asking for specific medications (particularly the case if this drug has high abuse potential)
  - Refusing other drug treatment(s) and/or changes in scheduled drug(s)
  - Refusing generic drug substitution or demanding short acting medications only
  - Stating a preference for the route of administration
  - Not accepting or following other non-opioid treatments

Collecting the Urine Sample

- Document all current medications so you can properly interpret the urine results. If a medication is taken on an as needed basis only, document this, it may/may not be in the urine depending on the last time it was taken.
  - Specifically ask about benzodiazepines and headache medications (patients may forget to mention prn medications)

- Document the last time the patient took their prescribed opiate and/or benzodiazepine for accurate interpretation of results
- Have a dedicated bathroom for sample collection
  - Should be in a location where the staff can monitor the activity
  - Patient should enter bathroom alone with no bags/drinks or coat/sweater which may be used to conceal urine they may have brought with them
  - Monitor for excessive time spent in restroom
  - Can use a blue dye in the toilet to prevent patient from diluting sample with toilet water
- If *patient is "unable to provide a urine sample"*
  - Advise patient not to leave the premise before giving sample
  - Provide drinking water and wait or consider oral swab for testing instead

Types of Urine Toxicology Testing [4]

1. **Immunoassay (IA)**
   (a) *Point of care testing (Immunoassay in office)*
     - Commonly referred to as "dip-stick" or "urine cup" testing
     - *Qualitative*: Reported as **present or absent** of the substance at a predetermined cutoff threshold
     - *Immediate results*
     - CLIA waiver required for performing in office
       - See website http://www.cms.gov/Regulations-and-Guidance/Legislation/CLIA/How_to_Apply_for_a_CLIA_Certificate_International_Laboratories.html for details
     - *Limited testing capability*
       - *Most cups are 12 panel testing including THC, Cocaine, Opiate (general screen), Amphetamine, Methamphetamine, PCP, MDMA, Barbiturates, Benzodiazepines, Methadone, TCAs, Oxycodone*
       - Important to know which opioid is covered in the opiate class because not all POC IA (manufacture dependent) detect semisynthetic or synthetic opioid [1]
     - Less costly
     - Cannot be used as confirmatory test
     - Sensitivity only 75 % for benzodiazepines [5]
   (b) *Immunoassay in laboratory*
     - Also qualitative
     - Benzodiazepine detection especially unreliable
     - Standard benzodiazepine screen does not test for alprazolam, lorazepam, or clonazepam
     - Sensitivity of 90–95 % and specificity of 85–90 % for standard screen

2. **Confirmatory testing in laboratory**
- Laboratories perform a confirmatory quantitative test if the IA is positive
- Specific drug (rather than class) can be identified
- Allow for identification and quantification of specific drug substances
- False positives/negatives still possible (sensitivity and specificity of around 99 %)
- Common methods
  - *Gas chromatography/mass spectrometry (GC/MS)* considered "gold standard" (i.e., use GC/MS result for final interpretation) [6]
  - *Liquid chromatography tandem mass spectrometry (LC/MS/MS)* or *high performance liquid chromatography (HPLC)* may also be used

Problems with Either Testing

- No way to tell from a urine drug test the exact amount of drug taken, when the last dose was taken, or the source of the drug
- Recent systematic review of the use of drug treatment agreements and urine drug testing to discourage misuse when opioids are prescribed for chronic non-cancer pain only found weak, heterogeneous evidence that these strategies were associated with less misuse [7]

- Processing errors (storage at extreme temperatures, low volume for testing due to bottle leakage, specimen contamination)
- Improper screens (especially for IAs)
  - Must know difference among natural, semisynthetic and synthetic opioid, as well as their metabolites (Fig. 6.1)
  - Must know expected metabolites for benzodiazepines (Fig. 6.2)
- **False negatives**
  - Taking less drug than prescribed (could be due to reduced need)
  - Taking medication on an irregular schedule (prn obviously ok but watch out for binging)
  - Adulterating or substituting urine sample to hide illicit use
  - Diverting the medication
  - Different rate of absorption (including route), distribution (body habitus/adipose tissue ratio), metabolism (either genetically or by concomitant exposure to enzyme inducers or inhibitors), and elimination (kidney function) of opioids/benzodiazepines [8]
  - Cross-reactivity
- **False positives** (Table 6.1)
  - The presence of small amounts of "process impurities," that is, other opioids that are created in acceptable amounts when manufacturing a different semisynthetic opioid

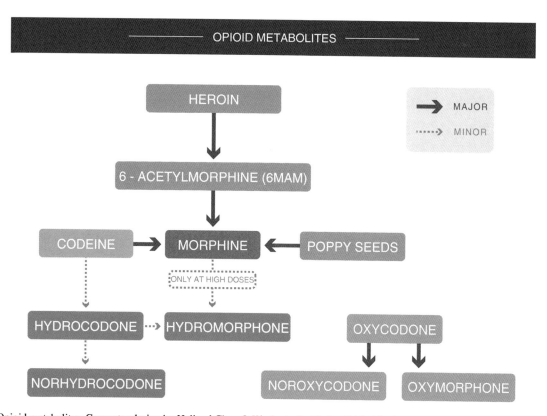

Fig. 6.1 Opioid metabolites. Computer design by Halland Chen © Kimberly Sackheim 2015. All Rights Reserved

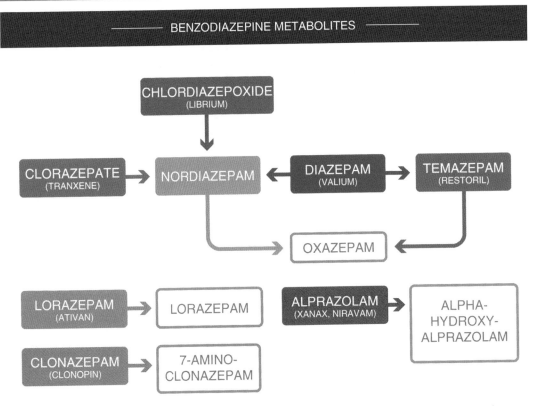

Fig. 6.2 Benzodiazepine metabolites. Computer design by Halland Chen © Kimberly Sackheim 2015. All Rights Reserved

- Different rate of absorption, distribution, metabolism, and elimination of opioids/benzodiazepines (see false negatives)
- Topical EtOH use
- Cross-reactivity

Some Examples of Cross-Reactivity [2]

- Multiple substances (including some diet pills, promethazine, and substances found in over-the-counter nasal inhalers such as Vicks® inhalers) cross-react with amphetamines
- A stereospecific chromatography test is recommended sometimes because standard laboratory GC/MS test will not differentiate the d-isomer (the stimulant) from the l-isomer (typically therapeutic) metabolites of methamphetamine
- Quinolone antibiotics can be misidentified as opiates
- Trazodone use can result in a false-negative test for fentanyl
- Venlafaxine use can produce a false-negative test for PCP
- Quetiapine can produce a false-negative test for methadone

- Proton-pump inhibitors may result in a false-negative test for THC
- Sertraline and oxaprozin can cause a false-negative benzodiazepine test

Interpreting Urine Toxicology Screen

- Ensure legitimate urine sample [6]
  - May need to visually monitor patient during specimen collection
  - Check temperature within 4 min of collection (should be 32–38 °C)
  - Check color and odor
  - Check pH (should be between 4.5 and 8.0)
    Influenced by diet, disease state, medication(s) [9]
    May affect results
    <3 or >11 inconsistent with human urine
  - Shake for bubbles (excessive bubbles created by additives such as detergents)
  - Check specific gravity (should be between 1.002 and 1.020)
  - Check creatinine

Table 6.1 Summary of agents contributing to positive results by immunoassay[a]

Substance tested via immunoassay	Potential agents causing false-positive result	Substance tested via immunoassay	Potential agents causing false-positive result
Alcohol	Short-chain alcohols (e.g., isopropyl alcohol)	Cannabinoids	Dronabinol
			Efavirenz
Amphetamines	Amantadine		Hemp-containing foods
	Benzphetamine		NSAIDs
	Bupropion		Proton pump inhibitors
	Chlorpromazine		Tolmetin
	Clobenzorex[b]	Cocaine	Coca leaf tea
	l-Deprenyl[c]		Topical anesthetics containing cocaine
	Desipramine	Opioids, Opiates, and Heroin	Dextromethorphan
	Dextroamphetamine		Diphenhydramine[e]
	Ephedrine[b]		Heroin
	Fenproporex[b]		Opiates (codeine, hydromorphone, hydrocodone, morphine)
	Isometheptene		Poppy seeds
	Isoxsuprine		Quinine
	Labetalol		Quinolones
	MDMA		Rifampin
	Methamphetamine		Verapamil and metabolites[e]
	l-Methamphetamine (Vick's inhaler)[d]	Phencyclidine	Dextromethorphan
	Methylphenidate		Diphenhydramine[e]
	Phentermine		Doxylamine
	Phenylephrine		Ibuprofen
	Phenylpropanolamine		Imipramine
	Promethazine		Ketadine
	Pseudoephedrine		Meperidine
	Ranitidine		Mesoridazine
	Ritodrine		Thioridazine
	Selegiline		Tramadol
	Thioridazine		Venlafaxine, O-desmethylvenlafaxine
	Trazodone	Tricyclic antidepressants	Carbamazepine[f]
	Trimethobenazmide		Cyclobenazprine
	Trimipramine		Cyproheptadine[f]
Benzodiazepines	Oxaprozin		Diphenhydramine[f]
	Sertaline		Hydroxyzine[f]
			Quetiapine

[a]MDMA-methylenedioxymethylamphetamine; NSAIDs = nonsteroidal anti-inflammatory drugs
[b]Approved in Mexico, not approved in the United States
[c]Converts to l-methamphetamine and l-amphetamine
[d]Newer immunoassays have corrected the false-positive result for Vick's inhaler
[e]Diphenhydramine and verapamil (including metabolites) have been shown to cause positive results in methadone assays only
[f]Reports of false-positive results occurred with serum only
Reprinted from Mayo Clinic Proceedings, 83/1, Karen E. Moeller, Kelly C. Lee, Julie C. Kissack, Urine Drug Screening: Practical Guide for Clinicians, 66–76, © 2013, with permission from Elsevier

Should be >20 mg/dL
<20 mg/dL: diluted, possibly by water loading
2.0 mg/dL: not consistent with human urine
- Check for medications prescribed and their metabolites
- Check for medications not prescribed and illicit substances
- Cross-reference with possible false positives and false negatives

Metabolism of Substances

Metabolism of Opiates [4, 10–13] (Fig. 6.1)

- Most metabolites stay in the system for 2–3 days except for much longer for methadone
- *If no metabolite(s), parent drug taken recently (not enough time for metabolism)*

Table 6.2 Major and minor substances and typical detection time in urine after opioid consumption

Opioid	Major substance(s) detected	Minor substance(s) detected	Typical detection time
Morphine	Morphine	Hydromorphone	3–4 days
Codeine	Codeine + Morphine	Hydrocodone + Hydromorphone	1–3 days
Hydrocodone	Hydrocodone + Norhydrocodone + Hydromorphone		1–2 days
Oxycodone	Oxycodone + Oxymorphone + Noroxycodone		1–3 days
Oxymorphine	Oxymorphone		2–3 days
Fentanyl	Fentanyl + metabolites with Fentanyl affix		1–3 days
Methadone	Methadone + EDDP		Up to 14 days
Buprenorphine	Buprenorphine + metabolites with Buprenorphine affix		2–4 days
Tramadol	Tramadol + metabolites with Tramadol affix		2–4 days
Tapentadol	Tapentadol + metabolites with Tapentadol affix		1–2 days
Meperidine	Meperidine + Normeperidine		2–3 days
Propoxyphene (no longer in US market)	Propoxyphene + Norpoxyphene		2–4 days
Heroin (not prescribed)	6-acetayl-morphine + Morphine		1–3 days
Poppy Seeds (not prescribed)	Morphine		1–3 days

EPPD = 2-ethylidene-1,5-dimethyl-3,3-diphenylpyrrolidine

Table 6.3 Substances and typical detection time in urine after benzodiazepine use

Benzodiazepine	Substance(s) detected	Typical detection time
Alprazolam	Alprazolam + Alpha Hydroxy Alprazolam	24–72 h
Clonazepam	Clonazepam + 7-Amino Clonazepam	24–72 h
Lorazepam	Lorazepam	1–5 days
Diazepam	Diazepam + Nordiazepam + Temazepam + **Oxazepam**	1–7 days
Nordiazepam	Nordiazepam + **Oxazepam**	1–7 days
Temazepam	Temazepam + **Oxazepam**	1–7 days
Chlordiazepoxide	Chlordiazepoxide + Nordiazepam + **Oxazepam**	1–7 days
Clorazepate	Clorazepate + Nordiazepam + **Oxazepam**	1–7 days
Flurazepam	Hydroxyethyl-flurazepam + Desalkyl-flurazepam	24–72 h
Midazolam	Midazolam + Alpha Hydroxy Midazolam + 4 Hydroxy Midazolam	24–72 h

- *If only metabolite(s), parent drug **not** taken "recently" (half-life dependent)*
- *See* Table 6.2

Metabolism of Benzodiazepines [14, 15] (Fig. 6.2)

- Not equally detectable on IAs due to different metabolic pathways
- May be insensitive even on GC/MS (particularly for lorazepam and clonazepam)
- Many degrade rapidly
- Oxazepam a common final metabolite that lingers (see Table 6.3)

Metabolism of Other Substances with Strong Addictive Potential [11, 12, 16–18]

- See Table 6.4

Other Commonly Tested Medications in UDS [11, 12]

- Gabapentin, pregabalin, amitriptyline (as amitriptyline + nortriptyline), nortriptyline, imipramine, and desipramine also commonly tested to establish compliant of the less addictive medications

Table 6.4 Substances detected and detection time in urine of other substances with strong addictive potential

Other Substance(s) with strong addictive potential	Substance(s) detected	Typical detection time
Amphetamine	Amphetamine	Up to 9 days
Methamphetamine (Speed, Crank, Crystal, Meth, Ice)	Methamphetamine + amphetamine	87 +/−51 h
Methylenedioxymethamphetamine (MDMA-Ecstasy)	MDMA	48 h
Methylenedioxyethylamphetamine (MDEA-Eve)	MDEA	~1.4–2.6 days
Modafinil	Modafinil + Modafinil acid	Up to 4 days
Armodafinil	Modafinil + Modafinil acid	Up to 4 days
Alcohol	Alcohol + ethyl glucoronide	7–12 h [Mayo]
Heroin	6-Acetayl-morphine + morphine + hydromorphone (if contained with codeine)	11–54 h
Cocaine	Cocaine + Benzolecgonine + Ecogonine methyl ester	22 days
PCP	PCP	2–7 days for casual use UP to 30 days [Christo]
Bath salts	Various, may include MDPV, Methylone and Mephedrone	Varies
Cannabis (Marijuana)	THC + 9-carboxy-THC	20–57 h in occasional users 3–13 days in regular users Up to 95 days
LSD	LSD + 2-Oxo-3-hydroxy-LSD	36–96 h
Amobarbital	Amobarbital	1–5 days
Pentobarbital	Pentobarbital	4–6 days
Butalbital	Butalbital	3–10 days
Secobarbital	Secobarbital	4–6 days
Phenobarbital	Phenobarbital	Up to 30 days
Carisoprodol	Carisoprodol + Meprobamate	2–4 days
Meprobamate	Meprobamate	2–4 days
Cyclobenzaprine	Cyclobenzaprine	
Methylphenidate	Ritalinic acid	2–4 days

Other Important Points of UDS

- Repeat UDS needed whenever results inconsistent
- Also useful in checking for the presence of other prescribed medications with no or less addictive potential (i.e., AED, TCA) to confirm general compliance in treatment
- Must have a plan for inconsistent UDS, especially on a repeat study
- Other ways of drug testing exist (blood, oral fluid, hair)

Recommendations

Low-risk individuals

- Such as an individual who takes only one short-acting opioid (especially one with lower addictive potential and/or street price) on as needed basis for flares (especially when the number taken is less than the maximum prescribed)
- A regular dipstick may be adequate but both qualitative and quantitative testing may be beneficial at least on first visit may be adequate

- Make sure the dipstick tests for the medication prescribed (confirmed with manufacture if in doubt)

Intermediate-risk individuals

- Everyone in between (i.e., an individual on long-acting opioid(s) or uses short-acting opioid(s) relatively frequently, an individual who may have associated depression but symptoms reasonably well managed)
- Qualitative and quantitative testing is recommended including medications prescribed every 3–4 months likely adequate performed
- A plan should be in place when there are questionable results for (repeated) testing(s)

High-risk individuals

- Qualitative and quantitative testing is recommended including medications prescribed and past medications/drugs misused may be adequate
- May expand on the panel if there are suspicions for misuse
- May need to perform on every visit or very frequently if needed

References

1. Tenore PL. Advanced urine toxicology testing. J Addict Dis. 2010;29(4):436–48.

2. Official Disability Guidelines (ODG), Treatment Index, 11th Edition (web), 2013, Pain (Chronic).

3. Chelminski PR, Ives TJ, Felix KM, Prakken SD, Miller TM, Perhac JS, Malone RM, Bryant ME, DeWalt DA, Pignone MP. A primary care, multi-disciplinary disease management program for opioid-treated patients with chronic non-cancer pain and a high burden of psychiatric comorbidity. BMC Health Serv Res. 2005;5(1):3.

4. Christo PJ, Manchikanti L, Ruan X, Bottros M, Hansen H, Solanki DR, Jordan AE, Colson J. Urine drug testing in chronic pain. Pain Physician. 2011;14(2):123–43.

5. Mikel C, Pesce AJ, Rosenthal M, West C. Therapeutic monitoring of benzodiazepines in the management of pain: current limitations of point of care immunoassays suggest testing by mass spectrometry to assure accuracy and improve patient safety. Clin Chim Acta. 2012;413(15–16):1199–202.

6. Moeller KE, Lee KC, Kissack JC. Urine drug screening: practical guide for clinicians. Mayo Clin Proc. 2008;83(1):66–76.

7. Starrels JL, Becker WC, Alford DP, Kapoor A, Wlliams AR, Turner BJ. Systemaitc review: treatment agreements and urine drug testing to reduce opioid misuse in patients with chronic pain. Ann Intern Med. 2010;152(11):712–20.

8. Markway EC, Baker SN. A review of the methods, interpretation, and limitations of the urine drug screen. Orthopedics. 2011;34(11):877–81.

9. Nafziger AN, Bertino Jr JS. Utility and application of urine drug testing in chronic pain management with opioids. Clin J Pain. 2009;25(1):73–9.

10. Smith HS. Opioid metabolism. Mayo Clin Proc. 2009;84(7):613–24.

11. Redwood Toxicolog Laboratory. Laboratory testing reference guide. http://www.redwoodtoxicology.com/documents/3034_refguide.pdf. Accessed 10 Feb 2013.

12. Ameritox Medication Monitoring Solutions. Drug test quick reference guide. Baltimore: Ameritox Ltd; 2010.

13. DuPont RL, Baumgartner WA. Drug testing by urine and hair analysis: complementary features and scientific issues. Forensic Sci Int. 1995;70(1–3):63–76.

14. Pesce A, West C, Egan City K, Strickland J. Interpretation of urine drug testing in pain patients. Pain Med. 2012;13(7):868–85. doi:10.1111/j.1526-4637.2012.01350.x. Epub 2012 Apr 11.

15. Fraser AD, Bryan W, Isner AF. Urinary screening for midazolam and its major metabolites with the Abbott ADx and TDx analyzers and the EMIT d.a.u. benzodiazepine assay with confirmation by GC/MS. J Anal Toxicol. 1991;15(1):8–12.

16. Verstraete AG. Detection times of drugs of abuse in blood, urine, and oral fluid. Ther Drug Monit. 2004;26(2):200–5.

17. McKinney AR, Suann CJ, Stenhouse AM. The detection of modafinil and its major metabolite in equine urine by liquid chromatography/mass spectrometry. Rapid Commun Mass Spectrom. 2005;19(10):1217–20.

18. Wong EC, Koenig J, Turk J. Potential interference of cyclobenzaprine with HPLC measurement of Amitriptyline and Nortriptyline: resolution by GC-MS analysis. J Anal Toxicol. 1995;19(4):2118–24.

Geet Paul

Abbreviations

ABG	Arterial blood gases
BMP	Basic metabolic panel
CBC	Complete blood count
CNS	Central nervous system
CVA	Cerebrovascular accident
CXR	Chest X-ray
Cx	Culture
EKG	Electrocardiogram
GI	Gastrointestinal
HEENT	Head, eyes, ears, neck, throat
IM	Intramuscular
IV	Intravenous
O_2	Oxygen
PCP	Phencyclidine
prn	As needed
UA	Urinalysis
UTOX	Urine toxicology

Opioid Overdose

Epidemiology

- The rate of exposure to analgesics including opioids and sedatives continues to rise each year [1].
- Rates of opioid abuse and deaths due to overdose are highest among non-Hispanic whites males, between 20 and 64 years old, from low socioeconomic and rural populations [2].

G. Paul, M.D. (✉)
Department of Rehabilitation Medicine, Mount Sinai
Medical Center, 257 Gold St. Apt 506, Brooklyn, NY 11201, USA
e-mail: gpaul26@gmail.com

History

- Know type of opioid used (if possible), route of exposure, amount taken, time ingested, possible co-ingestion of other substances, and prior history of opioid abuse. If the patient is not able to provide this information, it should be ascertained from family members/friends. Empty prescription bottles will also provide important information.

Serum Half-Life ($t_{1/2}$) of Commonly Prescribed Opioids (Table 7.1)

Serum half-life ($t_{1/2}$) of the drug ingested is an important factor in the length of duration and dosing of naloxone. Naloxone's $t_{1/2}$ and duration is shorter than most opioids; therefore, overdose of long acting or extended release opioids may require multiple IV boluses of naloxone or continuous infusion (see treatment).

Physical Exam Found in Opioid Overdose

- *Vitals*: Examine for hypothermia, bradycardia
- *Psych*: Possible euphoria
- *Neuro*: Depressed mental status, somnolence, decreased arousal, coma (e.g., especially with Tramadol/Meperidine) [3] can have restlessness, agitation, confusion, jerking, and/or seizures [4]
- *HEENT*: Miosis
- *Cardio*: Evaluate for hypovolemia
- *Resp*: Decreased respiratory rate (remember normal may be 8–12 breaths/min particularly at night), decreased tidal volume

  Pulmonary edema: Rales/hypoxia/frothy sputum seen in patients with overdose of heroin and other opioids [5]
- *GI*: Decreased bowel sounds
- *Skin*: Track/needle marks commonly found in the forearms and sometimes in feet

K.A. Sackheim, *Pain Management and Palliative Care: A Comprehensive Guide*,
DOI 10.1007/978-1-4939-2462-2_7, © Springer Science+Business Media New York 2015

Table 7.1 Serum half-life ($t_{1/2}$) of commonly prescribed opioids

Opioid	Half-life (h)
Morphine	1.5–4.5
Codeine	3–4
Hydromorphone	2–3
Oxycodone	2–4
Hydrocodone	3–4.5
Methadone	8–59
Tramadol	5–7
Fentanyl	2–4

Differential Diagnosis

- Ethanol/Benzo/Clonidine intoxication
- Hypoglycemia
- CVA (altered mental status)
- Pontine hemorrhage (presents with miosis)
- Ketamine overdose (CNS and respiratory depression)
- PCP overdose (CNS depression and miosis)
- Sepsis (hypovolemia/altered mental status)

Workup

- *Labs*
  - Blood glucose level: Rule out hypoglycemia
  - UTOX: Rule out ingestion of another toxic substance and know what substance they ingested
  - CBC, Blood Cx, UA, rule out infection
  - ABG: Assess respiratory status
  - BMP: Detect electrolyte abnormalities
- *EKG*: Methadone causes QTc prolongation/Torsades de Pointes [6]
- *Imaging*
  - CXR: Reserved for patient with hypoxia or abnormal lung sounds. May reveal opioid-induced pulmonary edema.
  - CT Head without contrast: Rule out CVA/mass effect/herniation

Treatment

If no respiratory depression and patient is arousable, with holding opioid along with IVF hydration and monitored vital signs may be adequate

In Severe Cases Consider

- *Naloxone*: μ-opioid receptor competitive antagonist
  - *Pharmacology*:
    Onset: IV: 2–3 min

Duration: 10–15 min as it quickly redistributes in adipose tissues [4]

Half-life: 45–100 min

*The effective dosing and length of naloxone administration will depend on the type of ingested opioid and its affinity to the mu receptor, amount of ingested opioid, patient's weight, and the degree of penetration into CNS. Most of the time this information is unattainable and dosing should be started empirically [7].

IV/IM naloxone is used to maintain adequate ventilation

- *If respiratory rate >12 and O2Sat >90 on RA* → closely monitor the patient's vital signs. Naloxone can be held, and opioid will be cleared by normal metabolism.
- *Significant hypoxemia, significant hypotension, or respiratory rate <6–8* can treat with naloxone [4].
  - Ensure adequate respiration with bag-valve mask prior to naloxone administration. Because of its possible side effects, naloxone use should be avoided if possible and only used when absolutely necessary.
- **IV bolus:**
  - Initial dose of naloxone should be 0.4–1 mg can be diluted with 10 ml saline and 0.1–0.2 mg IV bolus can be given every 1–2 min if required [4]. If patient respiratory status (O$_2$ saturation and respiratory rate) does not improve, consider increasing frequency to every 2 min until improvement is seen or a maximum dose of 15 mg is given [7]. Bolus dose increase should only be given if 0.1–0.2 mg is not effective after multiple doses to avoid side effects of naloxone [4].
  - If no improvement is seen after a few doses, especially after 15 mg total it is unlikely that the underlying etiology is opioid overdose. A total of 15 mg should be avoided if necessary as naloxone can cause serious complications.
  - If patient continues to have recurrent respiratory depression after IV bolus, then IV continuous infusion of naloxone should be considered.
- **IV continuous infusion:**
  - If patient overdosed on long acting or extended release opioid (i.e., Methadone, fentanyl patch), patient should be monitored in ICU setting and started on continuous naloxone infusion. Orotracheal intubation can be an alternate option especially if patient is found to have pulmonary edema [7].
  - Initial bolus dose of IV naloxone is given followed by continuous infusion of naloxone 4 mg diluted in 1 L of 0.45 % saline. The rate of infusion can be started at 100 cm^3/h (0.4 mg/h). The infusion rate, length of duration, and concentration can be adjusted depending on the resolution of patient's clinical symptoms [8]. Stop infusion when patient's saturation has improved

or if patient is having acute withdrawal symptoms. Observe for another 4–6 h.

- Stop naloxone administration if signs of opioid withdrawal are seen (see below)

Goal of treatment with naloxone → maintain adequate ventilation

Caution: Naloxone Use/Overdose Can Cause

- *Acute pain crisis* [4]
- *Acute withdrawal symptoms*: Seizures, cardiac arrhythmias, severe hypertension, nausea, vomiting, piloerection, diarrhea, yawning, lacrimation, rhinorrhea
- *Severe abdominal pain, psychosis, myocardial infarction* [4]
- *Pulmonary edema*: Most likely due to increased afterload secondary to catecholamine surge in the setting of iatrogenic reversal (naloxone) of opioid toxicity. This can cause interstitial edema [5, 9].

Opioid Withdrawal

Etiology

Natural: Chronic users of opioids develop physical dependence and are predisposed to withdrawal once they stop taking the drug, run out of medications or rapidly decrease their dose

Iatrogenic: High-dose or rapidly infused naloxone administered to a patient who is overdosed with an opioid may precipitate excess catecholamine release and consequently pulmonary edema and cardiac arrhythmias

History

Most patients experiencing withdrawal symptoms will have been on the opiates for at least several weeks but this can start earlier. Withdrawal symptoms can begin even with slight decreases in opioid doses in some patients [4]. Symptoms may present 6–12 h after last dose of short-acting opioid and 24–48 h after last methadone dose. Common symptoms/complaints are listed in Table 7.2.

Physical Exam

- *Vitals*: Tachycardia/arrhythmias (rare), hypertension, tachypneic
- *GI*: Hyperactive bowel sounds
- *Neuro/Psych*: Agitated, anxiousness, tremors
- *HEENT*: Mydriasis, lacrimation, rhinorrhea
- *Skin*: Piloerection, diaphoretic

Table 7.2 Symptoms seen in opioid overdose vs. opioid withdrawal

Opioid overdose	Opioid withdrawal
- Euphoria	- Dysphoria, restlessness, anxiety, hyperactivity, tachycardia, flushing, palpitations
- Depressed mental status (i.e., somnolence, decreased arousal, coma)	- Rhinorrhea
- Hypothermia	- Lacrimation
- Bradycardia	- Headache, myalgias
- Miosis	- Arthralgias
- Decreased respiratory rate, respiratory depression	- Diarrhea, nausea, vomiting
- Decreased bowel sounds	- Insomnia
	- Abdominal cramping

Differential Diagnosis

- Ethanol/Benzo withdrawal
- Sympathomimetic intoxication
- Cholinergic agent toxicity

Treatment

- Opioid withdrawal is usually not life threatening but patients especially those with comorbidities can be placed at heightened risk of increased intracranial pressure and unstable angina due to the sympathetic tone [4]
- Even to healthy patients, opioid withdrawal is very uncomfortable to experience [4]
- Outpatient management may be sufficient for most withdrawal symptoms
- In severe case—Continuous monitoring of vital signs and possible telemetry
- If patient is hypovolemic due to excessive vomiting/diarrhea, treat with IVF, and consider inpatient treatment
- If withdrawal accompanied by serious cardiopulmonary disease (i.e., cardiac arrhythmias, hypertension, pulmonary edema) or suicidal ideation or psychotic symptoms, then patient should be monitored in acute setting [10].

Opioid agonist therapy (not given in cases of iatrogenic produced withdrawal, should be treated by a trained specialist)

- Restart opiates in patients where this is appropriate, can consider IV or IM dose in severe cases
- Opiate taper can be initiated if goal is for patient to be off the opiates
  - *For example*: If a patient is chronically on Percocet 10/325 five times a day, instead of just stopping this medications abruptly, you can decrease the dose by 5–10 mg each week as tolerated

Table 7.3 Adjunctive agents for symptoms of opioid withdrawal

Symptom	Agent type	Agent to Consider
Overall withdrawal	Alpha2 agonist	Clonidine (0.1–0.3 mg PO q4–6 h)
Diarrhea	Bismuth products	Pepto-Bismol®
		Imodium (4 mg PO initially then 2 mg after each loose stool)
Rhinorrhea	Antihistamines	Diphenhydramine (25–50 mg PO q6 h)
		Loratidine (10 mg PO qDay)
Muscle aches	Muscle relaxants	Methocarbamol (1 g PO q6 h)
Abdominal cramps	Anticholinergics	Dicyclomine HCl (20 mg PO q6 h)
Insomnia	Antihistamines	Diphenhydramine (25–50 mg PO q6 h)
	Antidepressants	Trazodone (25–100 mg PO qHS)
		Doxepin (3–6 mg PO qHS)

Adapted with permission from Benzon HT, Raja SN, Molloy RE, Liu S, Fishman SM. Editors, Essentials of Pain Medicine and Regional Anesthesia, Second Edition, W.B. Saunders Company, New York, 2005

- – Opiate tapers are usually only given to compliant patients who are not at risk of suicide attempt, not using concurrent illicit substances, and not getting opiates from other doctors
- Other options to consider:
  - – Switch to long half-life pure opioid agonist such as methadone, sustained release morphine or oxycodone, and transdermal fentanyl patches [4]
  - – Methadone (can be dosed once daily): Long-acting synthetic opioid agonist; taper dose weekly by 3 % of the initial dose
  - – Use of partial agonist/antagonist opioids: Buprenorphine (4–16 mg PO daily) is another option. Taper over several weeks [10].

Non-opioid Adjunctive Medications
- Clonidine shown to reduce opioid withdrawal symptoms [11] (caution of hypotension)
  - – 0.1–0.2 mg every 4 h prn, taper after day 3 with total treatment lasting about 10 days [10].
- *Acute withdrawal symptoms due to naloxone treatment should be managed symptomatically. Naloxone should be stopped immediately if withdrawal symptoms are seen.

Symptomatic Treatment

Symptomatic treatment may not be necessary for mild symptoms in patients who will be restarted on opiates (Table 7.3)

Benzodiazepine Withdrawal

Many features of benzo withdrawal are similar to that of opioid withdrawal. Some signs of benzo withdrawal include hyperarousal, tremors, seizures, delirium, delusions, hallucinations, nausea, vomiting, tachycardia, and diaphoresis. Unlike opioid withdrawal, benzo withdrawal can be very dangerous, life threatening, and can cause seizures; these patients should be sent to an expert or managed in an inpatient setting [4].

References

1. Bronstein A, Spyker D, Cantilena L, Rumack B, Dart R. 2011 Annual report of the American Association of Poison Control Centers' National Poison Data System (NPDS): 29th annual report. Clin Toxicol (Phila). 2012;50(10):911–1164.
2. Centers for Disease Control and Prevention (CDC). CDC grand rounds: prescription drug overdoses—a U.S. epidemic. MMWR Morb Mortal Wkly Rep. 2012;61(1):10–3.
3. Jovanović-Cupić V, Martinović Z, Nesić N. Seizures associated with intoxication and abuse of tramadol. Clin Toxicol (Phila). 2006;44(2):143–6.
4. Benzon HT, Raja SN, Molloy RE, Liu S, Fishman SM, editors. Essentials of pain medicine and regional anesthesia. 2nd ed. New York: W.B. Saunders; 2005. p. 215–8, 531.
5. Sporer KA, Dorn E. Heroin-related noncardiogenic pulmonary edema: a case series. Chest. 2001;120(5):1628–32.
6. Mayet S, Gossop M, Lintzeris N, Markides V, Strang J. Methadone maintenance, QTc and torsade de pointes: who needs an electrocardiogram and what is the prevalence of QTc prolongation? Drug Alcohol Rev. 2011;30(4):388–96.
7. Boyer E. Management of opioid analgesic overdose. N Engl J Med. 2012;367(2):146–55.
8. Handal K, Schauben J, Salamone F. Naloxone. Ann Emerg Med. 1983;12(7):438–45.
9. Bansal S, Khan R, Tietjen P. Naloxone-induced pulmonary edema. Chest. 2007;132(4_meeting abstracts):692.
10. Kosten T, O'Connor P. Management of drug and alcohol withdrawal. N Engl J Med. 2003;348(18):1786–95.
11. Jasinski D, Johnson R, Kocher T. Clonidine in morphine withdrawal. Arch Gen Psychiatry. 1985;42(11):1063–6.

Detoxification from Opiates and Benzodiazepines

Clifford Gevirtz and Alan David Kaye

Abbreviations

AAOD   Anesthesia-assisted opiate detoxification
CES   Cranial electrostimulation
DEA   Drug enforcement agency
HBV   Hepatitis B
HCV   Hepatitis C
HIV   Human immunodeficiency virus
NSAIDs Non-steroidal anti-inflammatory drugs
UROD   Ultra rapid opiate detoxification

Introduction

Drug abuse is in epidemic proportions throughout the United States, with an estimated total economic cost of nearly 100 billion dollars [1]:

1. The illegal use of opiates, i.e., heroin and prescription drugs, is on the rise in the United States. In recent years, opiate-induced deaths have increased in particular because of more potent drugs and accessibility. Emergency rooms have reported an increase of 35 % in opiate-related morbidities and mortalities compared to 1995 [2].
2. The continuing rise in abuse of opiates has placed greater emphasis on treatment modalities.

C. Gevirtz, M.D., M.P.H.
LSU New Orleans Health Sciences Center, 627 West Street, Harrison, NY 10528, USA
e-mail: cliffgevirtzmd@yahoo.com

A.D. Kaye, M.D., Ph.D. (✉)
Department of Pharmacology, LSU School of Medicine, Anesthesia, 278 Citrus Road, River Ridge, LA 70123, USA
e-mail: alankaye44@hotmail.com

Definitions

It is important to carefully document addiction and to differentiate these behaviors from dependence:

Detoxification: clearance of the intoxicating drug from the body

Dependence: a physical or psychologic state in which a person displays withdrawal symptoms if drug use is halted suddenly

- **Withdrawal syndrome for opiates**: symptoms of restlessness, rhinorrhea, lacrimation, diaphoresis, myosis, piloerection, and cardiovascular changes associated with increased catecholamine levels (tachycardia, hypertension). See previous chapter for more details
- **Withdrawal syndrome for benzodiazepines**: symptoms of insomnia, irritability, increased tension and anxiety, panic attacks, hand tremor, sweating, difficulty in concentration, nausea, palpitations, headache, muscular pain and stiffness, perceptual changes and may progress to seizures and psychosis.

Withdrawal syndrome: refers to symptoms including restlessness, rhinorrhea, lacrimation, diaphoresis, myosis, piloerection, and cardiovascular changes associated with an increase in catecholamine levels [3–5].

- Catecholamine surge caused by induction of the withdrawal syndrome in UROD has life-threatening implications.
- Clonidine, an α-2 receptor agonist is used to reduce these catecholamine levels [6, 7].

Addiction: characterized by a pattern of behaviors which include an inability to consistently abstain from a drug, impairment in behavioral control, craving, diminished recognition of significant problems with one's behaviors and interpersonal relationships, and a dysfunctional emotional response.

Pseudoaddiction: a drug-seeking behavior that simulates true addiction, which occurs in patients with pain who are receiving inadequate pain medication.

K.A. Sackheim, *Pain Management and Palliative Care: A Comprehensive Guide*,
DOI 10.1007/978-1-4939-2462-2_8, © Springer Science+Business Media New York 2015

**It is important to realize that a patient that is on chronic opiates but following medical direction is dependent but not addicted. In contrast, a patient that does not follow directions and self-escalates drug dosages is demonstrating addictive behavior.*

Opioid Detoxification

Detoxification is the appropriate next step when a patient:
- Fails to achieve meaningful pain relief from opiates
- Fails to follow directions while on opiates
- Has illicit substances in their toxicology screens

Detoxification may be achieved by:
- Using a slow taper of the current opiate
- Conversion to methadone or buprenorphine and then tapering that medication
- Anesthesia-assisted detoxification
  - **Conventional treatments** for opiate abuse include a variety of treatment models, all of which have low success rates.
  - **Methadone and Buprenorphine** treatment involves substituting long-acting agents for the opiate of abuse; in effect substituting one opiate for another [3].
  - **Rapid opiate detoxification** is a 3-day process involving large amounts of an opiate antagonist, such as naloxone or naltrexone. However, there are problems associated with both of these treatments. Methadone and Buprenorphine treatment have high initial relapse rates, and rapid opiate detoxification elicits severe withdrawal symptoms [4].
  - **Ultra rapid opiate detoxification (UROD)** entails anesthetizing a patient and precipitating withdrawal while unconscious [3]. This procedure shortens the withdrawal period opiate addicts experience upon cessation, and allows the patient to avoid much of the subjective discomfort associated with withdrawal [5, 6]. One advantage of UROD is that the withdrawal period is markedly shortened to about 4–6 h versus up to several months for conventional treatments. The patient is anesthetized during the acute withdrawal period and thus does not experience the unpleasant consequences of acute detoxification.

When used regularly, opioids result in physical dependence and neural adaptation by their interaction with central nervous system and systemic opioid receptors.

Paradoxically, the treatment of opioid dependence can be carried out with:
- Opioid receptor agonists
- Partial agonists
- Antagonists

Methadone is an opioid agonist that meets the needs of neurons dependent on opioids. This compound has a long half-life and thus, occupies receptors longer than agents with short half-lives.

Buprenorphine, a partial agonists, may treat opioid dependency by not inducing a full clinical effect when binding to the opioid receptor.

Naltrexone, an orally administered opioid antagonist, blocks the opioid receptor and thus blunts opioid cravings and euphoria. Neural adaptation of the central nervous system due to exogenous opioids may be reversed with naltrexone or other antagonists [7, 8].

Traditional medical approach to detoxification from opiates: either gradual tapering of the current opiate or substitution with a long-acting opioid (e.g., methadone or buprenorphine) [9] and subsequent tapering, along with the use of non-opioids, such as clonidine along with NSAIDs, analgesics, hypnotics, and benzodiazepines.

Gradual Taper

- Success requires patient motivation and full awareness that the process is long and difficult.
- Most common cause of taper failure: dropping the dose too quickly
- Best success is obtained by dropping the dose by *no more than 5 % per week, which means a taper of over 20 weeks*.
- While most patients can reduce their intake by 40–50 % of their daily dose, there is often a plateau below which the patient has great difficulty. Getting the patient through this plateau is the most challenging part and requires both intense pharmacologic and psychological support.

Substitution with Long-Acting Opioid

1. Opiate rotation onto methadone or buprenorphine is actually a very challenging method with many reports of overdosage appearing in the literature [10] due to the use of conversion tables that were based on single dose testing and not chronic administration.
   - **Methadone**:
     - Start with 10 mg total daily dosage (typically 5 mg PO BID)
     - Slowly increase dosage by no more than 5 mg every 3 days, using additional short duration opiates to prevent withdrawal.
     - Once an equivalent level of methadone to the baseline medication is reached, a slow taper of 2 mg every 3 days is started.
     - The patient must be warned that this will be a long protracted course.

- **Buprenorphine**:
  - Actually easier to rotate onto, but in order to use it for detoxification, special training and a special DEA license must be obtained.
  - The National Alliance of Advocates for Buprenorphine Treatment (www.naabt.org) has a matching service that can locate appropriated trained and licensed physicians.
  - The basic process is to allow the patient to go into a moderate degree of withdrawal and incrementally administer buprenorphine which is a partial opiate agonist.

    Start with 4 mg increments administered SL until the objective and subjective signs of withdrawal abate.

    Typically, a patient on 100 mg of daily morphine equivalent will need 24 mg per day of buprenorphine to feel comfortable.

    Dosage is tapered slowly in 2 mg weekly increments.

2. In general, when a patient is fully detoxified, the gradual introduction [11] of oral mu-receptor antagonist such as naltrexone is recommended to maintain sobriety (50 mg PO daily for 2–5 months).

3. Substitution therapy with methadone has a high initial dropout rate (30–90 %) and an early relapse rate [12–14]. Alternative pharmacological detoxification programs include the use of clonidine with or without methadone, midazolam, trazodone, or buprenorphine [15]. Nonpharmacological programs, such as cranial electro-stimulation (CES), have reported varied success rates [16, 17].

Indications, Contraindications, and Prerequisites for Anesthesia-Assisted Opiate Detoxification (AAOD)

When patients fail multiple attempts at detoxification or are phobia about detoxification, then anesthesia-assisted opiate detoxification may be considered.

Indications

Patient-related factors:
- Only a highly selected subgroup of patients may benefit from this procedure. It is specifically NOT appropriate for all patients.
- Many patients who are seeking a "quick fix" to their problem are NOT appropriate candidates.

Appropriate Candidates Include

- Those who have been unable to abstain using opiates even with methadone substitution despite adequate motivation
- Those who are unable to completely stop methadone and who continue along with 10–20 mg/day
- Patients who are socially and occupationally active and cannot go through the usual long detoxification procedures without jeopardizing their jobs.
- Sports stars and celebrities, who need to achieve sobriety by a particular date, in order to continue their careers, may also be appropriate candidates if they are committed to long-term sobriety and not just a quick solution to their problems.
- Pain patients who have become physically dependent on opiates but are not receiving a significant amount of pain relief from them.
- Patient's preferences are an important variable to consider as some patients may have tried various approaches to detoxification multiple times.
- Its use should be restricted to patients with only opioid dependence as simultaneous dependence on other substances can complicate the procedure [18].

Contraindications

Contraindications include: [18]
- Pregnancy
- History of significant cardiac disease or evidence of the same on clinical examination
- End stage renal disease
- End stage liver disease
- Concurrent co-dependence on benzodiazepines, alcohol, or cocaine
- Current suicidal or homicidal ideation

Organizational Requirements

- *The procedure of anesthesia-assisted opiate detoxification (AAOD) requires*:
  - A setting where intensive care procedures are performed or an operating room (for administration of anesthesia/deep sedation and monitoring)
  - Ongoing care with a psychiatry or detoxification unit to facilitate continuity of care
  - Team should have an anesthesiologist and/or a specialist in intensive medicine, a psychiatrist, nursing staff, and a psychotherapist/counselor

    This would ensure attention to the procedure, the immediate post-procedure complications as well as later abstinence-oriented programs [19].

– Anesthesia-assisted opiate detoxification should not be performed in a store front or in a hotel room, where there is inadequate backup should difficulty be encountered.

There are a myriad of recipes for conducting AAOD, which differ in the exact procedure employed.

Essential Components for AAOD Regime

1. Initial assessment involves obtaining a detailed history regarding the drug-intake and general medical and psychiatric illness. A detailed history of past attempts at detoxification and the reason for failure. An assessment of the need for AAOD as opposed to methadone maintenance, buprenorphine maintenance, or tapering.
2. Formulating a treatment plan which addresses and effectively treats each element of the opiate withdrawal syndrome and the post-procedure follow-up, i.e., ongoing psychiatric care must be in place prior to starting detoxification.
3. Obtaining a detailed written informed consent. The patient should be clearly and adequately informed of the available treatment options, the comparative costs incurred for each and the relative risks/advantages inherent in them.

Methodology

Pre-anesthetic testing: key issue is to identify the damage that the substance abuse may have already caused
- Detailed physical examination
- Electrocardiogram
- Serum chemistry
- Liver function test
- Complete Blood Count
- Tests for HIV, HBV, and HCV
- Chest X-ray

Premedication: *Suppository, Vitamin C to enhance opioid elimination by acidifying the urine, and a sleeping aide are typical the night prior.*
- High-dose α_2-2 agonist is introduced incrementally [20] to reduce the sympathetically mediated effects of withdrawal.
  - Clonidine may be administered orally, transdermally, or intravenously.
  - Total dose used prior to induction is usually >0.5 mg and is determined by the patient's hemodynamic ability to tolerate the dosage. (It is important to understand

that trying to save a few dollars in costs by minimizing dosages leads directly to uncontrolled symptomatology including hypertensive crisis and elevations in the objective and subjective clinical withdrawal scales post-procedure).
  - Dexmedetomidine IV may be used as it is more selective, has a shorter duration of action, and is easier to titrate than clonidine.
- Antiemetic medications (droperidol or ondansetron) are given simultaneously in dosages usually used to treat chemotherapy-induced vomiting.
- Another approach uses prior induction onto buprenorphine for 1 week prior to AAOD which is believed to mitigate the intensity of the withdrawal syndrome [21].

Monitoring: Thorough anesthetic monitoring of the vital functions is needed. Hensel and Kox [22] used BIS monitoring to regulate the depth of anesthesia with the advantage of being able to significantly reduce the total dose of propofol required, time to recovery from anesthesia, and objective withdrawal symptoms.

Induction and maintenance:
- Anesthesia is induced with propofol or a barbiturate and succinylcholine or rocuronium can be used as the muscle relaxant in a rapid sequence induction and intubation.
- Intubation is needed since opiates decrease gastric emptying and vomiting can be a prominent component of the withdrawal syndrome if adequate antiemetic medications are not administered.
- Maintenance anesthesia is done with an infusion containing a combination of midazolam and propofol or any inhalational agent.
- A test dose of the opioid antagonist is used to gauge the adequacy of the α-2-mediated blockade and is followed by a high-dose intravenous infusion of naloxone [18–20], or nalmefene in normal saline or naltrexone via an orogastric tube into the stomach.
- Because a volume shift into the intestines is expected after administration of opiate antagonists, a liberal amount of lactated Ringer's solution is infused to maintain fluid balance [20]. Thereafter, patients are monitored for withdrawal signs.
  - *Major signs of withdrawal under anesthesia are*: piloerection and myoclonic jerking as the other signs are masked by the use of the α-2 agonist.
- Anesthesia is maintained until the patients respond negatively to another test dose of opioid antagonist. This is usually after 6–8 h but may be longer in cases of methadone-maintained patients [22].

Pearl: One technique involves substituting methadone with a short-acting agent such as hydromorphone (Dilaudid) over a 5–7-day period allowing washout of the methadone. UROD would require a shorter interval given the quicker washout period of hydromorphone, e.g., 24–36 h versus approximately 5 days for methadone.

Role of Clonidine in Mitigating Withdrawal

- Symptoms associated with the withdrawal syndrome, such as restlessness, rhinorrhea, lacrimation, diaphoresis, myosis, piloerection, and cardiovascular changes, are mediated through increased sympathetic activity.
- Thirtyfold increase in the levels of epinephrine and lesser increases in norepinephrine can be observed during withdrawal from opioids [23].
- During opioid withdrawal, neural activity in the locus ceruleus, the major noradrenergic nucleus in the brain, is greatly increased.
  - This surge is responsible for many of the symptoms seen during withdrawal [24, 25].
- Clonidine, an α_2-agonist, has been shown effective in suppressing noradrenergic hyperactivity, relieving withdrawal symptoms [26–29].
- Without clonidine or an equivalent α_2-agonist agent, UROD would result in large increases in both total and fractionated catecholamine levels.
- These increases would be associated with unacceptable morbidity and mortality.

Another Method for Determining Completion of the Procedure

- Measure spontaneous minute ventilation immediately after administration of the narcotic antagonist (obviously after the muscle relaxant effects have resolved).
- It has been observed to more than double from the normal volume.
- When the minute ventilation falls to 75 % of the peak value, the detoxification is usually complete.

Post-procedure Monitoring and Discharge

- Usual policy is to discharge the patient within 24 h
- Some patients who keep on complaining of persistent withdrawal symptoms may need to be kept for a few additional days and managed symptomatically.
  - Major complaints are usually insomnia, muscle aches, and abdominal discomfort.
  - Use of sedatives to treat insomnia must be tempered with the risk of starting a different dependency.

- Muscle aches or bone pain are usually treated with an NSAIDs
- Abdominal cramping is treated with Bentyl and with octreotide
- Number one reason for failure in the first few days post-detoxification is the inability to sleep and some short-term measures need to be taken to restore the circadian rhythm.
- A thorough physical examination for any anesthetic complications, persistent withdrawal symptoms, and psychiatric symptoms is needed before discharge to prevent "bounce-backs" to the emergency room.
- Patients who are transferred directly to an inpatient psychiatric facility to initiate aftercare abstinence-oriented program often have better success in maintaining abstinence.

Management of Complications

- **Emesis**:
  - Prominent feature of the withdrawal syndrome
  - Antacids and antiemetics, in high doses are used prophylactically
  - Ranitidine should be avoided as it may cause tachycardia, vomiting, insomnia, and elevation of liver enzymes in higher doses
- **Diarrhea**:
  - Another prominent feature of the withdrawal syndrome
  - Prophylactically treated with octreotide, a synthetic polypeptide
    It inhibits the anterior pituitary, suppressing the pancreatic secretions and thus inhibiting gastric acid, serotonin, and VIP secretion which, in turn, decreases gastrointestinal motility.
  - Loperamide should be avoided as it is absorbed into systemic circulation and may increase the signs of withdrawal post-procedure.
- **Sepsis**: Some centers also advocate the use of a single dose of an antibiotic, e.g., cephalozin to prevent infection.
- **Gastric ulcer**: Cushing's ulcer which can be prevented with H-2 Blocking agents.
- **Cardiovascular complications** [24]: These include cardiovascular stimulation, QT prolongation, bradycardia, bigeminy, and cardiac arrhythmia
- **Thyroid**: Suppression of hormones
- **Psychiatric complications**: include dysphoria and acute psychotic episode requiring haloperidol, suicide attempts on Day 3 and Day 5 post-procedure

- **Deaths**:
  - Deaths have been reported 16–40 h following the procedure.
  - In most of the cases, the cause has been found to be: Pulmonary edema, upper gastrointestinal ulceration, and aspiration
    One patient suffered from an intracerebral hemorrhage, presumably due to poor control of blood pressure.
  - It was also seen that in these cases, the use of clonidine was a very limited and it was not continued after the procedure. In most of these cases, the ASA basic monitoring standards were not followed.
- **Prolonged withdrawal symptoms**:
  - Many patients continue to experience moderate withdrawal symptoms hours after the anesthesia or sedation ended, including nausea, vomiting, diarrhea, and sleep disturbances.
  - Others report only mild to moderate symptoms only for the next 3–4 days.
  - In addition, the severity of withdrawal may also be related to the anesthetic used. It must be emphasized that aggressive control of these symptoms is necessary or the patient will immediately relapse. This means large doses of antiemetics, anti-spasmodics, and sedatives for sleep.
- **Induction onto an antagonist**: Both during the procedure and immediately following long-acting opiate antagonists are administered. Naltrexone pellets (vide infra) have been inserted subcutaneously and can last up to 6 months. Use of injectable nalmefene in large doses intramuscularly administered will provide mu receptor blockade for a week. A new preparation of intramuscular depot naltrexone, which was originally developed for to help in alcohol abstinence, has been demonstrated to last a month. The later three methods insure "enforced abstinence" as the mu receptor blockade is exceedingly difficult to overcome.

Benzodiazepine Detoxification

- Benzodiazepine use by the drug-abusing population consists of the combined use of benzodiazepines with other psychoactive drugs.
- They are used to enhance cocaine toxicity, as a secondary or tertiary drug to boost the effects of alcohol or heroin, and by those who have developed tolerance and dependence to sedative-hypnotic drugs.
- The presence of an anxiety disorder, a family history of addiction, or benzodiazepine polydrug use will significantly affect the type of withdrawal a patient will experience and its treatment course.

- Medical procedures accepted for benzodiazepine discontinuation include:
  - Gradual taper
  - Substitution of a long-acting benzodiazepine (diazepam)
  - Phenobarbital substitution
- The best clinical evidence suggests that the patient be switched to a long-lasting benzodiazepine and the dose then tapered by 5 % of the initial dose each week. Diazepam is the drug most often used in the framework.
- In opiate users, diazepam may raise special problems of misuse, as suggested by clinical and epidemiologic studies.
- Nonetheless, diazepam is the only benzodiazepine found to be effective for this withdrawal in controlled studies and some studies indicate that unprescribed diazepam use in heroin users is sometimes motivated by the desire to alleviate withdrawal symptoms and discomfort.
- More recently, Oxcarbazepine has been utilized [30] to ameliorate many of symptoms of benzodiazepine withdrawal.
- Typical and critical features specific to tapering of chronic benzodiazepines include a fractional decrease of no more than 10–20 % per week with constant focus on withdrawal features. These can include anxiety, insomnia, increase in heart rate and blood pressure, and seizures.

References

1. http://www.nida.nih.gov/Infofax/costs.html
2. http://www.nida.nih.gov/Infofax/heroin.html
3. Kaye AD, Gevirtz C, Bosscher HA, et al. Ultrarapid opiate detoxification: a review. Can J Anaesth. 2003;50:1–9.
4. Krabbe PF, Koning JPF, Heinen N, et al. Rapid detoxification from opioid dependence under general anaesthesia versus standard methadone tapering: abstinence rates and withdrawal distress experiences. Addict Biol. 2003;8:351–8.
5. McCabe S. Rapid detox: understanding new treatment approaches for the addicted patient. Perspect Psychiatr Care. 2000;36:113–9.
6. Gevirtz C, Frost E. Ultra rapid opiate detoxification. Curr Concepts Curr Opin Clin Exp Res. 2000;2:151–68.
7. Gerra G, Zaimovic A, Giusti F, et al. Lofexidine versus clonidine in rapid opiate detoxification. J Subst Abuse Treat. 2001;21:11–7.
8. Diaz A, Pazos A, Florez J, et al. Regulation of mu-opioid receptors, G-protein-coupled receptor kinases and beta-arrestin 2 in the rat brain after chronic opioid receptor antagonism. Neuroscience. 2002;112:345–53.
9. Pilling S, Strang J, Gerada C. Psychosocial interventions and opioid detoxification for drug misuse: summary of NICE guidance. BMJ. 2007;335:203–5.
10. Madden ME, Shapiro SL. The methadone epidemic: methadone-related deaths on the rise in Vermont. Am J Forensic Med Pathol. 2011;32:131–5. doi:10.1097/PAF.0b013e3181e8af3d.
11. Charney DS, Heninger GR, Kleber HD. The combined use of clonidine and naltrexone as a rapid, safe and effective treatment of

abrupt withdrawal from methadone. Am J Psychiatry. 1986;143: 831–7.

12. Jasinski DR. Tolerance and dependence to opiates. Acta Anaesthesiol Scand. 1997;41:184–6.

13. Kleber HD, Topazian M, Gaspari J, et al. Clonidine and naltrexone in the outpatient treatment of heroin withdrawal. Am J Drug Alcohol Abuse. 1987;13:4–17.

14. O'Brien CP, McLellan AT. Myths about the treatment of addiction. Lancet. 1996;347:237–40.

15. Broers B, Giner F, Dumont P, Mino A. Inpatient opiate detoxification in Geneva: follow-up at 1 and 6 months. Drug Alcohol Depend. 2000;58:85–92.

16. Fudala PJ, Jaffe JH, Dax EM, Johnson RE. Use of buprenorphine in the treatment of opioid addiction. II. Physiologic and behavioral effects of daily and alternate-day administration and abrupt withdrawal. Clin Pharmacol Ther. 1990;47:525–34.

17. Alling FA, Johnson BD, Elmoghazy E. Cranial electrostimulation (CES) use in the detoxification of opiate-dependent patients. J Subst Abuse Treat. 1990;7:173–80.

18. Gevirtz C. Anesthesia assisted opiate detoxification. Int Anesthesiol Clin. 2003;41:79–93.

19. Bell J, Kimber J, Lintzeris N. Guidelines for rapid detoxification from opioids. NSW Health, circular no. 2001/17, file no. 00/1287, issued on 23 February 2001.

20. Kaye AD, Gevirtz C, Bosscher HA, Duke JB, Frost EA, Richards TA, et al. Ultrarapid opiate detoxification: a review. Can J Anaesth. 2003;50:663–71.

21. Bochud Tornay C, Favrest B, Monnat M, Daeppen JB, Schnyder C, Bertschy G, et al. Ultra-rapid opiate detoxification using deep sedation and prior oral buprenorphine preparation. Drug Alcohol Depend. 2003;69:283–8.

22. Hensel M, Kox WJ. Safety, efficacy and long term results of a modified version of rapid opiate detoxification under general anesthesia: a prospective study in methadone, heroin, codeine and morphine addicts. Acta Anaesthesiol Scand. 2000;44:326–33.

23. Poshychinda V. Thailand: treatment at the Tam Kraborg Temple. In: Edwards G, Arif A, editors. Drug problems in the sociocultural context: a basis for policies and program planning. Geneva: World Health Organization; 1980. p. 121–5.

24. Kienbaum P, Scherbaum N, Thurauf N, Michel M, Gastpar M, Peters J. Acute detoxification of opioid-addicted patients with naloxone during propofol or methohexital anesthesia: a comparison of withdrawal symptoms, neuroendocrine metabolic and cardiovascular patterns. Crit Care Med. 2000;28:969–76.

25. Christie MJ, Williams JT, Osborne PB, Bellchambers CE. Where is the locus in opioid withdrawal? Trends Pharmacol Sci. 1997;18: 134–40.

26. Keinbaum P, Thurauf N, Michel M, et al. Profound increase in epinephrine concentration in plasma and cardiovascular stimulation after μ-opioid receptor blockade in opioid addicted patients. Anesthesiology. 1998;88:1154–61.

27. Langer SZ. Presynaptic regulation of release of catecholamines. Pharmacol Rev. 1981;32:337–62.

28. Gold MS, Redmond Jr DE, Kleber HD. Noradrenergic hyperactivity in opiate withdrawal supported clonidine reversal of opiate withdrawal. Am J Psychiatry. 1979;136:100–2.

29. Gold MS. Opiate addiction and locus ceruleus. The clinical utility of clonidine, naltrexone, methadone and buprenorphine. Psychiatr Clin North Am. 1993;16:61–73.

30. Croissant B, Grosshans M, Diehl A, Mann K. Oxcarbazepine in rapid benzodiazepine detoxification. Am J Drug Alcohol Abuse. 2008;34(5):534–40. doi:10.1080/00952990802149021.

Discharging the Non-compliant Pain Patient

Anjuli Desai

Abbreviation

GC/MS   Gas chromatography/mass spectroscopy

Introduction

This chapter will focus on how to address a patient who is non-compliant with the practice guidelines for safe opioid analgesic use and how to properly discharge them from the practice if necessary. Please keep in mind that practice guidelines cannot anticipate each individual patient's situation and must be adapted to the individual situation using the clinician's judgment.

Definitions

- *Physical dependence*: a physiologic state initiated by a sudden dose decrease or termination of opioid treatment which causes the patient to experience withdrawal symptoms, dependence does not necessarily mean a person is addicted [1, 2]
- *Tolerance*: a physiologic state created when a patient is treated with chronic opioids in which a higher dose may be needed to achieve the equivalent analgesic effect [1, 2]
- *Addiction*: a "neurobiological disease" [1] with psychological, social, genetic, and environmental factors in which the patient may exhibit drug seeking behaviors, diminished control over their drug use, cravings, compulsive behaviors, and repeated use despite negative consequences [1, 2].

A. Desai, M.D. (✉)
Capitol Pain Institute, Austin, TX, USA

Department of Pain Medicine, Temple University Hospital, 3401 N. Broad Street, Philadelphia, PA 19140, USA
e-mail: julidahiya@yahoo.com

- *Pseudoaddiction*: an iatrogenic condition of abnormal patient behavior, often exhibited as exaggerated pain behavior, which develops as a direct result of inadequate pain management

Patient Compliance

All clinicians must abide by a large spectrum of guidelines in healthcare in order to assure that they are practicing the safest medicine for their patients. Thus, it is essential that the clinician review their practice guidelines with every new patient so that they understand the practice philosophy and what is expected of both parties. The informed consent should be verbally discussed with the patient and all questions answered. In this way, you have clear communication from the beginning of your relationship with a new patient, and thus have increased patient compliance. Most facilities do this informed consent with the use of an opioid contract (see Appendix 1).

General guidelines of an opioid contract: *Each practice must take into account their individual patient population and the needs of this population when establishing their own practice guidelines.*

1. Explain opioid medications, possible side effects, tolerance, dependence, and withdrawal symptoms so patients understand what they will be taking.
2. Explain that they are not to drive, operate heavy machinery, or use a weapon on the job (in the case of a policeman) while taking these medications.
3. If a female patient becomes pregnant, she should inform her physician as soon as this is known in order to avoid medications that could be harmful to the fetus.

Patient must agree to the following:

4. I agree to show up for my follow-up appointments so I can be properly monitored while on opioid medications.
5. I agree not to increase my medication dose without discussing it with my pain physician

6. I agree to fill all prescribed opioid analgesics at one pharmacy. If I need to change to another pharmacy, I agree to notify my pain physician.
7. I agree not to refill my opioid analgesics early.
8. I agree not to alter my prescription or medication in any way.
9. I agree not to use any illicit substances such as marijuana, cocaine, and heroin.
10. I agree not to use alcohol with my medications.
11. I agree to do psychological testing, random urine/saliva drug screens, or blood tests if needed during my pain management treatment.
12. I agree to provide my pill bottle for random pill counts at any time during my pain management treatment at your office.
13. I agree not to share, trade, or sell any of my prescribed opioid analgesics.
14. I agree to bring any unused medications or patches into my pain physician's office or pharmacy to be properly discarded. This scenario may occur in the event that my medications are adjusted or discontinued by my pain physician or when a patient has previous left over medications at home.
15. I agree to only obtain my opioid analgesics from your pain practice. If I require treatment in an emergency department or hospital, I will notify the emergency department physician of my treatment at your pain practice and I will ask that they call your office before discharging me on any opioid analgesics.
16. I agree to keep my opioid medications locked away and out of reach from children or animals.

Monitoring Compliance

1. *Random urine drug immunoassays to screen for*:
   - Presence of the prescribed medications
   - Presence of non-prescribed medications
   - Presence of illicit drugs/alcohol
     - If a patient with no renal disease is unable to provide urine, have them sit in the waiting room and drink water until they can provide a sample. Consider oral swab if patient is unable to urinate.
     - If the patient refuses to provide a urine sample, do not prescribe opioids.
2. *Random pill counts*
   - Random pill counts provide the clinician with an assessment of whether the patient is taking their medications as prescribed. The patient is randomly selected via phone call, and instructed to bring in their opioid analgesics into the office at their next visit or sooner. If the patient is unable to bring these medications into the office within

this time frame, then caution should be taken when prescribing future opioids to this patient should be taken and possible taper/discharge should be considered.
- Some exceptions to presenting for the random pill count may include an emergency situation, or if the patient is hospitalized.
3. *Using only one pharmacy*
   - By requiring the patient to adhere to one pharmacy, the clinician provides a safeguard from the use of multiple pharmacies for filling medications.
   - Pharmacist will become accustomed to the signatures of your practice, and the usual prescribed opioid regimens
     - Maintain an open line of communication with the patient's pharmacy as well as the patient's other practitioners.
4. *Bring in all unused medications*
   - Have patients bring in all unused medication bottles or patches to be properly discarded so they are not laying around at the home. By doing so, the patient can avoid accidental or intentional use of these medications in the future.

Identifying the addict/practice guideline violations: *important to look for the following behaviors* [1]
- Appearing "drugged" or intoxicated, unsteady gait, slowed speech, etc.
- Unkempt appearance
- Obtaining medications on the "street"
- Using medications from friends/family
- Forging prescriptions
- Discharge from previous pain offices
- Criminal history (drug related)
- History of selling drugs/prescription medications
- History of drug use/abuse, injecting medications, evidence of track marks on physical exam
- Lost/stolen prescriptions
- Multiple self-dose increases
- Frequent requests for early refills
- Uses opioids to treat non-painful conditions (such as anxiety, depression, insomnia)
- Obtaining opioids from multiple prescribers
- Obtaining medications from multiple pharmacies
- Non-compliant with office visits
- Demanding only one certain opioids
- Demanding only immediate release opioids
- Unwilling to try adjuvant medications or other opioid options
- Inconsistent or negative urine drug screens
  - Inconsistent urine drug screens would be those that are positive for non-prescribed substances including medications and/or illicit drugs

– Urine drug screens that are negative for prescribed opioids shoulder be further investigated by the physician to determine if the patient is sharing or selling their medications, or not taking them as prescribed [5]

How to Manage the Non-compliant Pain Patient

After discussing the particular violation with the patient, it is necessary to explain to the patient how their action is a violation of the practice guidelines, which they signed on their opioid contract. The clinician should then decide how they would like to address this violation.

*Below are **some** options on how to deal with this patient: each situation is unique and should be approached appropriately for that specific patient*

1. *Discharge the patient with **no** opioid taper*
   - **Consider no opioid taper if**:
     – Patient is at risk of overdose with medications given
     – Patient is careless with medications (e.g., loses them or leaves them near children)
     – Patient has no opioid medications in urine
     – Patient has multiple opioids in urine and/or multiple prescribers
     – Patient has illicit drugs in urine
     – There is evidence of medication diversion/selling
     – Patient has forged or stolen a prescription
     – Patient threatens the physician/staff or is verbally abusive
2. *Discharge the patient **with** opioid taper*
   - Giving a taper is up to the clinician. Safety is always the primary concern. In trustworthy patients, who are not at risk to themselves or at risk of medication diversion, it is best to give a taper in order to avoid withdrawal symptoms/patient abandonment. Unfortunately, when discharging the patient, non-compliance is usually the reason for discharge and opioid taper may not be appropriate.

- The decision to provide a taper is often based on the patient's current dose, and how this can be safely decreased without having significant withdrawal. If the patient's violation was noted on a urine drug immunoassay or GC/MS confirmatory test, the clinician can use these results to determine how to proceed.
  – *No opioids in the urine?*
    Taper may not be necessary as the patient is not taking not taking the opioids
  – *Presence of multiple unprescribed medications or illicit drugs?*
    Taper may not be necessary as the patient is extremely non-complaint and most likely getting medications from multiple prescribers
  – *Patient exhibits signs of self-harm behavior?*
    Taper not necessary as this can actually place the patient at risk of harming themself with the medication. Psychiatry/psychology should be involved
  – *Patient has severe comorbidities and health may be threatened by withdrawal*
    Taper may be needed to avoid harmful effects in these patients
3. Taper the patient's opioid medications but continue to treat with non-opioid adjuvants and interventional procedures
4. Some clinicians allow one minor violation if the patient is well established and has a long history of compliance.
   - Major violations such as selling medications, abusing medications (multiple non-prescribed opioids in urine), or using heroin or cocaine are not acceptable in any office
5. By following the above recommendations, the clinician reduces the risk of abandonment felt by the patient. If a patient is officially discharged, a letter should be sent to the patient. This letter should clearly state the reason the patient is being discharged. This letter should also include a list of alternative pain practices the patient can contact. A sample of such a discharge letter can be seen at the end of the chapter (see Appendix 2).

Appendix 1: Sample opioid contract.
© Kimberly Sackheim 2015. All Rights Reserved

OPIOID CONTRACT

This is an agreement between _____ (the patient) and Dr. _____ (the doctor) concerning the use of opioid analgesics for the treatment of chronic pain. The opioid medication given will probably not completely eliminate my pain, but it is expected to reduce it enough that I may become more functional and improve my quality of life.

1. **SIDE EFFECTS:** I understand that opioid analgesics are strong medications of pain relief and I have been informed of the risks and side effects involved with taking them. Some of these side effects include sedation, sleepiness, dizziness, respiratory issues, nausea, vomiting, itching, and constipation. I will alert my doctor if I experience any of these.

2. **I understand it is my responsibility to inform the doctor of any and all side effects I have from this medication.**

3. **OVERDOSE:** Overdose on this medication may cause death by stopping my breathing; this can possibly be reversed by emergency medical personnel if they know that I have taken opioid medications. It is suggested that I wear a medical alert bracelet or necklace that contains this information.

4. **DRIVING/HEAVY MACHINERY:** While on these medications, I understand that I must not drive a motor vehicle or operate machinery that could put my life or someone else's life in jeopardy.

5. **COMPLIANCE:** I agree to take this medication as prescribed and not to change the amount or frequency of the medication without first discussing it with Dr. _____. Running out early, needing early refills, escalating doses without permission and losing prescriptions may be signs of misuse of the medication and may be reasons for Dr. _____ to discontinue prescribing this medication to me. Medication refills will not be made early if I run out of the medication, or if the medication is lost or stolen.

6. **PHARMACY:** I agree that the opioids will be prescribed by Dr. _____ or designated replacement at _____ (name of facility). I agree to fill my prescriptions at only one pharmacy. If I receive opioid medications from numerous pharmacies/ physicians, I understand that Dr. _____ may no longer prescribe opioid medications to me and I can be discharged from the practice.

7. **OTHER PHYSICIANS: I will not get pain medications from any other physician unless Dr. _____ is aware.** I agree not to take any pain medication or mind altering medication prescribed by any other physician without first discussing it with Dr. _____. I give permission for Dr. _____ to verify that I am not seeing other doctors for opioid medications or going to other pharmacies. If I receive opioid medications from a source other than Dr. _____ without first gaining approval from him/her or the office, I understand that Dr. _____ may no longer prescribe opioid medications to me and I can be discharged from the practice.

8. **SAFETY:** I agree to keep my medication in a safe and secure place. Lost, stolen, or damaged medication will not be replaced. I will make sure to keep my medications out of reach of any children.

9. **DIVERSION:** I agree not to sell, lend, or in any way give my medication to any other person. I agree not to take my medications by other routes or misuse them in any way.

Agreement – page 2

10. **ILLICIT SUBSTANCES:** I agree not to take any mind-altering illicit substances. **If I do, I understand that Dr. _____ will no longer prescribe opioid medications to me and I can be discharged from the practice.** I understand that this rule applies to marijuana, cocaine and all other illicit substances.

11. **ALCOHOL:** I agree not to drink alcohol while I am taking opioid analgesic medication. This can alter the effect of the pain medication and cause serious side effects, the worst being death.

12. **URINE TOXICOLOGY:** I understand that I will have a urine toxicology analysis performed prior to the prescribing of any opioid medications and that I will be periodically asked to perform additional urine toxicology analysis. If my urine test is not consistent with the manner in which my opioid medications are prescribed, or if other illegal drugs of abuse are found in the urine analysis, Dr. _____ will no longer prescribe my opioid medications. I agree to submit a urine specimen any time my doctor requests and give my permission for it to be tested for alcohol and drugs. **I understand that if at any time I refuse to give a urine sample I will automatically be discharged from the practice.**

13. **FOLLOW UP:** I agree that I will attend all required follow-up visits with the doctor to monitor this medication and I understand that failure to do so will result in discontinuation of this treatment. I also agree to participate in other chronic pain treatment modalities recommended by my doctor.

14. **DEPENDANCE/WITHDRAWAL:** In particular, I understand that opioid analgesics could cause physical dependence. If I suddenly stop or decrease the medication, I could have withdrawal symptoms (flu-like syndrome such as nausea, vomiting, diarrhea, aches, sweats, chills) that may occur within 24-48 hours of the last dose. I understand that opioid withdrawal is quite uncomfortable, but is not a life threatening condition.

15. **ADDICTION:** I understand that there is a risk that opioid addiction could occur. This means that I might become dependent on the medication, using it to change my mood or get high, or be unable to control my use of it. **People with past history of alcohol or drug abuse problems are more susceptible to addiction.** If this occurs, the medication will be discontinued and I will be referred to a drug treatment program for help with this problem.

I have read the above, asked questions, and understand the agreement. If I violate the agreement, I know that the doctor may discontinue this form of treatment.

Patient Signature _____ DATE: _____

PHARMACY NAME: _____

LOCATION: _____

PHONE NUMBER: _____

Appendix 2: Sample discharge letter.

Physician Letter head

Physician Name
Physician Title
Department of Pain Medicine
Physician address

Date

Patient Name
Patient address

Dear Mr/Mrs. _____,

This letter is to inform you that I and my associates of _____ (name of facility) will be ending our relationship with you as of _____ (date of practice guideline violation). You are being discharged from our practice because behaviors that we have observed prevent us from providing care that is safe and effective. We cannot continue to provide treament for your condition because _____ (state the specific violation here: eg. inconsistent urine drug screens, non-compliance, or verbally abusive/threatening behavior). This behavior prevents us from developing a therapeutic relationship with you and providing a safe treatment plan.

As a result, we are terminating our relationship with you and formally discharging you from our practice.

We believe that it is important that you obtain appropriate medical care. You may be able to identify a new physician or other health care professional to treat you through various hospital/insurance referral services. Alternatively, you may wish to explore whether other pain management programs in this area will accept your case.

Once you identify a new physician or other health care professional to treat you, we can provide a copy of your medical record upon receiving a written request from you. Should you require emergency care, the emergency department at _____ (list nearby hospitals) or any other hospital is available to you. It is unfortunate that we must terminate treatment at this time, but your actions have necessitated this course. We wish you the best in finding a new source of care.

Attached to this letter, you will find a list of alternative pain management practices that you can consider for your future care.

Sincerely,

Dr. _____

References

1. Webster L, Dove B. Avoiding opioid abuse: while managing pain. North Branch: Sunrise River Press; 2007. p. 21–50.
2. Manchikanti L, Trescot AM, Christo PJ, Falco FJE. Pain medicine & interventional pan management clinical aspects: pain relief in substance abusers. Paducah: American Society of Interventional Pain Physicians; 2011.
3. Owen GT, Burton AW, Schade CM, Passik S. Urine drug testing: current recommendations and best practices. Pain Physician. 2012; 15:ES119–33.
4. Katz N, Fanciullo GJ. Role of urine toxicology testing in the management of chronic opioid therapy. Clin J Pain. 2002;18: S76–82.
5. Foltz RL, Fentiman AF, Foltz RB. GC/MS assays for abused drugs in body fluids. NIDA Res Monogr. 1980;32:1–198.

Part II

Medication Management for the Pain Patient

Nonsteroidal Anti-inflammatory Drugs (NSAIDs)

10

SriKrishna Chandran

Abbreviations

CNS	Central nervous system
COX	Cyclooxygenase
FDA	Federal Drug Administration
NSAID	Nonsteroidal anti-inflammatory drug
PDR	Physician's desk reference
PGE_2	Protglandin E_2
PGI_2	Prostaglandin I_2
TXA_2	Thromboxane A_2

Introduction

- NSAIDs are a chemically heterogeneous group of compounds commonly used for the following properties:
  - *Anti-inflammatory*
  - *Analgesic*
  - *Antipyretic*
- Aspirin and acetaminophen, while used in certain cases for similar purposes, act differently.
- Unlike opioids, NSAID use does not result in tolerance and in certain cases can be more effective in terms of pain relief than opioids in certain circumstances [1].
- The information provided here is for educational purposes and is abridged. Please refer to product inserts/PDR for more detailed information.

S. Chandran, M.D. (✉)
Department of Physical Medicine and Rehabilitation,
Johns Hopkins Hospital, Baltimore, MD, USA
e-mail: srikchan@gmail.com

NSAID Categories

NSAIDs can be broadly categorized based on their site of action and molecular composition.

1. *Nonselective cyclooxygenase (COX) inhibitors*
   - NSAIDs that target both COX-1 and COX-2
   - Structural subclasses are listed in Table 10.1
2. *Selective cycloxygenase inhibitors*
   - NSAIDs that selectively target COX-2
   - Decreased risk of GI side effects as they do not affect COX-1
3. *Salicylates*
   - For the purposes of this chapter, we will discuss aspirin.

Acetaminophen
- Known for its antipyretic and analgesic properties, it is mostly devoid of anti-inflammatory activity.
- In certain cases it may be preferred due to its lack of platelet, gastric, bone, and renal effects [2].
- Caution with liver pathology

Generic Names by Class (Table 10.1)

Mechanism of Action

- NSAIDs inhibit COX enzymes
- Evidence shows that they inhibit the release of inflammatory mediators from neutrophils and macrophages as well as act at the level of the CNS [3].
- COX enzymes function to transform arachadonic acid to prostaglandins, prostacyclins, and thromboxanes.

Two isoforms of cycloogenase:
1. *COX-1*
   - COX-1 inhibition mainly, though not entirely, results in the gastrointestinal adverse side effects of NSAIDs.
   - Primarily constitutive, meaning it is found in most tissues and normal cells

K.A. Sackheim, *Pain Management and Palliative Care: A Comprehensive Guide,*
DOI 10.1007/978-1-4939-2462-2_10, © Springer Science+Business Media New York 2015

Table 10.1 Select generic NSAID names by class [2, 6]

Salicylates	Proprionic acid derivative
Aspirin	Ibuprofen
Para-aminophenol derivative	Naproxen
Acetaminophen	Fenoprofen
Acetic acid derivative	Ketoprofen
Indomethacin	Flurbiprofen
Sulindac	Oxaprozin
Etodolac	Enolic acid derivatives
Femanates	Piroxicam
Mefenamic acid	Meloxicam
Meclofenamate	Nabumetone
Tolmetin	COX-2 selective inhibitor
Diclofenac	Celecoxib
Ketorolac	Valdecoxib

2. *COX-2*
   - COX-2 inhibition is thought to mediate, to a large extent, the antipyretic, analgesic, and anti-inflammatory effects of NSAIDs.
   - COX-2 is both constitutively expressed (i.e., CNS and kidney) and inducible via inflammatory mediators and cytokines [4, 5].
   - Aspirin inhibits COX enzymes in a molecularly distinct manner from the competitive, reversible, active site inhibition of NSAIDs [6].
     - It acts by irreversibly acetylating COX
     - Therefore, the duration of aspirin's effects is correlated with the turnover rate of COX in different target tissues.

Side Effects/Adverse Effects

- *Caution in elderly*:
  - Age is usually associated with an increased probability of developing serious adverse reactions to NSAIDs, so caution should be exercised in the elderly population as well as consideration for a lower starting dose.
- *Gastrointestinal toxicity*
  - Abdominal pain, nausea, dyspepsia, anorexia, diarrhea, and hepatotoxicity
  - Inhibition of COX-1 results in decreased production of gastric mucosal cyto-protective prostaglandins (including PGI_2 and PGE_2).
    - These prostaglandins usually act to produce intestinal mucous, inhibit gastric acid production, and enhance mucosal blood flow.
    - Decreased production can thus increase the risk of ulceration [6].
  - Local irritation via oral consumption can contribute to ulceration.
  - GI ulcers can occur in 15–30 % of regular users.
    - Ulceration may be associated with blood loss resulting in anemia.
    - This has led to the Federal Drug Administration (FDA) issuing a warning for the general class of NSAIDs.
    - Associated risk factors include infection with *Helicobacter pylori*, heavy alcohol consumption, and the concurrent use of glucocorticoids [6].
  - Studies suggest that combining low-dose aspirin (for cardioprotection) with other NSAIDs synergistically increases the risk of gastrointestinal side effects [6].
  - Selective COX-2 inhibitors are less prone to induce endoscopically visualized gastric ulcers [7].
  - Transaminitis is considered by many to be a class effect of NSAIDs. The mechanism of toxicity appears to be metabolic or immunologic with dose-related toxicity associated with aspirin and acetaminophen. Most NSAIDs cause hepatocellular injury with only a few causing cholestatic or mixed injury [8].
- *Nephrotoxicity*
  - NSAIDs, including COX-2 inhibitors, can increase the risk of renovascular adverse events.
  - At-risk populations include those with congestive heart failure, hepatic cirrhosis, chronic kidney disease, hypovolemia, and other states of sympathoadrenal or renin-angiotensin system activation.
  - Within the kidneys, prostaglandins are associated with the inhibition of chloride reabsorption and antidiuretic hormone actions. Therefore, the inhibition of prostaglandin synthesis can result in salt and water retention [9].
  - NSAIDs may also increase the risk of hypertension resulting from the decreased production of vasodilatory prostaglandins (PGE_2 and PGI_2) [10].
  - Analgesic nephropathy is a condition of slowly progressive renal failure, decreased concentrating capacity of the renal tubule, and sterile pyuria.
    - Risk factors are the chronic use of high doses of combinations of NSAIDs and frequent urinary tract infections.
    - Early recognition and discontinuation of NSAIDs may permit recovery of renal tubules [6].
- *Hematologic toxicity*
  - Arachadonic acid is converted to prostaglandin endoperoxides by COX.
  - These endoperoxides are further converted to thromboxane A_2 (TXA_2) in platelets and prostaglandin I_2 (PGI_2) in vascular endothelium.

– TXA$_2$ functions as a platelet activator and vasoconstrictor, whereas PGI$_2$ functions as a platelet inhibitor and vasodilator.
– Platelet activity is thus dependent upon the homeostasis of these agents [2].
– NSAIDs increase the risk of bleeding at the platelet level by inhibiting platelet activation (via inhibiting TXA$_2$ formation). In the case of aspirin, the action on platelet COX is irreversible.
– The paucity of COX-2 within platelets gives COX-2 inhibitors an advantage in terms of decreasing bleeding risk when compared to nonselective NSAIDs [11, 12].

• **Cardiotoxicity**
– NSAIDs, unlike aspirin, do not provide cardio-protection [13].
– Patients at risk for cardiovascular disease and thrombotic events are at increased risk when taking COX-2 selective inhibitors.
  • One proposed reason is that selective inhibition of COX-2 depresses PGI$_2$ formation in endothelial cells without concomitant inhibition of platelet thromboxane.
  • Experiments in mice suggest that PGI$_2$ blunts the cardiovascular effects of TXA$_2$. This may cause an increased risk of thrombosis [6].
– The FDA has issued a warning on NSAIDs as a class.
  • Based on the review of long-term placebo and active controlled clinical trials, the FDA has concluded that a serious risk of adverse cardiovascular events may be a class effect of NSAIDs (excluding aspirin).
  • Furthermore, the FDA has issued a contraindication for NSAID use immediately post-operatively following coronary artery bypass graft surgery.
  • They have recommended careful consideration of the potential risks and benefits before a decision is made to use an NSAID [14].

• **Asthma**
– Termed aspirin-induced asthma, nonselective NSAIDs may produce bronchospasms, typically in diagnosed asthmatics.
  • The mechanism appears to stem from the NSAID-induced inhibition of COX.

• This allows for increased arachadonic acid substrate conversion to leukotrienes via the lipooxygenase pathway.
• The increased leukotrienes trigger bronchospasm [15, 16].

• **Bone healing**
– COX-1 and COX-2 have been shown to play a role in bone healing following fracture [17].
– In the setting of NSAID use, an important subgroup (those having undergone lumbar fusions) may be at risk for unsuccessful fusions [18].
– It appears that in the setting of lumbar fusions, it may be best to minimize NSAIDs, perhaps even COX-2 inhibitors, due to concerns for bone healing [2].
– It remains unclear whether other subgroups are at similar risks [2].

Select Precautions/Contraindications

• Allergy to specific medication or class of medications
• Pregnancy: (especially close to term) is a relative contraindication for the use of NSAIDs
  – Use must be weighed against potential fetal risk [6].
• Some individuals present with hypersensitivity to aspirin and NSAIDs.
  – *Hypersensitivity reaction* may manifest as rhinitis, angioedema, urticaria, bronchial asthma, laryngeal edema, bronchoconstriction, flushing, hypotension, and shock.
  – In cases of hypersensitivity, aspirin intolerance is a contraindication to therapy with any other NSAID because cross-sensitivity can provoke a life-threatening reaction reminiscent of shock [6].
• Celecoxib and valdecoxib are contraindicated in patients with known sulfa allergy.
• Caution should be used in patients on oral anticoagulants.
• Most NSAIDs potentiate the effects of warfarin either by displacing the protein-bound drug or by inhibiting the metabolism [19, 20].
• Contraindicated for use immediately post-operatively following coronary artery bypass graft surgery.

Example Medications/Doses (Table 10.2)

Table 10.2 Select anti-inflammatory agents [6, 21]

Medication	Preparations/half-life	Dosing	Usual adult daily range
Celecoxib (Celebrex)	6–12 h	100 mg qd-bid	200 mg/day (Canadian labeling 400 mg /day for up to 7 days) Contraindicated with sulfa allergy
Diclofenac	1–2 h	50 mg tid or 75 mg 2 bid	150–200 mg/day
Etodolac	7 h	200–400 mg tid-qid	400–1,200 mg/day
Ibuprofen	2–4 h	Analgesia: 200–400 mg every 4–6 h Anti-inflammatory: 300 mg every 6–8 h or 400–800 mg tid-qid	Analgesia: 1,200–2,400 mg/day Anti-inflammatory: 2,400–3,200 mg/day
Meloxicam	15–20 h	7.5 mg daily	7.5–15 mg/day
Indomethacin	2.5 h	25 mg bid-tid or extended release (ER) dose: 75–100 mg qhs	<200 mg/day
Ketorolac (Toradol)	4–6 h	*<65 years old*: 20 mg PO, then 10 mg PO every 4–6 h *>65 years old*: 10 mg orally every 4–6 h Commonly given parenterally (60 mg IM followed by 30 mg every 6 h or 30 mg IV every 6 h)	Oral: <60 mg/day Parenteral: 30–60 mg, then 15–30 mg/day

Note: Use the lowest effective dose for the shortest effective period of time

Doses listed above may be lowered when considering patient specifics

Caution when prescribing NSAIDs as they can cause GI and renal side effects

References

1. Parr G, Darekar B, Fletcher A, Bulpitt CJ. Joint pain and quality of life; results of a randomised trial. Br J Clin Pharmacol. 1989;27(2):235–42.
2. Katz J. NSAIDs and COX-2-selective inhibitors. In: Benzon H, Raja S, Molloy R, Liu S, Fishman S, editors. Essentials of pain medicine and regional anesthesia. 2nd ed. Philadelphia: Elsevier; 2005. p. 141–58.
3. Abramson S. Therapy with and mechanisms of nonsteroidal anti-inflammatory drugs. Curr Opin Rheumatol. 1991;3(3):336–40.
4. Seibert K, Zhang Y, Leahy K, Hauser S, Masferrer J, Isakson P. Distribution of COX-1 and COX-2 in normal and inflamed tissues. Adv Exp Med Biol. 1997;400A:167–70.
5. Breder CD, Dewitt D, Kraig RP. Characterization of inducible cyclo-oxygenase in rat brain. J Comp Neurol. 1995;355(2):296–315.
6. Burke A, Smyth EM, FitzGerald GA. Analgesic-antipyretic agents; pharmacotherapy of gout. In: Brunton L, Lazo J, Parker K, editors. Goodman & Gilman's the pharmacological basis of therapeutics. 11th ed. Columbus: McGrawHill; 2006. p. 671–716.
7. Deeks JJ, Smith LA, Bradley MD. Efficacy, tolerability, and upper gastrointestinal safety of celecoxib for treatment of osteoarthritis and rheumatoid arthritis: systematic review of randomised controlled trials. BMJ. 2002;325(7365):619.
8. Fry SW, Seeff LB. Hepatotoxicity of analgesics and anti-inflammatory agents. Gastroenterol Clin North Am. 1995;24(4):875–905.
9. Patrono C, Dunn MJ. The clinical significance of inhibition of renal prostaglandin synthesis. Kidney Int. 1987;32(1):1–12.
10. Qi Z, Hao CM, Langenbach RI, Breyer RM, Redha R, Morrow JD, Breyer MD. Opposite effects of cyclooxygenase-1 and -2 activity on the pressor response to angiotensin II. J Clin Invest. 2002;110(3):419.
11. Leese PT, Talwalker S, Kent JD, Recker DP. Valdecoxib does not impair platelet function. Am J Emerg Med. 2002;20(4):275–81.
12. Leese PT, Hubbard RC, Karim A, Isakson PC, Yu SS, Geis GS. Effects of celecoxib, a novel cyclooxygenase-2 inhibitor, on platelet function in healthy adults: a randomized, controlled trial. J Clin Pharmacol. 2000;40(2):124–32.
13. García Rodríguez LA, Varas-Lorenzo C, Maguire A, González-Pérez A. Nonsteroidal antiinflammatory drugs and the risk of myocardial infarction in the general population. Circulation. 2004;109(24):3000–6.
14. FDA website. Information for healthcare professionals: non selective non steroidal antiinflammatory drugs (NSAIDs). http://www.fda.gov/Drugs/DrugSafety/PostmarketDrugSafetyInformationfor PatientsandProviders/DrugSafetyInformationforHeathcare Professionals/ucm085282.htm. Page last updated 27 Jan 2010. Accessed 14 Jan 2013.
15. Szczeklik A, Nizankowska E, Mastalerz L, Szabo Z. Analgesics and asthma. Am J Ther. 2002;9(3):233–43.
16. Ivi SS, Krishna MT, Sampson AP, Holgate ST, Holgate ST. The anti-inflammatory effects of leukotriene-modifying drugs and their use in asthma. Chest. 2001;119(5):1533–46.
17. Gerstenfeld LC, Thiede M, Seibert K, Mielke C, Phippard D, Svagr B, Cullinane D, Einhorn TA. Differential inhibition of fracture healing by non-selective and cyclooxygenase-2 selective nonsteroidal anti-inflammatory drugs. J Orthop Res. 2003;21(4):670–5.

18. Maxy RJ, Glassman SD. The effect of nonsteroidal anti-inflammatory drugs on osteogenesis and spinal fusion. Reg Anesth Pain Med. 2001;26(2):156–8.

19. Schafer AI. Effects of nonsteroidal antiinflammatory drugs on platelet function and systemic hemostasis. J Clin Pharmacol. 1995;35(3):209–19.

20. Shorr RI, Ray WA, Daugherty JR, Griffin MR. Concurrent use of nonsteroidal anti-inflammatory drugs and oral anticoagulants places elderly persons at high risk for hemorrhagic peptic ulcer disease. Arch Intern Med. 1993;153(14):1665–70.

21. Buvanendran A, Lipman AG. Nonsteroidal anti-inflammatory drugs and acetaminophen. In: Fishman SM, Ballantyne JC, Rathmell JP, editors. Bonica's management of pain. 4th ed. Baltimore: Lippincott Williams & Wilkins; 2010. p. 67190–965.

Muscle Relaxants and Antispasticity Medications

Alan David Kaye and Laurie E. Daste

A.D. Kaye, M.D., Ph.D. (✉)
Department of Anesthesiology, Interim LSU Hospital and Ochsner Kenner Hospital, New Orleans, LA, USA

Department of Pharmacology, Interim LSU Hospital and Ochsner Kenner Hospital, New Orleans, LA, USA
e-mail: alankaye44@hotmail.com

L.E. Daste, M.D.
Department of Anesthesiology, Ochsner Medical Center, New Orleans, LA, USA
e-mail: lswind@lsuhsc.edu

Abbreviations

CBC   Complete blood count
CNS   Central nervous system
COOMBs   Indirect and Direct Antiglobulin testing
GABA   Gamma-aminobutyric acid
IV   Intravenous
LFT   Liver function tests
MAOI   Monoamine oxidase inhibitors
NMDA N-Methyl-D-aspartate
TCAs   Tricyclic antidepressants

Introduction

Muscle relaxants: drugs that alleviate painful stimuli generated from a muscle spasm or spasticity.

Muscle relaxant medications are chosen based upon their symptomatic need, side effect profile, and tolerability. Often patients with a primary pain issue may experience secondary muscle spasm; therefore, practitioners sometimes use muscle relaxants concurrently with other medications to adequately treat their patient's pain.

- *Muscle spasm:* an abrupt, involuntary contraction of a muscle fiber, or group of muscle fibers that is often associated with pain
- *Spasticity:* a sustained muscle fiber contraction that is also characterized by resistance to passive motion of an extremity

Most muscle relaxant agents act primarily as CNS depressants and often cause nonspecific side effects such as sedation and drowsiness. There is no clear evidence that one skeletal muscle relaxant is superior to another for musculoskeletal spasms. Tailor choice of medication based on specific patient situation.

Centrally Acting Skeletal Muscle Relaxants
- Effective in the treatment of muscle spasms/spasticity
- **Somnolence** is a common side effect [1]
- May largely produce effects by causing sedation, which reduces the firing of painful nerve stimuli without actually causing direct skeletal muscle relaxation [1, 2]
- Some of these agents, including metabolites, can be **addictive** (e.g., meprobamate) and carry a high risk for abuse potential [1]

Muscle Relaxant Medications

Chlorzoxazone (Parafon Forte, Lorzone)

- Treatment of muscle spasms
  - Little efficacy in treatment of spasticity [3]
- *Clinical:* May cause less side effects and food/drug interactions then other medication options.
- *Mechanism of action:* Unknown; believed to predominantly block polysynaptic reflex conduits in the spinal cord implicated in muscle contraction [2, 3]
- *Side effects:* Some patients may experience less side effects with the lower doses of this medication vs the other muscle relaxant choices. Uncommonly results in dizziness, stomach upset, lethargy, and hepatotoxicity [3]
- *Dosage:* 250–750 mg po tid prn, up to 3,000 mg/day

K.A. Sackheim, *Pain Management and Palliative Care: A Comprehensive Guide*,
DOI 10.1007/978-1-4939-2462-2_11, © Springer Science+Business Media New York 2015

Carisoprodol (Soma)

- Acute treatment of muscle spasms in severe cases
  - Little efficacy in treatment of spasticity [3]
- *Clinical:* Avoid in patients with possible addiction/misuse issues, ensure no concurrent use of alcohol and CNS depressants to prevent worsening of sedative effects
- *Mechanism of action:* Unknown; may interrupt the interneuronal communication in the spinal cord and descending reticular formation [2]
  - Produces **meprobamate**, a metabolite which interacts with GABA-A receptors and displays similarities to barbiturates [2]
- *Side effects:* Drowsiness, ataxia, tremor, irritability, insomnia, confusion, disorientation, tachycardia, and postural hypotension [3]
- *Potential for abuse*
  - Meprobamate is highly *addictive*; carisoprodol is not indicated for long-term use
  - Carisoprodol is never to be stopped suddenly following prolonged use, a taper should be used. Important to recognize *withdrawal symptoms,* such as restlessness, insomnia, anorexia, upset stomach, anxiety, seizures, and even death. If any withdrawal symptoms are experienced, taper should be done at a slower pace.
  - Taper examples are listed below, but this should be done according to your patient's needs/medical conditions to prevent the precipitation of withdrawal symptoms.
    Short taper (4 days): 350 mg tid×1 day → 350 mg bid×2 days → 350 mg qday×1 day
    Long taper (9 days): 350 mg tid×3 days → 350 mg bid×3 days → 350 mg qday×3 days
    If any issues with patient taper, can consider transitioning to the 250 mg dose prior to discontinuing
- *Dosage:* 250–350 mg po qday-tid (depending on patient's needs), up to 1,400 mg/day, no longer than 2–3 weeks, as cases of abuse, dependence, and withdrawal have been associated with prolonged use

Cyclobenzaprine (Flexeril, Amrix)

- Treatment of muscle spasms
  - Little efficacy in treatment of spasticity [3]
- *Clinical:* Has a role in acute or chronic pain states with muscle spasm or strain. This agent has a multitude of different roles related to its structure and efficacy. It is indicated as an adjunct for muscle spasm associated with any acute painful musculoskeletal state that limits motion, tenderness, pain, or limits activities of daily living.
- *Mechanism of action:* Blocks serotonergic receptors in the descending pathways of the brainstem and ventral

spinal cord, thus interfering with signals that travel to alpha-motorneurons and interact directly with skeletal muscles [2]
- *Side effects: Anticholinergic* symptoms such as sedation, dry mouth, blurred vision, elevated intraocular pressure, urinary retention, constipation, dizziness, increased heart rate, and arrhythmias [1, 3]
  - May lead to worsening of benign prostatic hyperplasia, angle-closure glaucoma, cardiac conduction abnormalities, and congestive heart failure [1]
  - Structurally similar to tricyclic antidepressants (TCAs) [2]
  - Should not be used in conjunction with monoamine oxidase inhibitors (MAOI)
- *Dosage:* 10 mg po qhs-tid prn (depending on patient's needs), up to 40 mg/day, if given once daily—usually dosed at night as drowsiness and somnolence are commonly experienced side effects

Metaxalone (Skelaxin)

- Treatment of muscle spasms
- *Clinical:* Metaxalone is less commonly associated with side effects such as sedation and somnolence. May be considered "weaker" by some patients, may be good in elderly patients with no liver pathology or patients who are very sensitive to other medications.
- *Mechanism of action:* CNS depression [2]
- *Side effects:* Possible hepatotoxicity, hemolytic anemia [1]
  - Avoid in patients with liver failure
  - Patients should be followed with LFTs and monitoring for side effects such as jaundice, dark urine, nausea/vomiting, and abdominal pain. Patients taking long-term metaxalone need an established baseline LFT and serial testing at least once a year and more frequently with preexisting liver pathology.
  - Regularly monitor CBCs and obtain a COOMBs test if a hemolytic process occurs
- *Dosage:* 400–800 mg po qday-qid prn up to 3.2 g/day

Methocarbamol (Robaxin)

- Acute and chronic treatment of muscle spasms or strain [2]
- *Clinical:* Consider in patients who are sensitive to medications where skelaxin and/or lorzone have been unhelpful but did not cause side effects.
- *Mechanism of action:* Uncertain; indirect CNS depression [3]
  - Blocks acetylcholinesterase inhibition by pyridostigmine
- *Side effects:* Drowsiness, dizziness, nausea, anaphylactic reactions, thrombophlebitis, dyspepsia, jaundice, leucopenia, blurred vision, metallic taste, and vertigo [2, 3]

- *Dosage:* 500 or 750 mg po tid-qid (depending on symptoms) × 2–3 days (up to 8 g/day may be given in severe conditions), then decrease to 4–4.5 g/day in 3–6 divided doses
- Lower/less frequent dosing can be used in other conditions

Orphenadrine Citrate (Norflex)

- Improves and serves as an adjuvant for joint pain, muscle spasms/myofascial pain, neuropathic pain, and certain forms of muscular attributed headaches; also possesses antimuscarinic activity and local anesthetic effects
- *Clinical:* utilized for muscle spasm associated with acute painful musculoskeletal conditions
- *Mechanism of action:* Postulated to work similarly to diphenhydramine by blocking histaminic and cholinergic receptors; may also cause some NMDA antagonism and sodium channel interference [1, 2]
- *Side effects* [1]*:* Anticholinergic symptoms such as; dry mouth, blurred vision, and urinary retention; rarely, may result in aplastic anemia
- *Dosage:* 100 mg q12 h, up to 400 mg/day

Tizanidine (Zanaflex)

- Treatment of muscle spasticity with various pain syndromes and as an adjuvant hypnotic for insomnia
- *Clinical:* Initially dosed at night as this is likely to cause sedation but can be dosed q6–8 h if needed, do not use in patients with hepatic impairment or history of hypotension
- *Mechanism of action:* Stimulation of alpha-2 adrenergic receptors → reduction of excitatory neurotransmitter release by pre-synaptic neurons → interference in transmission of polysynaptic and monosynaptic reflexes in the dorsal horn of spinal cord [1–5]
  - Also reduces unprompted CNS activity and blocks the action of the cerulospinal pathway by inhibition of the locus ceruleus (which normally enhances synaptic transmission in the spinal cord) [3]
- *Side effects* [1, 3]*:* Hypotension (avoid other alpha-2 agonists), asthenia, headache, weakness, sedation, dry mouth, hallucination, upset stomach, and liver injury (may cause elevated LFTs >3 × upper limit of normal)
  - Avoid in patients with impaired hepatic function
  - Monitoring of LFTs is recommended during first 6 months (Baseline, then at first, third, and sixth month of use, then yearly). Monitor for side effects such as jaundice, dark urine, or nausea and vomiting.
- *Dosage:* 2–6 mg po every qday-qid prn hrs, up to 36 mg/day

Other Drugs

Baclofen (Lioresal)

- Treatment of spasticity secondary to CNS pathology (e.g., multiple sclerosis or spinal cord injuries); also reduces incidence of flexor spasms and associated pain [1, 3]
- *Clinical:* May help patients experiencing increased tone and/or leg cramping.
- *Mechanism of action:* Binds to and activates GABA-B receptors, which inhibits the release of excitatory neurotransmitters [3, 4]; interferes with synaptic communication in the spinal cord [1]
- *Side effects:* Somnolence, dizziness, weakness, confusion, upset stomach, and hypotension [1]
- If on high doses, requires taper if discontinued to avoid serious withdrawal effects
- Intrathecal pumps allow direct delivery of the drug and decrease risk of unwanted systemic effects [3]
- *Dosage:* Start at 5 mg po qhs or tid and increase by 5 mg q3 days, up to 80 mg/day as needed.

Dantrolene Sodium (Dantrium)

- Peripherally acting skeletal muscle relaxant
- Treatment of spasticity associated with spinal cord injuries, multiple sclerosis, cerebral palsy, and stroke [3]; treatment of malignant hyperthermia; to reduce muscle rigidity secondary to neuroleptic malignant syndrome, preventing muscle deterioration and the release of creatine phosphokinase [3]
- *Clinical:* Not Recommended secondary to possible hepatotoxicity
- *Mechanism of action:* Blocks the release of calcium from the sarcoplasmic reticulum within muscle cells, which prevents the formation of the actin–myosin bridge and thus inhibits muscle contraction [3]
- *Side effects:* Drowsiness, dizziness, muscle weakness, malaise, and diarrhea [2, 3]; fulminant hepatotoxicity has been reported (females >35 years old)
  - Can cause a large decrease in muscle tone which may be detrimental to an ambulatory patient
- *Dosage:* 25 mg po BID, up to 400 mg/day × 3 weeks

Benzodiazepines (e.g., Diazepam)

- Treatment of muscle spasms and spasticity related to CNS pathology (e.g., cerebral palsy or cord injury) [1]
- *Clinical:* This agent can be utilized for any muscle spasm associated with acute painful musculoskeletal conditions but should be considered only in refractory states.

- *Mechanism of action:* Enhances the release of GABA and it's subsequent binding to GABA-A receptors → activation of chloride channels presynaptically, inhibiting the release of excitatory neurotransmitters [3]
  - Sedation may play a role in relief of muscle spasms
- **Potential for addiction and abuse** [1]
  - Benzodiazepines should *never be stopped abruptly*; it is important to implement a slow tapering dose over time [1]
  - *Withdrawal symptoms*: anxiety, dysphoria, insomnia, diaphoresis, vomiting, diarrhea, tremor, seizure, and possibly death [1]
- *Side effects:* Sedation, cognitive dysfunction, confusion, dizziness, behavioral changes, respiratory depression, hypoventilation, and hypotension [1, 2]
  - Flumazenil 0.1–1 mg IV may be used to help rapidly reverse effects of any benzodiazepine [2]
  - *Geriatric patients are at increased risk of becoming disoriented with longer acting benzodiazepines*
- *Dosage:* 2–10 mg po qday-qid prn, up to 40 mg/day

Clinical Pearls When Prescribing Muscle Relaxers

- If an elderly patient requires a muscle relaxer to control their pain, consider starting with skelaxin or lorzone as this may cause less side effects.
- In normal healthy adults, can consider starting with tizanidine if no hypotension or liver pathology. If pain is refractory, consider flexeril, norflex, or robaxin.
- More often, patients on flexeril can experience extreme sleepiness and a sensation of feeling "drugged." The editor finds that most patients will tolerate tizanidine more easily with less side effects.

- Patients experiencing spasticity along with spasm may do better on baclofen.
- Soma should be avoided or reserved for severe refractory cases as this medication is addictive.
- Benzodiazepines are best used in acute circumstances and not for long-term treatment as they are associated with severe life-threatening withdrawal effects.
- Dantrolene should be avoided secondary to severe liver consequences.
- When prescribing any muscle relaxant the physician should always dicuss all possible side effects with the patient: sleepiness, dizziness, etc. Patients should always first try these medications at night, as they may be sedating, and alert the physician of any untoward side effects.
- Patients should not drive or drink alcohol while on these medications.

References

1. Waldman HJ, Waldman SD, Waldman KA. Centrally acting skeletal muscle relaxants and associated drugs. In: Waldman S, editor. Pain management, vol. 2. Philadelphia: Saunders; 2007. p. 977–82.
2. Lindley DA. Muscle relaxants: overview of muscle relaxants in pain. In: Sinatra RS, Jahr JS, Michael Watkins-Pitchford J, editors. The essence of analgesia and analgesics. Cambridge: Cambridge University Press; 2011. p. 360–65.
3. Melen O, Benzon HT. Muscle relaxants. In: Essentials of pain medicine and regional anesthesia. New York: Churchill Livingstone; 1999. p. 78–82.
4. Simon O, Yelnik AP. Managing spasticity with drugs. Eur J Phys Rehabil Med. 2010;46:401–10.
5. Toth PP, Urtis J. Commonly used muscle relaxant therapies for acute low back pain: a review of carisoprodol, cyclobenzaprine hydrochloride, and metaxalone. Clin Ther. 2004;26:1355–67.

Neuropathic Antidepressant Medications

12

Jignyasa Desai

Abbreviations

ARDS	Acute respiratory distress syndrome
ASA	Aspirin
CNS	Central nervous system
EKG	Electrocardiogram
FM	Fibromyalgia
GABA	Gamma-aminobutyric acid
GI	Gastrointestinal
5-HT	5-Hydroxytryptamine
HTN	Hypertension
INR	International normalized ratio
MAOIs	Monoamine oxidase inhibitors
NMDA	N-Methyl-D-aspartate
NSAIDs	Non-steroidal anti-inflammatory drugs
SNRI	Serotonin–norepinephrine reuptake inhibitor
SSRIs	Selective serotonin reuptake inhibitors
TCA	Tricyclic antidepressants

Introduction

- Psychiatric medications are primarily used to treat major depression and anxiety disorders but also have uses in chronic pain disorders
- The below medications are not effective in the management of chronic muscular aches and pains
- Chronic pain uses are primarily related to neuropathic pain conditions
- *Neuropathic pain states include*:
  - Diabetic peripheral neuropathy
  - Post-herpetic neuralgia
  - Central post-stroke pain
  - Phantom limb pain
  - Peripheral neuropathy
  - Other neuralgias
- *Antidepressants may also treat*:
  - Fibromyalgia (FM)
  - Chronic tension headaches
  - Migraines
- Tricyclic antidepressants (TCAs) are the most commonly used antidepressants to treat pain
- SSRI, SNRI, and other atypical antidepressants have also been used in painful conditions
- Patients have varying responses and effectiveness to the medication, thus often times different classes will have to be trialed for good relief of pain.
- *Depression*: caused by the under activity of certain neurotransmitters in the brain
  - Neurotransmitters are generally monoamines, such as dopamine, serotonin, and norepinephrine [1].
- Mechanism of action of antidepressants in pain management is not entirely known, and multiple mechanisms are believed to be involved.
  - Most common theory is their effects upon serotonin and norepinephrine along the descending spinal pathways.
  - Antidepressants may be effective via their ability to modulate the sodium pathways involved in nerve conduction as well as histamine receptors [2].

Antidepressant Drug Categories (Table 12.1)

- Tricyclic antidepressants (TCAs)
- Selective serotonin reuptake inhibitors (SSRIs)
- Selective serotonin–norepinephrine reuptake inhibitors (SNRIs)
- Atypical antidepressants
- Monoamine oxidase inhibitors (MAOIs)

J. Desai, D.O. (✉)
1407 Tower Dr., Edgewater, NJ 07020, USA
e-mail: Desai4spine@gmail.com

K.A. Sackheim, *Pain Management and Palliative Care: A Comprehensive Guide*,
DOI 10.1007/978-1-4939-2462-2_12, © Springer Science+Business Media New York 2015

Table 12.1 Antidepressant medications. © Kimberly Sackheim 2015

Drug	Mechanism of action	Pharmacokinetics	Side effects/contraindications	Therapeutic indications	Preparations/dosing
Amitriptyline (Elavil)-3	TCA: mechanism is not established. Inhibits the membrane pump mechanism responsible for uptake of norepinephrine and serotonin in adrenergic and serotonergic neurons	Fat soluble, metabolized by the liver and excreted by the kidneys, requires plasma levels for efficacy	Weight gain. Anticholinergic effects greater than secondary (TCA), orthostatic hypotension, cardiovascular effects, lethality in overdose, coma, Seizures CI: avoid with MAOIs	Neuropathic pain disorders	Available strengths: 10 mg, 25 mg, 50 mg, 75 mg, 100 mg, 150 mg Typical adult dosage: 75 mg/day in divided doses Max daily dose: 150 mg/day
Doxepin (Silenor)-3	TCA: not established. Suspected to influence adrenergic activity at the synapses, preventing deactivation of norepinephrine by reuptake into nerve terminals	Fat soluble, metabolized by the liver and excreted by the kidneys, requires plasma levels for efficacy	Suicidality, unusual changes in behavior, drowsiness, dry mouth, blurred vision, constipation, urinary retention, N/V, indigestion, taste disturbances, diarrhea, anorexia, aphthous stomatitis, skin rash, decreased or increased libido. CI: Glaucoma, tendency to urinary retention	Neuropathic pain disorders	Available strengths: 10 mg, 25 mg, 50 mg, 75 mg, 100 mg, 150 mg; sol: 10 mg/mL [120 mL] Typical adult dosage: usual: 75–150 mg/day Max daily dose: 150 mg daily
Imipramine (Tofranil)-3 3-(Tertiary)	TCA: mechanism unknown. Suspected to potentiate adrenergic synapses by blocking uptake of norepinephrine at nerve endings	Fat soluble, metabolized by the liver and excreted by the kidneys, requires plasma levels for efficacy	Suicidality, unusual changes in behavior, clinical worsening, sleep disorders, tiredness, mild GI disturbances, orthostatic hypotension, HTN, confusion, hallucinations, numbness, tremors, dry mouth, urticaria, N/V CI: Acute recovery period following myocardial infarction, MAOI coadministration or use within 14 days after stopping MAOI therapy.	Neuropathic pain disorders	Available strengths: 10 mg, 25 mg, 50 mg Typical adult dosage: main: 50–150 mg/day Max daily dose: 200 mg/day
Nortriptyline (Pamelor)-2 2-(Secondary)	TCA: inhibits activity of histamine, 5-hydroxytryptamine, and acetylcholine; increases pressor effect of NE, blocks pressor response of phenethylamine, and interferes with transport, release, and storage of catecholamine	Fat soluble, metabolized by the liver and excreted by the kidneys, requires plasma levels for efficacy	Arrhythmias, hypotension, HTN, tachycardia, MI, heart block, stroke, confusion, hallucination, insomnia, tremors, ataxia, dry mouth, blurred vision, skin rash. CI: MAOI	Neuropathic pain disorders	Available strengths: 10 mg, 25 mg, 50 mg, 75 mg; sol: 10 mg/5 mL Typical adult dosage: 25 mg tid-qid Max daily dose: 150 mg/day
Desipramine (Norpramin)-2	TCA: mechanism is not established, suspected to restore normal levels of neurotransmitters (NE and 5-HT) by blocking their re-uptake from the synapse in the CNS	**Absorption:** Rapid (via GI tract). **Metabolism:** Liver. **Elimination:** Urine (70 %). Fat soluble, metabolized by the liver and excreted by the kidneys, requires plasma levels for efficacy	Arrhythmias, hypotension, HTN, tachycardia, confusional state, Suicidiation, disorientation, delusions, ataxia, tremors, dry mouth, anorexia, N/V, gynecomastia, breast enlargement. CI: with use of MAOIs	Neuropathic pain disorders	Available strengths: 10 mg, 25 mg, 50 mg, 75 mg, 100 mg, 150 mg Typical adult dosage: 25–100 mg qd Max daily dose: 100 mg/day

Drug	Mechanism	Onset/Half-life	Side effects/Contraindications	Indication	Dosing
Venlafaxine (Effexor)	SNRI; potentiates neurotransmitter activity in CNS by inhibiting neuronal serotonin and norepinephrine reuptake	Onset: T_{max} = 5.5 h; $T_{1/2}$: ODV: $T_{1/2}$ = 11 h	Asthenia, sweating, headache, N/V, constipation, anorexia, dry mouth, dizziness, insomnia, nervousness, somnolence, abnormal ejaculation/orgasm, abnormal dreams, pharyngitis. CI: with use of MAOIs	Neuropathic pain disorders. Studies show similar efficacy to TCA at doses 150 mg per day or higher (i.e., typical antidepressant doses, thus superior efficacy for the treatment of neuropathic pain	Available strengths: Cap. Extended-Release: 37.5 mg, 75 mg, 150 mg. Typical adult dosage: 150 mg per day or higher. Max daily dose: 225 mg/day
Duloxetine (Cymbalta)	Selective SNRI: not established. Believed to be related to potentiation of serotonergic and noradrenergic activity in the CNS	Onset: T_{max} = 6 h; $T_{1/2}$: 12 h	Nausea, dry mouth, constipation, diarrhea, decreased appetite, fatigue, dizziness, somnolence, hyperhidrosis, headache, insomnia, abdominal pain. CI: concomitant use of MAOIs	Management of neuropathic pain associated with diabetic peripheral neuropathy (DPNP), Management of fibromyalgia (FM) and chronic musculoskeletal pain	Available strengths: 20 mg, 30 mg, 60 mg. Typical adult dosage: initial: 60 mg qd or 30 mg qd for 1 week before increasing to 60 mg qd. Max daily dose: 60 mg day
Bupropion (Wellbutrin)	Aminoketone antidepressant; not established. Weak inhibitor of the neuronal uptake of norepinephrine and dopamine	Onset: 2 h; $T_{1/2}$: 21 h	Dry mouth, excessive sweating, headache/migraine, insomnia, tremor, agitation, weight loss, N/V, constipation, dizziness, sedation, blurred vision, decreased libido. CI: Seizure disorder, bulimia or anorexia nervosa, other medications that contain bupropion, use of MAOIs within 14 days and patients undergoing abrupt d/c of alcohol or sedatives (including benzodiazepines)	Neuropathic pain disorders	Available strengths: 75 mg, 100 mg; Tab, Sustained-Release (SR): 100 mg, 150 mg, 200 mg (Wellbutrin SR). Typical adult dosage: 100 mg bid. Max daily dose: 450 mg/day
Paroxetine (Paxil)	SSRI: inhibits CNS neuronal reuptake of serotonin	Onset: T_{max} = 6–10 h; $T_{1/2}$: 15–20 h	Suicidiality, somnolence, insomnia, nausea, asthenia, abnormal ejaculation, dry mouth, constipation, dizziness, diarrhea, decreased libido, sweating, abnormal vision, headache, tremor. CI: concomitant use with MAOI	Neuropathic pain disorders	Available strengths: 12.5 mg, 25 mg, 37.5 mg. Typical adult dosage: 25 mg daily. Max daily dose: 75 mg/day
Citalopram (Celexa)	SSRI: presumed to be linked to potentiation of serotonergic activity in the CNS, resulting from its inhibition of CNS neuronal reuptake of serotonin	Onset: T_{max} = 4 h; $T_{1/2}$: 35 h	N/V, dyspepsia, diarrhea, dry mouth, somnolence, insomnia, increased sweating, ejaculation disorder, rhinitis, anxiety, anorexia, tremor, agitation, sinusitis. CI: During or within 14 days of d/c of MAOI therapy, concomitant use of pimozide	Neuropathic pain disorders	Available strengths: 10 mg, 20 mg, 40 mg. Typical adult dosage: initial: 20 mg qd. Titrate: Increase dose to 40 mg at an interval of no less than 1 week. Max daily dose: 40 mg/day

(continued)

Table 12.1 (continued)

Drug	Mechanism of action	Pharmacokinetics	Side effects/contraindications	Therapeutic indications	Preparations/dosing
Milnacipran hcl (Savella)	Selective SNRI: not established. Potent inhibition of neuronal norepinephrine and serotonin reuptake without directly affecting uptake of dopamine or other neurotransmitters	Onset: T_{max}=2–4 h $T_{1/2}$: 6–8 h	N/V, headache, constipation, hot flash, insomnia, hyperhidrosis, palpitations, upper respiratory infection, increased HR, dry mouth, HTN, anxiety, dizziness. CI: uncontrolled narrow-angle glaucoma, concomitant use with MAOIs or within 14 days of stopping an MAOI	FM	Available strengths: 12.5 mg, 25 mg, 50 mg, 100 mg Typical adult dosage: 50 mg BID Max daily dose: 100 mg BID
Desvenlafaxine (Pristiq)	SNRI: potentiates neurotransmitter activity in CNS by inhibiting neuronal serotonin and norepinephrine reuptake	Onset: T_{max} = 7.5 h $T_{1/2}$: 11 h	Headache, N/V, dry mouth, diarrhea, dizziness, insomnia, somnolence, hyperhidrosis, constipation, anxiety, decreased appetite, male sexual function disorders, fatigue. CI: avoid with MAOIs	Neuropathic pain disorders	Available strengths: 50 mg, 100 mg Typical adult dosage: 50 mg Max daily dose: 100 mg

Tricyclic Antidepressants

Amitriptyline (Elavil), Desipramine (Norpramin), Imipramine (Tofranil), Nortriptyline (Pamelor)

- *Indications*
  TCAs are *second-line treatment for chronic pain*:
  Neuralgia or neuropathic pain, FM, chronic headache
- *Research*:
  - An evidence-based guideline sponsored by the International Association for the Study of Pain recommends nortriptyline as a first-line medication for neuropathic pain [3].
  - TCAs are the most studied antidepressants for the treatment of neuropathic pain and are a mainstay in the treatment for neuropathic pain [4].
  - Pain relief is independent of the antidepressant effects of these drugs and may be achieved at doses lower than those used in the treatment of depression [5].
- *Mechanism of action*: TCA affects many receptors: beta-adrenergic receptors, muscarinic acetylcholine receptors, peripheral alpha-adrenergic receptors, histamine receptors, central gamma-aminobutyric acid (GABA), *N*-methyl-D-aspartate (NMDA), and dopamine receptors [6–10].
  - Inhibit the presynaptic reuptake of biogenic amines, primarily serotonin and norepinephrine [6]
  - TCAs act to block the serotonin transporter and the norepinephrine transporter [7, 8]

Structurally divided into secondary and tertiary amines (Table 12.2):

Secondary amines
- More selective reuptake of norepinephrine inhibitors
- Desipiramine and nortriptyline have least orva inter

Tertiary amines
- More selective on the serotonin
- Cause more side effects having increased anticholinergic side effects
- Highly sedating because of their central effects on histamine [6]

Table 12.2 Tertiary and secondary amines

Tertiary amines	Secondary amines
Amitriptyline (Elavil, Endep, Vanatrip)	Desipramine (Norpramin, Pertofrane)
Imipramine (Tofranil)	Nortriptyline (Aventyl, Nortrilen, Pamelor)
Clomipramine (Anafranil)	Protriptyline (Vivactil) [11]
Doxepin (Adapin)	
Butriptyline (Evadene, Evadyne)	
Dosulepin (Prothiade)	
Lofepramine (Feprapax, Gamanil, Lomont)	
Trimipramine (Surmontil)	

- *Pharmacokinetics TCA*:
  - Large side effect profile
  - Highly metabolized by the cytochrome P450 hepatic enzymes
  - Highly plasma bound up to 95 % and lipophilic with large volume of distribution including the brain and has many drug to drug interactions with other highly protein-bound structures
  - Renal impairment will substantially affect clearance of TCA metabolites with an increase in plasma concentrations [9, 11, 12]
- *Drug interactions contraindications*
  - TCAs inhibit sodium and L-type calcium channels which lead to *cardiotoxicity* [13, 14]. Combining TCAs with drugs that also affect the heart's conduction system: disopyramide (Norpace), procainamide (Pronestyl, Procan SR, Procanbid) may increase the frequency and severity of an abnormal heart rate and rhythm.
  - Drugs that inhibit cytochrome P450 decrease TCA metabolism and increase blood concentrations and thus lead to toxicity: e.g., cimetidine, methylphenidate, fluoxetine, antipsychotics, and calcium channel blockers
  - TCAs may inhibit the antihypertensive effect of clonidine (Catapres). Therefore, combining TCAs with clonidine may lead to dangerous elevations in blood pressure.
  - Combining TCAs with carbamazepine (Tegretol) may result in lower TCA blood levels because carbamazepine increases the breakdown of TCAs, potentially reducing the effect of TCAs.
  - Drugs that prolong the QT interval: quinidine, astemizole, terfenadine, and some antipsychotics may increase the chance of ventricular dysrhythmias.
  - Avoid use with alcohol and barbiturates and other CNS depressants.
  - Avoid drugs with anti-muscarinic properties as this may potentiate the effects. TCAs should be avoided by individuals with prostatic hypertrophy, cognitive impairment, or narrow-angle glaucoma because of the anticholinergic side effects [15]
- *Dosing*: Lower doses may be used in treatment of pain conditions
  - **Nortriptyline (Pamelor)**: start with 25 mg qhs, titrate to desired effect as long as tolerated; doses above 150 mg/day are not recommended.
  - **Amitriptyline (Elavil)**: start with 25–75 mg of amitriptyline qhs. Titrate to desired effect as long as tolerated. If necessary, this may be increased to a total of 150 mg per day.
  - **Imipramine (Tofranil)**: start with 75 mg/day increased to 150 mg/day. Dosages over 200 mg/day are not recommended.

- **Desipramine** (**Norpramin**): Usual adult dose is 100–200 mg per day. Dosages above 300 mg/day are not recommended.
- *Side effects*
  - Cardiovascular toxicity is the most common cause of morbidity and mortality—can lead to severe hypotension, dysrhythmias, and conduction delays. *Avoid in patients with preexisting conditions.*
  - TCAs affect sodium conduction, therefore affecting cardiac conduction with delaying ventricular depolarization. EKG can present with prolonged QT_C and may lead to torsade de pointes and sinus tachycardia. Most common cause of death is refractory hypotension with bradycardia from the inhibition of alpha1-adrenergic receptors.
  - Anticholinergic effects: Dry mouth, altered mental status, psychotic behavior, agitation, hallucinations, generalized seizures, urinary retention, hyperthermia, decreased gastric motility/ileus
  - Severe side effects: Acute lung injury—(ARDS), hypoventilation related to ARDS, aspiration pneumonitis, tachycardia, hypothermia [15–19]
  - Best dose at night as somnolence is common

Selective Serotonin Reuptake Inhibitors

Fluoxetine (Prozac), Paroxetine (Paxil), Sertraline (Zoloft), and Citalopram (Celexa)

- *Indications*: SSRIs are most useful and first-line treatment of depression and other psychiatric illnesses; they are second-line treatment for chronic pain [20]
- *Mechanism of action*:
  - Inhibit the reuptake of the serotonin (5-hydroxytryptamine or 5-HT) into the presynaptic cell → increasing levels of 5-HT within the synaptic cleft [20, 21]
- *Research*:
  - *Paroxetine* and *citalopram* to demonstrate modest efficacy in the management of neuropathic pain
  - Fluoxetine has not demonstrated any efficacy at all for pain management [4].
  - As a category, SSRI are less effective than other types of antidepressants in treatment of neuropathic pain treatment [22–24].
- *Pharmacokinetics*:
  - Metabolized by liver [25]
  - Minimal affinity for histaminic, dopaminergic, alpha-adrenergic, and cholinergic receptors thus mild side effect profile, and relative safety in overdose
  - Paroxetine (most potent inhibitor of serotonin reuptake) > fluoxetine > sertraline > citalopram [25]
  - Antidepressant effect takes approximately 3 – 6 weeks after initial treatment [21]

- Renal disease and age → affects elimination of citalopram, paroxetine, but has no effect on fluoxetine or sertraline [25].
- *Side effects*
  - Sexual dysfunction [22], increased suicidal ideation, weight gain, GI abnormalities, dyspepsia, nausea, vomiting, diarrhea, initial anxiety, tremors, nervousness, dizziness, and headache [23]
- *Drug interactions/contraindications*:
  Certain drugs may increase toxicities of SSRIs:
  - Avoid use with drugs that affect the serotonergic neurotransmitter systems (e.g., triptans, linezolid, tramadol, or St. John's Wort); these may lead to serotonin syndrome.
  - Contraindicated with MAOIs, lead to fatal serotonin syndrome
  - Avoid alcohol, tryptophan, other SNRIs, SSRIs, TCAs, pimozide
  - May potentiate drugs metabolized by CYP2D6 (e.g., TCAs, Type 1C antiarrhythmics)
  - May induce metabolism of cisapride
  - May shift concentrations with plasma-bound drugs (e.g., warfarin, digitoxin)
  - Increased risk of bleeding with NSAIDs, ASA, warfarin [11, 24, 25]

Selective Serotonin–Norepinephrine Reuptake Inhibitors

Duloxetine (Cymbalta), Milnacipran (Savella), Venlafaxine (Effexor XR, Effexor), Desvenlafaxine (Pristiq)

- *Indications*:
  Venlafaxine (Effexor, Effexor XR) is indicated for the treatment of certain psychiatric disorders
  - Case reports [4, 26, 27] and empirical studies [28, 29] have indicated that venlafaxine is effective for the management of neuropathic pain at doses of 150 mg per day or higher (typical antidepressant doses).
  - In the treatment of neuropathic pain, venlafaxine is comparable to imipramine [27], suggesting that it may be comparable to other TCAs as well.
  - Despite a milder side effect profile than the TCAs, venlafaxine may elevate blood pressure and has a discontinuation syndrome with abrupt cessation [5].
  Duloxetine (Cymbalta) is indicated for the treatment of:
  - Certain psychiatric disorders, Diabetic Peripheral Neuropathic Pain, FM
  - Duloxetine has been confirmed in several studies as an effective agent in the treatment of neuropathic pain [27].
  - Doses for the treatment of neuropathic pain as well as depression are between 60 and 120 mg per day.

- *Pharmacodynamics*

  Second-generation SNRIs (Cymbalta and Effexor) have a mixed action on both major neuroamines of depression: norepinephrine and serotonin. They have limited adverse effects because they do not affect muscarinic, histaminic, α1-adrenergic receptors, and monoamine oxidase. They are better tolerated in comparison to the TCAs and MAOIs [30]. Neuropathic pain is thought to be related to increased levels of norepinephrine [31].

- *Pharmacokinetics*
  - Venlafaxine (Effexor, Effexor XR): at low dose (75 mg/day) it acts only on serotonin, at higher doses (150–225 mg/day) acts as SNRI. At very high doses (above 350 mg/day), may also weakly block the reuptake of dopamine.
  - Duloxetine (Cymbalta) is a strong, balanced inhibitor of both norepinephrine and serotonin reuptake.
  - Cymbalta is more noradrenergic than Effexor, with Effexor has almost 30 x higher higher affinity for the serotonin inhibition verses norepinephrine [32].
  - Venlafaxine—Metabolism: Hepatic via CYP2D6 Elimination: Urine (5 % unchanged), $T_{1/2} = 5$ h
  - Duloxetine—Metabolism: Hepatic via CYP1A2, 2D6; Elimination: Urine (70 %), feces (20 %); $T_{1/2} = 12$ h
- *Side effects*: Nausea, dizziness, fatigue or sleepiness, insomnia, anticholinergic effects, loss of appetite, nervousness, sweating, sexual side effects, constipation, increased blood pressure
- *Drug interactions/contraindications*
  - Avoid alcohol and tryptophan
  - Increased risk of bleeding with anti-coagulants
  - Caution with cimetidine in elderly, HTN, hepatic dysfunction
  - Decreases clearance of haloperidol
  - Caution with CNS-active drugs and serotonergic drugs
  - Effexor: Inhibitors of CYP3A4 and CYP2D6, Coadministration with tryptophan supplements and weight-loss agents are not recommended.
  - Cymbalta: Avoid CYP1A2 inhibitors (e.g., fluvoxamine, cimetidine, some quinolone antibiotics). Caution with drugs metabolized by CYP2D6 having a narrow therapeutic index (e.g., TCAs, phenothiazines, type 1C antiarrhythmics)
  - Venlafaxine (Effexor) is less likely than duloxetine (Cymbalta) to interact with co-administered medications [33].
- *Contraindications*: Do not use in patients taking concurrent MAOIs, and uncontrolled narrow angle glaucoma

Atypical Antidepressants

Not commonly used to treat pain conditions but these pain patients may be taking concurrent medications so practitioners should be familiar with them

Bupoprion (Wellbutrin), Trazodone (Desyrel)

- *Indications*:
  - Bupropion is less likely to cause sexual side effects. Prescribed for patients with fatigue and poor concentration, it is mildly stimulating. It also has been used with some success in the treatment of attention deficit hyperactivity disorder [34]. It is not an anxiolytic as it lacks serotonergic properties.
  - Mirtazapine may be useful if patient is experiencing insomnia or agitation.
  - Trazodone in small dosages is often used along with an SSRI to help with sleep disturbances.

Bupropion (Wellbutrin)

- *Mechanism of action*: Suspected to inhibit neuronal uptake of norepinephrine and dopamine. Bupropion SR was similar in efficacy to TCAs in a double-blind crossover study of patients with various forms of neuropathic pain at doses of 300 mg per day [35].
- *Pharmacokinetics*: Absorption: $T_{max} = 3$ h. Metabolism: liver, extensive, via CYP2B6 metabolite;
- *Contraindications*: *Absolute contraindications*—Seizure disorders, eating disorders [36]
  - MAOIs concomitantly
  - Patients undergoing abrupt d/c of alcohol
  - Sedatives (including benzodiazepines)
  - Patients with bulimia or anorexic nervosa
- Adverse effects: Dry mouth, excessive sweating, headache/migraine, insomnia, tremor, agitation, weight loss, nausea/vomiting, constipation, dizziness, sedation, blurred vision, decreased libido, anorexia, neuropsychiatric events.
- *Interactions*:
  - Extreme caution with drugs that lower seizure threshold (e.g., antidepressants, antipsychotics, theophylline, systemic steroids)
  - Increased seizure risk with opioids, cocaine, OTC stimulants, oral hypoglycemics, insulin
  - Inhibits CYP2D6; caution with drugs that are metabolized by CYP2D6 (e.g., SSRIs, TCAs, antipsychotics, β-blockers, type 1C antiarrhythmics

Trazodone (Desyrel)

- *Mechanism of action*: suspected to selectively inhibit serotonin uptake by brain synaptosomes and potentiate behavioral changes induced by the serotonin precursor, 5-hydroxytryptophan
- *Pharmacokinetics*: Absorption: Well absorbed; $T_{max} = 1–2$ h. Metabolism: liver via CYP3A4 to m-chlorophenylpiperazine (active metabolite)

- *Adverse reaction*: Dry mouth, edema, constipation, blurred vision, fatigue, nervousness, drowsiness, dizziness, headache, insomnia, N/V, musculoskeletal pain, hypotension, confusion, priapism.
- *Drug interactions*: CYP3A4 inhibitors (e.g., ritonavir, ketoconazole, indinavir, itraconazole, nefazodone) may increase levels; carbamazepine decreases levels
  - Increases digoxin and phenytoin serum levels
  - Caution with MAOIs
  - May enhance response to alcohol, barbiturates, and other CNS depressants
  - May affect PT in patients on warfarin
  - Avoid in concomitant use with antihypertensive therapy
  - Avoid electroshock therapy
  - May interact with general anesthetics
  - Increased INR with warfarin

Monamine Oxidase Inhibitors

These medications are associated with severe adverse reactions, dangerous drug–drug interactions, and are not used to treat pain disorders.

- *Drug interactions/contraindications*
  - Tyramine-containing foods: aged cheeses, yeast extract foods, beer, wine, smoked meats
  - Potential drug interactions

    Any drug that releases catecholamines may precipitate life-threatening events in individuals also using MAOIs ex. Dextromethorphan

    Tramadol and Meperidine produce a release of serotonin precipitating a potentially fatal outcome [37, 38].

    All serotonergic agents, SSRIs—fluoxetine, paroxetine can lead to serotonin syndrome [39]

Antidepressants are used to treat many psychological diseases; however, they also are useful to chronic pain management. Not only do they help stabilize any mood disorders, which can play an important role in the psychological basis of pain, but the direct affects they have on the neurotransmitters and hormones in the body may have a direct correlation to the decrease in the symptomatic management of the patients' painful condition.

References

1. Pomara N, Sidtis JJ. Brain neurotoxic amyloid-beta peptides: their potential role in the pathophysiology of depression and as molecular therapeutic targets. Br J Pharmacol. 2010;161(4):768–70.
2. Gallagher RM. Management of neuropathic pain: translating mechanistic advances and evidence-based research into clinical practice. Clin J Pain. 2006;22:S2–8.
3. Dworkin RH, O'Conor AB, Audette J, Baron R, Gourlay GK, Haanpaa ML, Kent JL, Krane EJ, LeBel AA, Levy RM, Mackey SC, Mayer J, Miaskowski C, Raja SN, Rice AS, Schmader KE, Stacey B, Stanos S, Treede RD, Turk DC, Walco GA, Wells CD. Recommendations for the pharmacological management of neuropathic pain: overview and literature update. Mayo Clin Proc. 2010;85(3):S3–14.
4. Jackson KC, St. Onge EL. Antidepressant pharmacotherapy: considerations for the pain clinician. Pain Pract. 2003;3:135–43.
5. Sansone RA, Sansone LA. Pain, pain go away: antidepressants and pain management. Psychiatry. 2008;5(12):16–9.
6. Nelson JC. Tricyclic and tetracyclic drugs. In: Schatzberg AF, Nemeroff CB, editors. The American Psychiatric Publishing textbook of psychopharmacology. Washington, DC: American Psychiatric Publishing; 2009. p. 263.
7. Tatsumi M, Groshan K, Blakely RD, Richelson E. Pharmacological profile of antidepressants and related compounds at human monoamine transporters. Eur J Pharmacol. 1997;340(2–3):249–58.
8. Gillman PK. Tricyclic antidepressant pharmacology and therapeutic drug interactions updated. Br J Pharmacol. 2007;151(6): 737–48.
9. Rudorfer MV, Potter WZ. Pharmokinetics of antidepressants. In: Meltzer HY, editor. Psycohpharmacology: the third generation of progress. New York: Raven Press; 1987. p. 1353–63.
10. Cusack B, Nelson A, Richelson E. Binding of antidepressants to human brain receptors: focus on newer generation compounds. Psychopharmacology (Berl). 1999;114(4):559–65.
11. Li N, Wallén NH, Ladjevardi M, Hjemdahl P. Effects of serotonin on platelet activation in whole blood. Blood Coagul Fibrinolysis. 1997;8(8):517–23.
12. Rudorfer M, Matthew V, Potter WZ. Metabolism of tricyclic antidepressants. Cell Mol Neurobiol. 1999;19(3):373–409.
13. Pancrazio JJ, Kamatchi GL, Roscoe AK, Lynch C. Inhibition of neuronal Na+ channels by antidepressant drugs. J Pharmacol Exp Ther. 1998;284(1):208–14.
14. Zahradník I, Minarovic I, Zahradníková A. Inhibition of the cardiac L-type calcium channel current by antidepressant drugs. J Pharmacol Exp Ther. 2008;324(3):977–84.
15. Shannon M, Merola J, Lovejoy Jr FH. Hypotension in severe tricyclic antidepressant overdose. Am J Emerg Med. 1988;6(5): 439–42.
16. Keis NA. Cardiotoxic side effects associated with tricyclic antidepressant overdose. AACN Clin Issues Crit Care Nurs. 1992;3(1): 226–32.
17. Rose JB. Tricyclic antidepressant toxicity. Clin Toxicol. 1977;11(4): 391–402.
18. Thornton WE. Tricyclic antidepressants and cardiovascular drug interactions. Am Fam Physician. 1979;20(1):97–9.
19. Jefferson JW. A review of the cardiovascular effects and toxicity of tricyclic antidepressants. Psychosom Med. 1975;37(2):160–79.
20. Garnock-Jones KP, McCormack PL. Escitalopram: a review of its use in the management of major depressive disorder in adults. CNS Drugs. 2010;24(9):769–96.
21. Maes M, Meltzer H. The serotonin hypothesis of major depression. In: Bloom FE, Kupfer DJ, editors. Psychopharmacology: the fourth generation of progress. New York: Raven Press; 1995. p. 933.
22. Ekselius L, Von Knorring L. Effect on sexual function of long-term treatment with selective serotonin reuptake inhibitors in depressed patients treated in primary care. J Clin Psychopharmacol. 2001; 21(2):154–60.
23. Fava M. Weight gain and antidepressants. J Clin Psychiatry. 2000; 6(11):37–41.
24. Schellander R, Donnerer J. Antidepressants: clinically relevant drug interactions to be considered. Pharmacology. 2010;86(4):203–15.

25. Gury C, Cousin F. Pharmacokinetics of SSRI antidepressants: half-life and clinical applicability. Encéphale. 1999;25(5):470–6.

26. Eckert A. Clinically relevant drug interactions with new generation antidepressants and antipsychotics. Ther Umsch. 2009; 66(6):485–92.

27. Jann MW, Slade JH. Antidepressant agents for the treatment of chronic pain and depression. Pharmacotherapy. 2007;27: 1571–87.

28. Sullivan MD, Robinson JP. Antidepressant and anticonvulsant medication for chronic pain. Phys Med Rehabil Clin N Am. 2006; 17:381–400.

29. Chong MS, Brandner B. Neuropathic agents and pain: new strategies. Biomed Pharmacother. 2006;60:318–22.

30. Lambert O, Bourin M. SNRIs: mechanism of action and clinical features. Expert Rev Neurother. 2002;2(6):849–58.

31. Sindrup SH, Otto M, Finnerup NB, Jensen TS. Antidepressants in the treatment of neuropathic pain. Basic Clin Pharmacol Toxicol. 2005;96(6):399–409.

32. Bymaster FP, Dreshfield-Ahmad LJ, Threlkeld PG, Shaw JL, Thompson L, Nelson DL, Hemrick-Luecke SK, Wong DT. Comparative affinity of duloxetine and venlafaxine for serotonin and norepinephrine transporters in vitro and in vivo, human serotonin receptor subtypes, and other neuronal receptors. Neuropsychopharmacology. 2001;25(6):871–80.

33. Spina E, Santoro V, D'Arrigo C. Clinically relevant pharmacokinetic drug interactions with second-generation antidepressants: an update. Clin Ther. 2008;30(7):1206–27.

34. Wender PH. Pharmacotherapy of attention-deficit/hyperactivity disorder in adults. J Clin Psychiatry. 1998;59(7):76–9.

35. Wolfe GI, Trivedi JR. Painful peripheral neuropathy and its nonsurgical treatment. Muscle Nerve. 2004;30:3–19.

36. Clinical pharmacology [database online]. Tampa, FL: Gold Standard, Inc.; 2008. http://cp.gsm.com. Revised July 2008. Accessed 20 Nov 2008.

37. Guo SL, Wu TJ, Liu CC, Ng CC, Chien CC, Sun HL. Meperidine-induced serotonin syndrome in a susceptible patient. Br J Anaesth. 2009;103(3):369–70.

38. Fox MA, Jensen CL, Murphy DL. Tramadol and another atypical opioid meperidine have exaggerated serotonin syndrome behavioural effects, but decreased analgesic effects, in genetically deficient serotonin transporter (SERT) mice. Int J Neuropsychopharmacol. 2009;12(8):1055–65.

39. Torre LE, Menon R, Power BM. Prolonged serotonin toxicity with proserotonergic drugs in the intensive care unit. Crit Care Resusc. 2009;11(4):272–5.

40. Gillman PK. Tricyclic antidepressant pharmacology and therapeutic drug interactions updated. Br J Pharmacol. 2007; 151(6):737–48.

Neuropathic Anticonvulsant Medications

Leena Mathew and Lisa Kilcoyne

Abbreviations

AEDs	Anti-epileptic drugs
AMPA	2-(Aminomethyl)phenylacetic acid
AV	Atrioventricular block
CBC	Complete blood count
GABA	Gamma-aminobutyric acid
HIV	Human immunodeficiency virus
HTN	Hypertension
IV	Intravenous
LV	Liver
MAOI	Monamine oxidase inhibitor
NMDA	N-Methyl-D-aspartate
PO BID	Per os *bis in die* (Latin), twice a day
PO TID	Per os *ter in die* (Latin), three times a day
TCAs	Tricyclic antidepressant/s

Introduction

Neuropathic pain: pain arising as a direct consequence of a lesion or disease affecting the somatosensory system [1]
- May have positive and/or negative symptoms
  Positive symptoms: pain, paresthesia, dysesthesia, hyperalgesia, allodynia [2]
  Negative symptoms: weakness, hypoesthesia, hypoalgesia, reflex changes [2]
- Common causes: nerve root/disc pathology causing radiculopathy, diabetes, trigeminal neuralgia, postherpetic neuralgia, post-stroke syndrome, multiples sclerosis, spinal cord injury, cancer, HIV [1]
- Diverse group of drugs used to treat neuropathic pain
  - Anticonvulsants

- Antidepressants
- Membrane-stabilizing agents
- Alpha 2 agonists
- Opioids and Tramadol
- NMDA receptor antagonists (Ketamine)
- Topical treatments (such as Capsaicin)

Anticonvulsants (Anti-epileptic Drugs)

- *Three generations of AEDs*
  - *First generation*: Carbamazepine, Phenytoin, Phenobarbital, Valproic acid [3]
  - *Second generation*: Gabapentin, Pregabalin, Topiramate, Felbamate, Lamotrigine, Levitiracetam, Oxcarbamezapine, Vigabatrin [4]
  - *Third generation*: Lacosamide, Eslicabazepine [5]
- The newer generations (second and third) have a better safety profile

Phenytoin (Dilantin)

- *Mechanism of action*: stabilizes neuronal membranes and blocks sodium channels [3]
- *Pharmacokinetics*
  - Structurally related to the barbiturates but with a five-membered ring
  - High bioavailability after oral dose but peak serum levels reached 3–12 h after first dose [6]
  - Induces hepatic enzymes [7]
  - 90 % bound to albumin [8]
- *Metabolism*
  - Hepatic metabolism and glucuronidation followed by excretion in urine [8]
  - Hypoalbuminemia (pregnancy, nephrotic syndrome, chronic illness) and uremia increase the free fraction and increase potential for toxicity [9]
  - Serum $T_{1/2}$ is variable: 12–36 h [6]

L. Mathew, M.D. (✉) • L. Kilcoyne, B.A. M.D.
Department of Anesthesiology, Division of Pain Medicine,
New York Presbyterian Hospital, Columbia University,
New York, NY, USA
e-mail: LM370@Columbia.edu

K.A. Sackheim, *Pain Management and Palliative Care: A Comprehensive Guide*,
DOI 10.1007/978-1-4939-2462-2_13, © Springer Science+Business Media New York 2015

- *Dosing*
  - Start with 100 mg po tid
  - Check phenytoin blood levels 3 weeks after initiation [9]
  - Dosage should be individualized to provide maximum benefit
  - Serum blood level determinations may be necessary for optimal dosage adjustments—*clinically effective serum level is usually 10–20 mcg/mL* [6]
  - Steady-state blood levels achieved with 7–10 days [6]
  - Changes in dosage should not be carried out at intervals < 7–10 days [9]
  - IV infusion of 15 mg/kg phenytoin has an analgesic effect in acute flare-ups of neuropathic pain and that this relief outlives both the infusion time and plasma $T_{1/2}$ of phenytoin [6]
  - Toxic levels: 20 mcg/mL [10]
- *Side effects*
  If mild-moderate side effects occur, decrease dose for several days and then gradually increase
  - *Hirsutism*: excessive hair growth mostly on trunk, face, and extensor surfaces of extremities [11]
  - *Vestibular dysfunction*: resulting in ataxia [6], nausea, vomiting, gastritis [12], rash [11], hepatotoxicity [12], folic acid deficiency [11]
  - *Gingival hyperplasia*: due to fibrocyte stimulation (avoided by careful monitoring and aggressively good oral hygiene); reported in up to 50 % of patients on long-term therapy [11]
  - *Hyperglycemia* due to inhibition of insulin secretion, improves with decreasing dose of phenytoin [13]
  - Horizontal gaze nystagmus: occurs at therapeutic doses [6], paradoxical seizures [12], teratogenicity [11]
  - *Cerebellar atrophy*: (chronic high dose Phenytoin accumulation in the cerebral cortex over long periods of time causing atrophy of the cerebellum) [12]
  - *Osteomalacia*: due to phenytoin's interference with vitamin D metabolism [11]

Points to Remember About Phenytoin

- Intravenous phenytoin may be considered in patients experiencing acute flare-ups or crescendo pattern of neuropathic pain
- IV infusion must be done slowly to avoid adverse reactions including sudden precipitous hypotension, which can result from an IV bolus [6]
- Phenytoin can be teratogenic
- Check for toxic levels because the therapeutic window is narrow (10–20 mcg/mL)

Carbamazepine (Tegretol)

- Analgesic of choice in trigeminal neuralgia
- May have benefit in other cranial nerve neuralgias
- *Mechanism of action*: blocks voltage-dependent sodium channels, also has some calcium channel blocking action [3]
- *Pharmacokinetics*
  - Structurally similar to imipramine and other TCAs [14]
  - Slowly and unpredictably absorbed after oral administration
  - Peak concentrations are reached after 2–8 h
  - $T_{1/2} = 10$–25 h [3]
- *Metabolism*
  - Can cause auto-induction of its own metabolism [8]
  - 75 % of the absorbed drug is protein-bound to albumin and alpha-1 acid glycoprotein
  - Main route of elimination is oxidation [7]
- *Dosing*
  - Start at 100 mg po bid
  - Increased by 200 mg/day until pain is relieved to a max dose of 1,200 mg/day [15]
  - Serum concentrations should be checked at 3, 6, 9 weeks with goal 4–12 mcg/mL [15]
- *Side effects*
  - Nausea, gastric irritation, vomiting [16], HTN, acute LV failure [15], sedation, diplopia, vertigo [16], aplastic anemia, agranulocytosis [16] oliguria [15]
  - Hepatic dysfunction, jaundice [15]
    Obtain CBC and liver function panel—baseline, q 2 weeks × 1 month and q month × 3 months and q 6 months × 1 year and then yearly
- *Contraindications*
  - AV block
  - Hepatic disease
  - Bone marrow depression
  - Acute intermittent porphyria or serious blood disorders
  - Hypersensitivity to carbamazepine or tricyclic antidepressants
  - Not to be given with, or within 14 days of starting or stopping MAOI therapy
- *Precautions*
  - Pregnancy, lactation
  - Elderly patients: increased risk of urinary retention, increased intraocular pressure, cardiovascular disorders, activation of behavioral disorders, and exacerbation of seizures [15]
    Perform periodic ophthalmic examinations, evaluations of renal, hepatic, and bone marrow function

- Abrupt cessation of carbamazepine may precipitate seizures
- Cross-hypersensitivity with phenytoin and oxcarbazepine [15]

Points to Remember About Carbamazepine

- Drug of choice in trigeminal neuralgia
- Aplastic anemia and agranulocytosis are the most devastating side effects
- Monitor CBC and liver function panel during ongoing therapy [15]

Valproic Acid (Depakote)

- Predominantly used in the treatment of seizure disorder and as a mood-stabilizing drug
- Treatment of neuropathic pain, chronic headaches, and migraine
- *Mechanism of action*: GABA transaminase inhibitor (indirect GABA agonist) [16]
  Blocks voltage-gated sodium and calcium channels [16]
- *Pharmacokinetics*
  - Nearly complete bioavailability [3]
  - Peak serum levels achieved in 1–4 h [3]
  - Protein bound (90–95 %), mainly to albumin [15]
- *Metabolism*
  - Undergoes oxidation and glucuronidation in liver [7]
  - $T_{1/2} = 10–20$ h [3]
- *Dosing*
  - Adult dose is 15 mg/kg/day in divided doses [1]
  - Increased by 5–10 mg/kg/day Q week to a maximum of 60 mg/kg/day [15]
  - Check serum level 1–2 weeks after start of therapy, therapeutic drug levels 50–150 mcg/mL [15]
- *Side effects*
  - Nausea, vomiting, anorexia, liver failure [15], sedation, tremor, ataxia [15], skin rash, alopecia [15], weight gain [15]

Points to Remember About Valproic Acid

- Good choice in chronic headache and migraine prophylaxis
- Check baseline and periodic liver function tests, since liver failure is a rare complication of Valproic acid

Gabapentin (Neurontin)

- Second-generation AED
- Widely used as first line in neuropathic pain states and as an adjuvant agent

- *Mechanism of action*: Binds to the alpha 2 delta subunit of the calcium channel [14]
- *Pharmacokinetics*
  - Structural relationship to GABA but its actions are not GABA-mediated [14]
- *Metabolism*
  - No appreciable metabolism [1]
  - Less than 60 % bioavailability [17]
  - Peak serum levels 2–3 h after first dose [18]
  - Circulates largely free since it's only 3 % protein-bound [17]
  - Gabapentin is eliminated from the systemic circulation by renal clearance as an unchanged drug [7]
  - Elimination half-life is 5–7 h and is not altered by multiple doses [18]
  - In patients with impaired renal function, gabapentin plasma clearance is reduced [17], please see renal chapter for specifics on dosing
  - No known drug interactions except for decreased absorption with aluminum and magnesium antacids [18]
- *Dosing*
  - Consider starting at 100–300 mg and titrated from qday - tid dosing [16]
  - Weekly dose escalation can be contemplated in the absence of side effects to a max of 1,800 mg/day in divided doses [15]
  - Analgesic effects are expected at 900 mg total daily dose [14]
- *Side effects*
  - Nausea, vomiting, GI irritation [15], confusion, sedation, dizziness (resolves and tolerance develops), tremors (no tolerance—must discontinue) [15], peripheral edema [15]

Points to Remember About Gabapentin

- Gabapentin can be removed from plasma by hemodialysis
- Gabapentin is secreted into human milk following oral administration [15]. Gabapentin should be used in women who are nursing only if the benefits clearly outweigh the risks.

Pregabalin (Lyrica)

- An AED designed to be a potent successor to Gabapentin
- Adjunct therapy for partial seizures and in generalized anxiety disorder
- Pregabalin is effective at treating chronic pain disorders such as fibromyalgia and neuropathic pain.
- *Mechanism of action*: Binds to the alpha2-delta subunit [16]
  - Reduces the calcium-dependent release of several neurotransmitters by modulating calcium channel function [16]

- *Pharmacokinetics*
  - Structurally related to GABA but does not bind directly to any of the receptors and does not augment GABA response [16]
  - Pregabalin is well absorbed after oral administration
- *Metabolism*
  - Hepatic metabolism is negligible [1]
  - Renal excretion [7]
  - Elimination $T_{1/2} = 6$–7 h [17, 18]
  - Steady state levels reached within 24–48 h [18]
  - Peak serum levels reached within 1–2 h [17]
- *Dosing*:
  - Start at 25–50 mg PO BID-TID depending on patient specifics with slow titration upwards to desired effect [15]
  - Escalate if tolerated
  - Maximum dose of 150 mg PO TID over 3–4 weeks
- *Side effects*:
  - Dizziness, somnolence, nausea, blurred vision [16], weight gain, peripheral edema [16], thrombocytopenia

Points to Remember About Pregabalin

- Pregabalin is effectively removed by hemodialysis; plasma pregabalin concentrations are reduced by approximately 50 % and the dosing has to adjusted
- Can cause angioedema
- There are no known drug interactions [15]

Clonazepam (Klonopin)

- Falls into the benzodiazepine group
- Popularly used as an anticonvulsant and anxiolytic agent
- *Mechanism of action*: Binds to the benzodiazepine site of the GABA receptor [16]
  - Increased influx of chloride ions into the neurons causing an inhibition of synaptic transmission [16]
- *Pharmacokinetics*
  - Good oral absorption [19]
  - Peak serum levels are attained in 1–4 h [19]
  - Moderately protein-bound drug [19]
- *Metabolism*
  - Hepatic metabolism [19]
  - No active metabolites [19]
  - Renal excretion
  - $T_{1/2}$ is 12–24 h [19]

- *Dosing*
  - Start 0.5 mg po qd to tid
  - Increase by 0.5 mg/day every 5 days
  - Max dose: 6 mg/day
- *Side effects*
  Sedation, fatigue, ataxia, dependence, and withdrawal [19]

Points to Remember About Clonazepam

- Associated with withdrawal
- Must be tapered and titrated down cautiously
- Dependence develops rapidly
- Avoid in nursing mothers, pregnant women, and in patients with liver and renal dysfunction
- Caution in elderly

Lamotrigine (Lamictal)

- Structurally unrelated to the current AEDs
- Predominantly used as an antiepileptic agent and maintenance therapy of bipolar disorder
- *Mechanism of action*: Stabilizes neuronal membranes by inhibiting voltage-sensitive sodium channels [14]
  - Modulates presynaptic transmitter release of excitatory amino acids such as glutamate [14]
- *Pharmacokinetics*
  - Rapidly and completely absorption orally [17]
  - High bioavailability [15]
  - Peak plasma levels in 1–3 h [17]
  - $T_{1/2} = 15$–25 h [17]
- *Metabolism*
  - Metabolized by hepatic glucuronidation [7]
  - Inactive metabolites
- *Dosing*
  - Start at 25 mg/day and titrate over 2 weeks to 25 mg po bid × 2 weeks 14
  - Increase by 25 mg/2 weeks to 100 mg po bid
  - Maximum: 200 mg po bid [14]
- *Side effects*
  - Dizziness, somnolence, ataxia, headache [14], diplopia, blurred vision [14], nausea, and vomiting [14]
  - Toxic epidermal necrolysis, Stevens–Johnson syndrome [15]
    - Nearly all cases appear in the first 2–8 weeks of therapy or if medication is suddenly stopped then resumed at the normal dosage
    - Patients should be advised to seek immediate medical attention in the setting of an unexpected skin rash.

Points to Remember About Lamotrigine

- Lamotrigine has a black box warning regarding Stevens–Johnson syndrome and Toxic Epidermal Necrolysis

Topiramate (Topamax)

- Primarily used in the treatment of seizure disorder, depression as well in the pediatric population for the management of Lenox Gastaut syndrome
- Indicated in pain medicine for the management of chronic migraine prophylaxis
- Anecdotal benefit in treatment of neuropathic pain of diabetic neuropathy, migraines, and cluster headache therapy
- *Mechanism of action*:
  - Blocks sodium channels [16]
  - Potentiates the inhibitory effects of GABA [16]
  - Antagonizes the ability of kainate to activate the kainate/AMPA [16]
- *Pharmacokinetics*
  - Structurally unrelated to all the antiepileptic agents.
  - Time to peak serum concentration is 2–4 h [17]

- *Metabolism*
  - It is minimally bound to serum proteins and is primarily excreted in urine with some hepatic oxidation [7]
  - Adult $T_{1/2}=20$–30 h [17]
- *Dosing*
  - Start at 25–50 mg/day [15]
  - Increase by 50 mg every 7 days to 400 mg BID dosing [15]
- *Side effects*
  The presence and severity of many of these adverse effects appear to be dose-related
  - Somnolence, anxiety, ataxia, dizziness, memory loss, confusion [15], nausea, vomiting, constipation, anorexia, weight loss [15], personality changes, insomnia [15], metabolic acidosis due to bicarbonate wasting [15], fatigue

Points to Remember About Topiramate

- Few drug interactions
- Anorexia causing weight loss is a serious side effect and care must be taken in patients with eating disorders (Table 13.1)

Table 13.1 Summary of anticonvulsants used in the treatment of neuropathic pain

Drug	Dosing	Time to peak effect (h)	Serum $T_{1/2}$ life (h)	Adverse effects
Phenytoin (Dilantin)	Start at 100 mg PO TID and check blood levels in 3 weeks (therapeutic level 10–20 mcg/mL), dose changes no more frequently than every week	3–12	12–36	Hirsutism, ataxia, nausea, vomiting, gastritis, rash, hepatotoxicity, folic acid deficiency, gingival hyperplasia, nystagmus, teratogenicity, cerebellar atrophy, osteomalacia
Carbamazepine (Tegretol)	Start at 100 mg PO BID and increase 200 mg/day until pain is relieved to a maximum of 1,200 mg/day	2–8	10–25	Nausea, vomiting, gastric irritation, HTN, acute LV failure, sedation, diplopia, vertigo, aplastic anemia, agranulocytosis, liver dysfunction, jaundice, oliguria
Valproic acid (Depakote)	Start at 15 mg/kg daily in divided doses then increase by 5–10 mg/kg/day every week to a maximum of 60 mg/kg/day	1–4	10–20	Nausea, vomiting, anorexia, liver failure, sedation, tremor, ataxia, skin rash, alopecia, weight gain
Gabapentin (Neurontin)	Start at 100–300 mg PO daily and titrate to TID dosing, weekly escalation if tolerated to a maximum of 1,800 mg/day	2–3	5–7	Nausea, vomiting, GI irritation, confusion, sedation, dizziness, tremors, peripheral edema
Clonazepam (Klonopin)	Start at 0.5 mg PO daily or TID and increase by 0.5 mg/day every 5 days to a maximum of 6 mg/day	1–4	12–24	Sedation, fatigue, dependence, ataxia, withdrawal
Lamotrigine (Lamictal)	Start at 25 mg PO daily and titrate over 2 weeks to 25 mg PO BID and increase by 25 mg daily every 2 weeks to a maximum of 200 mg POBID	1–3	15–25	Dizziness, somnolence, ataxia, headache, diplopia, blurred vision, nausea, vomiting, Toxic epidermal necrolysis, Stevens-Johnson Syndrome
Topiramate (Topamax)	Start 25–50 mg PO daily; increase by 50 mg every 7 days to a maximum of 400 mg PO BID dosing	2–4	20–30	Anorexia, weight loss, nausea, vomiting, constipation, somnolence, anxiety, ataxia, dizziness, memory loss, personality changes, insomnia, metabolic acidosis
Pregabalin (Lyrica)	Start at 25 mg PO Qday to BID and increase if tolerated to a maximum of 150 mg PO TID over 3–4 weeks	1–2	6–7	Dizziness, somnolence, nausea, blurred vision, weight gain, peripheral edema, thrombocytopenia, angioedema

References

1. Schestatsky P, Nascimento OJ. What do general neurologists needs to know about neuropathic pain? Arq Neuropsiquiatr. 2009;67(3A):741–9.
2. Vranken JH. Elucidation of pathophysiology and treatment of neuropathic pain. Cent Nerv Syst Agents Med Chem. 2012;12(4):304–14.
3. Perucca E. An introduction to antiepileptic drugs. Epilepsia. 2005;46(4):31–7.
4. LaRoche S. A new look at the second-generation antiepileptic drugs: a decade of experience. Neurologist. 2007;13(3):133–9.
5. Luszczki JJ. Third-generation antiepileptic drugs: mechanisms of action, pharmacokinetics, interactions. Pharmacol Rep. 2009;61(2):197–216.
6. Gallop K. Review article: phenytoin use and efficacy in the ED. Emerg Med Australas. 2010;22(2):108–18.
7. Thorn CF, Whirl-Carrillo M, Leeder JS, Klein TE, Altman RB. PharmGKB summary: phenytoin pathway. Pharmacogenet Genomics. 2012;22(6):466–70.
8. Perucca E. Clinically relevant drug interactions with antiepileptic drugs. Br J Clin Pharmacol. 2006;61(3):246–55.
9. Aronson JK, Hardman M, Reynolds DJ. ABC of monitoring drug therapy. Phenytoin. Br Med J. 1992;305(6863):1215–8.
10. Von Winckelmann SL, Spriet I, Williams L. Therapeutic drug monitoring of phenytoin in critically ill patients. Pharmacotherapy. 2008;28(11):1391–400.
11. Scheinfeld N. Phenytoin in cutaneous medicine: its uses, mechanisms, and side effects. Dermatol Online J. 2003;9(3):6.
12. Craig S. Phenytoin poisoning. Neurocrit Care. 2005;3(2):161–70.
13. Al-Rubeaan K, Ryan EA. Phenytoin induced insulin insensitivity. Diabet Med. 2009;8(10):968–70.
14. Backonja MM. Use of anticonvulsants for treatments of neuropathic pain. Neurology. 2002;59(5):S14–7.
15. Schachter SC. Pharmacology of antiepileptic drugs; 2012. www.uptodate.com. Retrieved 10 Dec 2012.
16. Tremont-Lukats IW, Megeff C, Backonja MM. Anticonvulsants for neuropathic pain syndromes: mechanisms of action and place in therapy. Drugs. 2000;60(5):1029–52.
17. Krasowski MD. Therapeutic monitoring of the newer anti-epilepsy medication. Pharmaceuticals. 2010;3(6):1909–35.
18. Johannessen SI, Tomson T. Pharmacokinetic variability of newer antiepileptic drugs: when is monitoring needed? Clin Pharmacokinet. 2006;45(11):1061–75.
19. Riss J, Cloyd J, Gates J, Collins S. Benzodiazepines in epilepsy: pharmacology and pharmacokinetics. Acta Neurol Scand. 2008;118(2):69–86.

Opioid Medications

14

Stephen Kishner and Juliet P. Tran

Abbreviations

CNCP	Chronic non-cancerous pain
COT	Chronic opioid therapy
ECGs	Electrocardiograms
ER	Extended release
GABA	Gamma-aminobutyric acid
IR	Immediate release
MHRA	Medicines and Healthcare products Regulatory Agency
QTc	Rate corrected QT
SL	Sublingual

Introduction

Opioid use for pain relief can be found in ancient Egyptian papyrus records [1]. Historically, opium was derived from the poppy seed. Morphine was first isolated by Freidrich Serturner, a German pharmacist, in 1804 [2].

Definitions

Opioids: group of compounds that interact at the opioid receptors

This includes natural occurring opioids derived from opium poppy seed, semisynthetic opioids (e.g., hydrocodone), and synthetic opioids (e.g., fentanyl) [2, 3]

S. Kishner, M.D. (✉)
Department of Physical Medicine and Rehabilitation,
Louisiana State University School of Medicine, New Orleans,
New Orleans, LA, USA
e-mail: skishn@lsuhsc.edu

J.P. Tran, M.D., M.P.H.
Department of Family Medicine, East Jefferson General Hospital,
Metairie, LA, USA
e-mail: tranjuliet@gmail.com

Opiates: derivatives of the nature alkaloids found in opium poppy that include morphine, codeine, and thebaine

Narcotics: a term used for all drugs that have psychoactive properties with a potential for abuse

Mechanism of action: Morphine-like opioid agonists act at several specific opioid receptor-binding sites in the CNS and other tissues, involving several neurotransmitter systems to produce analgesia. Opioids principally act on the presynaptic receptors of neurons that in turn inhibit the release of gamma-aminobutyric acid (GABA) [4].

Receptors: Three principle opioid receptors located in the central and peripheral nervous system.

1. *Mu*—analgesia at supraspinal levels, related to respiratory depression and to physical dependence with chronic use
2. *Kappa*—analgesia at spinal level, related to the sedative effects of opioid drugs
3. *Delta*—analgesia at supraspinal levels, related to respiratory depression and to psychomimetic and dysphoric effects

   Most of the clinically used opioids have their principal effect at the Mu receptor [5–7].

Opioid usage: Used in acute and chronic pain, with chronic pain defined as "pain that persists beyond normal tissue healing time, which is assumed to be 3 months" by the International Association for the Study of Pain.

Opioid Chemical Classification [2]

1. Phenanthrenes—morphine, codeine, oxycodone, hydrocodone, hydromorphone
2. Benzomorphans—pentazocine
3. Phenylpiperidines—meperidine, fentanyl
4. Diphenylheptanes—methadone, propoxyphene
5. Tramadol—does not fit into any of the four above chemical classes

K.A. Sackheim, *Pain Management and Palliitation Care: A Comprehensive Guide*,
DOI 10.1007/978-1-4939-2462-2_14, © Springer Science+Business Media New York 2015

Opioid Activity Classification

1. Agonists—most of the common opioids, e.g., codeine, hydrocodone
2. Partial agonists—buprenorphine
3. Agonists–antagonists—pentazocine
4. Antagonists—naloxone
5. Tramadol—an atypical opioid

The Controlled Substance Act

This act is a federal law as part of the federal US drug policy. This act classifies controlled drugs into five schedules overseen by the Drug Enforcement Administration (DEA) [8].

Schedule of Drugs

I—No medical use, high potential for abuse, e.g., heroin, LSD

II—Accepted medical use with high potential for abuse, e.g., hydrocodone, morphine, methylphenidate, oxycodone, fentanyl, hydromorphone

III—Accepted medical use with potential for abuse less than drugs in schedule I and II

Tylenol #3 (with codeine)

IV—Accepted medical use with potential for abuse less than drugs in schedule III, e.g., benzodiazepines

V—Accepted medical use with potential for abuse less than drugs in schedule IV, tramadol, carisoprodol, e.g., pregabalin and codeine-containing cough suppressants

Opioid Duration of Action

Opioids have varying half-lives and corresponding durations of action. Long $T_{1/2}$ agents are more beneficial in chronic pain conditions requiring around the clock medications.

- *Short duration of action (up to 4–6 h)*: Immediate release—tramadol, codeine, morphine, hydromorphone, hydrocodone, oxycodone, oxymorphone, and tapentadol
- *Long duration of action (approximately 8–12 h)*: Extended release—tramadol (Conzip), morphine (MSContin, Avinza, Kadian), oxycodone (OxyContin), oxymorphone (Opana ER), tapentadol (Nucynta ER), fentanyl patch (48–72 h), buprenorphine (Butrans, Suboxone *24–48 h*), methadone

Opioids in managing pain: The analgesic ladder was first presented by the World Health Association. This ladder attempts to match the severity of pain with the strength of analgesics that can be prescribed. Multimodal approach to pain treatment is emphasized

- *Mild pain*—treated with non-opioid mediations and adjuvants, with progressive use of milder, and then stronger opioids up the ladder as pain becomes more severe initiate treatment with NSAIDs and acetaminophen
- *Moderate pain*—consider tramadol, codeine, and hydrocodone
- *Severe pain*—consider morphine, methadone, hydromorphone, fentanyl, oxycodone, oxymorphone, tapentadol, and levorphanol

Patient selection [9]: Before initiating chronic opioid therapy (COT), physicians should assess the patient with a complete history, physical examination, and appropriate testing, including an evaluation of the risk of substance abuse, misuse, or addiction. Full details can be found in the chapter on obtaining a history for the pain patient.

- Trial of COT is an option to consider when alternative treatments fail to control moderate or severe pain that adversely affects a patient's function or quality of life and benefits outweigh risks
- Goal of opioid therapy for chronic non-cancerous pain (CNCP) is rarely the elimination of pain, but rather an improvement in function or a reduction of pain intensity by at least 30 % [10]

Initiation and titration of COT [11]: Opioid therapy for CNCP should be started at low dose and titrated slowly.

- Immediate release (IR) medications can be used to start to make sure they are well tolerated
- IR medications are also best when patients do not have pain everyday
- If a patient requires an IR medication >3–4 times everyday, consider treating the patient with a long-acting or extended release (ER) medication
- Some patients require both IR and ER medications to properly control their pain
- When possible, use the same class of opioid analgesic for long-acting (i.e., 24-h scheduled doses) and short-acting (i.e., PRN doses for breakthrough pain) pain relief
- For severe pain, first-line therapy may start with hydrocodone, oxycodone, oxymorphone, hydromorphone, tapentadol, or morphine, with second-line therapy leading to fentanyl and if absolutely necessary, the third-line therapy for severe pain with methadone or buprenorphine
- There is a correlation between increasing mortality with increasing doses

Adverse effects of opioids: Anticipation and treatment of adverse effects reduce the likelihood that patients will discontinue opioid due to intolerable adverse effects, and may allow use of higher opioid doses if needed for uncontrolled pain.

- **Constipation**: one of the most common side effects
  - Constipation secondary to opioids does *not* improve with time; stool softeners, laxatives, and increased fiber intake are commonly needed.

- *Medications to consider for treatment*: Colace 100 mg bid-tid, Senna 1–2 po qhs prn, Dulcolax 5–10 mg PO or PR prn. If conservative measures fail, methylnaltrexone (Relistor) 0.15 mg/kg SC every other day can also consider Amitiza.
  - In the elderly, controlled release oxycodone is 7× more likely to cause constipation than transdermal fentanyl [12]. Elderly patients should preemptively be placed on a bowel regimen when starting opioid medications to avoid constipation complications.
- **Urinary retention:** Elderly are at higher risk for developing opioid-induced urinary retention. Treatment is with catheterization and a reduction or discontinuation of the opioid [13].
- **Pruritis:** Mechanism of opioid-induced pruritis is unclear. It is more common with IV and intrathecal administration of opioids. Treatment with antihistamines is not very effective. Treatment is generally a change in opioid such as fentanyl or hydromorphone that have less histamine releasing issues, or with the use of naloxone. Naloxone may however, decrease the effectiveness of opioid analgesia [14].
- **Nausea and vomiting:** A common opioid-associated adverse effect that tends to diminish over days or weeks of continued opioid exposure. Available treatments include antiemetics, metoclopramide (Reglan), serotonin antagonists, antihistamines, and corticosteroids. It can be used alone or in combinations [15]. Commonly used antiemetics are Zofran 4–8 mg PO/IV q6 hours prn and/or Phenergan 12.5–25 mg PO/IM/IV q8 hours prn.
- **Sedation or impaired cognition:** This tends to wane over time. If severe, sedation can be treated with dextroamphetamine (Dexedrine) 2.5–5 mg PO BID or methylphenidate (Ritalin) 2.5–5 mg PO BID. Caution with these medications in patients with cardiac pathology, increased BP or increase HR. Delirium or reduced cognition can be treated with haloperidol (Haldol) 0.5–2 mg PO BID or other antipsychotic drugs at lose dose.
- **Respiratory depression:** Risk is highest in opioid-naïve patients and may occur when initial opioid doses are too high, opioids are titrated too rapidly, or opioids are combined with other drugs that are associated with respiratory depression or that may potentiate opioid-induced respiratory depression (such as benzodiazepines) [9]. Naloxone (Narcan) 0.4–2 mg IV every 2–3 min up to 10 mg total can be used to reverse the opioid effects of respiratory depression. Some patients may need intubation for mechanical respiration. More details on this subject can be seen in the dedicated chapter.
- **Opioid-induced hyperalgesia (OIH):** OIH is a less recognized side effect of chronic opioid treatment where paradoxically there is increased sensitivity to certain painful stimuli. The incidence or prevalence is not known.

The mechanism is not understood but there appears to be increased sensitization of the nociceptive pathway. There is no definitive treatment. Tapering of opioids for opioid free trial may help in the treatment of these symptoms. Methadone, as an NMDA receptor agonist, may prevent or reduce OIH [16].

Opioid rotation: Opioid rotation should be considered if there are excessive side effects, insufficient pain relief when using one opioid during dose titration, or extreme tolerance develops [17].

Overdose: Opioid overdoses can be reversed with an opioid antagonist, naloxone. More details on this subject can be seen in Chap. 7.

Changes in Therapy [9]
- Opioid therapy is continued if appropriate analgesia and functional status is achieved either with opioid therapy alone or in conjunction with other modalities.
- Patients who are unable to obtain adequate analgesia with high dosages and with other issues may be converted to SL buprenorphine.
- If opioids are to be discontinued for reasons not associated with non-compliance, then tapering should be a slow decrease of 10 % of the original dose per week. This regimen is generally well tolerated with minimal adverse physiological effects.
- Symptoms of mild opioid withdrawal may occasionally persist for 6 months after opioids have been discontinued.
- Benefit may be obtained from adjuvant agents such as antidepressants to manage irritability and sleep disturbances, or antiepileptics for neuropathic pain.
- The majority of treatment recommendations are based on evidence consensus and practice patterns, rather than high-quality evidence alone.

Therapy for the opioid-naïve patient: refer to initiation and titration of COT above and opioid equianalgesic doses table for potency comparison.

Therapy for Opioid-Tolerant Patients

With below doses around the clock ≥1 week, patient is considered "opioid tolerant":
- 60 mg PO morphine daily
- 25 mcg TD fentanyl/h
- 30 mg oxycodone daily
- 8 mg PO hydromorphone daily
- Equianalgesic of another opioid
  Opioid Equianalgesic Doses (Table 14.1) [17, 18]:
  Opiate Conversion Chart (Fig. 14.1)

Opioid metabolism: Most opioid metabolism occurs in the liver and not in the kidney. This is primarily through the cytochrome P450 or glucuronidation system [2].

Strong Full Agonists [19]

- *Fentanyl (Duragesic)*
  - Available as transdermal patch; approximately 80–100 times as potent as morphine

Table 14.1 Opioid equianalgesic doses [17, 18]

Opioid	Oral (mg)	IM/IV (mg)	Transdermal (µg/h)	Duration (h)
Morphine	30	10		2–4
Tramadol	450			4–6
Codeine	300	130		2.5–4
Meperidine	150	50		2.5–4
Hydrocodone	30			3–4
Oxycodone	20			3–4
Methadone	20	10		8–12
Oxymorphone	10			3–4
Hydromorphone	7.5	1.5		2.3–2.5
Levorphanol	4			4–8
Fentanyl		0.1	12.5	3–20

*There are variations in metabolization for intermediate release (2–6 h) and long-acting (8–12 h) forms
It is important to note that dosing may require TID instead of BID dosing

- Considered good option in patients with renal insufficiency or patients who cannot tolerate PO medication options
- Helpful when treating patient with abdominal issues as absorption bypasses the GI tract
- Patients should be educated never to leave the patches in a garbage can, where children can find them as this could be very dangerous.
- *Hydromorphone (Dilaudid)*
  - More soluble than morphine
  - Nausea, vomiting, and constipation may be less marked with hydromorphone than with morphine
  - High potential for abuse, use extra caution when prescribing
- *Levorphanol (Levo-Dromoran)*
  - Useful for patients who are unable to tolerate morphine and methadone
  - Do to its long half-life it can be useful in chronic pain and palliative care
- *Meperidine (Demerol)*
  - Causes little or no constipation and has antitussive activity only in analgesic doses
  - Not recommended in chronic pain settings or long-term use due to adverse neurological events resulting in confusion and seizures secondary to accumulation of toxic metabolite normeperidine

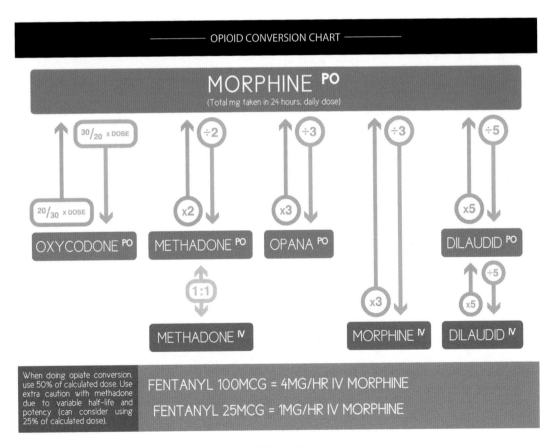

Fig. 14.1 Opioid conversion chart. © Kimberly Sackheim 2015. All Rights Reserved

- *Methadone*
  - Careful titration is necessary to avoid delayed adverse events, such as overdose, since methadone has a very long and highly variable half-life
  - Should not be used to treat breakthrough pain or as an as-needed medication
  - Good option in patients with renal insufficiency
  - Associated with multiple adverse consequences including prolonged QT interval; Avoid or use with caution and careful monitoring in patients who are at risk for development of prolonged QT syndrome
    - The Medicines and products Regulatory Agency (MHRA) advise electrocardiograms (ECGs) for patients on methadone with heart/liver disease, electrolyte abnormalities, concomitant QT prolonging medications/CYP3A4 inhibitors or prescribed methadone >100 mg daily [20]
    - Rate corrected QT (QTc) prolongation refers to the QTc interval extending beyond normal limits, >450 ms in men, and >470 ms in women [21]
    - A mechanism for methadone-related QTc prolongation has been proposed whereby methadone may block potassium channels, leading to prolonged repolarization and consequent QTc prolongation [22]
    - Clinically significant QTc prolongation and torsade de pointes are rare, and further research is required to determine the number of ECGs needed to prevent harm and the management of QTc prolongation if observed [23]
- *Morphine (MSContin, Avinza, Kadian)*
  - Can be administered in oral or suppository form
  - Prototype and standard of comparison for opioid analgesics
  - Morphine-6-glucuronide: active metabolite that appears to contribute to analgesic activity of morphine is eliminated by the kidney and will accumulate in patients with renal insufficiency
- *Oxycodone (OxyContin, Percocet)*
  - Second-line therapy for mild to moderate pain
- *Oxymorphone (Opana)*
  - Available in suppository form, as well as immediate and sustained release oral forms.

Weak Full Agonists [19]

- *Codeine (Tylenol #3, Tylenol #4)*
  - First-line therapy for mild to moderate pain
  - Can be administered in fixed combination with aspirin or acetaminophen
- *Hydrocodone (Lorcet, Lortab, Vicodin)*
  - First- and second-line therapy for mild to moderate pain
  - Administered in fixed combination with acetaminophen

- *Propoxyphene (Darvocet)*
  - Withdrawn from the market in the United States due to increased risk of serious cardiac toxicity even at therapeutic doses

Dual Mode of Action

- *Tramadol (Ultram) [24]*
  - First-line therapy for mild to moderate pain
  - Can be administered orally alone or in combination with acetaminophen
  - Also blocks reuptake of serotonin and norepinephrine; enhances neuronal serotonin release
  - Increases risk of seizures in patients taking SSRIs, TCAs, or other tricyclic compounds(e.g., cyclobenzaprine, promethazine), or other opiate agonists
- *Tapentadol (Nucynta)*
  - Tapentadol is a relatively new analgesic agent. It has a dual mode of action - mu receptor agonist as well as a norepinephrine reuptake inhibitor. This dual mode of action allows for analgesic effects with a lower side effect profile [25, 26]
  - Potentially life-threatening serotonin syndrome with SNRIs, including tapentadol, particularly with concurrent use of other serotonergic drugs (e.g., 5-HT1 receptor agonists ["triptans"], SSRIs, tricyclic antidepressants) or drugs that impair serotonin metabolism (e.g., MAO inhibitors) [27]

Partial Agonists and Mixed Agonist/Antagonists

- *Buprenorphine (Butrans, Suboxone, Subutex) [25]*
  - Administered transdermally for management of chronic pain only and administered sublingually as a single agent or in fixed combination with naloxone for management of opiate dependence
  - Acts as a partial agonist at μ-opiate receptors in the CNS and peripheral tissues, an antagonist at κ-opiate receptors, and an agonist at δ-opiate receptors
  - Certification required for its use in addiction medicine, but not if it is purely for pain control. To use buprenorphine in the treatment of opioid addiction, a special waiver is required for office-based treatment. This requires 8 h of specific training and notifying the Center for Substance Abuse Treatment. A special identification number is assigned to each certified physician from the Drug Enforcement Administration.
- *Butorphanol (Stadol) [19]*
  - Can be administered by nasal inhalation
    Most commonly used as an intranasal spray in the treatment of migraines
  - Opiate antagonistic effect may result from competitive inhibition at the opiate receptor and it exerts antagonistic effects at μ opiate receptor sites

– The manufacturer has discontinued production, but it is still available as a generic

Opioid Use with Renal or Hepatic Dysfunction

- Active agent or their metabolites may accumulate if renal or hepatic function is present
- Meperidine should be avoided with renal dysfunction
- In addition, the active metabolite of morphine, morphine-6-glucuronide may accumulate with around the clock use
- Combination products of opioids with acetaminophen are best avoided in hepatic dysfunction

Opioid use in the elderly: Opioids can be considered in the elderly. However, there are increased risks with an increased incidence of falls and fractures [28].

Route of Administration

- Oral route of administration is the most common and preferred
- Patients who are unable to swallow pills, other routes are available
  - *Transdermally*—Fentanyl, Butrans
  - *Rectal suppository*—morphine sulfate suppositories
  - *Buccal/transmucosal routes*—Ryzolt, Actiq, Subutex, Suboxone, Stadol, Sufenta
- The intramuscular route does not produce reliable absorption and is generally not recommended
- Intravenous or subcutaneous routes can produce a very rapid onset of analgesia [29]

Clinical Pearls

- Patients who are on a methadone maintenance program requiring opioid analgesics should continue their methadone maintenance dose and use short-acting opioid analgesics only if severe pain [30]. Caution is always used when prescribing opioids to these patients as they have history of drug abuse.
  - To decrease the total amount of opioid provided to these patients, multimodal analgesia (e.g., nonsteroidal anti-inflammatory drugs and acetaminophen) [31] and adjuvant analgesics that enhance opioid effects (e.g., tricyclic antidepressants) [32] may be coadministered [33].
- *Caution with combination medications*
  - In adults without liver or kidney disease who are taking opiates that are combined with other products
  Do not exceed total daily dosage of 4 g of acetaminophen
  Do not exceed total daily dosage of 400 mg/kg of ibuprofen
  Do not exceed total daily dosage of 150 mg/kg of aspirin
  Patients should be educated to not take additional over the counter medications that contain the combination medication in their opiate therapy

- Opiate-naïve patients
  - It is common to start with tramadol and progress with stronger medication to achieve adequate pain control. The next step in the progression can be a schedule III medication. Longer acting medication may be considered depending on patient requirements.

References

1. Breasted JG. Ancient records of Egypt. University of Chicago Oriental Institute Publications. vol. III. Chicago: University of Chicago Press; 1930. p. 217.
2. Trescot AM, Datta S, Lee M, Hansen H. Opioid pharmacology. Pain Physician. 2008;11:S5–62 [opioids special issue].
3. Warner EA. Opioids for the treatment of noncancer pain. Am J Med. 2012;125(12):1155–61.
4. Nestler EJ. Molecular basis on longterm plasticity underlying addiction. Nat Rev Neurosci. 2001;2:119–28.
5. Fukuda K. Intravenous opioid anesthetics. In: Miller RD, editor. Miller's anesthesia. 6th ed. Philadelphia: Elsevier; 2005.
6. Martell BA, O'Connor PG, Kerns RD, Becker WC, Morales KH, Kosten TR, Fiellin DA. Systematic review: opioid treatment for chronic back pain: prevalence, efficacy, and association with addiction. Ann Intern Med. 2007;146(2):116–27.
7. Noble M, Treadwell JR, Treager SJ, Coates VH, Wiffen PJ, Akafomo C, Schoelles KM. Long-term opioid management for chronic noncancer pain. Cochrane Database Syst Rev. 2010;1, CD006605.
8. Title 12, Chapter 13, Part B12: Schedules of controlled substances. DEA. www.ibt.tamhsc.edu/safety_office/pdf_stuff/DEA-Sch_%20of_Cont_Sub.Pdf
9. Chou R, et al. Clinical guidelines for the use of chronic opioid therapy in chronic noncancer pain. J Pain. 2009;10(2):113–30.
10. Manchikanti L, et al. American Society of Interventional Pain Physicians (ASIPP) guidelines for responsible opioid prescribing in chronic non-cancer pain: Part 1—evidence assessment. Pain Physician. 2012;15:S1–66.
11. Manchikanti L, et al. American Society of Interventional Pain Physicians (ASIPP) guidelines for responsible opioid prescribing in chronic non-cancer pain: Part 2—guidance. Pain Physician. 2012; 15:S66–116.
12. Ackerman SJ, Knight T, Schein J, et al. Risk of constipation in patients prescribed fentanyl transdermal system or oxycodone hydrochloride controlled-release in a California Medicaid population. Consult Pharm. 2004;19:118–32.
13. Verhamme KM, Sturkenboom MC, Stricker BH, Bosch R. Drug-induced urinary retention: incidence, management and prevention. Drug Saf. 2008;31(5):373–88.
14. Ganesh A, Maxwell LG. Pathophysiology and management of opioid-induced pruritus. Drugs. 2007;67(16):2323–32.
15. Swegle JM, Logemann C. Management of common opioid-induced adverse effects. Am Fam Physician. 2006;74(8):1347–54.
16. Lee M, Silverman S, Hansen H, Patel V, Manchikanti L. A comprehensive review of opioid-induced hyperalgesia. Pain Physician. 2011;14:145–61.
17. Kishner S. Opioid equivalents. eMedicine from WebMD, August 7; 2012.
18. Derby S, Chin J, Portenoy RK. Systemic opioid therapy for chronic cancer pain: practical guidelines for converting drugs and routes of administration. CNS Drugs. 1999;9(2):99–109.
19. Jaffe JH, Martin WR. Opioid analgesics and antagonists. In: Gilman AG, Goodman LS, Rall TW, et al., editors. Goodman and Gilman's

the pharmacological basis of therapeutics. 7th ed. New York: Macmillan Publishing Company; 1985. p. 491–531.

20. MHRA and Commission on Human Medicines. Risk of QT interval prolongation with methadone. Report no.: 31; 2006.

21. Moss AJ. Measurement of the QT interval and the risk associated with QTc interval prolongation: a review. Am J Cardiol. 1993; 72:23B–5B.

22. Katchman AN, McGroary KA, Kilborn MJ, et al. Influence of opioid agonists on cardiac human ether-a-go-go-related gene K(+) currents. J Pharmacol Exp Ther. 2002;303:688–94.

23. Mayet S, Gossop M, Lintzeris N, Markides V, Strang J. Methadone maintenance, QTc and torsade de pointes: who needs an electrocardiogram and what is the prevalence of QTc prolongation? Drug Alcohol Rev. 2011;30(4):388–96.

24. Kahn LH, Alderfer RJ, Graham DJ. Seizures reported with Tramadol. JAMA. 1997;278:1661.

25. Lewis JW. Buprenorphine. Drug Alcohol Depend. 1985;14: 363–72.

26. Tzschentke TM, Christoph T, Kögel B, Schiene K, Hennies HH, Englberger W, Haurand M, Jahnel U, Cremers TI, Friderichs E, De Vry J. Tapentadol HCl: a novel mu-opioid receptor agonist/norepinephrine reuptake inhibitor with broad-spectrum analgesic properties. J Pharmacol Exp Ther. 2007;323(1):265–76.

27. Boyer EW, Shannon M. The serotonin syndrome. N Engl J Med. 2005;352:1112–20.

28. Ferrel B, Argoff CE, Epplin J, Fine P, Gloth 3rd FM, Herr K, Katz JD, Mehr DR, Reid MC, Reisner L. American geriatrics society panel on the pharmacological management of persisting pain in older persons. Pain Med. 2009;10(6):1062–83.

29. Brookoff D. Abuse potential of various opioid medications. J Gen Intern Med. 1993;8(12):688–90.

30. Alford D, Compton P, Samet J. Acute pain management for patients receiving maintenance methadone or buprenorphine therapy. Ann Intern Med. 2006;144(2):127–34.

31. Kehlet H, Dahl JB. The value of "multimodal" or "balanced analgesia" in postoperative pain treatment. Anesth Analg. 1993;77: 1048–56.

32. Botney M, Fields HL. Amitriptyline potentiates morphine analgesia by a direct action on the central nervous system. Ann Neurol. 1983;13:160–4.

33. Mitra S, Sinatra RS. Perioperative management of acute pain in the opioid-dependent patient. Anesthesiology. 2004;101:212–27.

Topical Analgesic Medications

15

Russell K. McAllister and Christopher J. Burnett

Abbreviations

Ca^{++}	Calcium
CRPS	Complex regional pain syndrome
DMSO	Dimethyl sulfoxide
DPN	Diabetic peripheral neuropathy
EMLA	Eutectic mixture of local anesthetics
FDA	Food & Drug Administration
G6PD	Glucose-6-phosphate dehydrogenase
GABA	Gamma amino butyric acid
Na^+	Sodium
NMDA	*N*-methyl D-aspartate
NSAID	Nonsteroidal anti-inflammatory drug
PHN	Post-herpetic neuralgia
TCA	Tricyclic antidepressant
TRP	Transient receptor potential

Introduction

- **Topical Analgesics**: describes analgesics applied locally and directly to painful areas and whose site of action is local to the site of application [1]
  - This is in contrast to transdermal medication formulations which require systemic levels for their desired effects such as fentanyl [1]
- *Some chronic pain conditions with a discreet region or localized area of pain include*:

R.K. McAllister, M.D., D.A.B.P.M. (✉)
Department of Anesthesiology, Baylor Scott & White Health/Texas A&M College of Medicine,
6725 Las Colinas, Temple, TX 76502, USA
e-mail: rmcallister@sw.org

C.J. Burnett, M.D., D.A.B.I.P.P., FIPP
Department of Anesthesia and Perioperative Care, University of California San Francisco Medical Center, University of California San Francisco, 2401 South 31st Street, Temple,, TX 76502, USA
e-mail: cburnett@sw.org

- Muscle strain/sprain
- Arthritic conditions
- Complex regional pain syndrome
- Neuropathic pain conditions (radiculopathy, neuropathy, etc.)
- Peripheral nerve pathology

- Oral medications can result in significant unwanted side effects; therefore, topical medications are considered to avoid these untoward effects as they typically exert their effects locally with minimal systemic absorption.
- For patients with localized symptoms who do not tolerate oral formulations of these medications, topical agents can be both effective and much more tolerable, resulting in significant improvement in quality of life.
- In some cases, topical application of these medications can lead to detectable blood levels of the drug.
  - When this occurs, systemic effects of the drug can be seen Ex. Doxepin cream may cause drowsiness
- *Drug dosage and pharmacokinetics in topical analgesics can vary widely depending on*:
  - Area of treatment
  - Blood flow to the affected area
  - Skin temperature
  - Quantity of formulation applied
  - Type of dressing applied over the area (occlusive dressings increase the absorption of most topical drugs)
- *Topical medications desired effects*:
  - Anesthesia
  - Analgesia
  - Alteration of systemic blood flow
  - Decreased inflammation
  - Relief of distressful symptoms ex. pruritus

The available topical agents include over-the-counter preparations, Food & Drug Administration (FDA)-approved formulations, and a seemingly endless number of compounded formulations of drugs or drug combinations.

K.A. Sackheim, *Pain Management and Palliative Care: A Comprehensive Guide*,
DOI 10.1007/978-1-4939-2462-2_15, © Springer Science+Business Media New York 2015

Drug Classes Include the Following:

- **Menthol/Camphor**—Creams/balms containing menthol or camphor can cause the skin to feel warm or cold. Mechanism of action for pain relief is most likely counterirritant distraction mediated by the Transient Receptor Potential (TRP) channel. These agents may also modulate blood flow to the affected area and may provide temporary relief, but should not be applied more than 3–4 times a day.
  - *Ingestion or absorption of camphor through overuse or use on non-intact skin can lead to severe skin irritation, neurologic symptoms such as seizures, hepatotoxicity, or even death* [2].
- **Capsaicin**—Topical preparations derived from hot peppers that work by activation of TRP channels and by depleting substance P
  - Regarded as an adjunct to be used in combination with other agents [3].
  - Can give moderate relief of musculoskeletal-related pain.
  - Has been shown to provide modest pain relief, but no long-term benefit in neuropathic pain conditions such as PHN, DPN, and post-mastectomy pain syndrome [3, 4].
  - Severe burning of the skin may occur in as much as 80 % of patients and can lead to treatment failures [1].
    - Pretreatment with EMLA cream fails to reliably decrease the burning pain associated with application [5].
    - Patients must be educated to apply the cream with nitrile gloves (latex gloves provide inadequate protection), avoiding contact with other regions of the body, especially the eyes
- **Local Anesthetic**—Block voltage-gated sodium channels
  - **Lidocaine 5 % patch**—FDA approved for treatment of post-herpetic neuralgia
    - Mechanism thought to involve a decrease in ectopic discharges from peripheral sensory afferents, since pain relief occurs in the absence of anesthetic effects [5].
    - Patients typically get adequate amounts of absorption to provide analgesia, but not enough to provide complete sensory blockade [6].
    - May also have anti-inflammatory effects [7].
    - Excellent safety profile with little systemic effect [8].
    - Patients should be educated that the skin underlying the patch will become numb.
    - Limited studies have shown encouraging results in the use of EMLA cream in the treatment of neuropathic pain such as PHN and CRPS [1]

- **Nonsteroidal Anti-inflammatory Drugs**—Inhibition of cyclooxygenase activity with a resultant decrease in the conversion of arachidonic acid into prostaglandins and thromboxane [9]
  - **Methylsalicylate**—Readily available over the counter and has an anti-inflammatory mechanism
    - At least one death attributed to extreme overuse by a teen athlete with resulting salicylate toxicity [10].
  - **Trolomine Salicylate**—Over-the-counter topical NSAID
  - **Diclofenac**—Topical preparations of this NSAID are available for the treatment of arthritis-related musculoskeletal pain with moderate results when used short term.
    - Diclofenac solution 1.5 %(Pennsaid) contains DMSO 45.5 % as a carrier for the drug and is applied in drop form onto the affected joint
    - Also available in 1 % gel (Voltaren) or a 1.3 % patch (Flector).
    - A 3 % gel (Solaraze) is also available, but is indicated for treatment of actinic keratosis
    - Less efficacy than oral NSAIDs but with fewer systemic side effects [11]
  - **Piroxicam and Ketoprofen**—Topical NSAID preparations that are not yet FDA-approved in the United States, but may be available through compounding pharmacies
- **Tricyclic Antidepressants**—Primarily block reuptake of norepinephrine and serotonin, they also affect adenosine A receptors and sodium channels
  - **Doxepin 5 % Cream (Zonalon)**—Approved to treat pruritus associated with painful neuropathy [12]
    - Significant systemic absorption with drowsiness has been shown to occur in up to 20 % of patients treated, especially when >10 % of the body surface area is involved [12].
    - Combination with capsaicin may speed onset of relief [13].
  - **Amitriptyline Cream**—In animal studies, shown to have local anesthetic properties when applied peripherally in high doses [14, 15].
    - Frequently compounded as a single agent (2–10 %) or in combination with other agents
- **Opioids**
  - Topical application of morphine has been reported to alleviate burn pain, pain from epidermolysis bullosa, and morphine oral rinse has been shown to be helpful when applied topically for radiation-induced oral mucositis, suggesting a possible role for efficacy in topical application for peripheral analgesia [16–18].
    - The role of systemic opioids in pain medicine is discussed further in the opioid medication chapter.

- **Dimethyl Sulfoxide (DMSO)**—A free radical scavenging anti-inflammatory agent which is absorbed rapidly across the skin and greatly enhances percutaneous penetration when used in combination with other agents [19]
  - Has been used as a liniment for athletes and in veterinary medicine
  - It is excreted as a distinctive garlic taste in the breath when applied topically [19]
  - Care must be taken, since any impurities in the DMSO formulation can be carried across the skin and rapidly absorbed systemically.
  - FDA approved only for intravesicular bladder infusion for symptomatic treatment of interstitial cystitis.

There is insufficient evidence available on its effectiveness as a single agent in treating arthritis or any other pain syndrome, though it has been shown to have moderate efficacy in treating arthritis as a carrier agent for diclofenac [11]

Table 15.1 Prescription and over-the-counter topical medications

Prescription topical medications	Over-the-counter topical medications
Compounded formulations	Menthol—Biofreeze
	Methylsalicylate—Bengay; IcyHot, etc.
Lidocaine—Lidoderm 5 % patch, EMLA cream, etc.	Trolomine salicylate—Aspercream; Myoflex
Diclofenac—Pennsaid 1.5 % solution(applied as drops and contains DMSO as carrier), Voltaren 1 % gel, Flector 1.3 % patch, Solaraze 3 % gel (indicated for treatment of actinic keratosis)	Menthol and methylsalicylate—Salonpas
	Capsaicin—Zostrix, Capzasin
	Menthol and Camphor—Tiger Balm
Doxepin 5 % cream—Zonalon	

Compounded Products

- Compounding pharmacies are now capable of making topical cream or gel formulations of numerous classes of drugs.
  - *It must be remembered that these preparations have not been studied extensively for pharmacokinetics or efficacy. In addition, there is no proof of quality control or consistency from one batch to another and there have been many documented compounding pharmacy errors leading to significant morbidity and mortality related to drug dosing errors or contaminations* [1, 20].
  - One survey of pain physicians revealed that 27 % had prescribed a compounded topical agent and 47 % felt that their patient had responded favorably [21].
  - One study of an organogel preparation of combined baclofen, amitriptyline, and ketamine showed good relief of chemotherapy-induced peripheral neuropathy painful symptoms without systemic toxicity [22].
  - The combination of topical amitriptyline 2 % and topical ketamine 1 % was found to have mixed results in treatment of neuropathic pain in two studies. One showed no benefit while another showed pain reduction of 34 % [23, 24]. Compounded ketamine was suggested to be an effective topical analgesic in a study in the treatment of PHN [25].

    Compounding pharmacies are able to make topical formulations of a wide variety of medication classes.

    Examples of drugs available from large national compounding pharmacies can vary but may include:
    Membrane stabilizers (gabapentin 2 %, carbamazepine 2 %)
    Local anesthetics (lidocaine 5 %, tetracaine 5 %)
    Muscle relaxants (baclofen 2 %, cyclobenzaprine 2 %)
    NSAID's (piroxicam 2 %, ketoprofen 10–20 %, diclofenac 2 %)
    Corticosteroid anti-inflammatories (dexamethasone 2 %)
    Tricyclic antidepressants (amitriptyline 5 %),
    Alpha-2 agonists (clonidine 0.3 %)
    Antivirals (acyclovir 3 %)
    NMDA receptor antagonists (ketamine 50 mg/mL)

- These topical compounded formulations can be single drug or multiple drug formulations used to treat a wide variety of painful conditions including arthritis and neuropathic pain. These compounded formulations are poorly studied and efficacy is mostly anecdotal at the current time (Table 15.1).

References

1. Argoff CE. Topical agents for the treatment of chronic pain. Curr Pain Headache Rep. 2006;10(1):11–9.
2. Theis JG, Koren G. Camphorated oil; still endangering the lives of Canadian children. CMAJ. 1995;152(11):1821–4.
3. Watson CPN. Topical capsaicin as an adjuvant analgesic. J Pain Symptom Manage. 1994;9:425–33.
4. Rains C, Bryson HM. Topical capsaicin: a review of its pharmacological properties and therapeutic potential in post-herpetic neuralgia, diabetic neuropathy, and osteoarthritis. Drugs Aging. 1995;7:317–28.
5. Fuchs PN, Papagallo M, Meyer RA. Topical EMLA pre-treatment fails to decrease the pain induced by 1% topical capsaicin. Pain. 1999;80:637–42.
6. Yanigidate F, Strichartz GR. Local anesthetics. Handb Exp Pharmacol. 2007;177:95–127.
7. Hollman MW, Durieux ME. Local anesthetics and the inflammatory response. Anesthesiology. 2000;93:858–75.
8. Gammaitoni AR, Alvarez NA, Galer BS. Safety and tolerability of the lidocaine patch 5%, a targeted peripheral analgesic: a review of the literature. J Clin Pharmacol. 2003;43(2):111–7.

9. Brooks PM, Day RO. Nonsteroidal anti-inflammatory drugs-differences and similarities. N Engl J Med. 1991;324: 1716–25.

10. http://nbcsports.msnbc.com/id/19144600/. Last accessed 2/5/2013.

11. Nair B, Taylor-Gjevre R. A review of topical diclofenac use in musculoskeletal disease. Pharmaceuticals. 2010;3:1892–908.

12. Kastrup EK, editor. Drug facts and comparisons. St. Louis: Wolters Kluwer Health; 2013. p. 3147–9.

13. McCleane G. Topical application of doxepin hydrochloride, capsaicin and a combination of both produces analgesia in chronic human neuropathic pain: a randomized, double-blind, placebo-controlled study. Br J Clin Pharmacol. 2000;49(6):574–9.

14. Gerner P, Mujtaba M, Sinnott CJ, Wang GK. Amitriptyline versus bupivacaine in rat sciatic nerve blockade. Anesthesiology. 2001; 94:661–7.

15. Khan MA, Gerner P, Wang GK. Amitriptyline for prolonged cutaneous analgesia in the rat. Anesthesiology. 2002;96:109–16.

16. Long TD, Cathers TA, Twillman R, O'Donnell T, Garrigues N. Morphine-infused silver sulfadiazine cream for burn analgesia: a pilot study. J Burn Care Rehabil. 2001;22:118–23.

17. Cerchietti LC, Navigante AH, Bonomi MR, Zaderajko MA, Menendez PR, Pogany CE, Roth BM. Effect of topical morphine for mucositis-associated pain following concomitant chemoradiotherapy for head and neck carcinoma. Cancer. 2002;95(10): 2230–6.

18. Watterson G, Howard R, Goldman A. Peripheral opiates in inflammatory pain. Arch Dis Child. 2004;89:679–81.

19. Capriotti K, Capriotti JA. Dimethyl sulfoxide: history chemistry, and clinical utility in dermatology. J Clin Aesthet Dermatol. 2012;5(9):24–6.

20. Meyer T, Martin E, Prielipp R. The largest healthcare associated fungal outbreak in the U.S. APSF Newslett. 2013;28(1):4–7.

21. Ness TJ, Jones L, Smith H. Use of compounded topical analgesics-results of an internet survey. Reg Anesth Pain Med. 2002; 27:309–12.

22. Barton DL, Wos EJ, Qin R, Mattar BI, Green NB, Lanier KS, Bearden 3rd JD, Kugler JW, Hoff KL, Reddy PS, Rowland Jr KM, Riepl M, Christensen B, Loprinzi CL. A double-blind, placebo-controlled trial of a topical treatment for chemotherapy-induced peripheral neuropathy: NCCTG trial N06CA. Support Care Cancer. 2011;19(6):833–41.

23. Lynch ME, Clark AJ, Sawynok J, Sullivan MJ. Topical 2% amitriptyline and 1% ketamine in neuropathic pain syndromes: a randomized, double-blind, placebo-controlled trial. Anesthesiology. 2005;103(1):140–6.

24. Lynch ME, Clark AJ, Sawynok J, Sullivan MJ. Topical amitriptyline and ketamine in neuropathic pain syndromes: an open-label study. J Pain. 2005;6(10):644–9.

25. Quan D, Wellish M, Gilden DH. Topical ketamine treatment of post-herpetic neuralgia. Neurology. 2003;60:1391–2.

Headache

16

Alyssa Lettich and Sait Ashina

Abbreviations

5-HT	Serotonin
ANA	Antinuclear antibody
CAD	Coronary artery disease
CBC	Complete blood count
CGRP	Calcitonin gene-related peptide
CH	Cluster headache
CM	Chronic migraine
CNS	Central nervous system
CRP	C-reactive protein
CT	Computerized tomography
D2	D2 dopamine
DHE	Dihydroergotamine
DM	Diabetes mellitus
ECG	Electrocardiogram
ESR	Erythrocyte sedimentation rate
HA	Headache
HC	Hemicrania continua
HIV	Human immunodeficiency virus
HoTN	Hypotension
HTN	Hypertension
ICHD-2	International classification of headache disorders, second edition
ICP	Intracranial pressure
IM	Intramuscular
INR	International normalized ratio
IVF	Intravenous fluid
LP	Lumbar puncture
MA	Migraine with aura
MI	Myocardial infarction
MO	Migraine without aura
MOH	Medication overuse headache
MRI	Magnetic resonance imaging
MTC	Metoclopromide
NDPH	New daily persistent headache
NS	Nasal spray
NSAID	Nonsteroidal anti-inflammatory
PAD	Peripheral artery disease
PCZ	Prochlorperazine
PH	Paroxysmal hemicranias
PLT	Platelet count
PRES	Posterior reversible encephalopathy syndrome
PVD	Peripheral vascular disease
QTc	Corrected QT interval
RPR	Rapid plasma reagin
SAH	Subarachnoid hemorrhage
SUNA	Short-lasting unilateral neuralgiform headache attacks with autonomic features
SUNCT	Short-lasting unilateral neuralgiform headache attacks with conjunctival injection and tearing
TAC	Trigeminal autonomic cephalalgia
TTH	Tension-type headache
VDRL	Venereal disease research library

A. Lettich, M.D. (✉)
Intermountain Neurosciences Institute,
Intermountain Medical Center, Murray, Utah, USA

S. Ashina, M.D.
Department of Pain Medicine and Palliative Care, Neurology,
Beth Israel Medical Center, 10 Union Square East,
2Q-R, New York, NY 10003, USA
e-mail: sashina@chpnet.org

Introduction

Headache is the most common reason for medical consultation and the fourth most common reason for emergency room visits in the United States [1]. Migraine is a major cause of disability and remains a challenge for practitioners and afflicted patients alike [2]. Headache disorders, in general, can be subdivided into primary headache disorders and secondary headache disorders based on underlying cause or lack thereof.

K.A. Sackheim, *Pain Management and Palliative Care: A Comprehensive Guide*,
DOI 10.1007/978-1-4939-2462-2_16, © Springer Science+Business Media New York 2015

Evaluation of a Patient with Headache

The American Headache Society has created a mnemonic SNOOP for worrisome headache features or red flags, which should prompt further evaluation with various tests (Table 16.1).

History and Examination

Initial evaluation of a headache patient is based on history and examination and should include the following:

- *Headache onset*: sudden onset or thunderclap (less than 1 min)
- *Provoking factors*: maneuvers that increase intracranial pressure (Valsalva, sexual activity, exercise, coughing, sneezing, etc.), trauma, illness
- *Location of pain*:
  - Unilateral (side-locked) versus bilateral headache
  - V1-distribution pain: consider carotid dissection
- *Pain severity and course including duration and frequency of attacks*
- *Associated symptoms*:

- Abnormal neurologic signs including but not limited to level of arousal, visual changes, vertigo, speech difficulty, dysarthria, dysphagia, paresthesias, and/or motor weakness are red flags
- *Systemic signs/symptoms*: fever/chills, weight loss, etc. are red flags
- *Exacerbating Factors*: (position change) Headache worse upon standing might point to low ICP. Headache worse when lying down or upon awakening might point to increased ICP
- *Medical history*: consider vascular risk factors, systemic illness, malignancy, HIV, pregnancy, etc.
- *Medications*: previous headache treatments (both prescription and over the counter). CNS stimulants can exacerbate headache

Examination to Assess Headache Patient

- General appearance
- Head
  - Palpate for areas of tenderness
  - Listen for bruits
  - Temporal area tenderness
  - Temporal artery bruits can be consistent with temporal arteritis
  - Supraorbital or occipital area tenderness
- Eye examination/fundoscopic examination
- Temporomandibular joints: tenderness, range of motion, clicking, locking
- Neck and shoulders—range of motion, trigger points
- Neurologic exam
  - Cognition and level of arousal
  - Cranial nerve testing
  - Motor exam
  - Sensory Exam
  - Assess coordination and gait

Table 16.1 Use SNOOP to help identify patients with likely secondary headache

Mnemonic letter	Mnemonic words	Description
S	Systemic	Fever, weight loss, or decreased appetite often suggest systemic illness, including infection and malignancy
N	Neurological symptoms	Mental status changes, seizures, focal neurological signs or symptoms suggest possible brain pathology, e.g., CO poisoning, CVA, primary/secondary malignancy
O	Onset	New onset headaches that quickly reach peak intensity (thunderclap headaches) may occur in patients with subarachnoid hemorrhage or other secondary headaches, as well as cough or sex-related headaches
O	Older age	Headaches are more likely to be secondary in older patients. Any new headache in patients >50 years old will need an evaluation for secondary headaches, including giant cell arteritis, acute glaucoma, and primary/secondary malignancy
P	Progressive course	Headache progression may signify a worsening underlying illness, such as space occupying lesions

CO Carbon monoxide, *CVA* Cerebrovascular accident
With permission from: Marcus DA, Philip A. Bain PA. Getting Started. In: Marcus DA, Bain PA. Practical Assessment and Treatment of the Patient with Headaches in the Emergency Department and Urgent Care Clinic. Springer, 2011:21–52 [32]

Diagnostic Tests

1. Neuroimaging
   - *Computerized tomography (CT) best to evaluate for*:
     - Blood—95 % sensitive for SAH on day of presentation [3]
     - Bone (fracture)
     - Quick and readily available
     - When MRI is contraindicated (e.g., implantable devices such as pacemaker)
   - *MRI (Magnetic Resonance Imaging) to examine for*:
     - Vascular etiologies
     - Neoplasm
     - Posterior fossa pathology
     - Infectious etiologies

2. Laboratory testing
   - ESR and CRP to exclude temporal arteritis in patients >50 y/o
     - Elevated levels require prompt treatment and possible biopsy
     - Temporal arteritis can lead to permanent visual loss and stroke if not identified and treated early
   - Comprehensive metabolic profile, CBC, thyroid function tests, screen for autoimmune disease (ANA, RF), inflammatory markers (ESR, CRP), Lyme titers, HIV test, VDRL/RPR, drug screen
3. Lumbar Puncture (LP)
   - *Indications*:
     - Sudden onset, worst HA of patient's life
     - Headache with fever
     - HIV-infected patient
     - Cancer patient with subacute or progressive HA
     - Atypical chronic headache, HA not responsive to treatment
   - *Diagnostic for*:
     - SAH
     - Meningitis, encephalitis
     - Meningeal carcinomatosis
     - Low- or high-cerebrospinal fluid pressure (e.g., intracranial HTN, HoTN)
   - *Contraindications*:
     - Order CT head prior to exclude space occupying/obstructive lesion(s), if increased intracranial pressure or space occupying lesion, LP should not be done to avoid herniation
     - Coagulopathy
       - $INR \geq 1.3$
       - $PLT \leq 100$
     - Skin outbreak/infection at LP site
     - When in doubt, ask a neuroradiologist

In the evaluation of the headache patient, it is important to exclude all secondary causes. Secondary headaches are those attributed to underlying structural or systemic disease [4]. The patient's presentation, clinical history, and exam will guide further evaluation. An algorithm for headache diagnosis is presented in Fig. 16.1.

Secondary Headaches

Medication Overuse Headache (MOH): a secondary headache disorder formerly known as rebound headache brought on by the overuse of acute medications, namely triptans, simple analgesics, NSAIDs, butalbital-containing compounds and opioids [5]. In general, acute treatments should not be used more than two days per week.
- *Diagnostic criteria for MOH*:
  - Headache be present >15 days/month

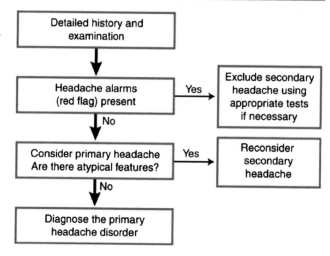

Fig. 16.1 Algorithm for headache diagnosis: flow assessment for patients with headache disorders. *Modified from* Evans R, Purdy A. Identification or exclusion of secondary headaches. In: Lipton RB, Bigal ME, editors. Migraine and other headache disorders. New York: Informa Healthcare; 2006;p131–144. [34]

- Patient who regularly overuses acute medications for >3 months
- Resolves within 2 months of overused medication(s) discontinuation [4]
  - Other examples of secondary headache disorders:
    - Headache attributed to head and/or neck trauma
    - Cerebral venous thrombosis and other vascular disorders
    - Primary and other brain neoplasms
    - Headache attributed to infectious and noninfectious inflammatory disease [4]

Primary Headaches

Once secondary causes have effectively been excluded, focus on the accurate diagnosis and treatment of the primary headache disorder. According to the International Classification of Headache Disorders (ICHD-2), there are four major categories of primary headache disorders: migraine, TTH, cluster headache, and other trigeminal autonomic cephalalgias, and other primary headaches [4].

Migraine

- Chronic condition with episodic manifestations
- Familial disorder with a genetic component
- Environmental and lifestyle triggers (stress, weather changes, menses, inconsistent sleep, alcohol, dehydration, etc.)
- Monogenic forms are rare and include hemiplegic migraine and other complicated migraine disorders
- Most important categories are migraine with and without aura

Table 16.2 International Headache Society (IHS) criteria for migraine without aura (MO) and migraine with aura (MA) [Headache Classification Subcommittee of the International Headache Society (HCC) 2004]

Migraine without aura

A. At least five attacks fulfilling criteria B–D

B. Headache attacks lasting 4–72 h (untreated or unsuccessfully treated)

C. Headache has at least two of the following characteristics:

    1. Unilateral location

    2. Pulsating quality

    3. Moderate or severe pain intensity

    4. Aggravation by or causing avoidance of routine physical activity (e.g., walking or climbing stairs)

D. During headache at least one of the following;

    1. Nausea and/or vomiting

    2. Photophobia and phonophobia

E. Not attributed to another disorder

Migraine with aura

A. At least two attacks fulfilling criteria B–E

B. Fully reversible visual and/or sensory and/or speech symptoms but no motor weakness

C. At least two of the following

    1. Visual symptoms including positive features (e.g., flickering lights, spots, or lines) and/or negative features (i.e., loss of vision) and/or sensory symptoms including positive features (i.e., pins and needles) and/or negative features (i.e., numbness)

    2. At least one symptom develops gradually over ≥5 min

    3. Each symptom lasts ≥5 min and ≤60 min

D. Headache fulfilling criteria B–D for migraine without aura begins during the aura or follows aura within 60 min

E. Not attributed to another disorder

With permission from de Vries B, Frants RR, Ferrari MD, van den Maagdenberg AMJM. Molecular genetics of migraine. Hum Genet 2009;126:115-132. (35) [4]

    – *Migraine without aura*: defined by the ICHD-2 as outlined in Table 16.2.

    – *Migraine with aura*:

        Aura is a transient focal neurologic symptom. A new or different focal neurologic symptom should prompt further investigation to exclude secondary causes.

        Migraine with aura is seen in 20 % of patients with migraine and is attributed to the phenomenon of cortical spreading depression [5].

        Aura may occur in the absence of headache. See Table 16.2 for the diagnostic criteria for typical aura

Prevalence: 18 % of women and 6 % of men, 12 % overall [2]

Migraine is divided into two groups determined by attack frequency:

1. **Episodic migraine** (<15 days of headache/month)

2. **Chronic migraine** (CM) (≥15 days of headache/month for at least 3 months) [6]

Pathophysiology: One proposed theory of migraine pathophysiology involves that activation of trigeminal nociceptive sensory fibers (i.e., first-order neurons) that convey pain signals from intracranial and extracranial blood vessels [7].

Once activated these trigeminal afferent fibers release proinflammatory and pronociceptive vasoactive neuropeptides including substance P, neurokinin A, and calcitonin gene-related peptide (CGRP) leading to peripheral sensitization [8, 9]. Activation of second- and third-order neurons, trigeminothalamic and thalamocortical neurons respectively, leads to central sensitization. Cutaneous allodynia is a marker of central sensitization, which plays an important role in the pathophysiology of chronic migraine [10, 11]. A second proposed theory of migraine pathophysiology suggests brain stem nuclei as the migraine initiation center [12, 13].

Migraine-Specific Treatment

- *Triptans* (e.g., sumatriptan, rizatriptan, almotriptan) are first-line treatments for moderate-to-severe attacks (See Table 16.3).
  - Specific 5-HT1 (serotonin) agonists at the neurovascular junction
  - Available subcutaneous (SC), PO, nasal spray (NS)
  - SC is most rapidly effective followed by NS followed by PO
  - Early treatment (at onset of headache) is believed to be key
  - Contraindicated in vascular disease (CAD, history of MI, PVD/PAD, history of stroke, DM, uncontrolled hypertension, uncontrolled hyperlipidemia), hemiplegic/basilar migraine, and pregnancy
  - Generic sumatriptan and rizatriptan are available
- *Ergots* (e.g., dihydroergotamine or DHE)
  - Nonspecific 5-HT1 agonist at the neurovascular junction
  - Available IV, IM, SC, NS
  - DHE nasal spray (0.5 mg/spray)—maximum dose 6 sprays/day, 8 sprays/week
  - Ergotamine/caffeine (1 mg/100 mg) tablets are also available (max dose ergotamine 6 mg/day, 10 mg/week)
  - Contraindicated in vascular disease, uncontrolled hypertension, hemiplegic/basilar migraine, and pregnancy
  - Do not use within 24 h of a triptan

Nonspecific Analgesics

- Aspirin 900–1000 mg (max 4 g/day)
- Acetaminophen 1000 mg (max 4 g/day)
- Ibuprofen 400–800 mg (2400 mg/day)
- Naproxen 500 mg (max 1 g/day)
- Diclofenac 50, 75, 100 mg (max 200 mg/day)
- Ketoprofen 100 mg (max 300 mg/day)

Treatment for Refractory Migraine/Status Migrainosus

- SC Sumatriptan 6 mg
- IV/IM antiemetic dopamine (D2) antagonists such as metoclopromide (MTC) 10–20 mg, prochlorperazine (PCZ) 5–10 mg chlorpromazine (0.1 mg/kg) 12.5–37.5 mg

Table 16.3 Triptans for treatment of migraine

	Strength, mg	Max mg/24 h	Half-life, h	Tmax, h	Efficacy, %[a]
First-generation triptans					
Sumatriptan PO	25, 50, 100	200	2.5	2	62/33
Sumatriptan NS	5, 20	40	2		64/31
Sumatriptan SC	6	12	2	12	80/40
Second-generation triptans					
Naratriptan	1, 2.5	5	6	1.5–3	58/27
Zolmitriptan	2.5, 5	10	3	2.3	67/33
Rizatriptan	5, 10	30	3	1.5	72/41
Frovatriptan	2.5	5	26	3	46/27
Almotriptan	6.25, 12.5	25	4	2	64/33
Eletriptan	20, 40	80	4	2	63/31

With permission from Lenaerts ME. Headache. Atlas of Clinical Neurology. Springer 2009; 565–597. [36]

Note: When multiple doses are listed, the highest dose is generally preferred except in the case of rizatriptan if patients also on a beta-adrenergic blocker

[a]Meta-analysis of patients at 2 h; first number = improvement from moderate or severe headache to mild or none; second number = pain free

- Drowsiness is the most common adverse effect [14]
- Risk of extrapyramidal effects including akathisia and dystonia is minimized by preadministration of IV or IM diphenhydramine 25 mg or IV or IM benztropine 1 mg
- 250–500 mL IVF bolus prior to administration of chlorpromazine to avoid postural hypotension
- Get an ECG first
  D2 antagonists, especially droperidol, can cause life-threatening QTc prolongation
  QTc must be <450 ms [15]
- IV DHE (0.5–1.0 mg up to every 8 h)
  - Maximum dose in a 24-h period is 2 mg
  - Preadministration of IV MTC 10 mg or IV PCZ 10 mg minimizes nausea/vomiting
  - Do not give within 24 h of a triptan
  - Other contraindications include severe hypertension, current use of macrolide antibiotics, and/or current use of retroviral therapy
- IV Valproic acid (500 mg up to every 8 h)
- Magnesium 1–2 g IV for migraine with aura
  - Caution in renal impairment
- IV/IM NSAIDs—ketorolac 30–60 mg
  - Monitor for renal toxicity
  - Caution with history of hepatic or renal impairment or history of GI bleed or PUD
- IV Corticosteroids (dexamethasone 4–10 mg) may help prevent headache recurrence [16]
- Nerve block with local anesthetic
  - Greater and lesser occipital nerve(s) (from upper cervical nerve roots)
  - Supraorbital nerve(s) and supratrochlear nerve(s) (branches of V1)
  - Auriculotemporal nerve(s) (branch of V3)
- Opioids are best avoided as they can sensitize the CNS to pain (hyperalgesia) [16]

Consider migraine prevention in patients with frequent and/or disabling headache attacks.

Migraine Preventive Drugs [17, 18]

Start at a low dose and titrate slowly. May take 2 or 3 months for clinical effect. Some refractory patients might require more than one preventive treatment.

- *Beta-adrenergic blockers*
  - Metoprolol (50–150 mg daily)
  - Propranolol (80–240 mg daily)
  - Timolol (10–20 mg daily)
  - Avoid in patients with high BMI, DM, and migraine with aura
  - Contraindicated in hemiplegic and basilar migraine
  - Monitor BP and HR
- *Antiepileptic drugs*
  - Divalproex sodium (250–1500 mg daily)
    Common side effects include weight gain, tremor, and hair loss
    Monitor for potential liver and blood abnormalities
    Avoid in women likely to become pregnant
  - Topiramate (25–150 mg/day total, divided BID)
    Limb paresthesias may occur early
    Cognitive side effects are dose dependent
    Avoid in women likely to become pregnant
    Higher dosages can decrease effectiveness of oral contraceptive
    Contraindicated in glaucoma and caution in patients with kidney stones
- *Antidepressants*
  - Venlafaxine (37.5–150 mg daily)
  - Amitriptyline (10–150 mg qhs)
    Generally effective at 5–25 mg at bedtime as this may cause sedation
    Anticholinergic side effects are dose limiting.
- *OnabotulinumtoxinA* (155U IM every 3 months)

– Only chronic migraine treatment approved by the FDA
– A second set of injections might be required for clinical benefit

Tension-Type Headache

- **Tension-type headache (TTH)** is a long-duration primary headache disorder with episodic (infrequent and frequent) and chronic (≥15 days of headache/month) forms. See Table 16.4 for the diagnostic criteria of episodic TTH.
- Most common of all primary headache disorders with lifetime prevalence estimated between 30 and 78 % [19, 20]
- Pathophysiology is poorly understood [20]. Pericranial myofascial mechanisms are likely as is central sensitization in the chronic form [21, 22].
- Genetic and environmental factors may also play a role [22]

TTH Acute or Attack Treatment

- Acute treatment with simple analgesics is generally effective
  – Acetaminophen 500–1000 mg
  – Aspirin 500–1000 mg
- *NSAIDs* are considered the acute treatment drug of choice [23]
  – Ibuprofen 200–800 mg, no more than every 6 h
  – Naproxen 375–550 mg, no more than every 12 h
  – Ketoprofen 25–50 mg, no more than every 8 h

TTH Prophylactic/Preventive Treatment

Consider headache prevention in patients with chronic TTH (≥15 days/month)

- Amitriptyline, a nonselective serotonin reuptake inhibitor, has consistently shown clinical efficacy for TTH prevention [24, 25]. Usual dose of amitriptyline is from 10 to 75 mg/day.

- Mirtazapine [26] and venlafaxine are other options for prevention [23].
  – Mirtazapine up to 30 mg/day at bedtime
  – Venlafaxine up to 150 mg/day

Cluster Headache

- Cluster Headache is a trigeminal autonomic cephalalgia (TAC), a group of primary headache disorders characterized by unilateral head pain and ipsilateral autonomic features.
  See Table 16.5 for the ICHD-2 diagnostic criteria for cluster headache (Table 16.5). Like migraine and TTH, there are both episodic and chronic cluster headache forms. Chronic cluster headache satisfies the condition that attacks occur for more than 1 year with remission periods of less than 1 month [4].

Cluster Headache (CH)

- One of the most painful conditions
- Rare with a population frequency of 0.1 % [23]
- As opposed to migraine, CH is more common in men with an approximate 3:1 male-to-female ratio [27].
- Circadian periodicity is a hallmark of the disorder with functional neuroimaging revealing activation of the posterior hypothalamus known to control circadian cycles [28].
- Alcohol is a well-established trigger for cluster headache attacks.

Treatment of cluster headache can be divided into acute and preventive (short-term and long-term) treatment. Because of the relatively short-duration and severity of attacks, acute treatment for this condition must be rapid in onset and effective.

Table 16.4 International Headache Society Criteria for tension-type headache

A. Headache lasting from 30 min to 7 days
B. Headache has at least two of the following characteristics
(a) Bilateral location
(b) Pressing/tightening quality
(c) Mild/moderate intensity
(d) No aggravation by physical activity
C. Both of the following
1. No nausea or vomiting
2. Photophobia and phonophobia are absent, or at least not present together
D. Not attributable to another disorder

With permission from Tepper J. Acute treatment of migraine. CONTINUUM: Lifelong Learning in Neurology: December 2006 - Volume 12 - Issue 6, Headache - pp 87–105 [33]

Table 16.5 Diagnostic criteria for cluster headache, ICHD-2

A. At least five attacks fulfilling criteria B–D
B. Severe or very severe unilateral orbital, supraorbital, or temporal pain lasting 15–180 min if untreated
C. The headache is accompanied by at least one of the following, ipsilateral to the pain:
1. Conjunctival injection and/or lacrimation
2. Nasal congestion or rhinorrhea
3. Eyelid edema
4. Forehead and facial sweating
5. Miosis and/or ptosis
6. A sense of restlessness and agitation
D. The attacks have a frequency from one every other day to three times per day
E. Not attributable to another disorder

Modified from: *ICHD-2: Headache Classification Subcommittee of the International Headache Society. The International Classification of Headache Disorders: 2nd edition. Cephalalgia 2004;24(suppl 1):9–160* [4]

Acute CH Treatment

- 100 % oxygen administered at 12–15 L/min via a 100 % non-rebreather mask for 15–20 min [27]
- SC Sumatriptan (6 mg) **or** zolmitriptan NS (5 mg) **or** sumatriptan NS (20 mg)
- Short-term prevention of CH can be accomplished with occipital nerve block with local anesthetic plus/minus steroid or a short tapering course of oral steroids

CH Preventive Treatment

- Verapamil is the mainstay of long-term CH prevention
  - 120–960 mg daily, divided
  - Monitor ECG for PR interval with dose change and 10–14 days after dose change
- Other long-term preventive options include
  - Melatonin 3–9 mg at bedtime
  - Topiramate 25–250 mg daily, divided
  - Gabapentin [27] 100–900 mg daily, divided
  - Lithium 600–1200 mg daily, divided

Other Primary Headache Disorders

Primary stabbing headache is characterized by brief paroxysms of head pain occurring as a single "stab" or a series of "stabs" [29]. This primary headache disorder often coexists with other primary headaches, especially migraine [30]. Triggered headaches are always a diagnosis of exclusion as a triggered headache is a red flag that possibly correlates with increased intracranial pressure. The following primary headaches are not attributable to another etiology:

- **Primary cough headache**
- **Primary exertional headache**
- **Primary headache associated with sexual activity**

Hypnic Headache

- Awakens patient from sleep
- Also known as the alarm clock headache
- Usual onset is after age 50 [29]

Primary Thunderclap Headache

- Sudden onset with maximum intensity reached in less than 1 min [4]
- Differential diagnosis of secondary thunderclap headache includes SAH and other intracranial bleeds, ischemic stroke, cerebral venous sinus thrombosis, arterial dissection, reversible cerebral vasoconstriction syndrome, posterior reversible encephalopathy syndrome (PRES), pituitary apoplexy, etc. [29, 31]

Hemicrania continua (HC) is characterized by constant unilateral head pain with superimposed exacerbations of pain and (often less prominent) ipsilateral autonomic features. The headache must be present for at least 3 months [4, 29]. Like paroxysmal hemicrania, by definition, this headache is responsive to therapeutic doses of indomethacin [4].

New Daily Persistent Headache (**NDPH**) is a daily headache persistent for at least 3 months. This primary headache is remarkable in that it is daily from onset or within 3 days of onset [29]. Other clinical features are consistent with chronic TTH (bilateral, nonpulsating quality, mild-to-moderate intensity, lack of associated features, and not aggravated by routine physical activity) [4].

Cervicogenic Headache is pain coming from an identifiable source in the neck and referred to the head and/or face generally in the distribution of the trigeminal nerve and/or upper cervical (C2, C3 nerves). Clinical or radiologic evidence (e.g., MRI cervical spine) of a lesion generally accepted as a cause of headache must be present. Treatment of the causative lesion results in relief of pain.

References

1. Kelley NE, Tepper DE. Rescue therapy for acute migraine, Part I: triptans, dihydroergotamine, and magnesium. Headache. 2012;52: 114–28.
2. Lipton RB, Bigal ME, Diamond M, et al. Migraine prevalence, disease burden, and need for preventive therapy. Neurology. 2007;68:343–9.
3. Silberstein SD, Lipton RB, Goadsby PJ. Headache in clinical practice. 2nd ed. New York: Taylor & Francis; 2002.
4. Headache Classification Subcommittee of the International Headache Society. The international classification of headache disorders: 2nd edition. Cephalalgia. 2004;24 suppl 1:9–160.
5. Ward TN. Migraine diagnosis and pathophysiology. Continuum: lifelong learning neurol. 2012;18(4):753–63.
6. Olesen J, Bouser MG, Diener HC, et al. New appendix criteria open for a broader concept of chronic migraine. Cephalalgia. 2006;26: 742–6.
7. Olesen J, Burstein R, Ashima M, et al. Origin of pain in migraine: evidence for peripheral sensitisation. Lancet Neurol. 2009;8:679–90.
8. Goadsby PJ, Edvinsson L, Ekman R. Release of vasoactive peptides in the extracerebral circulation of human and the cat during activation of the trigeminovascular system. Ann Neurol. 1988;23:193–6.
9. Edvinsson L, Brodin E, Jansen I, et al. Neurokinin a in cerebral vessels: characterization, localization and effects in vitro. Regul Pept. 1988;20:181–97.
10. Burstein R, Cutrer MF, Yarnitsky D. The development of cutaneous allodynia during a migraine attack clinical evidence for the sequential recruitment of spinal and supraspinal nociceptive neurons in migraine. Brain. 2000;123:1703–9.
11. Burstein R, Yarnitsky D, Goor-Aryeh I, et al. An association between migraine and cutaneous allodynia. Ann Neurol. 2000;47:614–24.
12. Weiller C, May A, Limmroth V, et al. Brain stem activation in spontaneous human migraine attacks. Nat Med. 1995;1:658–60.
13. Afridi SK, Matharu MS, Lee L, et al. A PET study exploring the laterality of brainstem activation in migraine using glyceryl trinitrate. Brain. 2005;128:932–9.

14. Siow HC, Young WB, Silberstein SD. Neuroleptics in headache. Headache. 2005;45:358–71.

15. Kelley NE, Tepper DE. Rescue therapy for acute migraine, Part 2: neuroleptics, anti-histamines, and others. Headache. 2012;52:292–306.

16. Kelley NE, Tepper DE. Rescue therapy for acute migraine, Part 3: opioids, NSAIDs, steroids, and post-discharge medications. Headache. 2012;52:467–82.

17. Rizzoli PB. Acute and preventive treatment of migraine. Continuum: lifelong learning neurol. 2012;18(4):764–82.

18. Silberstein SD, Holland S, Freitag F, et al. Evidence-based guideline update: pharmacologic treatment for episodic migraine prevention in adults: report of the Quality Standards Subcommittee of the American Academy of Neurology and the American Headache Society. Neurology. 2012;78(17):1337–45.

19. Rasmussen BK, Jensen R, Schroll M, et al. Epidemiology of headache in a general population – a prevalence study. J Clin Epidemiol. 1991;44:1147–57.

20. Schwartz BS, Stewart WF, Simon D, et al. Epidemiology of tension-type headache. JAMA. 1998;4:381–3.

21. Olesen J. Clinical and pathophysiological observations in migraine and tension-type headache explained by integration of vascular, supraspinal and myofascial inputs. Pain. 1991;46:125–32.

22. Kaniecki RG. Tension-type headache. Continuum: lifelong learning neurol. 2012;18(4):823–34.

23. Olesen J, Tfelt-Hansen P, Ramadan N, et al. The headaches. Philadelphia: Lippincott Williams & Wilkins; 2005.

24. Gobel H, Hamouz V, Hansen C, et al. Chronic tension-type headache: amitriptyline reduces clinical headache duration and pain sensitivity but does not alter pericranial muscle activity readings. Pain. 1994;59:241–9.

25. Diamond S, Baltes BJ. Chronic tension headache–treated with amitriptyline–a double-blind study. Headache. 1971;11(3):110–6.

26. Bendtsen L, Jensen R. Mirtazapine is effective in the prophylactic treatment of chronic tension-type headache. Neurology. 2004; 62(10):1706–11.

27. Goadsby PJ. Trigeminal autonomic cephalalgias. Continuum: lifelong learning neurol. 2012;18(4):823–34.

28. May A, Bahra A, Buchel C, et al. Hypothalamic activation in cluster headache attacks. Lancet. 1998;352(9124):275–8.

29. Newman LC, Grosberg BM, Dodick DW. Other primary headaches. In: Silberstein SD, Lipton RB, Dodick DW, editors. Wolff's headache and other head pain. New York: Oxford University Press; 2008. p. 431–47.

30. Piovesan EJ, Kowacs PA, Lange MC, et al. Prevalence and semiologic aspects of the idiopathic stabbing headache in a migraine population. Arq Neuropsiquiatr. 2001;59((2-A)):201–5.

31. Mortimer AM, Bradley MD, Stoodley NG, Renowden SA. Thunderclap headache: diagnostic considerations and neuroimaging features. Clin Radiol. 2013;68(3):e101–13 [Epub 2012 Dec 11].

32. Marcus DA, Philip A, Bain PA, Getting Started. In: Marcus DA, Bain PA, editors. Practical assessment and treatment of the patient with headaches in the emergency department and urgent care clinic. New York: Springer; 2011; p 21–52.

33. Tepper J. Acute treatment of migraine. Continuum: lifelong learning in neurology. Headache. 2006;12(6):87–105.

34. Evans R, Purdy A. Identification or exclusion of secondary headaches. In: Lipton RB, Bigal ME, editors. Migraine and other headache disorders. New York: Informa Healthcare; 2006. p. 131–44.

35. de Vries B, Frants RR, Ferrari MD, van den Maagdenberg AM. Molecular genetics of migraine. Hum Genet. 2009;126:115–32.

36. Lenaerts ME. Headache. In: Rosenberg RN, editor. Atlas of clinical neurology. New York: Springer; 2009. p. 565–97.

Facial Pain

17

Kathy Aligene, Marc S. Lener, David Spinner,
and Yury Khelemsky

Abbreviations

AKA	Also known as
CBC	Complete blood count
CT	Computed tomography
DIC	Disseminated intravascular coagulation
GN	Glossopharyngeal neuralgia
HFS	Hemifacial spasm
ICHD	International Classification of Headache Disorders
LFT	Liver function test
MC	Myoclonus
MSK	Musculoskeletal
MRI	Magnetic resonance imaging
PHN	Post-herpetic neuralgia
SIADH	Syndrome of inappropriate antidiuretic hormone
ST	Spasmodic torticollis
TENS	Transcutaneous electrical nerve stimulation
TN	Trigeminal neuralgia
W	With
W/O	Without

K. Aligene, M.D. (✉)
Department of Rehabilitation Medicine, Mount Sinai
School of Medicine, Physical Medicine and Rehabilitation,
One Gustave Levy Place, Box 1420, New York, NY 10029, USA
e-mail: kathy.aligene@mountsinai.org

Division of Pain Medicine, Department of Anesthesiology,
Icahn School of Medicine at Mount Sinai, One Gustave L. Levy
Place, KCC 8th Floor, Box 1010, New York, NY 10029, USA

M.S. Lener, M.D.
Department of Psychiatry, Icahn School of Medicine at Mount
Sinai, One Gustave L. Levy Place, New York, NY 10029, USA
e-mail: marc.lener@mountsinai.org

D. Spinner, D.O.
The Mount Sinai Hospital, Rehabilitation Medicine,
1425 Madison Avenue Box 1420, New York, NY 10029, USA

Beth Israel Deaconess Medical Center, Harvard Medical School,
Brookline, MA, USA
e-mail: davidspinner@mountsinai.org

Y. Khelemsky, M.D.
Division of Pain Medicine, Department of Anesthesiology,
Icahn School of Medicine at Mount Sinai, One Gustave L. Levy
Place, KCC 8th Floor, Box 1010, New York, NY 10029, USA
e-mail: yury.khelemsky@mountsinai.org

Overview of Facial Pain [1, 2]

Despite a broad array of training backgrounds and clinical approaches to the evaluation of a patient with facial pain, all clinicians should have a firm knowledge base of the overlapping anatomical structures of the face to aid in clinical diagnosis and management. Most commonly, anatomic localization of facial pain is oftentimes not obvious. Therefore, having a strong basic clinical evaluation will help in narrowing the differential diagnosis.

This chapter will briefly cover the following etiologies of facial pain:
1. Central causes of facial pain
2. Peripheral causes of facial pain
3. Musculoskeletal causes of facial pain
4. Other causes of facial pain

Central Causes of Facial Pain (*Also Referred As*: Craniofacial Pain) [2]

Classifications (Four Major Clinical Syndromes)
1. Anesthesia dolorosa
2. Central post-stroke pain
3. Persistent idiopathic facial pain
4. Facial pain attributed to multiple sclerosis (*see* section "Musculoskeletal Causes of Facial Pain")

Common Features
- **Definition**:
  - Lesion or dysfunction in the central nervous system that leads to a central neuropathy causing facial pain [3]

- **Etiology**:
  - Central neuropathic pain (*most common cause post-stroke*) [4]
  - Post stroke pain
- **Pathophysiology**:
  - Cortically mediated somatosensory dysfunction or spinothalamic tract dysfunction leading to a sensitized state causing persistent pain **without** progressive tissue injury [5].
- **Symptoms**:
  - Allodynia (increased pain response to non-painful stimuli) or hyperpathia (heightened response to pain stimuli)
  - Most common quality is burning, pricking, pins/needles/sting, sensation, shooting/lancinating, pressing, and muscle cramping or crushing
  - Intermittent or constant
  - Evoked pain (secondary to central stimuli) with paroxysm (brief attack) or steady pain (suggestion of brain lesion) [6]
  - Often variable pain character; with bizarre and vague [3]
  - Usually appears in association with abnormal neurological symptoms
  - Delayed onset from days to months, in some cases years
  - Exacerbating factors: mood change, temperature change (especially cold), light touch, and movement
  - Regional distribution, rather than corresponding to individual nerves
- **Work up** [3]
  - Diagnosis based on supporting clinical evidence of underlying central nervous system lesion or dysfunction with secondary facial pain [3]
  - Imaging (CT or MRI with and without contrast) of the brain may be necessary to identify location of the lesion
  - Some facial pain conditions are unclassifiable using strict diagnostic criteria of ICHD [7, 8]

1. **Anesthesia Dolorosa**
- **Description**:
  - *AKA* constant severe deafferentation pain
  - Uncommon complication of gasserian ganglion destruction (a treatment for trigeminal neuralgia) characterized by constant burning pain in facial area rendered insensate [9].
- **Pathophysiology**:
  - Transsynaptic degeneration resulting in deafferentation hypersensitivity of central trigeminal neurons or their connections.
- **Epidemiology**:
  - Incidence 0.3–2 %

- **Symptoms**:
  - Allodynia (increase pain response to non-painful stimuli) and/or hyperpathia (heightened response to pain stimuli) in trigeminal nerve distribution
- **Physical Exam**:
  - History of trauma or prior surgery
  - May encounter wounds or scars from prior surgery or trauma; may see facial paralysis on the ipsilateral side
- **Work Up**:
  - MRI with contrast to rule out a tumor as the cause of the pain
- **Treatment**:
  - **Pharmacologic** (*see* Table 17.1)
    - Opioids, antidepressants, and anticonvulsants have not shown to be successful treatment
    - May have mild benefit with gabapentin 1,200 mg daily in divided doses [10]
  - **Non-pharmacologic**
    - TENS
      - Chronic electrical stimulation of the gasserian ganglion
      - In refractory cases, trial of TENS, before considering invasive management [3]
  - **Surgical**
    - Deep brain stimulation
      - Implantation of an electrode to a specific part of the brain that is attached to a brain pacemaker, which sends electrical impulses to the brain in response to a brain signal.
    - Mesencephalotomy
      - Obliteration of the trigeminal tract and the periaqueductal gray junction
    - Dorsal root entry zone lesioning
      - Destruction of the sensory **nerve** fibers enters the dorsal root
    - Medial thalamotomy

2. **Central Post-stroke Pain (previously known as, Thalamic Pain)**
- **Description**:
  - Neuropathic pain syndrome, characterized by pain and sensory abnormalities in body regions that correspond to the brain territory injured by a cerebrovascular lesion [11, 12].
- **Pathophysiology**:
  - May be a combination of deafferentation and the subsequent development of neuronal hyperexcitability
- **Epidemiology**:
  - Prevalence between 1 and 12 % among stroke patients
- **Symptoms**:
  - Sensory loss
  - Hypersensitivity (e.g., Allodynia)
  - Pain can be spontaneous or evoked

Table 17.1 Medications for facial pain

Medication	Dosing	Indication	Side effects	Comments
Antiepileptics				
Gabapentin	1,200–2,400 mg daily; start single 300-mg dose on Day 1, 600 mg/day on Day 2 (divided BID), 900 mg/day on Day 3 (divided TID); titrate as needed	Seizures; post-herpetic neuralgia	Common: Dizziness, somnolence, and peripheral edema	Monitor kidney function in those who have pre-existing kidney condition; associated with an increased risk of suicidal acts
Lamotrigine	100–400 mg/day; start 25–50 mg daily, at week 3 increase to 100 mg/day, at week 5 increase 100 mg/day; max daily dose of 400 mg	Seizures; off-label: neuropathic pain and trigeminal neuralgia	Common: Sedation, blurred vision, headache, dizziness, insomnia, nausea, vomiting, benign rash Rare: Stevens–Johnson syndrome, toxic epidermal necrolysis, blood dyscrasias	Monitor CBC twice monthly for the first 2 months then every 3–6 months throughout treatment
Topiramate	25–800 mg/day with a suggested dose of 125–400 mg daily	Seizures, migraines; off-label neuropathic pain	Common: Dizziness, ataxia, speech problems, psychomotor slowing, abnormal vision, memory problems, paresthesia, diplopia, fatigue, nervousness, decreased appetite.	Monitor for changes in mental alertness and memory
Carbamazepine	400–1,200 mg/day; start 100 mg twice a day, increase weekly up to 200 mg/day; max daily dose of 1,200 mg	Seizures, trigeminal neuralgia	Common: Sedation, headache, dizziness, nausea, vomiting, rash, hyponatremia, benign leucopenia; Rare: aplastic anemia, Stevens–Johnson syndrome, SIADH	Monitor CBC, BMP, LFTs, Renal and Thyroid function tests; CBC twice monthly for the first 2 months then every 3–6 months throughout treatment. LFT, kidney, and thyroid function tests every 6–12 months
Oxcarbazepine	600–1,200 mg/day; start 150–300 mg/day and increase every 5 days by 150–300 mg/day	Partial seizures, trigeminal neuralgia	Common: Sedation, headache, dizziness, nausea, vomiting, rash, hyponatremia; rare: blood dyscrasias (leucopenia, thrombocytopenia) and dermatologic reactions (erythema multiforme, Stevens–Johnson syndrome, toxic epidermal necrolysis)	Monitor sodium levels within first 3 months; CBC twice monthly for the first 2 months then every 3–6 months throughout treatment
Pregabalin	100–600 mg/day; start 50 mg twice daily, double dose every 3–7 days up to desired effect, max daily dose of 600 mg	Diabetic peripheral neuropathy and spinal cord injury, post-herpetic neuralgia, fibromyalgia, trigeminal neuralgia	Common: Sedation, blurred vision, dizziness, weight gain, insomnia, nausea, constipation	Pregabalin should be reduced gradually tapered if discontinued; Withdrawal symptoms include difficulty sleeping, nausea, anxiety, diarrhea, flu or flu-like symptoms, headache, increased sweating, convulsions, pain, dizziness, nervousness, and depression.
Antispasmodics				
Baclofen	40–80 mg/day; start 5 mg three times daily, increase by 15 mg every 3 days	Spasticity and spasms	Common: Sedation, flaccidity, headache, dizziness, weakness, nausea, constipation, confusion Rare: Withdrawal	Avoid rapid withdrawal—fever, confusion, tachycardia, pruritis, seizures, DIC, rhabdomyolysis
Methocarbamol	1 g IV/IM; additional doses at q8h until PO; not to exceed 3 g/day; 1,500 mg PO q6h for 48–72 h; not to exceed 8 g/day then decrease to 4–4.5 g/day divided q4–8 h	Spasticity and spasms; tetanus	Common: Drowsiness, dizziness, leukopenia (IV), lightheadedness, blurred vision, headache, fever, nausea, anorexia, GI upset, nystagmus, diplopia, flushing, vertigo, mild muscular incoordination, syncope, hypotension, bradycardia urticaria, pruritus, rash	May cause drowsiness or dizziness; should not ingest alcohol or other CNS depressants; may take with food to avoid stomach upset
Cyclobenzaprine	Immediate-release: 5 mg q8h; may increase dose to 7.5–10 mg q8h PRN; Extended-release: 5 mg/day; may require up to 30 mg/day	Spasticity and spasms	Common: Drowsiness, dry mouth, headache, dizziness; less common: Pharyngitis, fatigue, palpitations, dysgeusia, GI upset, blurred vision, constipation, confusion, nausea, nervousness	Caution in patients in acute recovery phase of myocardial infarction, in patients with arrhythmia, heart block or conduction disturbances, or congestive heart failure; hyperpyretic crisis seizures and deaths concomitantly with MAO inhibitors

(continued)

Table 17.1 (continued)

Medication	Dosing	Indication	Side effects	Comments
Botulinum Toxin A	Cervical Dystonia: 198–300 units IM, divided among affected muscles (max: 50 units/site), may repeat in 3 months; Blepharospasm: 1.25–2.5 units/site IM q3 months (max: cum dose 200 units/30 days)	Cervical dystonia, hyperhidrosis, Blepharospasm, strabismus, spasticity, migraine	Common: Dysphagia, upper respiratory infection, neck pain, and headache; less common: increased cough, flu syndrome, back pain, rhinitis, dizziness, hypertonia, soreness at injection site, asthenia, oral dryness, speech disorder, fever, nausea, and drowsiness	Caution during injections if administered beyond the site of local injection; Must have close follow-up hours to weeks after injection; symptoms include asthenia, generalized muscle weakness, diplopia, ptosis, dysphagia, dysphonia, dysarthria, and breathing difficulties
Antidepressants				
Amitriptyline (TCA)	10–100 mg/day, suggested dose of 75 mg/day; start 10=25 mg/day, increase by 25 mg every 7 days	Major depressive disorder; TGA-labeled for migraine, neuropathic pain, fibromyalgia	Common: Orthostasis, conduction defects, ventricular arrhythmias, reflex tachycardia, anticholinergic effects, weight gain	Potential lethality in overdose due to cardiac conduction abnormalities—Monitor ECG for QTc prolongation at baseline and when increasing the dose; Monitor periodic potassium and Mg when patient is on a diuretic; should not use with MAOi as it may induce serotonin syndrome; activation of mania or suicidal ideation
Nortriptyline (TCA)	20–150 mg/day; start 10 mg/day, increase by 10=25 mg every 7 days	neuropathic pain, fibromyalgia		Monitor LFTs—has been associated with hepatotoxicity and/or elevated transaminases
Duloxetine (SNRI)	60–120 mg; start 30 mg/day, increase 30 mg every 3–5 days	Major depressive disorder, generalized anxiety disorder, diabetic neuropathic pain, fibromyalgia, chronic MSK pain	Common: Nausea, somnolence, dizziness, dry mouth, nervousness, tremor, insomnia, constipation, sexual dysfunction, sweating, anorexia, blood pressure elevation, orthostasis, conduction defects, ventricular arrhythmias,	
Benzodiazepines				
Clonazepam	0.5–2 mg/day (divided daily or BID); start 0.25 mg BID, increase by 0.25–9.5 mg/day	Epilepsy and panic disorder; clinically effective for various conditions including spasticity	Common: Sedation, ataxia, hypotonia, paradoxical agitation, memory changes, withdrawal syndrome	Withdrawal syndrome including seizures
Opioids				
Morphine (PO formulation)	10–30 mg PO q3–4 h PRN for pain; start at 10 mg PO q3–4 h and titrate as needed	Persistent moderate to severe acute and chronic pain	Common: Physical dependence, tolerance, opioid-induced hyperalgesia, pseudotolerance, addiction, aberrant behaviors, pseudoaddiction, opioid-induced constipation, nausea, vomiting, drowsiness, delirium, hypogonadism, urinary retention, edema, dermatologic	In rare cases, can cause respiratory depression
Oxycodone	5–80 mg/day; start 5 mg/day, increase 5–20 mg daily to three times daily, increase amount as needed			
Other				
Lidocaine 5 % patch	Each patch has 50 mg/g adhesive; maximum daily dose of 3 patches, on 12 out of 24 h	Post-herpetic neuralgia	Less common: Skin at the site of application: blisters, bruising, burning sensation, depigmentation, dermatitis, discoloration, edema, erythema, exfoliation, irritation, papules, petechia, pruritus, vesicles, or may be the locus of abnormal sensation	Minimal systemic absorption but possible if applied longer than recommended
Capsaicin 0.075 %	Up to 4 patches every 3 months or 3–4 times daily cream to affected areas	Post-herpetic neuralgia	Less common: Burning sensation, hyperalgesia, allodynia	For PHN: A single 1 h application of up to 4 patches can be used every 3 months as needed; For MSK pain requires 3–4 times per day dosing

– Spontaneous dysaesthesia is common (up to 85 % of patients)
- **Physical exam**:
  – Presence of sensory loss and signs of neuronal hypersensitivity in the painful area are common
- **Work up**:
  – Diagnosis of exclusion, no pathognomonic features of this syndrome
  – History of stroke should be confirmed by imaging (either CT or MRI) to visualize the lesion (type, location, and size) and to exclude other central causes of pain
- **Treatment**:
  – **Pharmacologic**:
    TCA (amitriptyline) as first line
    Lamotrigine and gabapentin as second line [13, 14]

3. Persistent Idiopathic Facial Pain [15, 16]

- **Description**:
  – *AKA* continuous neuropathic orofacial pain, atypical odontalgia, atypical facial pain, or phantom tooth pain
  – Constant, unremitting oral, or peri-orial pain (perceived to be within deep tissues) with variable and fluctuating intensity
- **Pathophysiology**:
  – Unknown; abnormal sensitization of trigeminal nociceptive system
- **Epidemiology**:
  – In the general population: 0.03–1 %
  – In patients who have undergone endodontic procedures: 3–12 %
  – More frequently reported by females in their 40s and 50s
- **Symptoms**:
  – Usually presents unilaterally
  – Heightened or reduced sensitivity, or a combination of both
  – Constant pain disproportionate to various stimuli
  – Pain may have started spontaneously (idiopathic) or due to an event, such as a traumatic injury, minor or major surgical procedure, or dental intervention.
- **Physical Exam**:
  – Common sites of onset are the nasolabial fold or the ipsilateral chin
- **Work Up**:
  – Imaging (CT and MRI) required to rule out central nervous system and hard/soft tissue pathology
  – Patients usually have seen multiple medical and dental practitioners without identified source and unsuccessful attempts at multiple interventions.
- **Diagnosis**:
  – Diagnosis of exclusion
- **Treatment**:
  – **Pharmacologic**
    First-line tricyclic antidepressants (preferred) [17]

SSRI or SNRIs
Some benefit reported with topiramate [18]
– **Nonpharmacologic**:
Cognitive behavioral therapy

Peripheral Causes of Facial Pain [2]

Classifications (Four Major Clinical Syndromes)
1. Trigeminal neuralgia
2. Glossopharyngeal Neuralgia
3. Nervus intermedius/geniculate ganglion neuralgia
4. Post-herpetic neuralgia (PHN)*

Common Features
- **Definition**:
  – Lesion or dysfunction in the peripheral nervous system that leads to a peripheral neuropathy and causing facial pain.
- **Etiology**:
  – Peripheral neuropathy (most common is trigeminal neuralgia)
- **Pathophysiology**:
  – Neurovascular compression or irritation of the involved peripheral nerve

1. Trigeminal Neuralgia (TN) [19–29]

- **Pathophysiology**:
  – Thought to be caused by neurovascular compression where an aberrant vessel (normally an artery) compresses the trigeminal nerve causing focal demyelination [29].
- **Classification**:
  – *Typical TN*: Lancinating sudden pain
  – *Atypical TN*: Burning constant pain
  – *Mixed TN*: Components of typical and atypical TN
  – *Secondary*: Factors which may increase risk for TN
- **Epidemiology**: [29, 30]
  – Female to male distribution, 2:1
  – Age distribution, after 40 years old (>90 % of cases)
- **Symptoms**: [2]
  – Severe paroxysmal pain in the distribution of one or more division of the trigeminal nerve
  – Usually unilateral
  – Abrupt in onset and termination that typically last from one to a few seconds
  – Sharp and electric in quality
- **Physical exam**: [29, 31]
  – Physical exam findings may be negative
- **Diagnosis primarily made by history**
  – Asymmetric jaw movements
  – Corneal reflex
  – Mild sensory changes with prolonged cases
  – Symptoms may be triggered by lightly stroking the affected TN nerve distribution
  – No tenderness, swelling, or erythema

- **Imaging**: [32]
  - High resolution MRI w/wo contrast to look for a neurovascular or other structural lesion at the root entry or exit zone from the brainstem causing compression
  - Potential causes of compression:
    - 60–90 % of neurovascular compression occur due to superior cerebellar artery
    - The remaining neurovascular lesions result from anterio-inferior cerebellar and basilar artery.
  - Must rule out multiple sclerosis as it can present similarly to TN
- **Diagnosis**: [30]
  - Clinical impression based upon the patient's age and history and physical exam, along with radiographic findings. Patients may complain of unilateral facial pain. This may present in association with multiple sclerosis.
- **Treatment**:
  - **Pharmacologic**: [30]
    - First-line oral therapy includes oxcarbazepine over carbamazepine secondary to safety profile. *Must obtain baseline CBC and LFTs and monitor periodically thereafter.*
    - Second-line oral therapy includes lamotrigine, baclofen, and/or pregabalin
  - **Nonpharmacologic**: [29, 30, 33–35]
    - Peripheral nerve injection of the desired trigeminal nerve distribution can be targeted blind or with ultrasound.
    - The supraorbital, infraorbital, or mental nerve is found by palpating or scanning the relative foramen.
    - An anesthetic, steroid, or alcohol can be injected.
    - Typical injections provide mild to moderate relief lasting a few weeks to a few months.
  - **Surgical**: [36]
    - Microvascular decompression has shown to have the greatest pain relief. Neurosurgeons are able to perform this skull-based surgery by placing a peace of Teflon between the abutting vascular structure and nerve.
    - Surgical referral can be made when conservative treatments are not effective, not tolerated, or MRI shows a clear neurovascular compression that can be decompressed.
    - Gamma knife directs a focused beam of radiation at the trigeminal root
    - Gasserian ganglion percutaneous radiofrequency thermocoagulation

2. Glossopharyngeal Neuralgia (GN)

- **Description**:
  - Can occur from compression by masses or vascular structures
- **Pathophysiology**:
  - Unclear etiology [37]

- **Epidemiology**:
  - May have higher incidence in men
- **Symptoms**: [38, 39]
  - Same clinical characteristics as Trigeminal Neuralgia except for preferential unilateral left-sided pain and distribution in cranial IX territory
  - Severe paroxysmal unilateral pain located in the posterior tongue, throat, ear, or angle of the mandible
  - Swallowing, chewing, talking, and sneezing are the most common triggers
  - Associated with anxiety and depression
  - Abrupt in onset and termination
  - Sharp and electric in quality
- **Physical exam**:
  - Assess location of pain in the glossopharyngeal nerve territory
  - Swallowing may trigger the pain
- **Imaging**:
  - MRI brainstem with further angiography may delineate the offending vessel, most commonly the posterior inferior cerebellar artery. It may also identify a cause such as tumor or other neurovascular compression.
  - CT vertebral angiography may help identify a primary cause such as an infarction or vertebral artery dissection.
- **Diagnosis**:
  - Clinical impression based upon the patient's age and history and physical exam
  - The patient should be seen by ENT to rule out other causes.
  - Stimulation of the nerve during surgery may help to confirm the diagnosis
- **Treatment**: [40]
  - **Pharmacologic**: [41]
    - Similar medical management to TN, although local anesthetic can be applied to the oropharynx with both therapeutic and diagnostic implications.
    - First-line oral therapy includes oxcarbazepine over carbamazipine, secondary to safety profile.
    - Second-line oral therapy includes lamotrigine, baclofen, and pregabalin.
  - **Surgical**: [42]
    - Neurosurgical treatment is usually indicated sooner than for TN
    - Craniotomy with rhizotomy or neurotomy or percutaneous surgery with radiofrequency rhizotomy, trigeminal tractotomy, or nucleotomy.

3. Nervus Intermedius/Geniculate Ganglion Neuralgia [43]

- **Description**:
  - Can occur from compression at its central-peripheral myelin junction by masses or vascular structures.
- **Pathophysiology**:

– Etiology unknown [44]
- **Epidemiology**: >50 years old
- **Symptoms**: [45]
  – Similar to that of TN, however, in the distribution of the nervus intermedius
- **Physical exam**:
  – Severe episodic lancinating pain in the posterior pharynx or ear canal
  – Unilateral
  – No motor or sensory findings
- **Imaging**:
  – High resolution MRI with and without contrast to look for a structural lesion or vascular compression
- **Diagnosis**:
  – Clinical impression based upon the patient's age and history and physical exam
- **Treatment**: [43]
  – **Pharmacologic**
    Same oral management as TN
  – **Surgical**
    - Microvascular decompression can provide long-term pain relief when impingement is identified and surgery is obtainable

4. PHN (Post Herpetic Neuralgia)
- **Description**:
  – Pain caused by the reactivation of the varicella-zoster virus in the affected nerves
- **Pathophysiology**: [46]
  – Current pathophysiologic mechanisms focus on sensitization and deafferentation as the primary mechanisms contributing to PHN
  – Injury to peripheral and central neurons via immune and inflammatory responses
  – Damaged peripheral nociceptors lead to central sensitization process in dorsal horn neurons
  – Abnormal reorganization to deafferentated spinal cord neurons and damaged peripheral neurons may lead to persistent pain
- **Epidemiology**: [47]
  – Main risk factor includes increasing age, >60 years old
- **Prevention**: [48]
  – Strategies include the varicella vaccine to decrease incidence of acute herpes zoster infection
  – Treating acute herpetic infection with antiviral medications and amitriptyline
- **Symptoms**:
  – Dermatomal burning pain following distribution of original infection or itching
- **Physical Exam**: [48]
  – Sensory deficits may include light touch, pinprick, and vibration
  – Myofascial pain can occur secondary to guarding

– Facial paralysis with facial nerve involvement
- **Diagnosis**: [49]
  – Clinical impression based upon the patient's age, history, and physical exam
  – Typically pain lasting >3 months following acute herpetic episode is considered PHN
  – More commonly occurs in the thoracic (T4–6), ophthalmic division of the trigeminal nerves and cervical levels.
  – Punch biopsy of affected skin shows loss of epidermal innervations (*not routinely performed*)
- **Treatment**: [48]
  – **Pharmacologic**
    - Multiple sites potentially causing PHN along the pain pathway, more than two therapies with complementary mechanisms of actions are often employed.
    - Lidocaine 5 % patch
    - Capsaicin 0.075 % cream
    - Pregabalin (dose-related risk of somnolence, dizziness, and peripheral edema)
    - First (Amitriptyline) or second generation TCAs (Nortriptyline) (less anticholinergic side effect profile)
    - Opioids (Oxycodone or Morphine) (adverse side effects include constipation and nausea)
  – **Invasive**
    - Sympathetic blocks may, provide temporary relief
    - Peripheral nerve blocks
    - Spinal cord stimulation

Musculoskeletal Causes of Facial Pain

Classifications (Three Major Clinical Syndromes): [2]
1. Temporomandibular disorders
2. Myofascial pain
3. Facial spasms:
   - *Hemifacial spasm*
   - *Torticollis*
   - *Myoclonus*
   - *Blepherospasm* (not discussed here)

1. Temporomandibular Disorders [50]
- **Description**:
  – Pain related to temporomandibular joint and muscles of mastication (masseter, temporalis, digastric, medial pterygoid, lateral pterygoid) or other muscles of the head and neck region.
- **Classification**
  – Classified by cause and symptoms; traumatic or idiopathic
- **Pathophysiology**: [51]
  – Muscular hyperactivity and dysfunction due to malocclusion

- Risk factors
  Predisposing factors: genetic, hormonal, and anatomical
  Precipitating factors: trauma, occlusal changes, parafunction (e.g., Bruxism)
  Prolonging factors: stress and parafunction
- TMD of articular origin, disc displacement is the most common cause and muscle spasm is secondary in nature.
- Other causes of TMD are: degenerative joint disease, rheumatoid arthritis, ankylosis, dislocations, infections, and neoplasia.
- **Epidemiology**:
  - 5–10 % of Americans
  - Highest incidence in young adults age 20–40; *highest in females*
  - About one third of patients have a history of psychiatric problems and patients with a chronic eating disorder have a higher prevalence.
  - Association with female smokers <30 years; and other factors (e.g., stress levels)
- **Symptoms**:
  - May also have neck and/or shoulder pain
  - Should inquire about daytime or nighttime clenching (daytime clenching has a stronger association with TMD than night time bruxism)
  - Pain usually periauricular, associated with chewing; "clicking, popping, and snapping" sounds
  - Described as a variable, deep ache with intermittent sharp pain with jaw movement
  - Unilateral, in TMD with articular origin
  - Bilateral, in TMD associated with myofascial pain or with rheumatoid arthritis
- **Physical exam**:
  - Comprehensive, focused facial MSK examination can usually elicit whether pain is related to the joint, muscles, or a combination of both
    Muscular or joint pain reproducible upon palpation or resistance against active muscle movement or passive movement.
- **Work up**:
  - Imaging: CT or MRI; fMRI can visualize anatomic structures during joint movement
  - If systemic illness is suspected:
    CBC to rule out infection
    Rheumatoid factor (RF), ESR, antinuclear antibody (ANA), and other specific antibodies are checked if rheumatoid arthritis, temporal arteritis, or a connective tissue disorder.
    Uric acid should be checked for gout
    Arthrocentesis is required to demonstrate specific crystals for gout or pseudogout
- **Treatment**:
  - **Pharmacologic**:
    NSAIDs, muscle relaxants, and tricyclic antidepressants (most common)

Botulinum toxin in conjunction with arthrocentesis
  - **Nonpharmacologic**:
    Occlusional splints (used at bedtime)
    Arthrocentesis.

2. **Myofascial Pain [52]**
- **Description**:
  - Pain that originates from myofascial trigger points (MTrPs) in skeletal muscle, either alone or in combination with other pain generators causing spasms and limited motion.
- **Pathophysiology**:
  - Continuous input from peripheral muscle nociceptors leads to changes in function and connectivity of sensory dorsal horn neurons and result in central sensitization.
- **Epidemiology**:
  - High prevalence among individuals with regional pain complaints
  - 21 % of patients seen in a general orthopedic clinic
  - 30 % of general medical clinic patients with regional pain
  - 85–90 % of patients presenting to specialty pain management centers
- **Symptoms**:
  - Local or regional deep aching sensations varying in intensity
  - Frequently, associated autonomic dysfunction may occur, including abnormal sweating, lacrimation, dermal flushing, and vasomotor–temperature changes
  - Cervical myofascial pain may be associated with neuro-otologic symptoms including impaired balance, dizziness, and tinnitus
  - Functional complaints include decreased work tolerance, impaired muscle coordination, stiff joints, fatigue, and weakness
- **Physical exam**:
  - Emphasis on posture, biomechanics, and joint function to identify underlying factors
  - Active MTrPs typically associated with a painful restricted range of motion
  - Trigger points should be identified by gentle palpation across the direction of muscle fibers
  - May appreciate "ropelike" nodularity within a taut band of muscle; palpation of area is painful and may reproduce the local and referred pain pattern
- **Diagnosis**:
  - Thyroid function tests to exclude thyroid dysfunction in patients with muscle pain
  - Imaging (radiographs, CT scan, MRI) to rule out osteoarthrosis or diskogenic changes
- **Treatment**:
  - **Pharmacologic**:
    NSAIDs

Botulinum toxin
  – **Nonpharmacologic**:
    Postural, mechanical, and ergonomic modifications

3. **Facial Spasms (Collectively)**: *Hemifacial Spasm, Spasmodic Torticollis*, and *Myoclonus*
  • **Description**: Sudden muscle contraction on one side of the face, muscle contraction that causes the neck to twist unnaturally, muscle twitching, or twitching of the eyelid (*respectively*).
  • **Pathophysiology**:
    – *Primary Hemifacial Spasm (HFS)*
      Most frequently caused by a blood vessel of the posterior circulation compressing the facial nerve as it exits the brainstem.
    – *Spasmodic Torticollis (ST)*
      Primary ST: genetics, associated with DYT7 locus on chromosome 18p and DYT13 locus on chromosome 1p36 studied in German and Italian: Autosomal dominant with reduced penetrance, for both loci.
      Secondary ST: perinatal cerebral injury, kernicterus, cerebrovascular diseases, drug-induced, central nervous system tumor, peripheral or central trauma, infectious or post-infectious encephalopathies, toxins, metabolic, paraneoplastic syndromes, central pontine myelinolysis.
      Common pathway for both Primary and Secondary ST: associated with abnormalities of the basal ganglia and hyper-activation of the cortical area leading to over-activity of the medial and prefrontal cortical areas and hypo-activity of the primary motor cortex during movement.
    – *Myoclonus (MC)*
      Typically one of several signs in Multiple Sclerosis, Parkinson's disease, Alzheimer's disease, Subacute Sclerosing Panencephalitis and Creutzfeldt–Jakob disease (CJD), serotonin toxicity, Huntington's disease, epilepsy, and intracranial hypotension.
      Most cases are due to dysfunction in brain areas involved with startle reflex.
      Involvement of GABA and Serotonin neurotransmitter systems.
  • **Epidemiology**:
    – HFS (extremely rare)
      More commonly seen in Asians
    – ST (congenital)
      Incidence in newborn infants: 0.3–2 %
    – MC
      Secondary to underlying condition (72 %); Epileptic myoclonus (17 %); and Essential myoclonus (11 %).
      Lifetime prevalence in 1990: 8.6 per 100,000 population.
  • **Symptoms**:
    – HFS:
      Pain can vary in intensity

Typically brief, irregular movements
Presents unilaterally; in severe cases, bilaterally.
Begins with intermittent twitching of the eyelid leading to forced closure of eye, gradually spreading to the muscles of the lower part of the face.
All the muscles on the affected side are involved.
  – ST:
    The head may turn or tilt in jerky movements or sustain a prolonged involuntary position.
    Involuntary spasm of the neck muscles will increase in frequency and strength until it plateaus.
    Symptoms can worsen while walking or during psychological stress.
    May also present with muscle hypertrophy, neck pain, dysarthria, and tremor.
  – MC:
    Rapid, alternating, contraction and relaxation of muscles
  • **Physical exam**:
    – Complete neurological examination with focus on the cranial nerves, sensory and motor exam of the face, and musculoskeletal exam in the head and neck.
  • **Diagnosis**:
    – may require Electromyography, MRI, CT, and Angiography to make or support the diagnosis
    – HFS: MRI is best option to visualize vascular anomaly.
    – ST (congenital): Toronto Western Spasmodic Torticollis Rating Scale (TWSTRS) is commonly used scale to rate the severity of spasmodic torticollis
    – MC: Physical exam findings c/w myoclonic jerking with or without evidence of associated illness
  • **Treatment**:
    – **Pharmacologic**:
      HFS: Carbamazepine or Botulinum toxin
      ST: Botulinum toxin, anticholinergic agents (e.g., cyclobenzaprine), clonazepam, baclofen
      MC: Clonazepam, sodium valproate, piracetam, and primidone alone or in combination with each other
    – **Nonpharmacologic**:
      ST: Physical therapy
    – **Surgical**:
      Primary HFS: Microvascular decompression, relieves pressure on the facial nerve, which is the cause of most hemifacial spasm cases
      ST: Deep brain stimulation

Other Causes of Facial Pain

Causes of Facial Pain that Should be Considered in the Differential (*Briefly listed, not discussed in this chapter*)
  • *Facial paralysis*
    – Bells palsy

- *Neoplastic*
  - Primary tumors
  - Metastatic disease
  - Distant, non-metastasized cancer
  - Hematologic cancer
- *Systemic conditions*
  - Sjogren's syndrome
  - Systemic lupus erythmatosis
  - Rheumatoid arthritis
  - Mixed connective tissue disease
- *Vascular conditions*
  - Giant cell/temporal arteritis
  - Carotid artery dissection
- *Dental/oral causes*
  - Dental caries
  - Tooth fracture
  - Dentin hypersensitivity
- *Primary headaches (other than TN)*
  - Migraine headaches
  - Tension headaches
  - Hemicrania continua
  - Cluster headaches

References

1. Zakrzewska JM. Differential diagnosis of facial pain and guidelines for management. Br J Anaesth. 2013;111(1):95–104.
2. Headache Classification Subcommittee of the International Headache Society. The International Classification of Headache Disorders: 2nd edition. Cephalalgia. 2004;24 Suppl 1:9–160.
3. Boivie J, Casey KL. Central pain in the face and head. In: Olesen J, editor. The headaches. Philadelphia: Lippincott Williams & Wilkins; 2006. p. 1063.
4. Haanpää M. A central neuropathic pain. In: Guide to pain management. Seattle International Association for the Study of Pain (IASP) Press; 2010. pp. 189–94.
5. Rowbotham MC. Mechanisms of neuropathic pain and their implications for the design of clinical trials. Neurology. 2005;65(12 Suppl 4):S66–73.
6. Tasker R. Central pain states. In: Warfield C, Bajwa ZH, editors. Principles and practice of pain medicine. New York: McGraw-Hill; 2004. p. 394.
7. Zebenholzer K, Wober C, Vigl M, Wessely P, Wober-Bingol C. Facial pain in a neurological tertiary care centre—evaluation of the International Classification of Headache Disorders. Cephalalgia. 2005;25(9):689–99.
8. Zebenholzer K, Wober C, Vigl M, Wessely P, Wober-Bingol C. Facial pain and the second edition of the International Classification of Headache Disorders. Headache. 2006;46(2):259–63.
9. Tatli M, Keklikci U, Aluclu U, Akdeniz S. Anesthesia dolorosa caused by penetrating cranial injury. Eur Neurol. 2006;56(3):162–5.
10. Rozen TD. Relief of anesthesia dolorosa with gabapentin. Headache. 1999;39(10):761–2.
11. Zakrzewska JM, Forssell H, Glenny AM. Interventions for the treatment of burning mouth syndrome. Cochrane Database Syst Rev. 2005;1, CD002779.
12. Klit H, Finnerup NB, Jensen TS. Central post-stroke pain: clinical characteristics, pathophysiology, and management. Lancet Neurol. 2009;8(9):857–68.
13. Vestergaard K, Andersen G, Gottrup H, Kristensen BT, Jensen TS. Lamotrigine for central poststroke pain: a randomized controlled trial. Neurology. 2001;56(2):184–90.
14. Frese A, Husstedt IW, Ringelstein EB, Evers S. Pharmacologic treatment of central post-stroke pain. Clin J Pain. 2006;22(3):252–60.
15. Obermann M, Holle D, Katsarava Z. Trigeminal neuralgia and persistent idiopathic facial pain. Expert Rev Neurother. 2011;11(11):1619–29.
16. Klasser G. Management of persistent idiopathic facial pain. J Can Dent Assoc. 2013;79:d71.
17. Agostoni E, Frigerio R, Santoro P. Atypical facial pain: clinical considerations and differential diagnosis. Neurol Sci. 2005;26 Suppl 2:s71–4.
18. Volcy M, Rapoport AM, Tepper SJ, Sheftell FD, Bigal ME. Persistent idiopathic facial pain responsive to topiramate. Cephalalgia. 2006;26(4):489–91.
19. Bair MJ, Robinson RL, Katon W, Kroenke K. Depression and pain comorbidity: a literature review. Arch Intern Med. 2003;163(20):2433–45.
20. Holzberg AD, Robinson ME, Geisser ME, Gremillion HA. The effects of depression and chronic pain on psychosocial and physical functioning. Clin J Pain. 1996;12(2):118–25.
21. Gameroff MJ, Olfson M. Major depressive disorder, somatic pain, and health care costs in an urban primary care practice. J Clin Psychiatry. 2006;67(8):1232–9.
22. Solomon S, Lipton RB. Headaches and face pains as a manifestation of Munchausen syndrome. Headache. 1999;39(1):45–50.
23. Mongini F, Ciccone G, Ibertis F, Negro C. Personality characteristics and accompanying symptoms in temporomandibular joint dysfunction, headache, and facial pain. J Orofac Pain. 2000;14(1):52–8.
24. Hayashi H, Sumino R, Sessle BJ. Functional organization of trigeminal subnucleus interpolaris: nociceptive and innocuous afferent inputs, projections to thalamus, cerebellum, and spinal cord, and descending modulation from periaqueductal gray. J Neurophysiol. 1984;51(5):890–905.
25. Linnman C, Moulton EA, Barmettler G, Becerra L, Borsook D. Neuroimaging of the periaqueductal gray: state of the field. Neuroimage. 2012;60(1):505–22.
26. Meerwijk EL, Ford JM, Weiss SJ. Brain regions associated with psychological pain: implications for a neural network and its relationship to physical pain. Brain Imaging Behav. 2013;7(1):1–14.
27. Rawdin BJ, Mellon SH, Dhabhar FS, et al. Dysregulated relationship of inflammation and oxidative stress in major depression. Brain Behav Immun. 2013;31:143–52.
28. Turner JA, Mancl L, Aaron LA. Short- and long-term efficacy of brief cognitive-behavioral therapy for patients with chronic temporomandibular disorder pain: a randomized, controlled trial. Pain. 2006;121(3):181–94.
29. Jannetta P. Trigeminal neuralgia. New York: Oxford University Press; 2011.
30. Obermann M, Katsarava Z. Update on trigeminal neuralgia. Expert Rev Neurother. 2009;9(3):323–9.
31. Obermann M, Yoon MS, Ese D, et al. Impaired trigeminal nociceptive processing in patients with trigeminal neuralgia. Neurology. 2007;69(9):835–41.
32. Lutz J, Linn J, Mehrkens JH, et al. Trigeminal neuralgia due to neurovascular compression: high-spatial-resolution diffusion-tensor imaging reveals microstructural neural changes. Radiology. 2011;258(2):524–30.

33. Spinner D, Kirschner JS. Accuracy of ultrasound-guided superficial trigeminal nerve blocks using methylene blue in cadavers. Pain Med. 2012;13(11):1469–73.

34. McLeod NM, Patton DW. Peripheral alcohol injections in the management of trigeminal neuralgia. Oral Surg Oral Med Oral Pathol Oral Radiol Endod. 2007;104(1):12–7.

35. Shah SA, Khan MN, Shah SF, Ghafoor A, Khattak A. Is peripheral alcohol injection of value in the treatment of trigeminal neuralgia? An analysis of 100 cases. Int J Oral Maxillofac Surg. 2011;40(4):388–92.

36. Ammori MB, King AT, Siripurapu R, Herwadkar AV, Rutherford SA. Factors influencing decision-making and outcome in the surgical management of trigeminal neuralgia. J Neurol Surg B Skull Base. 2013;74(2):75–81.

37. Brzustowicz RJ. Combined trigeminal and glossopharyngeal neuralgia. Neurology. 1955;5(1):1–10.

38. Bodal A. The vagus and glossopharyngeal nerves. In: Broda A, editor. Anatomy in relation to clinical medicine. New York: Oxford University Press; 1969. p. 363–74.

39. Pearce JM. Glossopharyngeal neuralgia. Eur Neurol. 2006;55(1):49–52.

40. Teixeira MJ, de Siqueira SR, Bor-Seng-Shu E. Glossopharyngeal neuralgia: neurosurgical treatment and differential diagnosis. Acta Neurochir (Wien). 2008;150(5):471–5. discussion 475.

41. Rushton JG, Stevens JC, Miller RH. Glossopharyngeal (vago-glossopharyngeal) neuralgia: a study of 217 cases. Arch Neurol. 1981;38(4):201–5.

42. Sampson JH, Grossi PM, Asaoka K, Fukushima T. Microvascular decompression for glossopharyngeal neuralgia: long-term effectiveness and complication avoidance. Neurosurgery. 2004;54(4):884–9. discussion 889-890.

43. Tubbs R, Steck DT, Mortazavi MM. The nervus intermedius: a review of its anatomy, function, pathology, and role of neurosurgery. World Neurosurg. 2013;79(5–6):763–7.

44. Yentur EA, Yegul I. Nervus intermedius neuralgia: an uncommon pain syndrome with an uncommon etiology. J Pain Symptom Manage. 2000;19(6):407–8.

45. Bruyn GW. Nervus intermedius neuralgia (Hunt). Cephalalgia. 1984;4(1):71–8.

46. Woolf CJ, Max MB. Mechanism-based pain diagnosis: issues for analgesic drug development. Anesthesiology. 2001;95(1):241–9.

47. Philip A, Thakur R. Post herpetic neuralgia. J Palliat Med. 2011;14(6):765–73.

48. Argoff CE. Review of current guidelines on the care of postherpetic neuralgia. Postgrad Med. 2011;123(5):134–42.

49. Fields HL, Rowbotham M, Baron R. Postherpetic neuralgia: irritable nociceptors and deafferentation. Neurobiol Dis. 1998;5(4):209–27.

50. Kumar A, Brennan MT. Differential diagnosis of orofacial pain and temporomandibular disorder. Dent Clin North Am. 2013;57(3):419–28.

51. Scrivani SJ, Keith DA, Kaban LB. Temporomandibular disorders. New Engl J Med. 2008;359(25):2693–2705.

52. Borg-Stein J. Treatment of fibromyalgia, myofascial pain, and related disorders. Phys Med Rehabil Clin N Am. 2006;17(2):491–510. 2.

Post-Herpetic Neuralgia

18

Phong Kieu and SriKrishna Chandran

Abbreviations

DNA	Deoxyribonucleic acid
GABA	Gamma-Aminobutyric Acid
HZ	Herpes Zoster
PHN	Post-herpetic neuralgia
PO	Per os (by mouth)
TCA	Tricyclic antidepressant
TID	Three in a day
VZV	Varicella zoster virus

Definitions

- *Varicella-zoster virus (VZV) infection*: [1]
  - *Primary infection*: chicken pox—vesicular lesions in different stages typically on face, trunk, and extremities
  - *Herpes zoster (HZ)*: shingles—reactivation of latent varicella-zoster virus within the sensory ganglia causes painful vesicular eruption usually restricted to a unilateral dermatomal distribution
- *Post-herpetic neuralgia (PHN)*: previously described as persistence of pain after 30 days from disappearance of rash, but a newer classification has since been devised [2]
  - *Acute herpetic neuralgia*: pain accompanying rash that persists up to 30 days
  - *Subacute herpetic neuralgia*: pain persisting after rash from 30 to 120 days
  - *PHN*: pain persisting after rash for > 120 days

P. Kieu, M.D.
John Peter Smith, Orthopedics and Sports Medicine,
11 White Ave., Worcester, MA, USA
e-mail: pkieu@rocketmail.com

S. Chandran, M.D. (✉)
Department of Physical Medicine and Rehabilitation, Johns Hopkins Hospital,
817 Lakewood Drive, Rochester Hills, MI 48309, USA
e-mail: krishchan79@gmail.com

Epidemiology and Risk Factors

- A Harvard study in 2008 found the annual incidence for herpes zoster to be 0.47 cases per 1,000 patients [3].
  - 17.6 % of those patients progressed to developing PHN [3]
- *Risk factors*
  - Age: Older age is the most consistent risk factor in most studies [4]
  - Greater acute pain: Severe pain with HZ is a strong predictor for PHN [4]
  - Severity of rash: Positive correlation with the number of lesions present initially [5]
  - Association with presence and duration of symptoms: Includes pain, dysesthesia, and allodynia [5]
  - Other risk factors—not strongly supported in the literature [2]:
    - Ophthalmic and thoracic zoster
    - Smoking
    - Psychosocial factors

Etiology

- Pathophysiology of HZ: Hemorrhagic inflammation of the peripheral nerve, dorsal root, and dorsal root ganglion with occasional extension into the spinal cord [6].
- Pathophysiology behind the development of PHN is still under debate:
  - Fibrosis is noted in the dorsal root ganglion, nerve root, and peripheral nerve upon resolution of the acute process [7].
  - Potential strengthening of synaptic connections between central pain pathways and peripheral fibers [8].
  - No consistent link between neurotransmitters and PHN has been found [9]
  - Suspected ongoing VZV viral replication [10]
- *An individual who has not been exposed to VZV may be able to contract the virus from an individual with cutaneous lesions via direct cutaneous contact or by aerosolized droplet [1].*

K.A. Sackheim, *Pain Management and Palliative Care: A Comprehensive Guide*,
DOI 10.1007/978-1-4939-2462-2_18, © Springer Science+Business Media New York 2015

Clinical Presentation

- PHN is often described as a continuation of the initial pain from HZ infection [2].
  - Rarely will recurrence occur after months to years of complete resolution of initial pain with the HZ infection [11].
    - If this occurs, it is usually triggered by a traumatic event to the area.
  - Can last months to years
- Typically follows a dermatomal pattern (Fig. 18.1)
- Most commonly affected dermatomes are [12]:
  - Thoracic (T4–T6)
  - Cervical
  - Trigeminal nerves
- **Symptoms**:
  - Pain is usually described as a "burning" sensation [13]
  - May be described as numbness, itching, or tingling
  - Most patients will develop other neurologic changes [14]:
    - Hyperaesthesia

- Allodynia
- Anesthesia: deficits in thermal, tactile, pinprick, and vibration sensation
- **Associated symptoms**: fatigue, impaired sleep, anorexia, and decreased libido [11]

Ocular Shingles can present with:
- **Symptoms**
  - Visual defects
  - May lead to glaucoma, scarring, and blindness
  - Pain
  - Sensitivity to light
  - Changes in vision
  - Foreign body sensation
- **Physical Exam**
  - Tenderness, vesicular distribution around the eye or eyelid, swelling, redness, blisters at the nose
  - If blisters at the nose are present, patient should see an ophthalmologist promptly

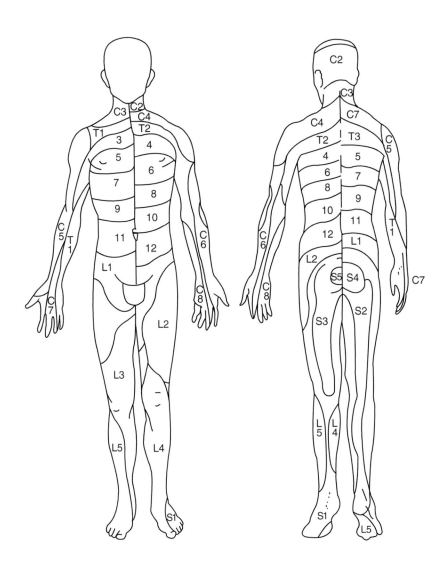

Fig. 18.1 Dermatomal map. Numbers indicate cervical, thoracic, lumbar, and sacral levels based on body location. With permission from Strasfeld L. Infectious complications. In: Maziarz RT, Slater S, eds. Blood and Marrow Transplant Handbook; Springer, New York, 2010:143. © Springer 2010 [50]

Treatment

Acute herpes zoster

1. Pain relief modalities:
   - Cold packs, cold water baths, cool wet cloths
   - Cover rash with loose nonsterile bandages
   - Loose fitting cotton clothing
   - Lotions containing Calamine may be used on blisters or open wounds to decrease pain and pruritis
   - Anesthetic ointments such as capsaicin and lidocaine patches may be used after lesions have crusted over
2. Oral medications: (see more details in medication chapters)
   (a) *Antivirals*:
      - DNA polymerase inhibitors
      - Studies show that during acute onset, *treatment started within 72 h of onset* may shorten duration of disease [1]:
         - Acyclovir (Zovirax) 800 mg PO 5×/day×7 days
            - May use 5 % ointment up to 6×/day×7 days for lesions, but avoid use in eyes
         - Famciclovir (Famvir) 500 mg PO TID×7 days
         - Valacyclovir (Valtrex) 1,000 mg PO q8 h×7 days
   (b) *Tricyclic antidepressants (TCA)*:
      - Inhibit the reuptake of norepinephrine and serotonin in the central nervous system and increase the inhibition of nociceptive signals from the periphery [15, 16].
      - It may take up to 3 weeks before TCAs begin to reduce pain.
      - Commonly used as a treatment PHN, but may be started during the acute process.
   (c) *Corticosteroids*:
      - Orally administered corticosteroids, such as prednisone, has been commonly used in conjunction with an antiviral if administered as early as possible in the disease process.
         - Prednisone 40–60 mg PO daily×7 days and then a rapid taper over 1–2 weeks (or an equivalent dose of another corticosteroid)
      - Studies have shown that they decrease pain at 3 and 12 months, but others also have shown no benefit.
      - Due to theoretical risk of immunosuppression and progression of disease, it has fallen out of favor except in cases with significant swelling.
   (d) *Opiates*:
      - Considered a part of the comprehensive treatment of acute herpes zoster infection.
      - Pain can range from mild to excruciating

   - Regular dosing schedules are recommended over "as needed" dosing during this phase.
   (e) *Special cases, ocular herpes zoster*:
      - Due to risk of glaucoma, scarring, and blindness, prompt ophthalmology referral is strongly recommended
   (f) Prevention (see below in prevention section)

PHN Treatment

1. Aspirin and NSAID medications have limited value.
2. *Tricyclic antidepressants (TCA)*:
   - Its efficacy for the treatment in PHN has been demonstrated in several studies [17, 18].
   - Several systematic reviews have proven that they are superior to SSRIs [19, 20].
   - Side effects are typically anticholinergic, sedation and dry mouth, which reduce patient compliance.
   - Side effects such as QT prolongation, blurred vision, and weight gain should be taken into consideration when prescribing TCAs.
   - In one study, nortriptyline was shown to be better tolerated than amitriptyline [21].
3. *Anticonvulsants*:
   Useful in treatment of PHN, has been noted to reduce the lancinating component of pain.
   (a) *Gabapentin*:
      - Immediate release gabapentin has been shown to be effective in treatment of PHN [22, 23].
      - Extended release gabapentin has had inconsistent data [24].
      - Divided doses of 1,800–3,600 mg daily given for 1–2 weeks have been effective in reducing pain, improving sleep, and quality of life [24].
      - Side effects are drowsiness, dizziness, ataxia, mild peripheral edema, and worsening cognitive impairment in the elderly population.
      - Side effects can be reduced with careful titration [25]
   (b) *Pregabalin*:
      - Structural analog of Gamma-aminobutyric acid (GABA) and similar mechanism to gabapentin.
      - Randomized controlled trials vs. placebo for PHN demonstrated a decrease in pain and improvement in sleep [26–28].
      - Recommended dosage is 150–600 mg daily in divided doses
      - Side effects are drowsiness, dizziness, dry mouth, peripheral edema, and weight gain.
   (c) *Divalproex sodium*
      - Not commonly used, but few studies have shown some effectiveness in treating PHN compared to placebo at dosages of 1,000 mg daily [29].

4. *Opioids*
   - Considered part of the comprehensive treatment for PHN
     - For moderate-to-severe pain, significantly impacted quality of life, and ineffective treatment with first-line agents [2, 30].
   - Opioids improve pain as well as TCAs, and are preferred by patients [31].
   - Other factors including development of tolerance, fear of addiction, and differences in governmental health policies may reduce the prescribing of opioids for PHN [32].
   - Investigated formulations include oxycodone, morphine, fentanyl, buprenorphine, methadone, dihydrocodeine, and tramadol.
   - Treatment should be started with a short-acting opioid and replaced after 1–2 weeks with a long-acting formulation [30].
     - Constipation, nausea, and sedation are common side effects.

5. *Topical agents*
   - Capsaicin:
     - Pungent ingredient in chilli peppers causes excitation of nociceptive afferents when applied topically.
       - Repeated application results in desensitization of unmyelinated epidermal nerve fibers and results in hypoalgesia [33].
     - Few studies have shown that low-concentration capsaicin cream (0.25–0.75 %) provide significant pain relief for PHN [33].
     - Recent studies have shown that a high-concentration capsaicin dermal patch (8 %) may provide rapid and long lasting relief [34].
   - Local analgesics
     - Local analgesics such as topical lidocaine patches (5 %) have been used for the treatment of PHN.
     - However, there is limited data support its use [35].

6. Interventional techniques
   - Sympathetic blocks:
     - Selective sympathetic nerve blocks are commonly used [36].
       - Complications are low, but may include pneumothorax, intraspinal/neuraxial injection, or neurologic injury [37].
     - Evidence is limited, but there are several small studies which have shown that sympathetic blocks are effective for treating PHN and preventing PHN [37–39].
     - After local administration of adrenergic agonists, there appears to be increased levels of pain and worsening of allodynia [40].

   - Intrathecal medications:
     - Intrathecal methylprednisolone has been shown to be effective in recalcitrant cases of PHN in several small studies [41, 43].
     - Other intrathecal medications have also been tried with varying success including morphine, lidocaine, and midazolam [44].
   - Spinal cord stimulator:
     - In extreme cases, spinal cord stimulators may be effective [41, 42, 45].

7. Other:
   - Pulsed radiofrequency, cryoanalgesia, *N*-methyl-D-ASPARTATE receptor antagonists, topical nonsteroidal anti-inflammatory drugs, topical TCAs, vincristine iontophoresis, botulinum toxin, minocycline, transcutaneous nerve stimulations have all been used but not established [2].

8. Surgery:
   - Electrical stimulation of the thalamus, anterolateral cordotomy, and electrocoagulation of the dorsal root, dorsal root entry zone lesions, mesencephalotomy, trigeminal neurectomy have all been described, but there is no consistent benefit and substantial risks [2].

Prevention

- Vaccination:
  - Vaccination for the HZ virus has been shown in multiple studies that it not only reduces the incidence of HZ infection but the incidence of PHN as well [2, 46].
    - It also reduces the pain, severity, and duration.
    - Currently recommended to everyone over the age of 50
  - Antivirals
    - Treatment of an acute HZ infection with antivirals has been described in the literature to reduce the incidence of PHN [47].
    - However, more recent studies have shown that antivirals reduce the severity and duration of PHN, but not its incidence [48, 49].
  - Corticosteroids and antidepressants have been shown to be ineffective in preventing PHN [2].
  - Interventional procedures including epidural steroid injections and sympathetic blocks have been described, but data is limited [2, 39].

References

1. Gnann Jr JW, Whitley RJ. Clinical practice. Herpes zoster. N Engl J Med. 2002;347:340.
2. Tontodonati M, Ursini T, Polilli E, Vadini F, Masi F, Volpone D, Parruti G. Post-herpetic neuralgia. Int J Gen Med. 2012;5:861–71.

3. Klompas M, Kulldorff M, Vilk Y, Bialek SR, Harpaz R. Herpes zoster and postherpetic neuralgia surveillance using structured electronic data. Mayo Clin Proc. 2011;86:1146–53.

4. Whitley RJ, Weiss HL, Soong SJ, Gnann JW. Herpes zoster: risk categories for persistent pain. J Infect Dis. 1999;179:9.

5. Jung BF, Johnson RW, Griffin DR, Dworkin RH. Risk factors for postherpetic neuralgia in patients with herpes zoster. Neurology. 2004;62:1545.

6. Denny-Brown D, Adams RD, Fitzgerald PJ. Pathologic features of herpes zoster: a note on "geniculate herpes". Arch Neurol Psychiatr. 1944;51:216.

7. Bartley J. Post herpetic neuralgia, schwann cell activation and vitamin D. Med Hypotheses. 2009;73:927–9.

8. Baron R, Saguez M. Postherpetic neuralgia: are C-nociceptors involved in signaling and maintenance of tactile allodynia? Brain. 1993;116:1477–96.

9. Watson CP, Morshead C, Van der Kooy D, et al. Post-herpetic neuralgia: post-mortem analysis of a case. Pain. 1988;34:129.

10. Gilden DH, Cohrs RJ, Hayward AR, Wellish M, Mahalingam R. Chronic varicella-zoster virus ganglionitis-a possible cause of postherpetic neuralgia. J Neurovirol. 2003;9(3):404–7.

11. Schott GD. Triggering of delayed-onset postherpetic neuralgia. Lancet. 1998;351:419.

12. Watson CP, Evans RJ, Watt VR, Birkett N. Post-herpetic neuralgia: 208 cases. Pain. 1988;35:289.

13. Johnson RW, Bouhassira D, Kassianos G, et al. The impact of herpes zoster and post-herpetic neuralgia on quality-of-life. BMC Med. 2010;8:37.

14. Bowsher D. Pathophysiology of postherpetic neuralgia: towards a rational treatment. Neurology. 1995;45:S56.

15. Dubner R, Bennett GJ. Spinal and trigeminal mechanisms of nociception. Annu Rev Neurosci. 1983;6:381.

16. Basbaum AI, Fields HL. Endogenous pain control mechanisms: review and hypothesis. Ann Neurol. 1978;4:451.

17. Argoff CE. Review of current guidelines on the care of postherpetic neuralgia. Postgrad Med. 2011;123:134.

18. Watson CP, Evans RJ, Reed K, et al. Amitriptyline versus placebo in postherpetic neuralgia. Neurology. 1982;32:671.

19. Hempenstall K, Nurmikko TJ, Johnson RW, A'Hern RP, Rice AS. Analgesic therapy in postherpetic neuralgia: a quantitative systematic review. PLoS Med. 2005;2(7):e164.

20. Attal N, Cruccu G, Baron R, Haanpaa M, Hansson P, Jensen TS, Nurmikko T. EFNS guidelines on pharmacological treatment of neuropathic pain. Eur J Neurol. 2006;13(11):1153–69.

21. Watson CP, Vernich L, Chipman M, Reed K. Nortriptyline versus amitriptyline in postherpetic neuralgia: a randomized trial. Neurology. 1998;51:1166.

22. Rowbotham M, Harden N, Stacey B, et al. Gabapentin for the treatment of postherpetic neuralgia: a randomized controlled trial. JAMA. 1998;280:1837.

23. Rice AS, Maton S, Postherpetic Neuralgia Study Group. Gabapentin in postherpetic neuralgia: a randomised, double blind, placebo controlled study. Pain. 2001;94(2):215–24.

24. Moore RA, Wiffen PJ, Derry S, McQuay HJ. Gabapentin for chronic neuropathic pain and fibromyalgia in adults. Cochrane Database Syst Rev. 2011;3, CD007938.

25. Mustafa MB, Arduino PG, Porter SR. Varicella zoster virus: review of its management. J Oral Pathol Med. 2009;38(9):673–88.

26. Dworkin RH, Corbin AE, Young Jr JP, et al. Pregabalin for the treatment of postherpetic neuralgia: a randomized, placebo-controlled trial. Neurology. 2003;60:1274.

27. Sabatowski R, Gálvez R, Cherry DA, et al. Pregabalin reduces pain and improves sleep and mood disturbances in patients with post-herpetic neuralgia: results of a randomised, placebo-controlled clinical trial. Pain. 2004;109:26–35.

28. Pregabalin (lyrica) for neuropathic pain and epilepsy. Med Lett Drugs Ther. 2005;47(1217):75–6.

29. Kochar DK, Garg P, Bumb RA, et al. Divalproex sodium in the management of post-herpetic neuralgia: a randomized double-blind placebo-controlled study. QJM. 2005;98:29.

30. Cohen SP, Raja SN. The middle way: a practical approach to prescribing opioids for chronic pain. Nat Clin Pract Neurol. 2006;2(11):580–1.

31. Raja SN, Haythornthwaite JA, Pappagallo M, et al. Opioids versus antidepressants in postherpetic neuralgia: a randomized, placebo-controlled trial. Neurology. 2002;59:1015.

32. Wu CL, Raja SN. An update on the treatment of postherpetic neuralgia. J Pain. 2008;9(1 suppl 1):S19–30.

33. Nolano M, Simone DA, Wendelschafer-Crabb G, Johnson T, Hazen E, Kennedy WR. Topical capsaicin in humans: parallel loss of epidermal nerve fibers and pain sensation. Pain. 1999; 81:135–45.

34. Backonja M, Wallace MS, Blonsky ER, et al. NGX-4010, a high-concentration capsaicin patch, for the treatment of postherpetic neuralgia: a randomised, double-blind study. Lancet Neurol. 2008;7:1106.

35. Khaliq W, Alam S, Puri N. Topical lidocaine for the treatment of postherpetic neuralgia. Cochrane Database Syst Rev. 2007;2, CD004846.

36. Janig W, Levine JD, Michaelis M. Interactions of sympathetic and primary afferent neurons following nerve injury and tissue trauma. Prog Brain Res. 1996;113:161–84.

37. Van Wijck AJ, Wallace M, Mekhail N, van Kleef M. Evidence-based interventional pain medicine according to clinical diagnoses. 17. Herpes zoster and post-herpetic neuralgia. Pain Pract. 2011;11(1):88–97.

38. Agarwal-Kozlowski K, Lorke DE, Habermann CR, Schulte am Esch J, Beck H. Interventional management of intractable sympathetically mediated pain by computed tomography-guided catheter implantation for block and neuroablation of the thoracic sympathetic chain: technical approach and review of 322 procedures. Anaesthesia. 2011;66(8):699–708.

39. Makharita MY, Amr YM, El-Bayoumy Y. Effect of early stellate ganglion blockade for facial pain from acute herpes zoster and incidence of postherpetic neuralgia. Pain Physician. 2012;15(6): 467–74.

40. Choi B, Rowbotham MC. Effect of adrenergic receptor activation on post-herpetic neuralgia pain and sensory disturbances. Pain. 1997;69:55–63.

41. Benzon HT, Chekka K, Darnule A, Chung B, Wille O, Malik K. Evidence-based case report: the prevention and management of postherpetic neuralgia with emphasis on interventional procedures. Reg Anesth Pain Med. 2009;34(5):541–21.

42. Philip A, Thakur R. Post herpetic neuralgia. J Palliat Med. 2011;14(6):765–73.

43. Kotani N, Kushikata T, Hashimoto H, et al. Intrathecal methylprednisolone for intractable postherpetic neuralgia. N Engl J Med. 2000;343:1514.

44. Nitescu P, Dahm P, Appelgren L, Curelaru I. Continuous infusion of opioid and bupivacaine by externalized intrathecal catheters in long-term treatment of "refractory" nonmalignant pain. Clin J Pain. 1998;14:17–28.

45. Lynch PJ, McJunkin T, Eross E, Gooch S, Maloney J. Case report: successful epiradicular peripheral nerve stimulation of the C2 dorsal root ganglion for postherpetic neuralgia. Neuromodulation. 2011;14(1):58–61.

46. Oxman MN, Levin MJ, Johnson GR, et al. A vaccine to prevent herpes zoster and postherpetic neuralgia in older adults. N Engl J Med. 2005;352(22):2271–84.

47. Dworkin RH, Boon RJ, Griffin DR, Phung D. Postherpetic neuralgia: impact of famciclovir, age, rash severity, and acute pain in herpes zoster patients. J Infect Dis. 1998;178 Suppl 1:S76–80.

48. Li Q, Chen N, Yang J, et al. Antiviral treatment for preventing postherpetic neuralgia. Cochrane Database Syst Rev. 2009;2.

49. Vander Straten M, Carrasco D, Lee P, Tyring SK. Reduction of postherpetic neuralgia in herpes zoster. J Cutan Med Surg. 2001;5(5):409–16.

50. Strasfeld L. Infectious complications. In: Maziarz RT, Slater S, editors. Blood and marrow transplant handbook. New York: Springer; 2010. p. 143.

Joint Pain

Niall G. Monaghan and James F. Wyss

Abbreviations

AAROM	Active assisted range of motion
AC	Acromioclavicular
ACL	Anterior cruciate ligament
ACR	American College of Rheumatology
AP	Anteroposterior
AROM	Active range of motion
BMP	Basic metabolic panel
CBC	Complete blood count
ESR	Erythrocyte sedimentation rate
FABER	Flexion, abduction, external rotation
FADIR	Flexion, adduction, internal rotation
FAI	Femoroacetabular impingement
GTN	Glyceryl trinitrate
ITB	Iliotibial band syndrome
LCL	Lateral collateral ligament
MCL	Medial collateral ligament
MRI	Magnetic resonance imaging
NSAID	Non-steroidal anti-inflammatory drug
OA	Osteoarthritis
OT	Occupational therapy
PCL	Posterior cruciate ligament
PFPS	Patellofemoral pain syndrome
PRICE	Protect, rest, ice, compression, elevation
PROM	Passive range of motion
PRP	Platelet-rich plasma
PT	Physical therapy
ROM	Range of motion
SLAP	Lesion superior labrum anterior to posterior lesion
TENS	Transcutaneous electric nerve stimulation
UCL	Ulnar collateral Ligament
US	Ultrasound

N.G. Monaghan, B.A., M.D. (✉)
Department of Rehabilitation Medicine, New York Presbyterian Hospital, Harkness Pavilion 1st Floor, Room 180, 180 Fort Washington Avenue, New York, NY 10032, USA
e-mail: nam2019@nyp.org

J.F. Wyss, M.D., P.T.
Department of Rehabilitation Medicine, Hospital for Special Surgery, Weill Cornell Medical College, 429 E 75th Street, 4th Floor, New York, NY 10021, USA
e-mail: wyssj@hss.edu

Joint Structure, Anatomy, Physiology [1–3]

This chapter will focus on the larger diarthroses (synovial joints). Synovial joints are composed of the joint capsule (the outer layer stratum fibrosum and the inner layer stratum synovium), the joint cavity, a synovial membrane that lines the joint capsule, synovial fluid that lubricates the joint, hyaline cartilage that covers the bony surfaces, and accessory structures adjacent to the joint capsule. Accessory structures include fibrocartilaginous discs, menisci and labrums, ligaments, tendons, fat pads, and bursae. Joints are richly innervated, particularly in the stratum fibrosum. Slow-conducting, unmyelinated C fibers transmit diffuse pain sensation. Nociceptors are located throughout the joint, having been identified via histopathology in the capsule, ligaments, menisci, periosteum, and subchondral bone (Fig. 19.1)..

Shoulder (Fig. 19.2) [2, 5–9]

Intra-articular Pathology

1. **Acromioclavicular (AC) joint sprain**: classified by Rockwood using types I–VI, type I being mild and VI being completely displaced inferiorly.
   - History
     - Often caused by a fall onto shoulder or outstretched arm
   - Examination
     - Step-off deformity if severe

K.A. Sackheim, *Pain Management and Palliative Care: A Comprehensive Guide*,
DOI 10.1007/978-1-4939-2462-2_19, © Springer Science+Business Media New York 2015

131

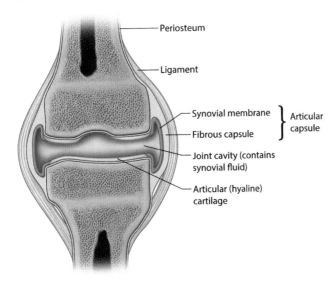

Fig. 19.1 Typical synovial joint anatomy

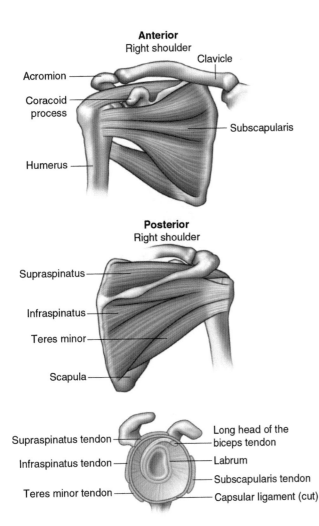

Fig. 19.2 Shoulder joint anatomy (anterior and posterior)

- Tenderness to palpation locally over AC joint
- Possible coexisting subacromial impingement and rotator cuff pathology
- Workup
  - X-ray
    - AP view with shoulder in neutral, internal, and external rotation
    - Transcapular Y view
    - Axillary view
    - 15° cephalic tilt view of the AC joint
- Treatment
  - Generally, types I–III are managed conservatively while types IV–VI (and type III that fails conservative management) require surgical repair
  - Types I–III: initially ice and immobilization in splint, then progressive ROM exercises, isometric strength training in PT when pain permits
  - Pain control with NSAIDs and topicals or stronger agents if required

2. **Glenohumeral subluxation**, **dislocation**: usually traumatic with anterior dislocation being most common, where arm is forced into excessive abduction and external rotation.

Anterior dislocations can result in an osseous defect in the posterolateral head of the humerus, known as a Hill–Sachs lesion. Often concomitant avulsion of the anterior glenoid rim (Bankart lesion).

Posterior dislocations are often associated with seizures. Recurrent subluxations without dislocation are often misdiagnosed as rotator cuff tendonitis.

Chronic atraumatic multidirectional instability of the shoulder can occur secondary to biomechanical factors such as shallow socket, lax ligaments, or weak muscles. Subluxation can be seen in stroke patients on the hemiparetic side.

- History
  - Often acute trauma
  - Sensation of arm "popping out"
  - Pain described as "dead arm"
- Examination
  - Obvious deformity if dislocated
  - Sulcus sign in subluxation
  - Examine for possible damage to axillary, radial, and/or musculocutaneous nerve causing weakness and paresthesias
  - May have concomitant supraspinatus tear
- Workup
  - X-ray prior to reduction, if not already done in the field, to rule out fracture
  - X-ray is usually normal in subluxation
  - MRI for investigation of damage to labrum and rotator cuff muscles

- Treatment
  - If dislocation exists, reduction as soon as possible as this procedure becomes more difficult to perform as time passes
  - After reduction, immobilization with sling, then PT focusing rotator cuff and scapular strengthening with gradual restoration of ROM
  - Surgical consultation for stabilization after reduction in young athletes might be considered as re-injury and disability is higher in this population
  - For stroke patients with a subluxed and painful shoulder, slings, arm troughs, lap boards, PT/OT, and electric stimulation can be used

3. **Labral tears**: labrum is a ring of fibrocartilaginous tissue attached to the glenoid fossa creating a deeper socket and therefore more stability for the glenohumeral joint. Plays a role in proprioception and load distribution. The joint capsule, glenohumeral ligaments, and the long head of the biceps tendon attach to the labrum. SLAP lesions (superior labrum anterior to posterior) are the most common labral tears and are graded from type I to IV.
   - History
     - Caused by sudden downward force on the long head of the biceps pulling on the labrum, for example, when catching a heavy object or falling on outstretched arm when shoulder is in abduction and slight forward flexion
     - Pain usually localized to the posterior–superior joint line, worse in abduction and overhead activities
     - Patient may report grinding, catching, and popping sensation with movement
   - Examination
     - Tenderness along posterior joint line
     - Decreased ROM in abduction and flexion secondary to pain
     - Joint laxity
     - Special maneuvers include dynamic labral shear test and O'Brien test (AKA active compression test)
   - Workup
     - If diagnosis is unclear after history and physical, MRI can confirm
     - MRI arthrogram in certain settings is considered to be more sensitive
   - Treatment
     - If patient is physically active and has an unstable tear (SLAP type II–IV), surgical repair should be considered
     - For type I tears and with older, less active patients, conservative treatment with NSAIDs, and PT focusing on scapular stabilization followed by

rotator cuff strengthening exercises should be pursued first

4. **Adhesive capsulitis (frozen shoulder)**: characterized by limited ROM with pain at end range. Typically, diffuse pain in the shoulder becomes progressively worse, followed by decreased ROM. Exact etiology is unclear but risk factors include diabetes, parkinsonism, thyroid disease, neoplasm near the shoulder, and CAD. It is often initiated by mild trauma. This trauma causes diffuse inflammation of the synovium and adherence to the joint capsule.
   Described in three stages:
   Stage 1: painful/freezing stage lasting weeks to several months
   Stage 2: adhesive/stiffening phase where pain decreases and lasts 4–12 months
   Stage 3: thawing stage lasting 2–26 months. This process is generally self-limiting, on average lasting 1.5 years.
   - History
     - Most common in females in their 40s and 50s
     - Pain described as dull ache around entire shoulder
     - Loss of motion over a few months
     - Discomfort when sleeping
   - Examination
     - Limited passive and active ROM particularly with passive external rotation with arm placed in 90° of abduction or while elbow is placed at the side
   - Workup
     - If minimal to no trauma, obtain CBC, ESR, BMP, thyroid function test to screen for metabolic and systemic risk factors
     - X-ray in AP, axillary and scapular Y view
     - Bone scan if there is suspicion of neoplasm
   - Treatment
     - Limit immobilization while also avoiding aggressive PROM in PT
     - Gentle A/AA/PROM, heat, TENS (transcutaneous electrical nerve stimulation), NSAIDs, and corticosteroid/lidocaine injections during stage I
     - Usually self-limiting, if detected early, strongly consider intra-articular corticosteroid injection performed with image guidance; if no improvement with conservative management in 6 months, consider manipulation under general anesthesia or surgical management especially if other pathology such as calcific tendonitis or impingement coexists

5. **Osteoarthritis (OA)**: not the most common site for OA, but when present in the shoulder, there is often a history of activities that cause repeated microtrauma, or any condition that can alter the articular cartilage to properly bear weight

- History
  - Insidious, dull ache
  - Pain with movement especially external rotation
- Examination
  - Pain with movement or limited ROM
  - Possible crepitus
- Workup
  - Radiographs may show joint space narrowing, osteophytes, sclerosis, or subchondral cysts
  - CT will be necessary if considering arthroplasty
- Treatment
  - Often responds well to conservative treatment
  - Acetaminophen is the first-line pharmacological treatment, followed by NSAIDs
  - PT to improve ROM and strengthening for joint stability
  - Can consider intra-articular anesthetic/corticosteroid injection and the authors recommend using image guidance (ultrasound or fluoroscopy)
  - Some clinicians are using off-label treatment with viscosupplementation to treat this condition; this has not yet been supported by the literature
  - If severe, arthroplasty

Extra-articular

1. **Rotator cuff impingement and tears**: very common cause of nontraumatic shoulder pain. Impingement is an overuse injury in the setting of encroachment on the rotator cuff muscles (supraspinatus, infraspinatus, subscapularis, and teres minor) by the acromion, coracoacromial ligament, coracoid process, and/or AC joint. Impingement can be external (subacromial) and internal (posterior–superior glenoid). Commonly, in primary external impingement, the supraspinatus outlet narrows due to acromion bone spur formation and degenerative changes in the AC joint. Impingement can lead to tearing of the rotator cuff muscles. Tears rarely occur nontraumatically in healthy patients; there is either history of acute trauma such as falling on an outstretched arm or underlying pathology such as RA, SLE, or frequent corticosteroid injections.
   - History
     - Usually insidious dull ache located in posterior and lateral shoulder
     - Worse with overhead activity
     - Discomfort while sleeping on affected side
     - History of repetitive shoulder motion or overuse injury
     - Tears can happen traumatically in an otherwise healthy shoulder
   - Examination
     - Pain with elevation between 70 and 110° described as a "painful arc"
     - Pain/weakness in abduction and external rotation

     - Limited internal rotation
     - Tenderness in supraspinatus outlet or at the greater tuberosity of the humerus
     - Special maneuvers include Neer's, Hawkin's, and empty can tests
   - Workup
     - X-ray may reveal hooked acromion, and in later stages narrowing of the of the acromiohumeral gap, superior subluxation of the humeral head, and are also useful in acute traumatic cases to rule out dislocation and fracture
     - US and MRI can evaluate rotator cuff muscles for tears
   - Treatment
     - Short period of rest (prolonged immobilization can predispose to adhesive capsulitis)
     - Then progressive rehabilitation effort to restore ROM, flexibility, especially of the posterior capsule, scapular mechanics, and strengthening
     - Ice
     - NSAIDs
     - Judicious use of subacromial corticosteroid/anesthetic injections can aid in pain relief and tolerance to PT
     - Consider OT ergonomic evaluation if overuse injury at work is suspected
     - Recent studies found topical glyceryl trinitrate (GTN) can improve pain, increase range of motion, and decrease shoulder impingement
     - For severe impingement, full-thickness tears, failure of 3–6 months of conservative management or symptomatic calcified tendonitis, surgical evaluation is warranted

2. **Biceps tendonitis**: often occurs where the long head of the biceps tendon passes through the bicipital groove while traversing to the superior glenoid
   - History
     - Pain in anterior shoulder
     - Often an overuse injury
   - Examination
     - Tenderness at bicipital groove which will move laterally as the arm is externally rotated in an adducted position
     - Special maneuvers include Yergason's and Speed's tests
   - Workup
     - Rule out concomitant injuries such as rotator cuff tear and/or labral tear
     - Can use US to examine the tendon in bicipital groove
   - Treatment
     - Acutely use ice, NSAIDs, topical patches, or creams
     - PT for decreasing pain and to restore ROM, strength, and function
     - Severe cases may warrant corticosteroid injection at the tendon sheath

Elbow [2, 5, 10–12]

Intra-articular

1. **Osteoarthritis (OA)**: the elbow is a rare site for OA, usually caused by trauma, crystal arthropathies, or repeated vibration exposure. See shoulder OA section for history, exam, workup, and treatment
2. **Ulnar collateral ligament (UCL) sprain**: commonly seen in overhead athletes, particularly baseball pitchers. The ligament can become inflamed, develop calcification and if severe, can rupture.
   - History
     – Usually occurs chronically when repetitive valgus stress is placed on the elbow (e.g., in the overhead throwing athlete), but on rare occasions may occur acutely or can have an acute-on-chronic presentation
   - Examination
     – Tenderness at medial elbow
     – Laxity/pain when valgus stress is placed on elbow
   - Workup
     – MRI may help confirm and determine severity of sprain, but visualization and stress tests at the time of arthroscopy are considered the gold standard to assess for UCL insufficiency
   - Treatment
     – Acutely use rest, ice, and NSAIDs
     – Then strengthening of forearm flexors and pronators
     – Some athletes undergo reconstruction

Extra-articular

1. **Lateral epicondylitis (tennis elbow)**: caused by forearm extensor tendinosis, most commonly the extensor carpi radialis brevis. These muscles stabilize the wrist while gripping and can become injured when a force pushes the wrist into flexion against resistance, as in hitting a tennis ball with the backhand technique (by far not the most common mechanism of injury). This is a common overuse injury that can be caused from a wide range of activities, from racquet sports to typing on a computer.
   - History
     – Usually occurs insidiously over several hours or days of repetitive manual activity, but can also happen acutely, i.e., after one single force is loaded on the extensor tendons
     – Pain is localized to the lateral elbow
     – Made worse with flexion/extension of the wrist and elbow
     – Patient may report pain while carrying heavy objects
   - Examination
     – Tenderness over the lateral epicondyle
     – Pain with resisted wrist extension especially when the elbow is fully extended

– Pain with passive full flexion of the wrist
– Special maneuvers include Cozen's and Mill's test
   - Workup
     – Typically a clinical diagnosis, but X-rays can be taken to rule out fractures, osteochondritis dissecans, degenerative joint disease, and heterotopic ossification
     – US can be used to confirm tendinosis
   - Treatment
     – Acutely use rest, ice, counterforce bracing; the role of NSAIDs has been questioned and corticosteroid injections may actually make the condition worse long term
     – Correction of ergonomics (or technique if incurred during sports)
     – PT focusing on pain-free ROM, and concentric followed by eccentric strengthening of wrist extensors
     – Some studies show platelet-rich plasma (PRP) injections are superior to corticosteroid injections for pain reduction in patients with chronic lateral epicondylosis
2. **Medial epicondylitis (golfer's elbow)**: similar to lateral epicondylitis, but the flexors tendons of the forearm are affected and is much less common. The pronator teres is most commonly implicated.
   - History/examination/workup/treatment
     – Similar to lateral epicondylitis, although obviously the medial epicondyle will have tenderness to palpation
     – Pain is elicited by having the patient flex the wrist and/or pronate against resistance
     – The ulnar nerve passes close to the medial epicondyle and can therefore be compressed by surrounding inflammation so neurovascular exam of the elbow, forearm, and hand should be performed
     – If instability is present or suspected, ulnar collateral ligament insufficiency should be considered in the differential
3. **Olecranon bursitis**: trauma can lead to inflammation of this subcutaneous bursa, which may then fill with serosanguinous fluid. Infection can occur via normal skin flora entering the bursa through breaks in the skin.
   - History
     – Acute trauma (i.e., falling onto posterior elbow)
     – Chronic repetitive trauma (i.e., prolonged weight bearing on elbows)
   - Examination
     – Visible swollen bursa may be noted
     – Tenderness, bogginess at posterior elbow
     – Excessive warmth, erythema, and pain suggest infection
   - Workup
     – US can confirm excess fluid in the bursa
     – If infection or crystal arthropathy is suspected, perform fluid aspiration with Gram stain and culture

- Treatment
  - Rest, ice, NSAIDs, compression
  - If conservative treatment fails, aspiration, then injection of local anesthetic and corticosteroid as long as infection is not suspected

Hip (Fig. 19.3) [2, 5, 13–16]

Intra-articular

1. **Osteoarthritis (OA):** this is the most prevalent pathology of the hip and a common site for OA largely because the hip bears a significant amount of body weight, which usually presents as unilateral, but can have a bilateral presentation in up to 42 % of cases. This is a degenerative process primarily affecting the articular cartilage. Hip OA can be primary/idiopathic, once considered to be the most common form, resulting from wear and tear, or secondary where the etiology such as history of major trauma, intra-articular infection, dysplasia, and femoroacetabular impingement (FAI) can be identified. With better understanding of FAI, secondary hip OA might be more common than primary (Tables 19.1 and 19.2).
   - History
     - Pain localized to the groin
     - Stiffness
     - Increased pain with weight bearing
   - Examination
     - Antalgic gait
     - Painful/loss of ROM especially internal rotation
     - Special maneuvers include Stinchfield, FABER, and FADIR tests
   - Workup
     - X-ray, preferably taken while weight bearing

- Changes in usual order of appearance: joint space narrowing, subchondral sclerosis, osteophytes, subchondral cysts
- Treatment
  - Start patient on exercise program as guided by a physical therapist
  - If overweight, add goal of weight reduction
  - For analgesia, start with acetaminophen, followed by NSAIDs, and then tramadol if pain is not controlled
  - Opioids can be cautiously considered if pain is still poorly controlled, or if patient is not a surgical candidate in severe cases
  - Fluoroscopically or US-guided corticosteroid and anesthetic injections delivered intra-articularly have been shown to improve pain and ROM
  - Hip resurfacing or total hip arthroplasty is necessary in severe cases

2. **Labral tears:** the acetabular labrum is a ring of fibrocartilagenous tissue that deepens the hip socket, providing more stabilization. Only the outer one-third is

Table 19.1 American College of Rheumatology (ACR) non-pharmacologic recommendations for the management of hip osteoarthritis (OA)

ACR strongly recommends:
Participation in cardiovascular and/or resistance land-based or aquatic exercise
Weight loss (for persons who are overweight)
ACR conditionally recommends:
Participation in self-management programs
Receiving manual therapy in combination with supervised exercise
Receiving psychosocial interventions
Instruction in the use of thermal agents
Walking aids, as needed
ACR has no recommendations regarding the following:
Participation in balance exercises, either alone or in combination with strengthening exercises
Participation in tai chi
Receiving manual therapy alone

Table 19.2 American College of Rheumatology's (ACR) pharmacologic recommendations for the initial management of hip OA

ACR conditionally recommends:
Acetaminophen
Oral NSAIDs
Tramadol
Intra-articular corticosteroid injections
ACR conditionally recommends against the following:
Chondroitin sulfate
Glucosamine
ACR has no recommendations regarding the following:
Topical NSAIDs
Intra-articular hyaluronate injections
Duloxetine
Opioid analgesics

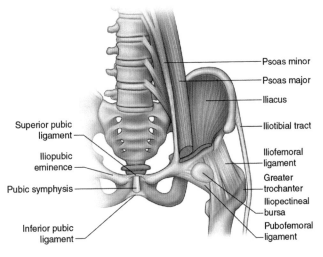

Fig. 19.3 Hip joint anatomy

vascularized, but nociceptive fibers are found throughout the structure. It is thinnest anteriorly, and this is where most tears occur. FAI and developmental dysplasia of the hip are risk factors. There are type I tears (labrum is detached from the articular cartilage) and type II (cleavage tears).

- History
  - Hip pain and/or bothersome clicking, catching, or popping sensations with movement
  - Often seen in athletic/active populations
- Examination
  - Pain and/or clicking with PROM
  - Special maneuvers include FADIR and FABER tests
- Workup
  - Properly sequenced MRI or MR arthrogram is the best noninvasive imaging study to confirm a labral tear
  - Arthroscopy is the gold standard for diagnosis
- Treatment
  - Activity modification, such as avoiding activities that require excessive flexion with internal rotation
  - PT focusing on neuromuscular control and strengthening of deep stabilizing muscles
  - If conservative measures fail, active patients might require hip arthroscopy for repair or debridement and to address possible causative factors (e.g., FAI)

Extra-articular

1. **Greater trochanteric bursitis**: AKA Greater Trochanteric Pain Syndrome because gluteus medius tendinosis may be more common than bursitis; it is a common cause of lateral hip pain. The trochanteric bursa, the gluteus medius bursa, or the tendinous insertions at the greater trochanter can become painful and possibly inflamed secondary to direct trauma, prolonged weight bearing on one leg, overuse, and sporting injuries. Also consider proximal hamstring tendinosis when pain is near the ischial tuberosity, or iliopsoas tendinosis/bursitis when pain is located more anteriorly.

- History
  - Pain at the lateral hip
  - Worse with activity
  - Pain at night when side-lying
  - History of vigorous activity or recent activity patient is not accustomed to
- Examination
  - Pinpoint and severe tenderness over the greater trochanter
  - +/− Trendelenburg gait
  - FABER test is often positive
- Workup
  - US can show enlarged bursa or tendinosis
  - MRI can determine if there is accompanying tendinopathy, tear, or intra-articular pathology

- Treatment
  - Minimize compression of area
  - Activity modification
  - Ice and NSAIDs
  - PT focusing on strengthening the gluteal muscles and restoration of muscle balance at the pelvis
  - Some studies show that corticosteroid injections reduce pain and increased tolerance to PT, while others show no long-term benefits; alternative injection-based treatments, such as PRP, are currently being investigated

Knee (Fig. 19.4) [2, 4, 5, 13, 17–19]

Intra-articular

1. **Osteoarthritis (OA)**: a progressive, degenerative disorder that initially affects cartilage, then later bone, resulting from idiopathic and mechanical factors. 10 % of people

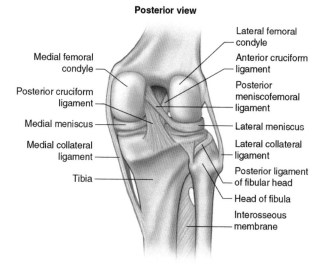

Fig. 19.4 Knee joint anatomy

older than 65 have symptomatic knee OA. Male to female ratio is equal from ages 45–55, after 55 more common in women. Risk factors for knee OA include obesity, malalignment, previous injury, and high-impact vigorous sports. Knee OA can occur in the medial compartment (most common), lateral compartment, the patellofemoral joint (10 % of knee OA), and can progress to tricompartmental involvement.

- History
  - Insidious, dull achy pain, increasing with weight-bearing activity
  - When severe, pain at rest
  - Joint stiffness <30 min, usually after periods of immobility, i.e., upon waking
  - Crepitus, catching, locking, knee giving way
- Examination
  - Possible biomechanical factors such as leg length discrepancy, genu-varum (could indicate medial compartment OA), genu-valgum (could indicate lateral compartment OA)
  - Antalgic gait
  - Swelling/effusion
  - Decreased ROM, crepitus with motion
  - On palpation, joint-line tenderness, warmth
- Workup
  - X-ray is imaging modality of choice, preferably taken while weight bearing; obtain AP, lateral, and merchant views
    - Changes in usual order of appearance: joint space narrowing, subchondral sclerosis, osteophytes, subchondral cysts
- Treatment (Tables 19.1 and 19.2)
  - Initially PRICE (protect, rest, ice, compression, elevation)
  - Tylenol, NSAIDs, Topicals
  - Assistive device to off load weight
  - In PT, aerobic conditioning for long-term improvement, strengthening (with focus on the quadriceps) for short-term pain control
  - Lateral wedge orthotics can be given for medial compartment OA
  - Flexible knee sleeves for mild OA
  - Corrective hinged bracing, also known as unloader braces, for moderate to severe unicompartmental OA
  - Consider aspiration if effusion is affecting ROM and causing pain
  - Trial acetaminophen first, then NSAIDs, tramadol if necessary for pain relief
  - Corticosteroid vs. viscosupplementation injections can be considered to reduce pain
  - Severe cases both clinically and radiologically that are refractory to conservative care require knee arthroplasty

2. **Ligament sprains/tears (ACL, PCL, MCL, LCL)**: these four ligaments, along with the musculature of the knee, stabilize the joint.
   - History
     - Often an acute injury, although can be from overuse
   - Examination
     - Local swelling
     - Point tenderness
     - Ecchymosis
     - Joint laxity
     - Special maneuvers include anterior/posterior drawer, Lachman's test, varus/valgus stress tests
   - Workup
     - MRI is the imaging modality of choice
   - Treatment
     - NSAIDs, topical medications, ice
     - PT (early progressive ROM, strengthening)
     - Hinged bracing
     - Can consider corticosteroid injection at the ligament in severe cases but this can compromise the integrity of the ligament

3. **Patellofemoral pain syndrome (PFPS)**: umbrella term to describe peripatellar and retropatellar pain, this is an overuse injury from repetitive overload at the patellofemoral joint causing maltracking of patella over femoral trochlear groove.
   - History
     - Anterior knee pain
     - Diffuse, vague ache
     - Insidious onset
     - Pain after prolonged sitting or "theater sign"
     - Pain with ascending/descending stairs, downhill running
   - Examination
     - Tenderness to palpation at medial and lateral patellar retinaculum
     - Clicks/crepitus during ROM
     - Restricted movement of patella
     - Special maneuvers include patellar tilt test, patellar mobility test, patellar apprehension test
   - Workup
     - PFPS is a clinical diagnosis
     - Imaging is generally not needed, but can obtain X-rays to better evaluate Q-angle, patella alta/baja, maltracking
   - Treatment
     - Natural history of PFPS is to resolve, but if untreated and does not resolve, chronic symptoms, or even patellofemoral OA can develop
     - Initially, activity modification, icing, NSAIDs
     - Strengthening, taping, and bracing to maintain medial glide

4. **Meniscal tears**: the meniscus is a fibrocartilaginous structure in the knee that helps evenly spread force

between the tibial plateau and the femoral condyles and also provides joint stability and lubrication. The outer third is vascularized while the inner two thirds are not, making central tears less likely to heal. Types of tears include flap, radial, degenerative, longitudinal, and bucket handle tears.

- History
  - Can occur with trauma, often during sudden twisting or cutting motions, but can also occur without inciting injury, particularly in patients with knee OA
  - Pain is often intermittent (the result of an unstable meniscus fragment)
  - Pain localized to the joint line
  - Sensation of clicking, catching, locking, knee giving way
- Examination
  - Joint line tenderness in up to 86 % of cases
  - Effusion
  - Special maneuvers include McMurray's, Apley's, and Thessaly's tests
- Workup
  - Can confirm with MRI, although arthroscopy is the gold standard for diagnosis
- Treatment
  - Initially PRICE (protect, rest, ice, compression, elevation) and crutches/cane to offload weight
  - Acetaminophen, NSAIDs for analgesia
  - PT to strengthen surrounding muscles
  - Partial-thickness longitudinal tears, <5 mm full-thickness tears in the outer third, and minor degenerative tears often do not require surgical intervention

Extra-articular

1. **Iliotibial band (ITB) syndrome**: an overuse injury secondary to impingement or friction of the distal ITB over the lateral femoral epicondyle. It is the most common cause of lateral knee pain in runners.
   - History
     - Pain is usually localized to the lateral epicondyle or Gerdy's tubercle
     - Occurs after repetitive activity such as running and biking
     - Activity that requires more time in the "impingement zone," i.e., at 20–30° of flexion is particularly painful such as downhill running, end of downstroke in cycling
   - Examination
     - Antalgic gait
     - Over pronation or supination
     - Tenderness at the lateral epicondyle, Gerdy's tubercle, and along the ITB
     - Special maneuvers include Thomas's, Ober's, and Noble compression tests
   - Workup
     - Imaging rarely required, can consider US, best used dynamically (during motion)
   - Treatment
     - Activity modification: decrease intensity/duration, usually can avoid complete stoppage of exercise
     - Icing and NSAIDs
     - In PT, stretch tight muscle groups, strengthen hip abductors and extensors
     - Can give corticosteroid injection to anatomic pouch at lateral femoral epicondyle for severe pain

2. **Quadriceps and patellar tendinitis**: AKA jumper's knee, this is a chronic overuse injury of the tendons responsible for knee extension. It is often seen in athletes required to perform repetitive jumping, running, and kicking. Along with patellofemoral pain syndrome, these are the two most common sources of anterior knee pain.
   - History
     - Repetitive loading of the extensor complex
     - Pain with activity, but often diminishes during course of activity, becoming more apparent after completion
     - Pain localized to the inferior or superior pole of the patella
   - Examination
     - Inspection is usually normal
     - Effusions/swelling very rare
     - ROM is usually normal
     - Tenderness at inferior and superior poles of patella
     - Reproducible pain with activity, i.e., jumping
   - Workup
     - Imaging generally not required, particularly in acute phase
     - Could consider US
     - MRI can show tendinopathy, but generally not ordered when considering this diagnosis
   - Treatment
     - Initially activity modification until pain resolves
     - Pain control with icing and NSAIDs
     - Eccentric muscle strengthening in PT
     - Corticosteroid injections have shown to decrease pain
     - In European studies, polidocanol injections have shown to decrease pain and improve function in patients with patellar tendinopathy
     - PRP is an emerging treatment for tendinopathies

Rheumatoid arthritis diagnosis and workup (Table 19.3) [20]

Table 19.3 2010 ACR/EULAR classification criteria for rheumatoid arthritis: score-based algorithm for classification in an eligible patient (cutoff point for RA: 6 or more out of 10)

Joint involvement	0–5
1 medium to large joint	0
2–10 medium to large joints	1
1–3 small joints	2
4–10 small joints	3
>10 joints with at least one small joint	5
Serology	0–3
Negative RF and negative ACPA	0
Low-positive RF or low-positive ACPA	2
High-positive RF or high-positive ACPA	3
Acute-phase reactants	0–1
Normal CRP and ESR	0
Elevated CRP or ESR	1
Duration of symptoms	0–1
<6 weeks	0
≥6 weeks	1

References

1. Levangie PK, Norkin CC, editors. Joint structure and function: a comprehensive analysis. Philadelphia: F.A. Davis; 2005.
2. Firestein GS, editor. Kelley's textbook of rheumatology. 8th ed. Philadelphia: Saunders Elsevier; 2009.
3. McDougall JJ. Arthritis and pain: neurogenic origin of joint pain. Arthritis Res Ther. 2006;8:220.
4. Woolf AD, Pfleger B. Burden of major musculoskeletal conditions. Bull World Health Organ. 2003;81:646–56.
5. Brukner P, Khan K, editors. Brukner and Khan's clinical sports medicine. 4th ed. Sydney: McGraw-Hill; 2012.
6. Reid D, Polson K, Johnson L. Acromioclavicular joint separations grade I-III: a review of the literature and development of best practice guidelines. Sports Med. 2012;42(8):681–96.
7. Stolzenberg D, Siu G, Cruz E. Current and future interventions for glenohumeral subluxation in hemiplegia secondary to stroke. Top Stroke Rehabil. 2012;19(5):444–56.
8. Neviaser AS, Neviaser RJ. Adhesive capsulitis of the shoulder. J Am Acad Orthop Surg. 2011;19(9):536–42.
9. Lin JC, Weintraub N, Aragaki DR. Nonsurgical treatment for rotator cuff injury in the elderly. J Am Med Dir Accoc. 2008; 9(9):626–32.
10. Safran M, Ahmad CS, Elattrache NS. Ulnar collateral ligament of the elbow. Arthroscopy. 2005;21(11):1381–95.
11. Gosens T, Peerbooms JC, van Laar W, den Oudsten BL. Ongoing positive effect of platelet-rich plasma versus corticosteroid injection in lateral epicondylitis: a double-blind randomized controlled trial with 2-year follow-up. Am J Sports Med. 2011;39(6):1200–8. Epub 2011 Mar 21.
12. Coombes BK, Bisset L, Brooks P, Khan A, Vicenzino B. Effect of corticosteroid injection, physiotherapy, or both on clinical outcomes in patients with unilateral lateral epicondylalgia. JAMA. 2013;309(5):461–9.
13. Walter F, editor. Hip osteoarthritis (Chapter 48). In: Essentials of physical medicine and rehabilitation, 2nd edn. Philadelphia: Saunders; 2008.
14. Kullenberg B, Runesson R, Tuvhag R, et al. Intraarticular corticosteroid injection: pain relief in osteoarthritis of the hip? J Rheumatol. 2004;31:2265–8.
15. Hochberg MC, Altman RD, April KT, et al. American College of Rheumatology 2012 recommendations for the use of nonpharmacologic and pharmacologic therapies in osteoarthritis of the hand, hip, and knee. Arthritis Care Res (Hoboken). 2012;64(4): 465–74.
16. Rompe JD, Segal NA, Cacchio A, et al. Home training, local corticosteroid injection, or radial shock wave therapy for greater trochanter pain syndrome. Am J Sports Med. 2009;37(10): 1981–90.
17. Golightly YM, Allen KD, Caine DJ. A comprehensive review of the effectiveness of different exercise programs for patients with osteoarthritis. Phys Sportsmed. 2012;40(4):52–65.
18. Segal NA. Bracing and orthoses: a review of efficacy and mechanical effects for tibiofemoral osteoarthritis. PM R. 2012;4(5 Suppl): S89–96.
19. Hoksrud A, et al. US-guided sclerosis of neovessels in painful chronic patellar tendinopathy. Am J Sports Med. 2006;34(11): 1738–46.
20. Aletaha D, Neogi T, Silman AJ, et al. Rheumatoid arthritis classification criteria: an American College of Rheumatology/European League Against Rheumatism collaborative initiative. Arthritis Rheum. 2010;62:2569–81.

Post-Amputation Pain

Jason W. Siefferman

Abbreviations

ADL	Activities of daily living
CBC	Complete blood count
CRP	C reactive protein
DBS	Deep brain stimulation
DM	Diabetes mellitus
DRG	Dorsal root ganglion
ESR	Erythrocyte sedimentation rate
LE	Lower extremity
MCS	Motor cortex stimulation
NMDA	N-methyl-D-aspartate
PLP	Phantom limb pain
PLS	Phantom limb sensation
RCTs	Randomized controlled trials
RLP	Residual limb pain
ROM	Range of motion
SCS	Spinal cord stimulation
SNRI	Serotonin-norepinephrine reuptake inhibitors
TCA	Tricyclic antidepressant/s
TENS	Transcutaneous electrical nerve stimulation
UE	Upper extremity
WDR	Wide dynamic range

Definitions

- *Phantom limb pain* (*PLP*)—Uncomfortable or bothersome sensation felt in an absent structure (may not be a limb)
- *Phantom limb sensation* (*PLS*)—Non-painful sensation felt in an absent structure

J.W. Siefferman, M.D. (✉)
Division of Pain Medicine, Department of Anesthesiology,
New York University School of Medicine, New York, NY, USA

Manhattan Pain Medicine, New York, NY, USA
e-mail: jsiefferman@gmail.com

- *Residual limb pain* (*RLP*)—Discomfort localized to the distal portion of the residual limb (Stump pain)
- *Other Pain*—May include back, contralateral leg, or other site of pain related to altered biomechanics after amputation

Epidemiology

- Prevalence of Pain from selected cross-sectional studies [1–12] (Table 20.1)
- *Reason for amputation* [1] (Table 20.2)
- *Risk factors*
  - *Age*
    - 42 % of amputations occurred in those >65 years old [1]
    - Intensity of PLP or RLP does not vary by age group [2]
  - *UE vs. LE*
    - PLP is more likely to be severe in the LE [2]
    - PLP and RLP may also be more bothersome in the LE than in the UE [2]
    - PLP more common after bilateral amputations and when amputation is more proximal [13]
  - *Reason for amputation*
    - Vascular may have more intense pain [2]
    - Traumatic may be more likely to have pain [2, 6]
  - *Pre-amputation pain*
    - Pre-amputation pain has been related to incidence, type, and severity of PLP
    - Some believe that pre-amputation pain or the memory of pain may contribute to the development and maintenance of PLP [14, 15].
  - *RLP*
    - 48–58 % have both PLP and RLP [2, 4, 10]
    - RLP is a risk factor for PLP [8]
  - *Prosthetic use*
    - Myoelectric prosthetic use correlated with less PLP and less somatosensory reorganization [16]
    - Use is associated with less RLP [2]

Table 20.1 Prevalence of pain from selected cross-sectional studies [2, 4–12]

Prevalence	PLS (%)	PLP (%)	RLP (%)	Back pain (%)	PLP+RLP+back pain (%)
Range	54–80	43–80	43–76	52–71	36–47
Weighted average	74	75	60	61	37

PLP phantom limb pain, *RLP* residual limb pain, *PLS* phantom limb sensation

Table 20.2 Prevalence of amputation by etiology [1]

Etiology	UE (%)	LE (%)	Total (%)
Vascular all	2	51	54
Vascular–DM	1.1	15	16
Vascular+DM	1.4	36	38
Trauma	32	13	45
Cancer	0.2	0.9	1.1
Total	34	65	100

UE upper extremity, *LE* lower extremity, *DM* diabetes mellitus

- *Medical co-morbidities*
  - Amputees with 2+ co-morbidities have more intense pain [2]
- *Mood*
  - Depression is associated with more intense pain [2]
  - Catastrophizing and passive coping are associated with PLP [17]

Pathophysiology

- Peripheral
  - Fibers from the end of the transected nerve grow into nodules, known as neuromas, which generate abnormal impulses and respond to low-threshold stimuli [18].
  - *Deafferentiation hyperexcitability*: Changes within the dorsal root ganglion (DRG) in response to a lowered depolarization threshold and generation of spontaneous impulses which sensitize wide-dynamic-range (WDR) neurons in the spinal cord, triggering wind-up.
  - Sympathetic fibers grow around the neuroma and DRG.
- Central
  - *Wind-up phenomenon*—As WDR neurons become sensitized, low-threshold input of other uninvolved mechanoreceptors or thermoreceptors which synapse with them may be interpreted as painful stimuli [19, 20].
  - The increased spinothalamic input triggers neuroplastic changes, including somatotopic reorganization of the primary sensory cortex [21].
  - These changes are primarily mediated by *glutamate* and the *NMDA receptor*.

Evaluating Patients Post-amputation

History

Goal: Tease out different sites and sources of pain (PLP *vs.* RLP *vs.* other)

- Amputation history (sites and dates of all amputations, surgical complications)
- Quality and location of pain(s)
- Onset and evolution of pain(s)
- Exacerbating factors (positions, prosthetic use, pressure on residual limb, cold, etc.)
- Alleviating factors (positions, medications, procedures)
- Limitations in function (ambulation, ADL's) and quality of life

Physical Examination

- Mental status
  - Patients with vascular disease may also have cognitive impairment, which must be considered when prescribing pain medications
- Inspection
  - Residual limb skin condition (inspect for possible skin breakdown, infection, edema, verrucous hyperplasia suggesting poor prosthetic fit)
  - Gait (stability, prosthetic function, effects of pain)
- Palpation
  - Incision sites/scars for neuroma(s) which may trigger PLP or RLP
  - Residual limb for bony changes/osteophytes which may cause pain with pressure (X-ray may be helpful)
- Range-of-Motion (ROM)
  - Muscle/Joint contractures are common and alter biomechanics, leading to pain
    Hip commonly flexed and externally rotated
    Knee commonly flexed
- General musculoskeletal examination for other causes of pain

Work-up

- *Infection*
  - Suspect if terminal limb is red, hot, swollen, tender, or has ulceration
  - Labs: CBC, CRP, ESR
  - Consult infectious disease specialist, consider 3-phase bone scan for osteomyelitis
  - Consult vascular surgeon for possible need for more proximal amputation
- *Heterotopic Ossification*
  - Suspect if terminal limb or proximal joint is red, hot, swollen, tender, has decreased ROM, or if abnormal density is felt within soft tissues
  - Labs: Alk phos, CRP, ESR

– Imaging: X-ray (may be normal in acute phase), 3-phase bone scan
- *Poor prosthetic fit*
  – Visualized during prosthetic use, or if residual limb has hypertrophic or erosive skin changes
  – Consult a prosthetist and/or physiatrist

Treatment

- Pharmacological
  – *Gabapentin or Pregabalin*
    ↓ Release of glutamate, substance p, and norepinephrine
    Side effects: Dizziness, sedation, weight gain
  – *Tricyclic antidepressants*
    Desipramine or Nortriptyline considered safer than amitriptyline [22]
    Activate descending spinal inhibitory pathways
    Side effects: Arrhythmias, agitation, dizziness, drowsiness, urinary retention, glaucoma, dry mouth
  – *Serotonin-Norepinephrine reuptake inhibitors (SNRI)*
    Duloxetine, Venlafaxine, or Milnacipran
    Activate descending spinal inhibitory pathways
    Side effects: Headache, somnolence, nausea, dry eyes
  – *NMDA antagonists*
    Memantine may be easiest to prescribe
    Likely only helpful for acute PLP—May prevent wind-up and central sensitization
    Side effects: Dizziness, nausea
  – *Opioids*
    Tramadol—A μ-opioid agonist with SNRI activity [23]
    Morphine use associated with reduced cortical reorganization [24]
    Methadone (racemic mixture of opioid agonist and NMDA antagonist) was helpful in patients who failed opioid therapy [25]
    Side effects: Dizziness, apnea, hallucination, tolerance, dependence, addiction, diversion, constipation, falls, lack of long-term efficacy, hyperalgesia
- Guided imagery
  – Visual feedback and imagery activate the motor cortex and thus may alter pain sensation and affect cortical plasticity [26].
  – *Mirror therapy*—A mirror box is used to display an image of the intact limb superimposed where one would expect to see the amputated limb [27, 28].
  – *Graded motor imagery*—Combines digital image recognition, imagined movements, and mirror box activities [29].
  – *Virtual reality*—An avatar with an intact limb can be manipulated by movements of the subject's residual limb [30, 31].
- Sensory discrimination training of the residual limb
  – Flor et al. reduced chronic PLP by 60 % and reversed somatosensory reorganization [32]

– Huse et al. reduced pain, increased sensory discrimination, and 5/6 showed evidence of reversal of somatosensory reorganization [33]
- Physical Modalities
  – TENS—2010 Cochrane review found that there was inadequate evidence for the use of TENS in PLP or RLP [34]
  – Auricular TENS—Reduced PLS and PLP [35]
- Interventional
  – Selective DRG block of affected nerve roots [1].
  – *Pulsed radiofrequency neuromodulation* of neuroma [36].
  – *Peripheral nerve stimulation*—Series of five patients with chronic PLP had decreased pain and improved quality of life over 20 years [37].
  – *Spinal cord stimulation (SCS)*, *deep brain stimulation (DBS)*, and *motor cortex stimulation (MCS)*—Evaluated in a series of 19 patients with PLP [38, 39].
    6/19 (32 %) had >80 % pain relief with SCS lasting 2+ years
    6/10 (60 %) had pain relief with DBS
    1/5 (20 %) had pain relief with MCS
  – *Nerve sling procedure*—Residual nerve is transected, bifurcated, and split ends are apposed to connect the axonal tracts so that neuromas cannot form [18]

Treatment Strategy

1. Evidence for PLP or RLP treatment is limited to small RCT's, retrospective studies, and case reports.
   - Due, in part, to highly varied nature of post-amputation pain
2. If RLP is present, or PLP is triggered by manipulation of the residual limb, treating it may also improve PLP.
   - Ensure proper prosthetic fit
   - Neuroma injection with steroid and/or pulsed radiofrequency
   - If allodynia/hyperalgesia present, suggesting wind-up:
     – Start gabapentinoid with TCA and/or NMDA antagonist and titrate as tolerated
     – May consider opioids for short-term (<3 months) use:
     – Tramadol 50–100 mg q6h prn
     – Methadone 2.5 mg q8–12 h
     – Sympathetic block
     – Consider spinal cord or peripheral nerve stimulation
3. For PLP only:
   - Conservative options: Mirror box, virtual reality, sensory training of residual limb, TENS
   - May try medications as above, but are less likely to be helpful with chronic PLP
   - DRG block
4. Psychological therapy for adjustment disorder and coping strategies.

References

1. Ziegler-Graham K, et al. Estimating the prevalence of limb loss in the United States: 2005 to 2050. Arch Phys Med Rehabil. 2008;89(3):422–9.

2. Ephraim PL, et al. Phantom pain, residual limb pain, and back pain in amputees: results of a national survey. Arch Phys Med Rehabil. 2005;86(10):1910–9.

3. Adams PF, Hendershot GE, Marano MA. Current estimates from the National Health Interview Survey, 1996. Vital Health Stat. 1999;10(200):1–203.

4. Desmond DM, Maclachlan M. Prevalence and characteristics of phantom limb pain and residual limb pain in the long term after upper limb amputation. Int J Rehabil Res. 2010;33(3):279–82.

5. Kern U, et al. Prevalence and risk factors of phantom limb pain and phantom limb sensations in Germany. A nationwide field survey. Schmerz. 2009;23(5):479–88.

6. Schley MT, et al. Painful and nonpainful phantom and stump sensations in acute traumatic amputees. J Trauma. 2008;65(4):858–64.

7. Ehde DM, et al. Chronic phantom sensations, phantom pain, residual limb pain, and other regional pain after lower limb amputation. Arch Phys Med Rehabil. 2000;81(8):1039–44.

8. Kooijman CM, et al. Phantom pain and phantom sensations in upper limb amputees: an epidemiological study. Pain. 2000;87(1):33–41.

9. Smith DG, et al. Phantom limb, residual limb, and back pain after lower extremity amputations. Clin Orthop Relat Res. 1999;361:29–38.

10. Sherman RA, Sherman CJ. Prevalence and characteristics of chronic phantom limb pain among American veterans. Results of a trial survey. Am J Phys Med. 1983;62(5):227–38.

11. Shukla GD, Sahu SS, Tripathi RP, Gupta DK. Phantom limb: a phenomenological study. Br J Psychiatry. 1982;141:54–8.

12. Siefferman JW. Post-amputation pain in the geriatric population. Top Pain Manage. 2013;28(7):1–9.

13. Dijkstra PU, et al. Phantom pain and risk factors: a multivariate analysis. J Pain Symptom Manage. 2002;24(6):578–85.

14. Flor H. Maladaptive plasticity, memory for pain and phantom limb pain: review and suggestions for new therapies. Expert Rev Neurother. 2008;8(5):809–18.

15. Hanley MA, et al. Preamputation pain and acute pain predict chronic pain after lower extremity amputation. J Pain. 2007;8(2):102–9.

16. Lotze M, et al. Phantom movements and pain. An fMRI study in upper limb amputees. Brain. 2001;124(Pt 11):2268–77.

17. Richardson C, et al. A prospective study of factors associated with the presence of phantom limb pain six months after major lower limb amputation in patients with peripheral vascular disease. J Pain. 2007;8(10):793–801.

18. Prantl L, et al. Surgical treatment of chronic phantom limb sensation and limb pain after lower limb amputation. Plast Reconstr Surg. 2006;118(7):1562–72.

19. Woolf CJ, Salter MW. Neuronal plasticity: increasing the gain in pain. Science. 2000;288(5472):1765–9.

20. Ji Y, Traub RJ. Spinal NMDA receptors contribute to neuronal processing of acute noxious and nonnoxious colorectal stimulation in the rat. J Neurophysiol. 2001;86(4):1783–91.

21. Garraghty PE, Muja N. NMDA receptors and plasticity in adult primate somatosensory cortex. J Comp Neurol. 1996;367(2):319–26.

22. Dworkin RH, et al. Pharmacologic management of neuropathic pain: evidence-based recommendations. Pain. 2007;132(3):237–51.

23. Wilder-Smith CH, Hill LT, Laurent S. Postamputation pain and sensory changes in treatment-naive patients: characteristics and responses to treatment with tramadol, amitriptyline, and placebo. Anesthesiology. 2005;103(3):619–28.

24. Huse E, et al. The effect of opioids on phantom limb pain and cortical reorganization. Pain. 2001;90(1–2):47–55.

25. Bergmans L, et al. Methadone for phantom limb pain. Clin J Pain. 2002;18(3):203–5.

26. Ramachandran VS, Altschuler EL. The use of visual feedback, in particular mirror visual feedback, in restoring brain function. Brain. 2009;132(Pt 7):1693–710.

27. Ramachandran VS, Rogers-Ramachandran D, Cobb S. Touching the phantom limb. Nature. 1995;377(6549):489–90.

28. Chan BL, et al. Mirror therapy for phantom limb pain. N Engl J Med. 2007;357(21):2206–7.

29. Moseley GL. Graded motor imagery for pathologic pain: a randomized controlled trial. Neurology. 2006;67(12):2129–34.

30. Cole J, et al. Exploratory findings with virtual reality for phantom limb pain; from stump motion to agency and analgesia. Disabil Rehabil. 2009;31(10):846–54.

31. Mercier C, Sirigu A. Training with virtual visual feedback to alleviate phantom limb pain. Neurorehabil Neural Repair. 2009;23(6):587–94.

32. Flor H, et al. Effect of sensory discrimination training on cortical reorganisation and phantom limb pain. Lancet. 2001;357(9270):1763–4.

33. Huse E, et al. Phantom limb pain. Lancet. 2001;358(9286):1015.

34. Mulvey MR, et al. Transcutaneous electrical nerve stimulation (TENS) for phantom pain and stump pain following amputation in adults. Cochrane Database Syst Rev. 2010;5, CD007264.

35. Katz J, Melzack R. Auricular transcutaneous electrical nerve stimulation (TENS) reduces phantom limb pain. J Pain Symptom Manage. 1991;6(2):73–83.

36. Higuchi Y, et al. Exposure of the dorsal root ganglion in rats to pulsed radiofrequency currents activates dorsal horn lamina I and II neurons. Neurosurgery. 2002;50(4):850–5; discussion 856.

37. Kupers R, et al. Multimodal therapeutic assessment of peripheral nerve stimulation in neuropathic pain: Five case reports with a 20-year follow-up. Eur J Pain. 2011;15(2):161.e1–9.

38. Katayama Y, et al. Motor cortex stimulation for phantom limb pain: comprehensive therapy with spinal cord and thalamic stimulation. Stereotact Funct Neurosurg. 2001;77(1–4):159–62.

39. Vaso A, et al. Peripheral nervous system origin of phantom limb pain. Pain. 2014;155(7):1384–91.

Spinal Pain

Jonathan S. Kirschner and Kiran Vadada

Abbreviations

ALL	Anterior longitudinal ligament
COG	Center of gravity
CT	Computed tomography
DDD	Degenerative disc disease
DRG	Dorsal root ganglia
HIZ	High intensity zone
HNP	Herniated nucleus pulposus
IDD	Internal disc disruption
IDET	Intradiscal electrothermal therapy
LE	Lower extremity
MBB	Medial branch blocks
MRI	Magnetic resonance imaging
PLL	Posterior longitudinal ligament
PSIS	Posterior superior iliac spine
RFA	Radiofrequency ablation
SI	Sacroiliac
SLR	Straight leg raise
UE	Upper extremity
Z-joint	Zygapophyseal joint

J.S. Kirschner, M.D. (✉)
Department of Physiatry, Hospital for Special Surgery, Assistant Professor of Clinical Rehabilitation Medicine, Weill Cornell Medical College, 535 East 70th Street, New York, NY 10021, USA
e-mail: kirschnerj@hss.edu

K. Vadada, M.D.
Interventional Spine and Sports Medicine, Spine Center and Orthopedic Rehabilitation of Englewood, Englewood, NJ, USA
e-mail: KVadadaMD@gmail.com

Primary Pain Generators

Intervertebral Disc: Internal Disc Disruption (IDD) or Degenerative Disc Disease (DDD)

- Ages 30–40 years old
- Most common levels: L4–5=L5–S1>C5–6
- Roughly 75 % have resolution of symptoms in 1 year with conservative care
- **Anatomy (Fig. 21.1)**
  - Innervation of the Discs:
    - *Posterior annulus:* sinuvertebral nerve
    - *Anterior and lateral annulus:* gray rami communicans
- **Pathophysiology**
  - **Nucleus pulposus**: the central core composed of type II collagen, proteoglycans, and water, normally lacks nociceptive innervation
  - **Annulus fibrosus**: the surrounding band-like outer layer composed of type I collagen arranged in overlapping lamellae, innervated with nociceptive fibers, *particularly in its outer 1/3rd layer*
    - *Three types of tears at the annulus* [1]:
      - *Peripheral* tears: occur at the outermost layer, can result in surrounding inflammatory-mediated nociceptor activation in adjacent structures such as the dura and nerve roots
      - *Radial* tears: begin in the innermost layer and gradually progress to the periphery as the defect fills with pressurized nucleus pulposus
      - *Circumferential* tears: result in separation of adjacent outer lamellae—picture two outer layers of an onion dislodging from each other
  - **Vertebral endplates** form the roof and floor of the disc and are anchored by hyaline cartilage. There is a central clearing at the interface of each endplate allowing the passage of nutrients from the bone marrow into the normally avascular disc. End plate fracture can

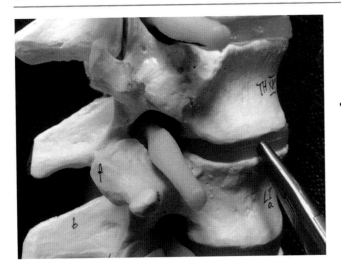

Fig. 21.1 Intervertebral Disc on spine model

result in malnutrition to the disc in addition to a local inflammatory response resulting in subsequent degeneration of healthy matrix.

- Chronically injured discs have been shown to undergo neovascularization, nerve ingrowth, and expression of substance P, correlating to painful discs as diagnosed by discography [2].
- Pressure analysis studies have shown there to be particularly high stresses in the posterolateral discs during axial loading activities, correlating with the high incidence of injury in this region [3].
- **Symptoms**
  - *Onset*: during transition from flexion to extension particularly during axial loading, amplified further if a rotatory component is present.
  - Axial pain predominates and referral patterns are usually limited to the lower gluteal folds and upwards.
  - *Pain description*: burning, electric, dull, and vague. It can have radicular components if exiting nerve roots are affected (see radiculopathy section)
  - *Exacerbating factors*: Valsalva (coughing, sneezing), sustained spine flexion, i.e., prolonged sitting, and any activity which increases the internal disc pressure, i.e., bending and lifting.
  - *Relieving factors*: (center around lowering the compressive forces) standing and walking, and laying prone is best
- **Physical Exam**
  - Focal tenderness over midline and paraspinal region
  - Dural tension maneuvers (SLR, slump, reverse SLR) elicit concordant back pain (and radicular pain if present).
  - Patients in severe pain avoid sitting in the examination room and have frequent position changes.
- **Workup**
  - XR Spine: loss of disc height is typical in chronic DDD, but it can also occur in acute HNP

- MRI Spine Discs with DDD appear dark (T2) due to decreased water content
- HIZ (T2) is indicative of an annular tear
- Discography is controversial but may be used for surgical planning in chronic refractory cases.
- **Treatment**
  - PT: extension based core strengthening, avoid sitting, lifting, bending, and reaching for objects (which subjects the discs to maximal pressure), gentle spinal traction.
  - ESI: reduces the inflammatory-mediated response surrounding the disc and is generally more effective when there is resultant radicular pain
  - Intradiscal injections: steroids have shown mixed results; regenerative biologic therapy is currently being investigated
  - IDET applies heat to the annulus with the intention of denervation and creating a stabilizing scar
  - Surgical discectomy and fusion is an option in refractory cases.

Zygapophyseal Joint (aka Z-Joint, Facet Joint): Facet Arthropathy

- Paired diarthrodial articulations of the posterior elements connecting adjacent spinal segments
- Function is to limit rotation and extension
- Orientation varies based on vertebral level
- *Lumbar facet arthropathy*:
  - 30 % of axial low back pain (Manchikanti)
  - Most common levels affected are L4–L5 and L5–S1.
  - Most common cause of LBP in adults > 55 years [4]
- *Cervical facet arthropathy*:
  - Single levels are usually affected rather than multiple levels in the cervical spine [5]
  - Most common level affected in cadaver studies C4–5 in the C-spine but clinically C2-3 and C5-6 are most affected [5]
- **Anatomy (Fig. 21.2a–c)**
  - Innervation:
    - Each joint is supplied by the medial branches of the dorsal rami of two consecutive nerve roots:
      - *Cervical*: the two levels denoted by the joint's name
        Ex. *C3–4 joint*: C3 and C4 MBs
      - *Thoracic and lumbar*: the two levels denoted by the joint *above's* name
        Ex. *T3–4 joint*: T2 and T3 MBs
        Ex. *L2–3 joint*: L1 and L2 MBs
    - This offset between the cervical and thoracolumbar innervation pattern occurs because the C8 root exits between the C7 and T1 vertebral bodies.

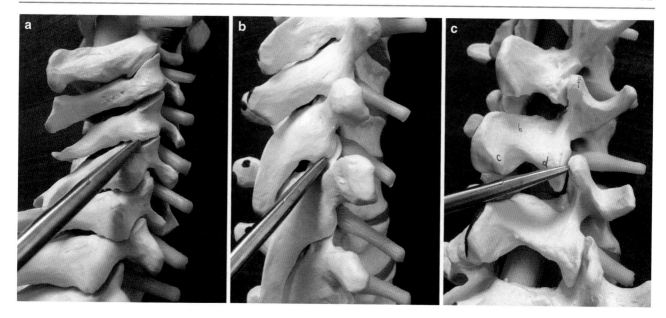

Fig. 21.2 (a–c) Z joints (facet joints) on spine model: (**a**) cervical, (**b**) thoracic, (**c**) lumbar

- **Pathophysiology**
  - Loss of disc height due to herniation or degeneration increases compressive forces at the corresponding Z-joints.
  - Postural imbalances resulting in excess lordosis (extension) can also result in increased Z-joint loading.
  - Increased loading of the facets can lead to degeneration of the cartilage and painful bone on bone contact.
  - (d)Subchondral bone in osteoarthritic Z-joints has been shown to contain substance P expressing nerve fibers [7].
  - The joint capsule is highly innervated with both nociceptive and autonomic fibers.
  - Z-joint hypertrophy can result in neuroforaminal encroachment and resultant radicular syndromes (see radiculopathy section)
- **Symptoms**
  - Injury mechanism usually involves extension and rotation to the ipsilateral side
  - The pain is generally axial and follows characteristic referral patterns (Fig. 21.3).
  - *Pain description*: dull and achy, but can be sharp with certain movements
  - *Exacerbating factors*: extension and oblique extension, however movement in any plane can stretch and aggravate the joint capsule, sometimes worsened by laying down flat
  - *Relieving factors*: flexion of the spine, unless the capsule is highly irritable in which case all movements result in pain

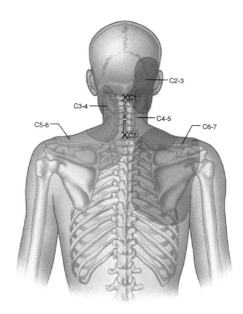

Fig. 21.3 Cervical Z joint (facet joint) pain referral pattern by specific level

- **Physical Exam**
  - Tenderness to palpation over Z-joints
  - + Kemps Maneuver—Ipsilateral extension and rotation results in facet loading, and if non-provocative can try extension, and furthermore with oblique extension. This resembles a Spurling's maneuver in the C-spine; however, the pain remains axial and follows the mentioned referral patterns without any radicular quality.
- **Workup**
  - XR Spine: can show sclerotic facets, excess lordosis, and loss of disc or vertebral body height

- MRI Spine: can reveal joint hypertrophy, irregularity of chondral surfaces increased fluid (if bilateral think spondylolisthesis), or cysts.
- Imaging is unreliable: pathologic lumbar Z-joint findings have been seen in up to 34 % of asymptomatic patients [8].
- LMBBs using the comparative two-block paradigm have the highest diagnostic value.
- Intra-articular facet injections can be both diagnostic and therapeutic, however can result in false-negative results in advanced degenerative disease.

• **Treatment**
- PT: flexion based core strengthening program and postural correction. Aggressive ROM is to be avoided—ROM and strengthening should be done in the pain-free range.
- Intra-articular facet and MBB injections are both diagnostic and therapeutic and help facilitate exercise program.
- Once the comparative two-block paradigm is satisfied, RFA can provide up to 1 year of relief.
- Surgical fusion is offered for refractory cases. This can lead to adjacent level disease. LBP after lumbar fusion has been shown to come from the Z-joints in 12.5 % of the patients. Of these patients, the affected joint was adjacent to the fusion level 80 % of the time [9].

Nerve Root: Radiculopathy

1. **Radiculopathy** is used to describe radiating pain in a characteristic dermatomal distribution of a nerve root, accompanied by one or more of the following: abnormal sensation, motor weakness, and diminished muscle stretch reflexes corresponding to that nerve distribution.
2. **Radiculitis** implies the presence of inflammatory mediators resulting in activation of nociceptive pathways. Often used interchangeably with the term "radicular pain."
   • **Anatomy (Fig. 21.4)**
   • **Pathophysiology**
   - The most important function of the bony spine is to stabilize and protect the spinal cord and nerve roots.
   - Sources of mechanical compression of the neural elements include a herniated disc, hypertrophic/sclerotic or cystic facet joint, osteophytic lipping/spurring/bony hypertrophy, bone fracture fragment, spondylolisthesis, and hematoma or mass formation resulting in central, subarticular (lateral recess) or neuroforaminal stenosis.
   - Animal studies have shown that chronic compression of the DRG results in sustained, spontaneous neural firing, which may contribute to pain [10].

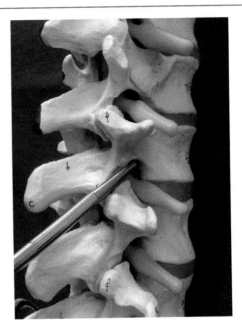

Fig. 21.4 Lumbar neuroforamina on spine model

- There is evidence that exposure of the nerve roots to HNP results in an inflammatory cascade.
- Compressed nerve roots have been shown to be more susceptible to pain in the presence of inflammation [11].

• **Symptoms**
- Injury mechanism usually involves nerve compression from disc herniation and/or bony overgrowth; however, nerve irritation can occur in the absence of any findings on imaging.
- Pain follows a dermatomal distribution, but can vary in location within a given dermatome. For example, L5 radicular pain can present as any combination of buttock pain, lateral thigh pain, or dorsal foot pain.
- *Pain description*: typically electrical, burning, sharp, shooting, and may be associated with numbness, tingling, cramping, and/or weakness
- *Exacerbating factors*: Lumbar flexion, sitting, bending, and lifting exacerbate symptoms in cases of central or subarticular disc herniations. Lumbar extension worsens pain associated with neuroforaminal compression and spinal stenosis. In the cervical spine, extension and oblique extension worsen radicular pain due to direct neuroforaminal compression.
- *Relieving factors*: laying down, rest, and standing
• **Physical Exam**
- Dural tension maneuvers are positive when they result in concordant pain:
  ▪ *SLR and slump/seated root*: tests the lower lumbar roots
  ▪ *Crossed SLR*: most specific, least sensitive
  ▪ *Reverse SLR/femoral stretch*: tests the upper lumbar roots

- *Spurling's maneuver*: compresses the cervical roots
- *Upper limb tension test*: limb is positioned in shoulder depression and abduction, forearm supination, wrist and finger extension, shoulder external rotation, and elbow extension. With this positioning, contralateral cervical lateral flexion worsens symptoms while ipsilateral cervical lateral flexion ameliorates them.
- *Bakody's sign*: placing the hand of the symptomatic side on the head relieves symptoms by reducing nerve root traction.

- **Workup**
  - Oblique XR: can show bony stenosis, but is of limited clinical value. Flex/Ex XR: can help detect positional changes in anatomy as seen in spondylolisthesis, which can aggravate symptoms.
  - Electrodiagnostic evaluation is the most objective method of diagnosing and localizing radiculopathy. It is highly specific and moderately sensitive.
  - MRI reveals cause and location of nerve root compression; however, it has been shown that roughly 50 % of asymptomatic patients have abnormal findings.
- **Treatment**
  - PT should initially avoid activities that exacerbate the symptoms and progress towards incorporating those lost activities into the program. Mechanical diagnosis and treatment (Mackenzie method) may be helpful.
  - Anti-inflammatories should be used in short courses during flare-ups.
  - For severe symptoms, consider an oral steroid taper; however, this is controversial due to a lack of evidence combined with the large side effect profile.
  - Opioid analgesics should be reserved for when mobility and function are severely impaired due to pain.
  - Muscle relaxants and sedatives can be considered in cases of pain induced insomnia.
  - ESI delivers steroid and anesthetic to the suspected location of pathology. They can provide both diagnostic and therapeutic benefits by flushing out the build up of toxic metabolites, and blocking nociceptive and inflammatory pathways.
  - Surgical consultation is indicated when there is a progressive neurologic deficit, spinal instability, cauda equina syndrome or severe intractable pain that is not amenable to conservative care.

Muscle-Tendon Complex and Ligament: Acute Muscular Strains and Chronic Muscular Overload

Muscle

- Injury often occurs at the musculotendinous junction during eccentric contraction.

- *Lumbar*: Although lumbar strain is considered a common cause of mechanical low back pain, much of the knowledge of its pathophysiology is applied from studies on peripheral muscles.
  - **Lower Crossed Syndrome** (sequence of events can vary) is associated with low back pain
    - Tight and shortened hip flexors result in anterior pelvic tilt (or vice versa)
    - Anterior displacement of COG results in increased lumbar lordosis to maintain upright posture
    - Gluteal and abdominal muscles are inhibited and weak
    - Increased lumbar lordosis can lead to increased Z-joint loading and resultant pain
- *Cervical*: Neck pain has been associated with decreased strength, imbalance between flexors and extensors, fatty infiltration of the extensors, decreased ROM, decreased bulk, and increased activation of accessory muscles [12–18].
  - **Upper Crossed Syndrome** is associated with neck pain.
    - Tightness of pectoralis minor and major, upper trapezius, and levator scapulae
    - Inhibition of deep neck flexors and lower scapular stabilizers and retractors (middle and lower trapezius, rhomboids)
    - Shoulder and scapular protraction
    - Increased thoracic kyphosis and decreased cervical lordosis
    - Anterior displacement of head results in increased contraction of the extensors and paraspinals to maintain upright position.
    - Sustained neck extensor contraction can lead to increased Z-joint loading and resultant joint and/or muscle pain.
- **Symptoms**
  - *Pain description*: dull and achy, but well localized.
  - *Exacerbating factors*: overuse and under activity. Patients generally report improvement of symptoms after light exercise, and then worsening of symptoms after prolonged or strenuous activity. Heat and massage can also provide temporary relief.
- **Physical Exam**
  - Trigger points are often found in dysfunctional muscles, and palpation can elicit characteristic patterns of radiation into the extremities, mimicking radicular pain.
  - Stretching, palpation, and activation of the suspected muscles reproduce symptoms.
- **Workup**
  - If multiple muscle groups are involved, consider systemic illness like fibromyalgia, neuromuscular, or rheumatologic disease.
- **Treatment**
  - Restoration of optimal muscle length, flexibility, strength, and posture

- Focus on strengthening through the entire ROM for the given muscle
- Trigger point injections are used primarily for mechanical disruption of tight muscle fibers and promotion of blood flow.

Ligament

- There is mixed evidence that the ligaments of the spine can be primary pain generators.
  - *Cervical*:
    - Studies have shown decreased strength of all cervical ligaments after whiplash injury [19].
    - Ligamentous laxity leads destabilization and subsequent abnormal mechanical loading of surrounding structures, leading to other painful conditions.
  - *Lumbar*:
    - Nociceptive fibers have been found in the PLL [20].
    - The PLL is connected to the outer annulus fibrosus, also known to be nociceptive.
    - Differentiating between PLL-mediated pain and annular pain is a challenge.
- **Workup**
  - MRI has not been shown to be reliable in identifying pathologic ligaments.
  - Diagnostic injections may be the best method for localizing pathology.
- **Treatment**
  - Relative rest and immobilization.
  - Prolotherapy may help in chronic cases.

Sacroiliac Joint

- **Anatomy (Fig. 21.5)**
  - Auricular shaped, diarthrodial
  - Hyaline cartilage on the sacral facet
  - Fibrocartilage on the iliac facet
  - Variable innervation [20]
    - *Anteriorly*: L3–S2 and superior gluteal n.
    - *Posteriorly*: dorsal rami of L5, S1, S2, +/− L4 and S3
- **Pathophysiology**
  - Cadaveric studies have found Substance P and Calcitonin G-Related Peptide (CGRP) in the anterior capsular and interosseous ligaments [21].
  - Degenerative changes in the joint have been found in 91 % of males and 77 % of females aged >40 [22].
  - Decreased ROM in the lumbosacral spine and/or hips can lead to increased shear forces across the SI joint, resulting in pain.
- **Symptoms**
  - Etiology typically pregnancy, seronegative spondyloarthropathies a fall onto the buttocks, forceful or awkward heel strike, for example jumping and landing on one leg.

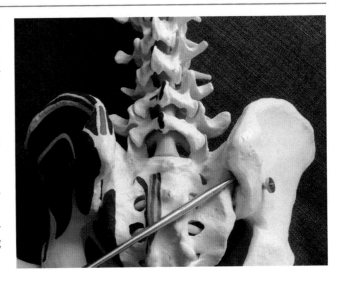

Fig. 21.5 Sacroiliac joint on spine model

- The pain localizes over the buttock and lower back—usually below the waistline. It can refer to the lower limbs in a pseudoradicular fashion.
- *Pain description*: Vague, dull, and achy, often with a catching sensation associated with sharp flare-ups. Some describe a feeling that the pain is on the verge of dramatically increasing with any movement. Can have referral pattern to the buttock groin and thigh, usually stays above the knee.
- *Exacerbating factors*: transitional movements (like arising from a seated position or shifting around in bed).
- *Relieving factors*: can vary, but usually involve repositioning and stretching maneuvers that release the catching sensation.
- **Physical Exam**
  - Unreliable, therefore one should maximize the number of provocative maneuvers used in order to increase sensitivity.
  - Tenderness at posterior SI joint line. Palpation of the PSIS creates rotational sheer and elicits pain.
  - Fortin finger: patient points to the SI joint region to show area of maximal discomfort/pain.
  - Other maneuvers include Sacral Compression, Iliac Compression, Gaenslen's, Gillette, Faber, Posterior Shear, Resisted Abduction, and Yeoman.
- **Workup**
  - XR: may be used to assess for fracture or seronegative spondyloarthropathies affecting the SIJ but are usually not helpful.
  - Image-guided contrast-enhanced injections are the gold standard for diagnosis.
- **Treatment**
  - Lumbopelvic and hip conditioning to restore normal mechanics and decrease shear forces across the SI joint.

- Manipulation to reset the joint
- Bracing for external stabilization
- Intra-articular steroid injections can provide lasting relief
- RFA at various lumbosacral levels has also been shown to provide long-term relief. L5–S3 is usually targeted.
- Topical and oral medications when needed
- Surgical fusion can be performed in refractory cases.

Coccyx: Coccygodynia

- **Anatomy (Fig. 21.6)**
  - Innervated by the ganglion impar
- **Pathophysiology**
  - Abnormal movement in the coccygeal segments, often post-traumatic, can be acute or chronic
- **Symptoms**
  - Onset is usually after a fall or childbirth; some cases are idiopathic
  - *Pain description*: sharp and well localized over the coccyx
  - *Exacerbating factors*: direct pressure or release of pressure to the region—sitting, rising from the seated position, straining during bowel movements
  - *Relieving factors*: center around avoiding movement in the region.
- **Physical Exam**
  - Focal tenderness to palpation
  - Pain can also be provoked with sitting—other areas such as the ischial bursae, piriformis should also be palpated and ruled out.
- **Workup**
  - XR: standing and while seated on a hard surface to check for movement
- **Treatment**
  - Wedge pillow with cut-out was shown to be the most effective pressure off-loading cushion, not a donut cushion
  - Coccygeal manipulation to re-align displaced segment is controversial.
  - Ganglion impar injection can provide long-term relief. If needed, RFA can also be performed [23].
  - Sacrococcygeal junction and coccygeal disc injections may be helpful, especially when abnormal motion at a particular segment is isolated and targeted.

Vertebral Bodies: Compression Fractures

- **Etiology**
  - Pain has been reported in up to 84 % of patients with vertebral fractures [24].

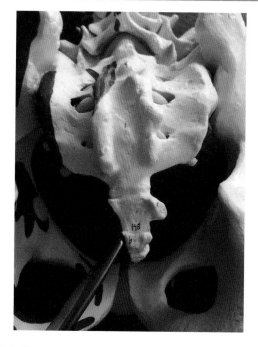

Fig. 21.6 Coccyx on spine model

- Female vertebrae cross-sections are 25 % smaller than males and have to withstand 30–40 % higher forces for a given axial load. This may explain the higher incidence of compression fractures in elderly women [25].
- T8 is most commonly involved because it is the transition point from the restricted thoracic spine to the highly mobile lumbar spine [26, 27].
- A history of compression fracture results in a fivefold increase in the probability of having another one [28].
- The most common area for second fracture is at the superior adjacent vertebra [29, 30].
- **Symptoms**
  - Injury usually occurs during bending and lifting, but can occur spontaneously in underlying pathological conditions.
  - Pain generally localizes to the level of the involved vertebra, but can radiate to the flanks, chest, and refer up to four levels from the site of fracture. Secondary radicular pain is not common [27].
  - *Pain description*: intense and deep aching
  - *Exacerbating factors*: valsalva, spinal flexion, and weight bearing
  - *Relieving factors*: lying supine
- **Physical Exam**
  - Local tenderness to palpation and percussion
  - Pain exacerbated by flexion
  - Loss of height, Kyphotic deformities in severe cases and/or with multiple fractures
- **Workup**
  - XR
  - CT
  - Bone scan
  - MRI

- **Treatment**
  - Conservative management is emphasized with topicals and medications for pain control, bracing, and judicious bed rest.
  - PT is initiated when patient is able to tolerate upright posture
  - Vertebroplasty is the injection of cement into the fracture defect in an attempt to stabilize the structure. Proposed mechanisms of pain relief include mechanical nerve disruption, ablation by the hot cement, and stabilization of micro-fractures. Cement injected levels have been shown to be more likely to resist continued deformation compared to native bone [31].
  - Kyphoplasty is the injection of cement after using a balloon to expand the area of the fracture defect in an attempt to restore vertebral height.
  - Adjacent segment fractures are a concern with both treatments.
  - Topical and oral medications when needed.

Multifactorial Pain Syndromes

1. **Spondylosis, Spondylolysis, and Spondylolisthesis**
   - **Spondylosis** describes a cascade of degeneration of the 3 joint complex formed through an intervertebral disc and its two corresponding Z-joints. Loss of disc height leads to increased forces across the Z-joints, which in turn degenerate. Conversely, increased motion due to Z-joint instability can lead to increased disruptive forces across a disc, resulting in subsequent degeneration. The Kirkaldy-Willis cascade describes the cycle of dysfunction leading to instability followed by eventual stabilization and has been a landmark concept in the mechanism of the degenerating spine.
   - **Spondylolysis** describes fracture, or lysis, of the pars interarticularis, which is the segment connecting the lamina to its underlying pedicle.
   - **Spondylolisthesis** is described as the slippage of a vertebral body over the adjacent segment below. It can result in spinal stenosis, discogenic pain, Z-joint-mediated pain, and radicular pain syndromes. Spondylolisthesis of L4 over L5 as well as L5 over S1 usually results in compromise of the L5 nerves.

2. **Spinal Stenosis**
   - **Central stenosis** can be caused by a multitude of factors, including disc herniation, spondylolisthesis, tumor, hematoma, Paget's disease, and a congenitally narrowed canal. Claudication describes the presence of extremity symptoms that improve with spine flexion. Neurological examination can be completely normal; however, patient may have dramatic intermittent symptoms during episodes of claudication. One way to differentiate neurogenic from vascular claudication in the LEs is the ability to tolerate bicycling, which would not be seen in vascular disease. Intuitively, it is also the best exercise to maximize aerobic efficiency of the lower extremity muscles and therefore improve function. In studies, ESIs have shown mixed results but they still may provide significant clinical benefit. Surgery is indicated for refractory cases.
   - **Foraminal stenosis** can result in nerve impingement and radicular syndromes. Provocation of concordant radicular pain with lumbar extension rather than flexion-based dural tension maneuvers points towards neuroforaminal compromise. It is important to distinguish this from symptoms of claudication, which are generally more vague and diffuse. Radicular symptoms with flexion, which are elicited by the standard dural tension maneuvers such as the SLR and slump tests, are more typical of central herniations.

3. **Chronic Postsurgical Pain**
   - Rates vary from 10 to 40 % [32–39]
   - **Causes** [27]
     - Recurrent disc herniation/retained fragment (4.6–63 %)
     - Epidural scar formation (0–12.3 %)
     - Instability of vertebral segment (3.1–6.5 %)
     - Facet joint mediated (16.9–23.1 %)
     - Myofascial (7.4–26.1 %)
     - Failed Back/Neck Syndrome
   - Other causes include hardware failure, malalignment, re-herniation, adjacent level disease, infection, and complex regional pain syndrome.
   - Note that patients are still prone to the same variety of painful etiologies as the nonsurgical population—a common pitfall is to relate all new symptoms to the prior operation.
   - Treatment options still include oral medications, ESI, MBB, and RFA. In refractory cases, consider spinal cord stimulation, intrathecal drug delivery systems, and reoperation.

4. **Spinal Infections**
   - 2–7 % of all musculoskeletal infections [40–42]
   - Can be bacterial, viral, or fungal
   - Can be caused by hematogenous spread, trauma, or surgical contamination
   - Fever and leukocytosis are not always present
   - Usually involves two adjacent vertebrae and the intervening disc due a common segmental arterial supply [43]
   - Lumbar spine is most commonly infected followed by thoracic, cervical, then sacral [44]
   - Pyogenic spondylitis is a blanket term for a variety of infectious conditions including spondylodiscitis, vertebral osteomyelitis, and epidural abscess

- Intradural infections include meningitis, encephalitis, and neurosyphilis
- **Symptoms**
  - Pain, fever, nausea, visual changes, lethargy, altered mental status, and neurological deficits
- **Workup**
  - Erythrocyte sedimentation rate and C-reactive protein are nonspecific diagnostically, but useful in monitoring treatment
  - X-rays can show bony destruction at the endplates and loss of disc height
  - Lumbar puncture is used when intradural involvement is suspected
  - Bone scans are sensitive but not specific
  - MRI is the gold standard
  - CT is useful for surgical planning to better assess the degree of bone necrosis
  - Percutaneous or open biopsy is needed to confirm diagnosis and determine the causative agent
- **Treatment**
  - Nonsurgical candidates are treated with antibiotics for 1–3 months
  - Bed rest is recommended during the initial acutely painful stage
  - Bracing is used to decrease pain and minimize deformity
  - Surgical debridement and fusion is needed for advanced cases

References

1. Osti OL, Vernon-Roberts B, Moore R, Fraser RD. Annular tears and disc degeneration in the lumbar spine. A post-mortem study of 135 discs. J Bone Joint Surg Br. 1992; 74(5):678–82.
2. Freemont AJ, Peacock TE, Goupille P, Hoyland JA, O'Brien J, Jayson MI. Nerve ingrowth into diseased intervertebral disc in chronic back pain. Lancet. 1997;350(9072):178–81.
3. Schmidt H, Kettler A, Heuer F, Simon U, Claes L, Wilke HJ. Intradiscal pressure, shear strain, and fiber strain in the intervertebral disc under combined loading. Spine. 2007;32(7):748–55.
4. DePalma MJ, Ketchum JM, Queler ED, et al. What is the etiology of LBP and does age affect prevalence. Best paper presentation. International Spinal Intervention Society Annual Meeting, Toronto. 2009.
5. Cooper G, Bailey B, Bogduk N. Cervical zygapophysial joint pain maps. Pain Med. 2007;8(4):344–53.
6. Lee MJ, Riew KD. The prevalence cervical facet arthrosis: an osseous study in a cadaveric population. Spine J. 2009;9(9): 711–4.
7. Beaman DN, Graziano GP, Glover RA, Wojtys EM, Chang V. Substance P innervation of lumbar spine facet joints. Spine. 1993;18(8):1044–9.
8. Boden SD, Davis DO, Dina TS, Patronas NJ, Wiesel SW. Abnormal magnetic-resonance scans of the lumbar spine in asymptomatic subjects. A prospective investigation. J Bone Joint Surg Am. 1990; 15(6):453–7.
9. DePalma MJ, Ketchum JM, Kouchouk A, et al. What is the etiology of low back pain in patients having undergone lumbar fusion?

An interim analysis of a cross-sectional analytic study. PMR J. 2009;1:S183.
10. Howe JF, Loeser JD, Calvin WH. Mechanosensitivity of dorsal root ganglia and chronically injured axons: a physiological bases for the radicular pain of nerve root compression. Pain. 1977;3:25–41.
11. Murphy RW. Nerve roots and spinal nerves in degenerative disk disease. Clin Orthop Relat Res. 1977;129:46–60.
12. Prushansky T, Gepstein R, Gordon C, Dvir Z. Cervical muscles weakness in chronic whiplash patients. Clin Biomech (Bristol, Avon). 2005;20(8):794–8.
13. Elliott J, Jull G, Noteboom JT, Darnell R, Galloway G, Gibbon WW. Fatty infiltration in the cervical extensor muscles in persistent whiplash-associated disorders: a magnetic resonance imaging analysis. Spine. 2006;31(22):E847–55.
14. Falla D, Bilenkij G, Jull G. Patients with chronic neck pain demonstrate altered patterns of muscle activation during performance of a functional upper limb task. Spine. 2004;29(13):1436–40.
15. Cusick JF, Yoganandan N, Pintar F, Gardon M. Cervical spine injuries from high-velocity forces: a pathoanatomic and radiologic study. J Spinal Disord. 1996;9(1):1–7.
16. Nakama S, Nitanai K, Oohashi Y, Endo T, Hoshino Y. Cervical muscle strength after laminoplasty. J Orthop Sci. 2003;8(1):36–40.
17. Vasavada AN, Brault JR, Siegmund GP. Musculotendon and fascicle strains in anterior and posterior neck muscles during whiplash injury. Spine. 2007;32(7):756–65.
18. Fernández-de-las-Peñas C, Albert-Sanchís J, Buil M, Benitez JC, Alburquerque-Sendin F. Cross-sectional area of cervical multifidus muscle in females with chronic bilateral neck pain compared to controls. J Orthop Sports Phys Ther. 2008;38:175–80.
19. Tominaga Y, Ndu AB, Coe MP, et al. Neck ligament strength is decreased following whiplash trauma. BMC Musculoskelet Disord. 2006;7:103.
20. Solonen KA. The sacroiliac joint in the light of anatomical, roentgenological and clinical studies. Acta Orthop Scand Suppl. 1957;27:1–127.
21. Szadek KM, Hoogland PV, Zuurmond WW, de Lange JJ, Perez RS. Nociceptive nerve fibers in the sacroiliac joint in humans. Reg Anesth Pain Med. 2008;33(1):36–43.
22. Sashin D. A critical analysis of the anatomy and the pathologic changes of the sacro-iliac joints. J Bone Joint Surg. 1930;12A: 891–910.
23. Usta B, Gozdemir M, Sert H, Muslu B, Demircioglu RI. Fluoroscopically guided ganglion impar block by pulsed radiofrequency for relieving coccydynia. J Pain Symptom Manage. 2010;39:e1–2.
24. Silverman SL. The clinical consequences of vertebral compression fracture. Bone. 1992;13 Suppl 2:S27–31.
25. Gilsanz V, Boechat MI, Gilsanz R, Loro ML, Roe TF, Goodman WG. Gender differences in vertebral sizes in adults: biomechanical implications. Radiology. 1994;190(3):678–82.
26. Cooper C, Atkinson EJ, O'Fallon WM, Melton III LJ. Incidence of clinically diagnosed vertebral fractures: a population-based study in Rochester, Minnesota, 1985–1989. J Bone Miner Res. 1992; 7(2):221–7.
27. Patel U, Skingle S, Campbell GA, Crisp AJ, Boyle IT. Clinical profile of acute vertebral compression fractures in osteoporosis. Br J Rheumatol. 1991;30(6):418–21.
28. Ross PD, Davis JW, Epstein RS, Wasnich RD. Pre-existing fractures and bone mass predict vertebral fracture incidence in women. Ann Intern Med. 1991;114(11):919–23.
29. Kayanja MM, Togawa D, Lieberman IH. Biomechanical changes after the augmentation of experimental osteoporotic vertebral compression fractures in the cadaveric thoracic spine. Spine J. 2005; 5(1):55–63.
30. Trout AT, Kallmes DF, Layton KF, Thielen KR, Hentz JG. Vertebral endplate fractures: an indicator of the abnormal forces generated in the spine after vertebroplasty. J Bone Miner Res. 2006;21(11):1797–802.

31. Dean JR, Ison KT, Gishen P. The strengthening effect of percutaneous vertebroplasty. Clin Radiol. 2000;55(6):471–6.

32. Andrews DW, Lavyne MH. Retrospective analysis of microsurgical and standard lumbar discectomy. Spine (Phila Pa 1976). 1990;15:329–35.

33. Caspar W, Campbell B, Barbier DD, Kretschmmer R, Gottfried Y. The Caspar microsurgical discectomy and comparison with a conventional standard lumbar disc procedure. Neurosurgery. 1991;28:78–87.

34. Frymoyer JW, Hanley E, Howe J, Kuhlmann D, Matteri R. Disc excision and spine fusion in the management of lumbar disc disease. A minimum ten year follow-up. Spine (Phila Pa 1976). 1978;3:1–6.

35. Rodríguez-García J, Sánchez-Gastaldo A, Ibáñez-Campos T, Vázquez-Sousa C, Cantador-Hornero M, Expósito-Tirado JA, Cayuela-Domínguez A, EchevarríaRuiz de Vargas C. Related factors with the failed surgery of herniated lumbar disc. Neurocirugia (Astur). 2005;16:507–17.

36. Ross JS, Robertson JT, Frederickson RC, Petrie JL, Obuchowski N, Modic MT, de Tribolet N. Association between peridural scar and recurrent radicular pain after lumbar discectomy: magnetic resonance evaluation. ADCON-L European Study Group. Neurosurgery. 1996;38:855–61.

37. Fritsch EW, Heisel J, Rupp S. The failed back surgery syndrome: reasons, intraoperative findings, and long-term results—a report of 182 operative treatments. Spine (Phila Pa 1976). 1996;21:626–33.

38. Manchikanti L, Singh V, Cash KA, Pampati V, Datta S. Preliminary results of randomized, equivalence trial of fluoroscopic caudal epidural injections in managing chronic low back pain: part 3. Post surgery syndrome. Pain Physician. 2008;11:817–31.

39. Bokov A, Isrelov A, Skorodumov A, Aleynik A, Simonov A, Mlyavykh S. An analysis of reasons for failed back surgery syndrome and partial results after different types of surgical lumbar nerve root decompression. Pain Physician. 2011;14(6):545–57. PubMed PMID: 22086096.

40. Tyrrel PNM, Cassar-Pollucino VN, McCall IW. Spinal infection. Eur Radiol. 1999;9:1066–77.

41. Stabler A, Reiser MF. Imaging of spinal infection. Radiol Clin North Am. 2001;39:115–35.

42. Danner RL, Hartmann BJ. Update of spinal epidural abscess: 35 cases and review of the literature. Rev Infect Dis. 1987;9:265–74.

43. Sapico FL, Montgomerie JZ. Vertebral osteomyelitis. Infect Dis Clin North Am. 1990;4(3):539–50.

44. Jaramillo-de la Torre JJ, Bohinski RJ, Kuntz C. Vertebral osteomyelitis. Neurosurg Clin N Am. 2006;17:339–51.

Chronic Pelvic and Abdominal Pain

22

Joslyn Gober, Melanie Howell, Sovrin M. Shah, and Kimberly A. Sackheim

Abbreviations

CBC	Complete blood count
CT	Computed tomography
DKA	Diabetic ketoacidosis
IC	Interstitial cystitis
GERD	Gastroesophageal reflux disease
GI	Gastrointestinal
GU	Genitourinary
HTN	Hypertension
LLQ	Left lower quadrant
LUQ	Left upper quadrant
MMT	Manual muscle testing
MRI	Magnetic resonance imaging
NSAIDS	Nonsteroidal anti-inflammatory drugs
PID	Pelvic inflammatory disease
PNA	Pneumonia
PTX	Pneumothorax
RLQ	Right lower quadrant
RUQ	Right upper quadrant
SI	Sacroiliac
UA	Urinalysis
UCx	Urine culture
UTI	Urinary tract infection

J. Gober, D.O. (✉)
Nova Southeastern University College of Osteopathic Medicine,
Fort Lauderdale, FL, USA
e-mail: jgober9@gmail.com

M. Howell, D.O. • K.A. Sackheim
Department of Rehabilitation Medicine, New York University
Langone Medical Center, New York, NY, USA
e-mail: melanie.howell@nyumc.org

S.M. Shah, M.D.
Department of Urology Female Pelvic Medicine and
Reconstructive Surgery, Icahn School of Medicine at Mount Sinai
Mount Sinai Beth Israel, New York, NY, USA
e-mail: sshah@chpnet.org

Introduction

Patients suffering from chronic abdominal and pelvic pain syndromes can be very complicated and difficult to diagnose and treat. These patients often end up visiting numerous physicians and undergo an abundance of tests and imaging prior to their physician establishing an accurate diagnosis. Unfortunately, some of the patients undergo unnecessary surgical interventions and continue to have their pain syndrome afterwards. It is important to establish a proper and detailed history, physical examination, and assure they have had all acute and surgical pathologies ruled out prior. Chronic abdominal and pelvic pain can be disabling and drastically effect a patient's quality of life.

Pelvic/Groin Pain

Acute pelvic pain: pain lasting <3 months
Chronic pelvic pain: pain lasting >3–6 months

Some Differential Diagnosis

- *Gynecological etiologies*
  - Adhesions
  - Endometriosis
  - Leiomyoma
  - Dysmenorrhea
  - Pelvic congestion syndrome
  - Pelvic inflammatory disease
  - Adenomyosis
  - Adenexal pathology (torsion, cyst)
  - Ovarian cancer
  - Vulvodynia
  - Vaginal vestibulitis
  - Vaginismus
- *Genitourinary etiologies*
  - Interstitial cystitis/bladder pain syndrome
  - Chronic prostatitis/chronic pelvic pain syndrome

- Bladder neoplasia
- Urinary tract infection
- Chronic prostatitis
- *Gastrointestinal etiologies*
  - Irritable bowel syndrome
  - Inflammatory bowel disease
  - Diverticulitis/osis
  - Colon cancer
  - Chronic constipation
  - Celiac disease
- *Musculoskeletal/spinal etiologies*
  - Pelvic floor dysfunction
  - Fibromyalgia
  - Coccydynia
  - Piriformis syndrome
  - Myofascial pain syndrome/trigger points
  - Osteitis pubis
  - Hip pathology
  - Inguinal neuralgia
  - Pudendal neuralgia
  - Upper lumbar radiculopathy
  - Facet arthropathy radiating to groin
  - Sacroiliac joint pathology
- *Mental health etiologies*
  - Somatization disorder
  - Opiate dependency
  - Physical and sexual abuse
  - Depression [1, 2]

Above etiologies can cause chronic pelvic pain. When dealing with acute pelvic pain other etiologies should be considered; this list is not all-inclusive.

If patient is unstable, has acute abdomen, or signs of infection they should be sent to ER.

General History for Pelvic Pain

- *Symptoms*:
  - Pain below umbilicus, may cause functional disability; pain may be generalized in chronic conditions
    - Quality (dull/sharp), Crampy: endometriosis, Hot/burning/numbness/tingling pain: can indicate nerve entrapment
    - Location of pain
      - *Lateralized*: adhesions, ectopic pregnancy, ovarian torsion
      - *Bilateral*: PID, pelvic congestion syndrome
      - *Midline*: dysmenorrhea
      - *Lower abdominal/pelvic*: endometriosis, adenomyosis
      - *Suprapubic/Perineal*: Interstitial cystitis/prostatitis
      - *Radiation to back, flank, or groin*: ovarian torsion, high lumbar radiculopathy, facet arthropathy

- Radiation of pain—typically to low back, sometimes urethra
- Association with: bowel or urinary voiding symptoms (frequency of daytime voids, nocturia, urgency, dysuria—incontinence is not typical in IC/BPS), vaginal discharge or bleeding
- Association with foods/drink—acidic or spicy foods may increase bladder pain
- Impact on sexual function—dyspareunia is often seen especially with deep penetration
- Exact date of last menstrual cycle, history of unprotected sex or more than one sexual partner
- Timing and onset of pain:
  - *Cyclic pain*: endometriosis or adenomyosis
  - *Between menstrual periods*: mittleschmerz
  - *Sudden onset*: ruptured ovarian cyst, ovarian torsion
- *Associated symptoms*: Abnormal menstruation (seen with Endometriosis),
- Dysmenorrhea (endometriosis); urinary urgency, frequency (interstitial cystitis, prostatitis); Paresthesias (nerve entrapment); nausea and vomiting (bowel obstruction); pregnancy symptoms (ectopic pregnancy); vaginal discharge (PID); **Red flags**: rectal bleeding and/or weight loss (malignancy) [2]
- *Exacerbating factors*: menstruation, intercourse, ejaculation, voiding, exercise, association with diet, sitting, bending forwards or backwards
- *Additional information*: menstrual status with timing of last menstrual period and relation to onset of pain, sexual history [3]

Past Medical/Surgical History

- *History of abuse*
- *History of STDs*: seen with PID
- *History of unprotected sex/more than one sexual partner*
- *"Negative" psychological features*: depression, anxiety (seen with chronic pain) [2]
- *Fibromyalgia/irritable bowel syndrome (IBS)*
- *Hyperuricemia*: can be prone to renal calculi
- *Diabetes*: consider DKA
- *Prior abdominal/pelvic surgery*: consider adhesions and obstruction
- *Prior inguinal surgery*: can lead to inguinal neuralgia
- *Family history*: cancer, inflammatory disorders

General Physical Exam for Pelvic Pain

- *Vital signs*: fever indicates infection (consider appendicitis or PID depending on localization of pain; tachycardia and hypotension suggest septic shock, (possibly due to ectopic pregnancy, septic abortion, uterine rupture, appendicitis, or ruptured ovarian cyst, etc.)

- *In chronic pelvic pain patients, vitals should be stable. If unstable vitals send to ER for immediate treatments*
- *Inspection*
  - Skin for rashes, ulcerations, discoloration, masses or hernias
- Orthopedic and postural abnormalities (e.g., Increased lumbar lordotic curve and anterior pelvic shift; scoliosis; uneven iliac crests heights), gait
- *Palpation abdomen/pelvic regions*
  - Localized or generalized tenderness
    - Suprapubic: UTI, interstitial cystitis
    - RLQ or LLQ: ectopic pregnancy, ovarian cyst or torsion, appendicitis
    Generalized: pelvic congestion syndrome
  - Presence of masses, surgical scars, hernias
  - Abdominal and pelvic muscle abnormalities, trigger points
  - *Vaginal exam*: Inspect external genitalia for lesions, trauma, inspect meatus (caruncle, urethral mucosal prolapse) quality of vaginal epithelial tissue, palpate distal anterior vaginal wall (rule out urethral diverticulum or urethritis), palpate deep anterior vaginal wall (cystitis), palpate apex of vagina/cervix for extreme tenderness (PID), check for associated vaginal prolapse, inspect for vaginal discharge (which if present should be swabbed), palpate for adnexal masses or tenderness, evaluate the cervix for shape, size, mobility, and tenderness
- *Male genitalia exam*: Check for lesions on penis, palpate urethra at ventral surface of penis to rule out mass or much less commonly—an impacted urethral stone or urethral diverticulum, check testes and epididymis for masses, induration, tenderness, rule out inguinal hernias
- *Rectal exam (only if clinically indicated)*: Inspection of anus (check for external hemorrhoids, fissures, skin lesions; rule out rectal mass; palpate anterior rectal wall to check for prostatic tenderness or fluctuance
- *MMT*: Rule out spinal pathology which can radiate pain to groin, strength testing should be normal, may be limited by severe pain, pelvic pain should not present with abnormal reflexes unless involvement of the spine is contributing
- *Provocative maneuvers*
  - *"Carnett's" sign*: *Incr*eased local tenderness during muscle tensing
    - Patient, laying supine, raises both legs off the table simultaneously while the examiner's fingers are placed on site of pain. If there is myofascial pain, this maneuver will increase pain. However, if the pain is associated with visceral pain, there will be less tenderness with the tensed abdominal muscles.

- *FABER test*: assessment of hip and SI joint
  - Examiner flexes, abducts, externally rotates, and extends the affected leg on top of the other knee and then slowly lowers the leg toward the examining table. Pain with maneuver indicates hip disease or iliopsoas spasm. Pain at SI joint indicates SI join pathology.
- *FADIR test*: assessment of hip
  - With patient supine, examiner flexes leg and knee to 90 degrees, adducts, and internally rotates hip. Pain with maneuver suggests hip impingement or labral tear.
- *Ganslens test*: Assessment of lumbar spine and SI joint
  - With patient supine, hip is flexed on one side and extended on opposite side. Pain with maneuver is indicative is SI joint instability and/or L4 nerve root lesion.
- *Psychological assessment*: screen for depression and physical/sexual abuse [1–3]

General Workup for Pelvic Pain
- *Labs*:
  - CBC, ESR, CRP: rule out infectious etiology
  - UA, UCx, Chlamydia/Gonorrhea
  - B-HCG: rule out pregnancy in all patients of childbearing age
  - Urine cytology (if family history of GU cancer, hematuria, or tobacco history)
- *Diagnostic studies*:
  - Cytoscopy: inspect bladder urothelium to rule out bladder cancer or ulceration
  - Laparoscopy: identify endometriomas; check for adhesions
- *Imaging*
  - X-ray: Pelvis, hips, lumbosacral spine: to rule out fracture or arthritis which can refer pain to pelvic region
  - Pelvic ultrasound
  - Ideal for imaging of gynecologic organs (ovarian cysts, fibroids, endometrial lesions)
  - CT abdomen/pelvis: evaluate abdominal/pelvic anatomy, rule out masses, inflammatory lesions, genitourinary stones, GI/GU/Gyn malignancy
  - MRI pelvis: an option for imaging if IV contrast for CT is contraindicated; ideal to check for urethral diverticulum, may consider for imaging of ovaries or better define cystic appearing lesions [1, 2]

Chronic Endometriosis

Presence of endometrial tissue out side of the uterus—can cause a chronic inflammatory response
- *Symptoms*: Chronic dull or crampy pain in the lower abdominal or pelvic region that typically cycles with menses

- *Associated symptoms*: Abnormal uterine bleeding, infertility, chronic Pelvic pain, Infertility, hematuria, dysuria, hematochezia, bowel pain, dyspareunia, dysmenorrhea, low back pain, chronic fatigue
- *Physical exam*: Pain or tenderness on pelvic exam, most common when palpating the posterior vaginal fornix; fixed uterus due to adhesions; lateral displacement of cervix: fixation of adnexa or uterus in a retroverted position, palpable tender nodules on pelvic exam; possible palpable adnexal mass
- *Labs*: normal (serum CA 125 >35 U/mL, but is not a sensitive indicator)
- *Imaging*:
  - Transvaginal ultrasound (first line) to help visualize uterine cysts and nodules
  - MRI or CT Pelvis with contrast to visualize endometrial tissue within pelvic and abdominal cavity
  - Laparoscopy (gold standard for direct visualization) in order to obtain biopsy and establishes definitive diagnosis
- *Treatment*:
  - First line: NSAIDs, oral contraceptives
  - If refractory can consider Medroxyprogesterone acetate, Leuprolide (GnRH agonist which will decrease FSH and LH production due to chronic stimulation, monitor bone mineral density, postmenopausal symptoms), Danazol (GnRH antagonist)
  - Surgery if medically necessary: laparoscopy with removal of lesions or hysterectomy if fertility is not an issue and conservative measures do not help
  - Patients who have undergone numerous surgeries and do not have an immediate surgical need but suffer from pain can be treated with opiates and possible addition of neuropathic agents (see opiate and neuropathic medication chapters for more details). These patients should have continued regular follow up with their Gynecologist to assure no further surgical intervention is needed. [1, 4, 5]

Interstitial Cystitis/Bladder Pain Syndrome

Chronic inflammation at bladder wall

- *Symptoms*: pelvic pain and discomfort or pressure-sensation perceived to be related to the bladder for >6 weeks; may be increased with bladder filling and improved with voiding. It is often associated with urinary frequency, urgency, dysuria, or nocturia. [6] symptoms of recurrent UTIs yet negative urine cultures
- *Associated symptoms*: may have dyspareunia (especially with deep penetration, but may be diminished with voiding), ejaculatory pain, suprapubic or low back pain; often coexists with vulvodynia [7, 8]

- *Physical exam*:
  - Abdomen: location of pain, typically suprapubic tenderness to palpation, location of scars (previous pelvic surgery may cause internal scarring which can be source of chronic pelvic pain) Musculoskeletal: hip girdle, gait—instability or pain induced by walking or body position may imply associated musculoskeletal pain, trigger points
  - Vaginal exam: No specific finding. It is important to rule out other conditions that may be a cause for chronic pelvic pain since IC is a diagnosis of exclusion.
- *Labs*:
  - Urine culture, and STD testing is negative with Interstitial Cystitis/Bladder Pain Syndrome
  - Post-void residual volume to screen for voiding dysfunction
  - Interstitial cystitis/chronic pelvic pain syndrome is a diagnosis of exclusion and is best made by a urologist/gynecologist with specialty training
- *Imaging*:
  - No specific imaging is required
  - Bladder ultrasound with report of post-void urine can be done if in-office bladder scan device is unavailable.
  - Cystoscopy is used to exclude bladder tumors. Cystoscopy is essential if there is associated hematuria, family history of genitor-urinary malignancy, abnormal urine cytology, or history of tobacco use. The presence of glomerulations (fine petechiae seen with bladder distention) or ulceration (Huner's ulcer, seen in 10 % of patients with IC) supports the diagnosis of IC/BPS but is not required for diagnosis; bladder biopsy should be considered if there is a suspicious lesion
- *Treatment*:
  - Education: an explanation of interstitial cystitis/bladder pain syndrome validates patients' symptoms and concerns. There is no single diagnostic test; treatment may involve multiple modalities
  - Stress/anxiety reduction and exercise: can help reduce exacerbation of symptoms
  - Behavioral changes
    - Application of local heat or cold to painful region of pelvis
    - Avoidance of dietary triggers (caffeine, alcohol, and spicy or acidic foods and drinks)
    - Patients may manage with increased cranberry juice or cranberry extract tablets, which are acidic and can exacerbate IC symptoms (cranberry juice is acidic and may exacerbate IC symptoms).
    - Fluid management: some patients experience worse symptoms with concentrated urine so increasing

fluids may be helpful while other patients experience worse symptoms with bladder filling in which case fluid restriction is beneficial to avoid the extremes

- Physical therapy
  - Evaluation and treatment by specialized pelvic floor physical therapist can help patient relax pelvic floor muscles and reduce trigger point pain, massage of scar tissue can improve pain, exercises to increase pelvic floor tone should be avoided (Kegel's exercises) since this will increase pain. [9, 10]
- Pharmacologic
  NSAIDs
  - Tricyclic antidepressant/neuropathic agents (Nortriptyline, Amitriptyline, Gabapentin, Lyrica): central analgesic effect [11]
  - Elmiron (pentosan polysulfate sodium, the only FDA-approved medication specifically approved for IC) 100 mg p.o. tid, which re-establishes the proposed defective glycosaminoglycan layer that coats the bladder urothelium (can be associated with mild hair loss that is reversible with cessation of medication) [12]
  - Antihistamines (Hydroxyzine-25–50 mg qhs, drowsiness is the most common side effect due to the hypothesis that mast cell release is responsible for bladder symptoms [13]
  - Muscle relaxant/anxiolytic: diazepam (Valium) 1–5 mg once or twice daily prn can reduce pelvic muscle tone [13]
  - Topical anesthetic: Pyridium 100 mg po q8hours prn acts as a topical anesthetic on the urothelium; limit use to 3–5 days due to potential for liver toxicity, inform patient that urine will be bright orange color
- Intravesical instillation of DMSO or a "cocktail" of lidocaine, bicarbonate, a steroid, and heparin or Elmiron (heparin and Elmiron are analogues of glycosaminoglycan that forms the layer that protects the urothelial cells from noxious stimuli in urine), typically done once weekly for 6 weeks. May be repeated depending on severity of symptoms [14]
- Cauterization of bladder ulcer (Huner's ulcer) with cystoscopy, improves pain
- Bladder hydrodistention—Distending the bladder under anesthesia can disrupt fine urothelial nerve fibers reducing transmission of pain stimuli. Some may see improvement last up to 6 to 9 months. If successful, it can be repeated [15]
- Sacral neuromodulation (Interstim therapy): unilateral or bilateral stimulation of the S3 nerve root with a four-lead electrode placed percutaneously under fluoroscopic guidance. Not FDA approved for IC but with failure of other therapies may result in symptom improvement [16]

- Bladder Botox can improve associated urinary frequency and urgency but no effect on pain [17]
- Bladder cystectomy and ileal conduit is a procedure of last resort for symptom control. Persistence of pain is common but may improve quality of life (reduce urinary urgency/frequency) [18]

Prostatitis/Chronic Pelvic Pain Syndrome

- *Symptoms*: pain in perineum, groin, testicles, penis, symptoms present for >3months, dull and achy pain typically at perineum and urethra or penis [19]
- *Aggravating factors*: full bladder, sexual activity, exertion (heavy lifting or exercise), bicycle riding (perineal trauma) or stress and anxiety.
- *Alleviating factors*: voiding, hot water Sitz bath, anxiety and stress reduction.
- *Associated symptoms*: painful ejaculation, irritative (urgency, frequency, dysuria) or obstructive (hesitancy, intermittent stream, weak stream) urinary symptoms, sexual dysfunction [20]
- *Physical exam*:
  - Vitals: if febrile, tachypneic, tachycardic consider acute prostatitis, prostate abscess, bacteremia, sepsis; with chronic prostatitis, vitals should be stable
  - Inspection: check general appearance, posture, sitting position, some may have trouble sitting on perineum
  - Genitalia: some patients may experience pain referred to urethra so rule out urethral pathology: palpate urethra at ventral surface of penis to rule out mass or much less commonly—an impacted urethral stone or urethral diverticulum–Rectal exam: palpate prostate for bogginess (soft, fluid-like feeling—suggesting an abscess) or tenderness (omit DRE if acute prostatitis is likely)
- *Labs*
  - UA and urine culture to r/o UTI
  - PSA not indicated—may be falsely elevated
  - Consider CBC
  - Consider Mears-Stamey 2 glass urine test: [2]
  - Send urine analysis with microscopy and culture
  - Perform prostatic massage
  - Send first 10 cc urine for analysis and microscopy and culture after prostatic massage
  - Can help determine chronic inflammatory prostatitis (+WBC and negative culture on post massage UA and culture) or chronic bacterial prostatitis (increased WBC with + culture on post massage UA and culture) or noninflammatory prostatitis (negative WBC and negative culture on post massage UA and culture)

- *Imaging*
  - Bladder scan or pelvic ultrasound: screen for voiding dysfunction, check for post-void residual, rule out prostatic abscess.
  - Transrectal ultrasound may be too painful
  - Pelvic CT: if suspect prostatic abscess, if treatment failure
- *Treatment*
  - Education about prevalence, triggers, proposed pathophysiology
  - Warm water Sitz bath, consider pelvic floor physical therapy especially if associated voiding symptoms, anxiety/stress reduction, relaxation exercises/yoga [21–23]
  - NSAIDS: ibuprofen
  - Oral antibiotics: Quinolones (Levoquin better than Cipro) are probably better than sulfonamides: both categories have good penetration into prostate, macrodantin is excreted in urine but has poor tissue penetration, may require 2–4 weeks or longer of antibiotic treatment.
  - Analgesics
  - Antipyretics as needed
  - Alpha-blockers: tamsulosin 0.4 mg po qhs (Flomax), alfuzosin 10 mg po qhs (Uroxatral), silodosin 4 or 8 mg po qhs (Rapaflo)—caution about orthostatic hypotension and retrograde ejaculation [23]
  - Antiandrogen: finasteride 5 mg po once daily (Proscar), dutasteride 0.5 mg po once daily (Avodart)—if associated BPH symptoms
  - Treatment of associated sexual dysfunction
  - Treat according to post massage urine culture results if positive
  - Consider treatment of atypical uropathogens: (Chlamydia, *Mycobacterium*, *Cryptococcus*) with doxycycline 100 mg p.o. b.i.d.
  - Transurethral microwave thermotherapy (TUMT) of prostate—heat causing necrosis of prostatic tissue [24]
  - Transurethral resection of prostate (TURP)—resection of prostatic tissue using cautery

Pelvic Venous Congestion

Congestion of pelvic veins, increases with multiparous women [2]
- *Symptoms*: often asymptomatic when this becomes symptomatic patients present with chronic pelvic pain of unknown etiology for over 6 months, vulvar discomfort and swelling worsened with prolonged standing and exercise and coitus; often manifests initially during or after pregnancy

- *Associated symptoms*: dyspareunia, dysuria, dysmenorrhea, menorrhagia
- *Aggravating factors*: menses
- *Physical exam*: normal pelvic exam, as laying down often relieves pressure from ovarian veins; vulvar varicosities on gynecological exam, cervical motion tenderness, uterine tenderness, and ovarian tenderness on direct palpation [2]
- *Labs*: normal
- *Imaging*: Not necessary to confirm diagnosis
  - Pelvic MRI or CT with contrast (preferred) can be used to evaluate pelvic and gonadal veins
  - Pelvic venography to visualize varices >4 mm
  - Transabdominal, transperineal or transvaginal ultrasound showing ovarian vein >6 mm, or tortuous venous plexus this also helps to exclude other potential etiologies
- *Treatment*:
  - Medroxyprogesterone Acetate
  - Embolization or sclerotherapy of ovarian veins
  - Surgical: Laparoscopic or open ligation of ovarian veins; hysterectomy; bilateral oophorectomy.
  - In patients refractory to surgical treatments, opiates or neuropathic agents can be used to help control pain. [2, 25]

Pelvic Trigger Points

- *Symptoms*: pain of the pelvic floor
- *Associated symptoms*: existence of coexisting musculoskeletal abnormalities i.e., SI dysfunction), often cause pain in a referred pattern, vulvodynia, dyspareunia, bowel/bladder dysfunction, pain during ambulation in more severe cases
- *Physical exam*: levator ani/perineal stiffness on pelvic exam, often times palpation of hypersensitive muscle fiber or taut on exam; trigger points can lead to shortening of muscle fibers, which causes significant pain on pelvic pain
- *Labs*: normal
- *Imaging*: normal
- *Treatment*: Pelvic floor rehabilitation, including Biofeedback therapy, as well as muscle stretch and relaxation exercises
  - Pelvic trigger point injections using dose of 1–5 mL of local anesthetic (lidocaine most commonly used); Common pelvic pain generators in women are anterior inferior levator ani, and bulbospongiosus in women, pubococcygeus, sphincter ani, and adductor magnus in both men and women
  - Saline injection, dry needling, as well as use of botulinum Toxin A have been found to treat symptoms

- Diazepam can also be helpful in treating tight pelvic floor muscles, oral or suppository formulation can be used
- Manual release techniques
- Acupressure [5, 26]

Pelvic Floor Abnormalities

Can be secondary to trauma, childbirth, postural abnormalities, or previous pelvic surgeries; may lead to involuntary spasming of pelvic floor muscles [2]
- *Symptoms*: Perineal pain
- *Associated symptoms*: Dyspareunia, vaginismus, dyschezia
- *Physical exam*: Point tenderness on vaginal or rectal examination; may have urine flow abnormality
- *Labs*: normal
- *Imaging*: normal
- *Treatment*:
  - Warm Sitz baths
  - Pelvic rehabilitation—biofeedback
  - Trigger point injections/Botulinum toxin into pelvic floor muscles
  - Anticholinergics (i.e., Tricyclic antidepressants)
  - Muscle relaxants
  - Bladder analgesics- Defecating program [5, 26]

Pudendal Neuralgia

Pudendal nerve stems off the sacral plexus (S2-4)
Compression can occur as a consequence of abdominal surgery or childbirth
- *Symptoms*: pain/paresthesias in distribution of pudendal nerve, which include groin, abdomen, pelvic and lower extremity, as well as perineal and gluteal regions (Fig. 22.1)
- *Associated symptoms*: Pain is often associated with concomitant pain in SI joint, coccyx, and piriformis; Pain often associated with sitting; relief associated with standing or lying on unaffected side; urinary frequency
- *Exacerbating factors*: sitting
- *Mitigating factors*: standing and laying on unaffected side
- *Physical exam*: perineal sensation and muscle tone are normal
- *Labs*: normal
- *Imaging*: MRI neurography or Ultrasound can be helpful to rule out a compressive lesion, however, diagnosis is largely clinical
- *Treatment*:
  - Rehabilitation of hip rotator, gluteal, lumbosacral, abdominal, and pelvic floor muscles
  - Pudendal nerve mobilization techniques
  - Diagnostic nerve block with local anesthetic

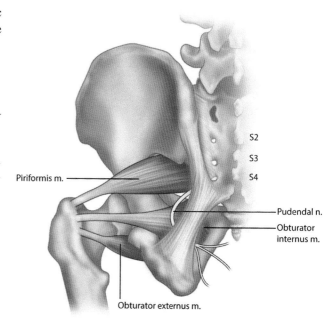

Fig. 22.1 Pelvic anatomy showing the course of the pudendal nerve which is effected with pudendal neuralgia

- Botulinum injection into pelvic floor muscles in spasm secondary to pudendal neuralgia (most common are obturator internus and levator ani)
- Refractory cases consider Gabapentin, Lyrica, Muscle relaxants, or low-dose antidepressants, Tramadol, and Opioids
- Surgical decompression [27]

Inguinal Neuralgia

Can be associated with previous abdominal surgeries or pregnancies, although incidence has decreased due to the advent of laparoscopic procedures
- *Symptoms*: pain/paresthesias over lower abdomen with radiations into scrotum or labia; hypo or hyperesthesias along inguinal ligament (Fig. 22.2)
- *Physical exam*: + Tinel's with tapping over ilioinguinal nerve; possible sensory deficit in the inner thigh, scrotum or labia in distribution ilioinguinal nerve; pain with hip extension; reproducible pain with palpation medial to the ASIS
- *Labs*: normal
- *Imaging*: MRI neurography or Ultrasound can be helpful to rule out a compressive lesion, however, diagnosis is largely clinical
- *Treatment*:
  - Diagnostic ilioinguinal nerve block with anesthetic
  - Trigger point injections
  - NSAIDs, COX-2 inhibitors; Anticonvulsants, Capsaicin cream, topical lidocaine [2]

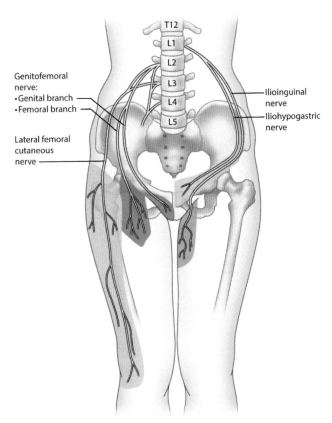

Genitofemoral
nerve:
• Genital branch
• Femoral branch

Lateral femoral
cutaneous
nerve

Ilioinguinal
nerve

Iliohypogastric
nerve

Fig. 22.2 Pelvic anatomy showing pelvic peripheral nerves that can be implicated in pelvic pain

Abdominal Pain

Acute abdominal pain: sudden onset of severe abdominal pain that may persist from hours to days and may be life threatening

Acute abdominal pain can be categorized with visceral or somatic etiologies
- *Visceral*: presents with diffuse, poorly localized pain
- *Somatic*: caused by stimulation of the peritoneum, pain is precisely localized

Chronic abdominal pain: "constant or recurrent pain over a 3-month period" [2] inconsistent localization
- Functional gastrointestinal disorders (FGID) usually present with diffuse abdominal pain in atypical locations [2]. May be associated with weight loss, nausea rarely vomiting
- Functional GI disorder vs. Chronic organic disease vs. functional abdominal pain syndrome
- Exacerbations and remissions
- Bloating (better in AM, worse at night)
- Increased with psychological stress (IBS, GERD, FGID)

Abdominal Differential Diagnosis
- **General differential**: Gastroenteritis, IBS, PUD, GERD, Constipation, UTI, Pyelonephritis, diverticulosis, diverticulitis, cholangitis, pancreatitis, hepatitis, choledocholithiasis, Infection, spontaneous bacterial peritonitis, Primary malignancy vs metastasis, fibromyalgia
- **Additional differential in women**: PID, Dysmenorrhea, Ovarian Cyst, Endometriosis, Ectopic Pregnancy
- **Differential requiring surgical evaluation**: Appendicitis, Acute Cholecystitis, Intestinal Obstruction, Perforated viscera, Dissecting Aortic Aneurysm, Embolic Mesenteric Ischemia, ectopic pregnancy (Table 22.1) [28]

It is important to differentiate between acute and chronic abdominal pain. The above medical conditions should always be ruled out prior to diagnosing a patient with chronic abdominal pain and treating with opioids or adjuvant medications. In addition it is necessary to rule out acute etiologies in patients with known chronic abdominal pain syndromes. Below is a general approach to assure the surgical and acute pathologies are ruled out before proceeding.

General History for Abdominal Pain
- *Symptoms*:
  - *Location of pain and referred pain*
    - *Localized*: somatic
    - *Diffuse*: FGID
    - *Epigastric*: stomach, duodenum, pancreas, biliary tree
    - *Periumbilical*: jejunum and ileum, ascending colon
    - *Suprapubic*: descending colon, sigmoid, rectum
    - *Radiating to back*: pancreatitis, PUD, spinal etiology
  - *Frequency and onset of pain*
    - Constant pain: etiology of parietal inflammation or capsule distention (ref bonica [2])
    - Colicky pain: etiology of visceral obstruction
      - Small or large bowel "repeatedly over seconds or minutes" (ref bonica [2])
      - Biliary or renal "hours to days" [2]
  - *Quality of pain*:
    - Burning: GERD
    - Tearing: aortic aneurysm
- *Associated symptoms*: Nausea, vomiting (Bowel obstruction—SBO—immediately after food intake, LBO—feculent vomit), diarrhea, changes in stool (blood (distal GI tract disease), melena (upper GI pathology), steatorrhea, etc.), loss of appetite, Avoidance of food (found with liver congestion and ureteric obstruction), autonomic symptoms such as sweating and nausea should be considered pathologic until otherwise noted, hematemesis (upper GI disease), hematuria and loin pain (ureteric obstruction and renal calculus), fever (acute

Table 22.1 Extra-abdominal causes of abdominal pain

Cardiopulmonary
Aortic dissection
Aortic aneurysm
Unstable angina
Acute myocardial infarction
Ischemic heart disease
Pericarditis
Pneumonia
Pneumothorax
Pulmonary empyema
Pulmonary embolism/infarction
Hematological
Henoch–Schonlein purpura
Sickle cell crisis
Metabolic/endocrinological
Acute intermittent porphyria
Addison's disease
Diabetic ketoacidosis
Hypercalcemia
Lead poisoning
Uremia
Genitourinary
Kidney stones
Pyelonephritis
Urinary retention
Gynecological
Ovarian rupture
Musculoskeletal
Inguinal/ventral hernia, strangulated
Osteomyelitis
Vertebral/spinal disorders
Thoracic compression fracture
Muscle injury
Neurocutaneous
Radiculopathy
Intercostal neuralgia
Herpes zoster
Tabes dorsalis
Injection abscess (in diabetics)
Miscellaneous
Lead poisoning with herbal medicines
Familial Mediterranean fever
Narcotic withdrawal
Fractured ribs
Liver pathology

abdomen possibly requiring surgical intervention), weight loss (chronic pathology), early satiety, back pain (pancreatitis), bloating
- *Mitigating factors*:
  - Posture
    - Leaning forwards: relieves retroperitoneal pain (e.g., Pancreas)
    - Fetal position: relieves retroperitoneal pain

  - Food intake:
    - Upper GI pathology relieved with food intake (gastroduodenal ulcers
  - Relief after vomiting: stomach or proximal small bowel pathology
  - Relief after bowel movement: colon disease
- *Exacerbating factors*:
  - Movement/Inspiration/coughing: parietal pain, abdominal wall muscle pain
  - Posture
    - Supine: worsens retroperitoneal pain
  - Food intake: worsens GI tract pain
    - Exacerbations with food mostly with functional disease and GERD
    - Specific foods: oil, milk, spicy
  - Temporal relationship between food and possible worsening of pain
    - GI tract pain: worsens within minutes
    - Small bowel or colon: worsens hours later
  - Associated with bowel movements (lower GI involvement, IBS) [29]

Past Medical/Surgical History
- *Alcoholics*: more likely to have hepatitis or pancreatitis
- *Hyperuricemia*: can be prone to renal calculi
- *CAD/PAD/HTN*: increased risk of aortic aneurysm or mesenteric ischemia
- *Diabetes*: consider DKA
- *Prior Abdominal surgery*: consider adhesions and obstruction
- *Chronic NSAID use*: consider PUD, GERD. *colitis*
- *Bisphosphonate use*: consider GERD
- *Recent antibiotics*: consider C. Diff
- *Antispasmodics*
- *Psychosocial factors*:
  - Stress can increase symptoms with IBS, GERD, and FGID
  - Also consider psychiatric comorbidities (anxiety, depression, etc.)
- *Drugs*: IVDA related to Hepatitis B and C or HIV—these place patient at risk for hepatoma and infections)
- *Family history*: cancer, inflammatory disorders (IBD, celiac disease)

General Physical Exam for Abdominal Pain
- *Inspection*:
  - Initial appearance
    - Alert, diaphoretic, tachypneic (alert physician to more acute and threatening etiologies, if present send to ER)
    - Writhing around in pain—visceral etiology
      - Patients unable to find a pain relieving position consider intestinal obstruction or renal colic

- Fetal position or lying still (peritoneal irritation
- Weight loss (chronic disease)
- Inspect for scars, ecchymosis and possible hernia
- Jaundice—seen with hepatobiliary disease
- Signs of chronic liver disease: palmar erythema, spider nevi, duputryens contracture
  - Chronic liver pathology and pancreatitis often coexist especially in alcoholics [2]
- Abdominal distention: bowel obstruction, ascites
- *Vital signs*: r/o hypotensive shock (secondary to sepsis or hypovolemia)
- *Palpation*: Begin exam away from painful region to avoid guarding, examine for tenderness located to specific quadrant vs generalized tenderness
  - *RUQ*: hepatobiliary disease
  - *LUQ*: splenic disorders
  - *RLQ*: ovarian cyst or mass, chronic appendicitis, ectopic pregnancy
  - *LLQ*: constipation, ovarian cyst or mass, ulcerative colitis
  - *Suprapubic*: menses, UTI
  - *Guarding, rigidity, rebound tenderness*: indicated peritonitis
  - *Costovertebral angle tenderness*: UTI, pyelonephritis
  - Masses (organomegaly, carcinoma)
- *Percussion*:
  - Painful percussion: perotinitis
  - Tympany: distended bowel and obstruction
  - Dullness: mass
    - Shifting dullness: ascites
- *Auscultation/bowel sounds*:
  - Normal
  - Absent: ileus
  - Hyperactive: early bowel obstruction, gastroenteritis
  - Hypoactive: late bowel obstruction
  - Tinkling: obstruction
  - Also auscultate for bruits found in aneurysms and hematoma
- *Provocative maneuvers*:
  - + Murphy's sign indicative of cholecystitis
  - + Psoas sign (hyperextension of hip indicates inflammation of psoas muscle, possible abscess
- *Neurological exam*: usually normal in abdominal pain patients,
- *Rectal exam and obtain stool for occult blood*: fecal impaction, masses, blood can indicate superficial or deep fissures, polyps, IBD, or malignancy;
- *Vaginal exam*: inspect external genitalia, look for skin lesions, inspect meatus (caruncle, Urethral mucosal prolapse) quality of vaginal epithelial tissue, palpate distal anterior vaginal wall (rule out urethral diverticulum or urethritis), palpate deep anterior vaginal wall (cystitis), palpate apex of vagina/cervix (PID), check for associated vaginal prolapse, inspect for vaginal discharge
- *Systemic exam*: to rule out extra-abdominal causes
  - Cardiac: HTN, evaluation for murmurs and/or A fib (predispose to embolic-associated ischemia)
  - Respiratory: evaluation for PTX, PNA
- *Psychological assessment* [27, 29]

General Workup for Abdominal Pain

- *Labs*:
  - CBC (iron deficiency anemia can be associated with colon cancer, increase WBC can indicate infection)
  - Calcium (malignancy)
  - Aminotransferases, alkaline phosphatase, bilirubin (hepatitis or other liver disorders)
  - Lipase (pancreatitis)
  - Ferritin (iron deficiency anemia)
  - Antitissue transglutaminase (Celiac disease)
- *Diagnostic studies*:
  - Upper GI series
  - Colonoscopy (IBS, colon ca)
  - Flexible sigmoidoscopy (IBS)
  - UA (UTI, pyelonephritis)
  - Vaginal swab (gonorrhea, Chlamydia, and bacterial vaginosis)
  - Stool culture (gastroenteritis)
  - Laparoscopy (endomeriosis, malignancy)
- *Imaging*:
  - Abdominal XR/KUB (obstruction)
  - Abdominal US (cholecystitis, appendicitis)
  - Renal US (nephrolithiasis, appendicitis)
  - Transvaginal US (PID, ectopic pregnancy, ovarian cysts, malignancy)
  - MRI
  - CT (obstruction) [27]

Chronic Painful Cholecystitis

- *Symptoms*: Epigastric pain localizing to the right upper quadrant (RUQ), pain may radiate to the right shoulder or scapula;
- Associated symptoms: nausea/vomiting with or without fever, abdominal cramping and bloating; symptoms usually occur after meals, especially those high in fat content
- *Physical exam*: RUQ tenderness with guarding or rebound; jaundice; lack of palpable RUQ fullness (as opposed to acute, which is usually associated with the presence of gallstones); + Murphy's sign
- *Labs*: leukocytosis with left shift, amylase and lipase to determine involvement of pancreas, liver function tests to evaluate the liver

- *Imaging*: Abdominal Ultrasound and abdominal CT revealing gallbladder wall thickening of greater than 4–5 mm along with edema, along with + physical exam findings can confirm diagnosis; HIDA scan
- *Treatment*:
  - Bowel rest
  - Medications: treatment with NSAIDs or Opioids for pain, such as Morphine, Hydromorphone or Meperidine
  - Surgical: ERCP, cholecystectomy [30]

Pancreatitis

- *Symptoms*: Epigastric pain with radiations to the back, pancreatic insufficiency-associated nausea and vomiting; possible dyspnea; Glucose intolerance
- *Physical exam*: Tenderness of fullness in the epigastric region, which may indicate a pseudocyst; abdominal distention, and hypoactive bowel sounds; fever, tachypnea, hypotension; patient with steatorrhea may exhibit signs of malnutrition, such as temporal wasting or decreased subcutaneous fat
- *Labs*: Usually associated elevated amylase and lipase; CBC, electrolytes, and liver function tests are usually normal
- *Imaging*:
  - X-ray shows calcification within pancreatic duct
  - Abdominal US shows enlarged and hypoechoic pancreas
  - Abdominal CT with contrast
  - MRI surrounding edema, pancreatic duct dilation, as well as pseudocysts
- *Treatment*:
  - *Acute pancreatitis*: Initially, treat with fluid resuscitation 5–10 mL/kg/h NS and pain control, often with IV opiates. Meperidine is favored over morphine in cases of pancreatitis because studies show that morphine causes an increase of pressure in the sphincter of Oddi. If an infection is suspected, antibiotics should be initiated as well while the source is being determined.
  - *Chronic pancreatitis*: Pain management with NSAIDS, Opiates, Amitriptyline; lifestyle modification with cessation of alcohol and smoking and implementation of small low-fat meals into diet; pancreatic enzyme supplementation (theory is suppression of feedback loops in duodenum, which may decrease release of cholecystokinin, suppressing of pancreatic exocrine secretion, resulting in decreased pain); surgery is considered for patients who fail medical therapy. [31]

Table 22.2 Rome III diagnostic criteria for irritable bowel syndrome

Recurrent abdominal pain or discomfort[b] at least 3 days/month in the last 3 months associated with two or more of the following
1. Improvement with defecation
2. Onset associated with change in frequency of stool
3. Onset associated with change in form (appearance) of stool

*Criterion fulfilled for the last 3 months with symptom onset at least 6 months prior to diagnosis

[b]Discomfort means uncomfortable sensation not described as pain

Used with permission from The Rome Foundation

Irritable Bowel Syndrome

- *Symptoms*: Chronic abdominal pain, gastroesophageal reflux, nausea, alternating constipation/diarrhea, impaired sexual dysfunction, increased urinary frequency, dysmenorrhea, dyspareunia; relieved by bowel movements (Table 22.2).
- *Physical exam*: Nonspecific abdominal tenderness; exam findings are generally normal
- *Labs*: Routine labs are normal in this condition
- *Imaging*: Routine imaging normal in this condition
- *Treatment*:
  - Diet modification
  - Antidepressants, probiotics, antidiarrheal agents, serotonin receptor agonists/antagonists
  - Psychosocial treatment [32]

Malignancy/Metastasis

- *Symptoms*: weight loss. Pain occurs late in disease due to capsular stretching from tumor growth, pain progresses over time and may be constant
- *Physical exam*: Anemia, abdominal mass, jaundice, organomegaly
- *Labs*: Leukocytosis, anemia
- *Imaging*: pelvic/abdominal ultrasound helps rule out masses
- *Treatment*: Chemotherapy/radiation treatment specific to cancer type

Functional Gastrointestinal Disorders

- *Symptoms*: classified by symptoms; diagnosis of exclusion
  - Functional esophageal disorders (reflux, dysphagia)
  - Functional colonic disorders (constipation, diarrhea)
  - Functional dyspepsia

- Noncardiac chest pain
- Chronic functional abdominal pain
- Irritable bowel syndrome
- *Physical exam*: Normal
- *Labs*: Normal
- *Imaging*: Normal
- *Treatment*:
  - Dietary management
  - *Anxie*ty management; symptomatic relief [33]

References

1. Howard F. Causes of chronic pelvic pain in women. In: Barbieri RL, editor. UpToDate. UpToDate, Inc. Accessed 4Jan 2014.
2. Vincent K, Moore J. Pelvic pain in females. In: Fishman SM, Ballantyne JC, Rathmell JP, editors. Bonica's management of pain. 4th ed. New York: Lippincott, Williams & Wilkins; 2009. p. 925–38.
3. Singh, Manish K. Chronic Pelvic Pain in Women Clinical Presentation. 2012. http://emedicine.medscape.com/article/258334-clinical.
4. Howard F. Treatment of chronic pelvic pain in women. In: Barbieri R, editor. UpToDate. UpToDate, Inc. Accessed 4 Jan 2014.
5. Bonder J, Rizzo JR, Chowdhury N, Sayegh S. Musculoskeletal pelvic pain and pelvic floor dysfunction. In: Sackheim K, editor. Rehab clinical pocket guide: rehabilitation medicine. New York: Springer; 2013. p. 467–85.
6. Hanno P, Dmochowski R. Status of international consensus on interstitial cystitis/bladder pain syndrome/painful bladder syndrome: 2008 snapshot. Neurourol Urodyn. 2009;28(4):274–86.
7. Hanno PM, Landis JR, Mathews-Cook Y, Kusek Jr NL. The diagnosis of interstitial cystitis revisited: lessons learned from the National Institutes of Health Interstitial Cystitis Database study. J Urol. 1999;161(2):553–7.
8. Driscoll A, Teichman JM. How do patients with interstitial cystitis present? J Urol. 2001;166(6):2118–20.
9. Anderson RU, Wise D, Sawyer T, Chan C. Integration of myofascial trigger point release and paradoxical relaxation training treatment of chronic pelvic pain in men. J Urol. 2005;174(1):155–60.
10. FitzGerald MP, Anderson RU, Potts J, Payne CK, Peters KM, Clemens JQ, Kotarinos R, Fraser L, Cosby A, Fortman C, Neville C, Badillo S, Odabachian L, Sanfield A, O'Dougherty R, Halle-Podell R, Cen L, Chuai S, Landis JR, Mickelberg K, Barrell T, Kusek JW, Nyberg LM. Urological Pelvic Pain Collaborative Research Network. Randomized multicenter feasibility trial of myofascial physical therapy for the treatment of urological pelvic pain syndromes J Urol. 2009;182(2):570–80.
11. Foster Jr HE, Hanno PM, Nickel JC, Payne CK, Mayer RD, Burks DA, Yang CC, Chai TC, Kreder KJ, Peters KM, Lukacz ES, FitzGerald MP, Cen L, Landis JR, Propert KJ, Yang W, Kusek JW, Nyberg LM. Interstitial Cystitis Collaborative Research Network. Effect of amitriptyline on symptoms in treatment naïve patients with interstitial cystitis/painful bladder syndrome J Urol. 2009; 183(5):1853–8.
12. Holm-Bentzen M, Jacobsen F, Nerstrom B, Lose G, Kristensen JK, Pedersen RH, Krarup T, Feggetter J, Bates P. Barnard. A prospective double-blind clinically controlled multicenter trial of sodium pentosanpolysulfate in the treatment of interstitial cystitis J Urol. 1987;138(3):503–7.
13. Rovner E, Propert KJ, Brensinger C, Wein AJ, Foy M, Kirkemo A, Landis JR, Kusek JW, Nyberg LM. Treatments used in women with interstitial cystitis data base (ICDB) study experience. The Interstitial Cystitis Data Base Study Group Urology. 2000;56(6):940–5.
14. Chong M, Hester J. Pharmacotherapy for neuropathic pain with special reference to urogenital pain. In: Baranowski A, Abrams P, Fall M, editors. Urogenital pain in clinical practice. New York: Informa Healthcare; 2008.
15. Welk BK, Teichman JM. Dyspareunia response in patients with interstitial cystitis treated with intravesical lidocaine, bicarbonate, and heparin. Urology. 2008;71(1):67–70.
16. Ottem DP, Teichman JM. What is the value of cystoscopy with hydrodistention for interstitial cystitis? Urology. 2005;66(3):494–9.
17. Peters KM, Konstandt D. Sacral neuromodulation decreases narcotic requirements in refractory interstitial cystitis. BJU Int. 2004;93(6):777–9.
18. Giannantoni A, Porena M, Costantini E, Zucchi A, Mearini A, Mearinin E. Botulinum A toxin intravesical injection in patients with painful bladder syndrome: 1-year followup. J Urol. 2008; 179(3):1031–4.4.
19. Hughes OD, Kynaston HG, Jenkins BJ, Stephenson TP, Vaughton KC. Substitution cystoplasty for intractable interstitial cystitis. Br J Urol. 1995;76(2):172–4.
20. Mears Jr EM. Prostatitis. Med Clinic North Am. 1991;75(2):405–24.
21. Nickel JC. Practical approach to the management of prostatitis. Tech Urol. 1995;1(3):162–7.
22. Pewitt EB, Schaeffer AJ. Urinary tract infection in urology, including acute and chronic prostatitis. Infect Dis Clin North Am. 1997;11(3):623–46.
23. Nickel JC. Effective office management of chronic prostatitis. Urol Clin North Am. 1998;25(4):677–84.
24. Nickel JC, Sorensen R. Transurethral microwave thermotherapy of nonbacterial prostatitis and prostatodynia: initial experience. Urology. 1994;44(3):458–60.
25. Ignacio EA, Intervent S. Radiol. Dec. 2008;25(4):361–8.
26. Moynihan, Leah K. Treatment of myofascial pelvic pain syndrome in women. In: Brubaker L, editor. UpToDate. UpToDate, Inc. Accessed 4 Jan 2014.
27. Fishman, M., Aronson, M., Chacko, M. Chronic abdominal pain in children and adults: Approach to evaluation. In: Middleman A, Ferry G, Drutz J, editors. UpToDate. UpToDate, Inc. Accessed 21 Feb 2014.
28. Fishman, M., Aronson, M. Differential Diagnosis of abdominal pain in adults. In: Fletcher, R., editor. UpToDate. UpToDate, Inc. Accessed 21 Feb 2014.
29. Fishman, M., Aronson, M. History and physical examination in adults with abdominal pain. In: Fletcher R, editor. UpToDate. UpToDate, Inc. Accessed 21 Feb 2014.
30. Zakko S, Afdhal N. Acute cholecystitis: pathogenesis, clinical features, and diagnosis. In: Chopra S, editor. UpToDate. UpToDate, Inc. Accessed 21Feb 2014.
31. Freedman S. Clinical manifestations and diagnosis of chronic pancreatitis in adults. In: Whitcomb D, editors. UpToDate. UpToDate, Inc. Accessed 21 Feb 2014.
32. Wald A. Clinical manifestations and diagnosis of irritable bowel syndrome in adults. In: Talley N, editor. UpToDate. UpToDate, Inc. Accessed 21 Feb 2014
33. Drossman D. The functional gastrointestinal disorders and the Rome III process. Gastroenterology. 2006;130(5):1377–90; Review.

Neuropathic Pain

23

Robin Iversen

Abbreviations

ACE	Angiotensin-converting enzyme
ANA	Antinuclear antibodies
CMAP	Compound muscle action potential
CBC	Complete blood count
CIDP	Chronic inflammatory demyelinating polyneuropathy
CRP	C reactive protein
CT	Computed tomography
EMG	Electromyography
ESR	Erythrocyte sedimentation rate
HIV	Human immunodeficiency virus
HNP	Herniated nucleus pulposis
INR	International normalized ratio
MMT	Manual muscle testing
MRI	Magnetic resonance imaging
NCV	Nerve conduction velocity
OTC	Over the counter
RF	Rheumatoid factor
ROM	Range of motion
SNAP	Sensory nerve action potential
SPEP	Serum protein electrophoresis
TENS	Transcutaneous electrical nerve stimulation
TFT	Thyroid function tests

Introduction

Neuropathic pain is a problem, which is usually chronic and severe and can be debilitating for patients. Neuropathic pain oftentimes affects a limb or body region, which on physical exam may appear normal. Patients with neuropathic pain report that their quality of life, mood, ability to continue working, and activities of daily living all suffer because of their pain [1].

Neuropathic pain is caused by a primary lesion or disease in the somatosensory system (Table 23.1) [2].

Pathophysiology

There is no single mechanism resulting in neuropathic pain. *A combination of concepts results in these basic tenets:*

1. Damaged peripheral nerves result in abnormal sodium channel activity which causes ectopic firing of these nerves [3]
2. Loss of inhibitory neurons [4]
3. Central sensitization results in spread of nociceptive activity to uninjured tissue-mediated through glutamate [5]
4. Wallerian degeneration results in abnormal myelin sheaths [4]

History

Obtain history including onset of the symptoms, duration of the symptoms, location, and severity.

Symptoms: (depend on which sensory nerves are damaged)
- *Large sensory fibers*—(myelinated fibers) these mediate vibratory sensation, light touch, and position sense
  Damage to these fibers cause:
  - Numbness of hands and or feet
  - Balance issues
  - Decreased dexterity and strength
- *Small sensory fibers*—these mediate temperature and pain sensation

R. Iversen, M.D. (✉)
Rutgers New Jersey Medical School, The Valley Hospital, Ridgewood, NJ 07450, USA
e-mail: galrbd2@aol.com

Table 23.1 Common neuropathic classes and examples [2]

Neuropathic category	Neuropathic conditions
Autoimmune	Multiple sclerosis
Metabolic	Diabetic peripheral neuropathy
Infectious	Post-herpetic neuralgia, HIV related
Vascular	Poststroke syndrome
Toxic	Chemotherapy-induced neuropathy
Traumatic	Herniated nucleus pulposis
Acquired	Trigeminal neuralgia
Postsurgical	Phantom limb, scar neuroma, failed
	Back syndrome, post mastectomy
Genetic	Charco Marie–Tooth
Idiopathic	No etiology found

Damage to these fibers cause:
- Allodynia (painful response to a non-noxious stimulus)
- Hyperalgesia (exaggerated pain response)
- Altered temperature sensation
- Hypoalgesia (numbness)

- Patients' pain descriptors for neuropathic pain:
  - Pins and needles
  - Stinging/cutting
  - Electric/tingling/numbness
  - Crawling/asleep

Physical exam:

Inspection: examine for skin changes—color changes/discoloration, scarring/hyperpigmentation from shingles lesions, sweat, hair growth/diminished hair growth, temperature changes, edema, or diabetic skin changes, nail fungus/thickening

Palpation: may be extremely painful to light touch in the affected area, examine for allodynia, hypoalgesia, hyperalgesia

ROM: may be limited by pain in the affected area

MMT: some weakness may be found surrounding involved nerves, but usually weakness is secondary to pain and not actual weakness unless severe progressed neuropathy is present

Reflexes: may be decreased or absent at affected nerves

Neurological:

Light touch and pin prick may be decreased or absent (decrease/absence may be in glove and stocking distribution)

Vibratory sensation with a 128 Hz tuning fork may be decreases in a glove and stocking areas [4, 6]

Decreased proprioception

Abnormal temperature sensation (ice cube to skin may feel like abnormal sensation "burning")

Aberrant extension of sensory disturbance beyond dermatome [1]

Workup

A diagnosis is based on symptom description, physical exam, and a clinical history that matches a neuroanatomical or dermatomal pattern [7]. Workup can be done to aide diagnosis and rule out other etiologies.

Labs to Evaluate Small Fiber Neuropathy

CBC, SMA20, ESR, CRP, Vitamin B12, Folate, TSH, serum and urine immunofixation, serum and urine electrophoresis, HgA1c, ACE levels, ANA, RF

Labs to evaluate for toxic/metabolic causes:

Autoimmune: lumbar puncture, rheumatologic markers, SPEP, TFT

Metabolic: HgbA1C, Vit B12, B1, folate, liver profile INR

Inflammatory/infectious: lyme titers, ESR, Hep B&C serology, HIV

Toxic: heavy metal screen

Hereditary: genetic testing

Imaging to Rule Out Other Etiology: Most Likely Normal with Neuropathic Pain

X-ray, CT, or MRI may be indicated if trying to identify location of an obstructive or traumatic cause (i.e., trigeminal neuralgia or HNP, tumor)

Electrodiagnostic Testing

- **EMG**: only evaluates large fiber-mediated neuropathic pathology. For a credible evaluation, three limbs must be tested (Table 23.2).
- **NCV**: only evaluates large fiber damage and can determine axonal disease vs. myelin degeneration. Abnormalities of small fibers may be associated with autonomic dysfunction may not be seen with standard NCS and may demand special tests [8].

Biopsy

- *Nerve biopsy*: can determine exact degree of nerve damage but has little use in helping treatment, it is a difficult, invasive procedure that does not change treatment or course of the condition; it is useful for determining amyloid neuropathies or chronic inflammatory demyelinating polyneuropathy (CIDP) [9]

Table 23.2 Summary

Condition	EtoH neuropathy	Diabetic neuropathy	Charcot Marie–Tooth	PHN	Lead neuropathy	HIV	Cis-Platinin	Trigeminal neuralgia
Class	Toxic	Metabolic	Genetic	Infectious	Toxic	Infectious	Toxic	Acquired
Symptoms	Gait disturbance	Abnl sensation	Abnl vibratory sensation	Painful paresthesias	B/L UE weakness	Painful paresthesia in extremities	Impaired sensation	Facial pain
	Abnl sensation	Painful paresthesia in extremities in stocking glove distribution	Pes cavus	In dermatomal distribution in location of herpetic eruption	Abdominal		Painful paresthesia	Allodynia
	Muscle spasm	Hypoalgesia	Sensory loss lower extremity>upper		Pain			hyperalgesia
	Korsakoff psychosis	Abnl vibratory sensation	Abnl proprioception		Wrist drop			
Workup	Vitamin levels	HgbA1C	CSF=↑protein	EMG=NL	Heavy metal screen	Viral load	CBC	CT or MRI to assess compression of CN V
	EMG=abnl	FBS		SNAP=abnl	RBC basophilic stippling EMG=Abnl radial muscles		Bun/Cr	
	SNAP=abnl CMAP=abnl	Nerve Bx=small and large fiber involvement		CMAP=Abnl	SNAP=Nl CMAP=Abnl			
Nerve Involvement	Sensorimotor Axonal loss	Sensorimotor with demyelination and axonal loss	Demyelination with sensory loss		Axonal loss with more motor than sensory	Sensorimotor with axonal loss	Pure sensory with axonal loss	
Intervention	Addiction counseling	Glycemic control	Membrane stabilizers	Membrane stabilizers		Membrane stabilizers	Membrane stabilizers	Membrane stabilizers
	Vitamin supplement	Membrane stabilizers	PT	Topical capsaicin		Topical lidocaine		Surgical decompression
	Membrane stabilizers	Foot care	braces	Topical lidocaine				

CMAP compound muscle action potential [11], *SNAP* sensory nerve action potential [12]

- *Skin biopsy*: can show small fiber damage. It is easy to perform and can direct treatment [3].
- *Muscle biopsy*: can aide in diagnosis of hereditary neuropathies

Treatment

Please see details on medications in the topical analgesic and neuropathic medication chapters

Modalities

- *TENS unit*: transcutaneous electrical stimulation has a position as a supplementary treatment in neuropathic pain. Stimulation across the affected area can provide transient relief [10]
- *Acupuncture*: has a position in treatment although success is considered anecdotal for lack of randomized controlled evaluations [10]

Psychological Treatment

As neuropathic pain patients report both decreased mood and anxiety and difficulty coping with their pain, cognitive behavioral therapy may be helpful [10]

Surgical Options

- *Decompression*: trigeminal neuralgia
- *Nerve ablation*: has risk of deafferentation
- *Nerve modulation*: i.e., *spinal cord stimulation*: based on the gate control theory good results in DPN and Failed Back Syndrome [10]
- *Anodyne monochromatic infrared photoenergy*: this is becoming a somewhat popular treatment also referred to as "red light" therapy. There are home kits patients may buy, but mostly this is administered by nonphysician health care providers. It is the application of infrared light directly to the areas of neuropathy daily. Theory is that this energy will result in increased circulation and with it an increase in nitric oxide, thus reducing pain and promoting healing of the nerves. Studies have shown no real effectiveness [11].

References

1. Gilron I, Watson CP, Cahill CM, Moulin DE. Neuropathic pain: a practical guide for the clinician. CMAJ. 2006;175(3):265–75.
2. Treed RD, Jensen TS, et al. Neuropathic pain redefinition—a grading system for clinical and research purposes. Neurology. 2008;70(18):1630–5.
3. Baron R, Binder A, Wasner G. Neuropathic pain: diagnosis, pathophysiological mechanisms and treatment. Lancet. 2010;9:807–19.
4. Bridges D, Thompson SW, Rice AS. Mechanisms of neuropathic pain. Br J Anaesth. 2001;87(1):12–26.
5. Dworkin RH, Backonja M, Rowbotham MC, Allen RR, Argoff CR, Bennett GJ, et al. Advances in neuropathic pain: diagnosis mechanisms and treatment recommendations. Arch Neurol. 2003;60(11):1524–34.
6. Vink T. Approach to the management of the patient with neuropathic pain. J Clinical Endocrinology Metabolism. 2010;95(11):4802–11.
7. Freynhagen R, Bennett MI. Diagnosis and management of neuropathic pain. BMJ. 2009;339:b3002. doi:10.1136/bmj.b3002. Review.
8. England JD, Gronseth GS, Franklin G, Carter GT, Kinsella LJ, Cohen JA, et al. Practice Parameter: evaluation of distal symmetric polyneuropathy: role of autonomic testing, nerve biopsy, and skin biopsy (an evidence-based review). Report of the American Academy of Neurology, American Association of Neuromuscular and Electrodiagnostic Medicine, and American Academy of Physical Medicine and Rehabilitation. Neurology. 2009;72(2):177–84. doi:10.1212/01.wnl.0000336345.70511.0f. Epub 2008 Dec 3.
9. Curullo S, editor. Physical medicine and rehabilitation board review. New York: Demos Medical Publishing; 2004. p. 304–89.
10. Xu B, Descalzi G, Ye HR, Zhuo M, Wang YW. Translational investigation and treatment of neuropathic pain. Mol Pain. 2012;8:15. doi:10.1186/1744-8069-8-15.
11. Lavery LA, Murdoch DP, Williams J, Lavery DC. Does anodyne light therapy improve peripheral neuropathy in diabetes? A double-blind, sham-controlled, randomized trial to evaluate monochromatic infrared photoenergy. Diabetes Care. 2008;31(2):316–21.

Complex Regional Pain Syndrome (CRPS)

24

Richard G. Chang and Houman Danesh

Abbreviations

ANA	Antinuclear Antibodies
CBT	Cognitive Behavioral Therapy
CRP	Creactive protein
CRPS	Complex regional pain syndrome
CT	Computed tomography
DMSO	Dimethyl sulfoxide
ECT	Electroconvulsive therapy
EMG	Electromyography
ESR	Erythrocyte sedimentation rate
HbA1c	Hemoglobin A1c
IV	Intravenous
IVIG	Intravenous immunoglobulin
MMT	Manual muscle testing
MRI	Magnetic resonance imaging
NMDA	N-methyl-D-aspartate
PVD	Peripheral vascular disease
RCT	Randomized controlled trial
ROM	Range of motion
RSD	Reflex sympathetic dystrophy
SNRI	Selective norepinephrine reuptake inhibitor
SNS	Sympathetic nervous system
TENS	Transcutaneous Electrical Nerve Stimulation

R.G. Chang, M.D., M.P.H. (✉)
Department of Physiatry, Hospital for Special Surgery,
429 East 75th Street, 3rd floor,
New York, NY 10021, USA
e-mail: changr@hss.edu

H. Danesh, M.D.
Division of Pain Medicine, Department of Anesthesiology,
Icahn School of Medicine at Mount Sinai, New York, NY, USA

- **Definition**: Neuropathic pain syndrome that is out of proportion to inciting event, characterized by the presence of the following:
  - **Allodynia**: pain response to a normally non-painful stimulus
  - **Hyperalgesia**: increased pain response to a noxious stimulus
  - **Sudomotor changes**: edema and/or sweating
  - **Vasomotor changes**: skin color and/or temperature changes
  - **Trophic changes**: hair, nail, and/or skin changes
  - **Motor changes**: decreased ROM, immobility, and/or motor dysfunction (weakness, tremor, dystonia)

- CRPS is a diagnosis of exclusion
- Diagnosis criteria is still debated, but most recent based on 2003 Budapest criteria

Classification

- **Type I**: reflex sympathetic dystrophy (RSD), absence of direct nerve injury. Usually caused by a noxious event such as crush injury or period of immobilization (e.g., cast).
- **Type II**: causalgia (Greek—kausis + algos, meaning "burning pain"), direct nerve injury

Pathophysiology

It is still not clearly understood, but a number of mechanisms have been proposed.
- Alterations in central and peripheral sensitization
- Changes in sympathetic nervous system (SNS) outflow with disturbed catecholamine response
- Exaggerated inflammatory response
- Genetic factors
- Biopsychosocial factors
- Reorganization of somatotopic maps in the brain

K.A. Sackheim, *Pain Management and Palliative Care: A Comprehensive Guide*,
DOI 10.1007/978-1-4939-2462-2_24, © Springer Science+Business Media New York 2015

Epidemiology and Causes [1–5]

- Women at greater risk than men; 3.5:1 ratio
- Most cases between 50 and 70 years old, but may develop in children
- Often occurs after trauma to an extremity. Commonly develops after minor soft tissue trauma (sprains, contusions), fractures, and surgery involving an extremity (e.g., post-fracture reduction/fixation, carpal tunnel release, knee surgery/arthroscopy, hip arthroplasty), but may commonly occur after long periods of immobilization (e.g., tight casts). For CRPS type II, the reported incidence secondary to peripheral nerve injuries varies from 2 to 14 % [6].

Clinical Diagnostic Criteria (Budapest Criteria) 2003 [7, 8]

Clinical Diagnosis can be made when the following criteria are met:

- Continuing pain that is disproportionate to any inciting event
- **At least 1 symptom reported in at least 3 of the 4 following categories:**
  - *Sensory*: hyperesthesia or allodynia
  - *Vasomotor*: temperature asymmetry, skin color changes, skin color asymmetry
  - *Sudomotor*: edema, sweating changes, or sweating asymmetry
  - *Motor/trophic*: decreased range of motion, motor dysfunction (e.g., weakness, tremor, dystonia), or trophic changes (e.g., hair, nail, skin)
- **At least 1 sign at time of evaluation in at least 2 of the following categories:**
  - *Sensory*: evidence of hyperalgesia (to pinprick), allodynia (to light touch, temperature sensation, deep somatic pressure, or joint movement)
  - *Vasomotor*: evidence of temperature asymmetry (>1 °C), skin color changes, or asymmetry
  - *Sudomotor/edema*: evidence of edema, sweating changes, or sweating asymmetry
  - *Motor/trophic*: evidence of decreased range of motion, motor dysfunction (e.g., weakness, tremor, dystonia), or trophic changes (e.g., hair, nail, skin)
- No other diagnosis better explaining the signs and symptoms

For research diagnostic criteria, the only difference compared to the clinical diagnostic criteria is that the patient should have **at least 1 symptom in ALL 4-symptom categories.** All other criteria are the same as above.

Types and Severity

(No Evidence to Suggest the Following Stages Occur Sequentially) [9]

Stage 1: Early stage (0–3 months post onset)
- Primarily characterized by hyperalgesia, allodynia, vasomotor dysfunction, prominent edema, and sudomotor disturbance

Stage 2: Dystrophic stage (3–6 months post onset)
- Marked pain/sensory dysfunction, continued evidence of vasomotor dysfunction, with development of significant motor/trophic changes

Stage 3: Atrophic stage (6–12 months post onset)
- Decreased pain/sensory disturbance, continued vasomotor disturbance, and markedly increased motor/trophic changes

Physiologic Staging [10]

- **"Hot" CRPS**: representing high blood flow state, clinically extremity is warm, swollen with burning/tearing pain (ischemic pain suggestive of inappropriate arteriovenous shunting) with no contractures. Often presents early, is generally sympathetically mediated and responds poorly to opiates.
- **"Cold" CRPS**: representing low blood flow state, clinically extremity is cool, atrophic, stiff, with decreased ROM. Pain may also be of burning/tearing quality.

Symptoms

- Persistent pain that is disproportionate to initial suspected insult (e.g., sprain, fracture, stroke, surgery)
- Pain may occur spontaneously without any identifiable injury
- No set time frame, but may occur immediately after injury
- *Acute CRPS*: < 2–3 months, *Chronic CRPS*: >2–3 months [8, 11]
- Pain quality may vary, but usually burning, throbbing, numbing, tingling, shooting, and/or aching
- Tends to affect distal extremity, but may spread to any other extremity or body part
- Difficulty in using affected body part, with accompanied decreased ROM and function
- Temperature changes: warm or cold compared to unaffected regions—"warm, acute" phase does not need to transition to "cold, chronic" phase [9]
- Skin color changes (reflecting autonomic dysfunction)
- Fatigue

Differential Diagnosis

- Peripheral neuropathy
- Radiculopathy
- Plexopathy
- Mononeuritis multiplex
- Thoracic outlet syndrome
- Autoimmune disorder
- Rheumatoid arthritis
- Infectious etiologies (Lyme, fungal, viral, tuberculosis)
- Peripheral vascular disease
- Deep vein thrombosis
- Conversion disorder
- Factitious disorder

Physical Exam

- Must fulfill at least 2 of the 4 categories mentioned in Budapest criteria
- **Typically unilateral limb involvement, but may spread to other body parts-no set pattern**
  - *Inspection*:
    - Skin discoloration ("acute" = red; "chronic" = blue)
    - Edema
    - Skin, hair, nail changes (e.g., increased/decreased/abnormal skin texture, hair growth, or nail quality)
    - Muscle atrophy secondary to disuse/avoidance
  - *Palpation*:
    - Allodynia, hyperalgesia; may be measured via Von Frey testing, which uses fine gauge metal wires to test response to mechanical stimuli [12]
    - Trigger points (myofascial pain syndrome)
    - Temperature differences between affected part (>1 °C difference) and surrounding tissue or unaffected regions; may use temperature taper or infrared thermometer
  - *ROM*: Decreased and painful ROM of affected extremity; measured with goniometer
  - *MMT*: Possible motor weakness
  - *Sensory*:
    - Allodynia, Hyperalgesia
    - Altered response to light touch (via cotton swab/brush), pinprick, and/or vibration
    - Temperature differences between affected part (>1 °C difference) and surrounding tissue or unaffected regions; may use temperature taper or infrared thermometer
  - *Reflexes*: may have exaggerated deep tendon reflexes on affected side
  - *Neurological*: [12]
    - Neglect or extreme favoring of affected extremity
    - Tremor
    - Dystonia

Labs

- No specific tests to confirm CRPS
- May perform basic inflammatory arthropathy workup (e.g., Rheumatoid factor, ANA, ESR, and CRP) to exclude rheumatologic conditions, *but often these values are normal in CRPS*
- HbA1c and thyroid function tests may also be done to rule out undiagnosed diabetes or hypothyroidism, respectively

Diagnostic Studies

- *EMG and Nerve conduction studies:* useful to perform to determine if there is an underlying nerve injury (for CRPS type II or to rule out peripheral neuropathy since CRPS has no characteristic EMG or nerve conduction pattern)
- *Vascular studies:* may be considered if PVD is suspected—used to exclude other differential diagnoses

Imaging

Not required for diagnosis, but may be used to support diagnosis and to assess severity of chronic disease. Controversy still exists in the utility of imaging alone in diagnosis given poor sensitivity, but high specificity—making such tools poor choices for screening. The clinical history and exam remain the gold standard [13].

- **X-ray of affected region**
  - *Acute*: generally not useful as initial imaging may be unremarkable
  - *Chronic*: patchy demineralization with subperiostal bone resorption and/or osteoporosis [13–16]
- **Triphasic bone scan**: In a 2012 meta-analysis by Ringer et al., they found that studies using clearly defined diagnostic criteria had a pooled mean sensitivity of 80 % and specificity 73 %. They concluded that this type of imaging alone does not confirm or exclude the presence of CRPS type I [17].
  - *Acute*:
    - Appears useful in acute phase up to 3–6 months with sensitivities ranging from 19 to 97 % (depending on study cited), but with fairly consistent high specificities, 95–99 % [13, 18]
    - Sensitivity decreases as time goes by [19, 20]
    - Positive findings consistent with CRPS type I show increased blood flow and periarticular activity during blood pool and delayed static phases of affected limb due to increased bone metabolism, neurogenic inflammation, or decreased sympathetic activity [17, 18, 21]
  - *Chronic*:
    - Pathologic findings noted above may show decreased activity in all three phases or may not reveal any distinguishing features [19, 22]

- **MRI**:
  - May show osteoporosis in affected limb, but are typically not of diagnostic value or may be misleading [13, 23]
- **CT**: Not useful in establishing diagnosis
- **Ultrasound**: Not routinely considered since it has not been widely studied and does not have same utility compared to plain radiographs or bone scan
  - Increased echogenicity with decreased muscle architecture (muscle outlines indistinct or obliterated)
  - Decreased muscle thickness irrespective of duration of disease
  - Flexors and forearm extensors maximally affected [24]
  - Pekindi et al. showed that arterial dopplers of posttraumatic CRPS may reveal loss of arterial triphasic waveforms in some cases of acute CRPS type I, but is not diagnostic for the disease [25].

Prognosis

The condition is treatable, but there exists no gold standard treatment. There are multiple options available, but emphasis is placed on early recognition, treatment, and immediate initiation of rehabilitation program.

- As many as 80 % of patients with the initial symptoms of CRPS type I are cured within 18 months from its onset, either spontaneously or with treatment [8]
- Other cases may progress to chronicity due to intolerance to therapy or delay in diagnosis

Treatment [26, 27]

Basic Principles

- Functional restoration is mainstay of treatment
- Begin aggressive physical therapy and other treatments as soon as possible
- Medications, psychotherapy, and anesthetic blocks in patients who do not respond to functional restoration techniques (therapy)
- Medications and injections can also be used to help patient have increased tolerance to physical therapy program
- Multidisciplinary approach
- **Preventive Measures**
- High-dose Vitamin C: beneficial in preventing CRPS incidence post-wrist and foot/ankle fractures. Mechanism not totally understood, but believed to be from ascorbate's antioxidant properties in stabilizing free radical activity.
  - According to existing studies, benefits appear to be seen with at least 500 mg daily of Vitamin C for 45–50 days post injury [28–33].

- **Physical and Occupational therapy** [26, 34]
  General Principles: Functional Restoration Is Goal
  - Early mobilization, but avoid aggressive ROM exercise and strengthening programs to prevent worsening of existing kinesiophobia/fear avoidance of involved extremity with activity, worsening pain
  - Avoid static splinting
  - In both cases, treatment of possible myofascial trigger points whether by dry needling before therapy or myofascial release may aid in recovery process
  - Concurrent CBT program may be beneficial
  - Medications and/or sympathetic blocks may have to be used earlier to facilitate therapy program
  - Edema control with specialized garments (e.g., stockings) and manual techniques (e.g., lymph massage)
  - Desensitization techniques
  - Slow, graduated weight-bearing exercises (isometric later to isotonic or isokinetic)
  - Aquatic/pool therapy
  - No consensus for TENS application (electrical stimulation may worsen allodynia through large myelinated fiber stimulation)
  Posture and movement retraining
- **Recreational therapy**
  - Incorporating a new leisure skill with emphasis on community reintegration
- **Vocational rehabilitation and counseling**
- **Alternative therapies**
  - Acupuncture
  - Electroconvulsive therapy (ECT)
  - Transcranial direct current stimulation
- **Medications** [35, 36]
  1. *Corticosteroids*: potentially effective in controlling pain. No consensus as to duration and dosage. Greatest efficacy during acute phase. Benefits may be seen up to 1 year. Long-term therapy not recommended given its many systemic side effects.
     - Consider oral prednisone 30 mg daily with taper over 2–12 weeks
     - For stroke patients with suspected "shoulder-hand syndrome," a recent randomized controlled trial by Kalita et al., showed that oral prednisolone 40 mg/day for 2 weeks, followed by 10 mg/week taper had greater improvement in pain, edema, shoulder ROM, and ADLs compared to patients on piroxicam 20 mg/day [37].
     - In Grundberg's 1996 prospective study of patients with CRPS of the UE followed for 1 year, the author found that IM methylprednisolone 80 mg administered every 2 weeks for a maximum total of 4 doses alleviated rest and night pain in 47 out of 69 patients [38–42]

2. *Anticonvulsants*: although not FDA approved for CRPS, they are often used given neuropathic component of the pain syndrome. Please refer to neuropathic pain chapter for more detailed dose and frequencies.

- *Gabapentin*: consider titration to 600 to 1800 mg by mouth daily in the first 8 weeks to help improve pain. In van de Vusse's randomized double blind placebo controlled crossover study of 58 chronic CRPS type I patients refractory to sympathetic blocks, mannitol infusions, and transcutaneous neuromodulation, they found that gabapentin 600 mg TID by mouth titrated within 3 weeks only showed a mild improvement in pain compared to placebo, but did improve sensory abnormalities over a 2-month period [43].
- *Pregabalin*: may be considered, start with 25 mg by mouth daily, may titrate up to 75 mg BID if tolerated. Though, no evidence for treatment of CRPS type I [35].
- *Phenytoin and carbamazepine*: (theoretically may help CRPS type II, peripheral nerve injuries alter sodium channel distribution on axons) can potentially be used, but there is insufficient evidence for effectiveness for CRPS type I [35, 44].

3. *Antidepressants*: although commonly used for neuropathic conditions, there is not enough literature to guide therapy in respect to CRPS. They may be considered as an adjunct to anticonvulsants. Please refer to neuropathic pain chapter for standard dosage and frequencies [45]

- SSRIs (selective serotonin reuptake inhibitors)
- TCA (tricylic antidepressants), e.g., Amitriptyline

4. *Opioids*: lack of evidence from literature demonstrating any consistent benefit. Tramadol may be considered an option given its selective norepinephrine reuptake inhibitor (SNRI) properties, which may help with neuropathic pain [8, 35, 36, 44, 45].

5. *Bisphosphonates*: believed to exert is effects via anti-osteoclast activity and modulating inflammatory cytokines. The existing evidence appears to support is use, but it is still unclear which bisphosphonate (if any) is preferred and optimal dosing and frequency of therapy [27, 46–50]

- Compared to placebo, bisphosphonates appear to improve pain, swelling, and range of motion.
- For oral therapy, in Manicourt et al.'s 2004 RCT study of 39 patients, patients assigned to alendronate 40 mg orally daily for 8 weeks showed marked improvement in pain, joint mobility, and pressure tolerance [48]. Avoid in patients with creatinine clearance <35.

- For IV therapy, the following has been used with improvement in pain and ROM compared to placebo:
  - Adami et al., 1997: IV alendronate 7.5 mg daily administered in 3 consecutive days [47]
  - Varenna et al., 2000: Clodronate 300 mg IV daily for 10 days [49]
  - Robinson et al., 2004: Pamidronate 60 mg IV in single dose with improved physical function and pain in 3-month follow-up [50]
- *Calcitonin*: limited and conflicting evidence; however, may prove to be beneficial similar to bisphosphonates, by inhibiting osteoclast activity and unexplained analgesic properties [35, 36].

6. *Vasodilators,* e.g., Tadalafil, Diltiazem

7. *Oral antioxidants and free radical scavengers,* e.g., DMSO

8. *Topicals*:
- Lidocaine
- Clonidine
- Ketamine

Interventional Treatment Options

- *IV NSAIDs*: e.g., 60 mg Ketorolac with lidocaine as IV regional blockade—questionable benefit and mixed results overall in treatment of neuropathic pain complaints [51, 52]
- *IV regional blockade* (e.g., guanethidine, reserpine, and/or droperidol): limited efficacy, but regional blockades with bretylium or Ketanserin can improve pain [35, 36]
- *Sympathetic blocks*: (e.g., stellate ganglion or lumbar sympathetic blocks)
- *Spinal cord stimulators*
- *Epidural/intrathecal clonidine*
- *Intrathecal baclofen*
- *IV Ketamine*: thought to decrease central sensitization, which is believed to play a role in pathophysiology of CRPS. Ketamine has been used traditionally as a general anesthetic, but as a noncompetitive antagonist for the NMDA (N-methyl D-aspartate) receptor, it prevents the influx of calcium through the voltage-gated receptor, decreasing the process of central sensitization. Appears to show promise, but few studies and RCTs have not clarified optimum dosage, frequency, and duration [53, 54].
- *IVIG (intravenous immunoglobulin)*: consider for chronic refractory cases; more studies needed for optimal dose and duration [55]

Surgical

- Sympathectomy
- Motor cortex stimulation [56]

Pediatric CRPS

Epidemiology [57]

- Occurs most commonly in girls, around later childhood and adolescence
- Tends to affect lower extremities more compared to adults

Pathophysiology and Causes

- Believed to be same as above, but significant trauma as the precipitating event is a less frequent cause when compared to adults
- Establishing diagnosis with symptoms and physical exam is similar to adults.

Labs/Imaging

- Generally same guidelines as above
- Bone scans used to rule out orthopedic abnormalities or infectious cases (e.g., osteomyelitis)

Treatment

- Greater response to noninvasive treatment, primarily physical therapy and/or intensive multidisciplinary rehabilitation [58–60]
- **Alternative Therapies**
- Acupuncture—high acceptance rate and case reports demonstrating benefit [58]
- **Medications**
- *Intense physical therapy*: Case series and reports have shown benefits with TCAs, anticonvulsants, e.g., gabapentin, corticosteroids, NSAIDs, and opioids, but again not routinely recommended in view of side effects and limited data [59, 60].
- **Interventional Treatment Options**—reserved for patients who do not respond to multidisciplinary and/or pharmacologic treatment [58]
  - *Spinal cord stimulators*—mixed results
  - *Sympathectomy*—consider carefully; indicated for sympathetically mediated portion of pain complaints.

- *Disadvantages*: irreversible and may cause sympathalgia; long-term physiologic effects of lumbar sympathectomy on adolescent girls not well studied.

References

1. Shipton EA. Complex regional pain syndrome-mechanisms, diagnosis, and management. Curr Anaesth Crit care. 2009;20:209–14.
2. De Mos M, Sturkenboom MC, Huygen FJ. Current understandings on complex regional pain syndrome. Pain Pract. 2009;9(2):86–99.
3. Sandroni P, Benrud-Larson LM, McClelland RL, Low PA. Complex regional pain syndrome type I: incidence and prevalence in Olmsted county, a population-based study. Pain. 2003;103:199–207.
4. Allen G, Galer BS, Schwartz L. Epidemiology of complex regional pain syndrome: a retrospective chart review of 134 patients. Pain. 1999;80:539–44.
5. De Mos M, De Bruijn AG, Huygen FJ, et al. The incidence of complex regional pain syndrome: a population-based study. Pain. 2006;1:12–20.
6. Hsu ES. Practical management of complex regional pain syndrome. Am J Ther. 2009;16(2):147–54.
7. Harden RN, Bruehl S, Stanton-Hicks M, Wilson PR. Proposed new diagnostic criteria for complex regional pain syndrome. Pain Med (Malden, Mass). 2007;8(4):326–31.
8. Wheeler AH. Complex regional pain syndromes. In: Berman SA, (Ed.) eMedicine. 2012. http://emedicine.medscape.com/article/1145318-overview. Accessed 12 Oct 2012.
9. Bruehl S, Harden RN, Galer BS, Saltz S, Backonja M, Stanton-Hicks M. Complex regional pain syndrome: are there distinct subtypes and sequential stages of the syndrome? Pain. 2002;95(1–2):119–24.
10. Patterson RW, et al. Complex regional pain syndrome of the upper extremity. J Hand Surg Am. 2011;36(9):1553–62.
11. Mathur S, Harden N. Complex regional pain syndrome part 1: essentials of assessment and diagnosis [Internet]. 2012 [updated 11/9/12] http://now.aapmr.org/pain-neuro/pain-medicine/Pages/CRPS-Part-1.aspx.
12. Albazaz R, Wong YT, Homer-Vanniasinkam S. Complex regional pain syndrome: a review. Ann Vasc Surg. 2008;22(2):297–306.
13. Schurmann M, et al. Imaging in early posttraumatic complex regional pain syndrome: a comparison of diagnostic methods. Clin J Pain. 2007;23(5):449–57.
14. Bickerstaff DR, Charlesworth D, Kanis JA. Changes in cortical and trabecular bone in algodystrophy. Br J Rheumatol. 1993;32:46–51.
15. Bickerstaff DR, O'Doherty DP, Kanis JA. Radiographic changes in algodystrophy of the hand. J Hand Surg Br. 1991;16:47–52.
16. Stengel M, Binder A, Baron R. Updates on the diagnosis and management of complex regional pain syndrome. Adv Pain Manage. 2007;1:96–104.
17. Ringer R, et al. Concordance of qualitative bone scintigraphy results with presence of clinical complex regional pain syndrome 1: meta-analysis of test accuracy studies. Eur J Pain. 2012;16(10):1347–56.
18. Wuppenhorst N, Maier C, Frettloh J, et al. Sensitivity and specificity of 3-phase bone scintigraphy in the diagnosis of complex regional pain syndrome of the upper extremity. Clin J Pain. 2010;26:182–9.
19. Lee GW, Weeks PM. The role of bone scintigraphy in diagnosing reflex sympathetic dystrophy. J Hand Surg Am. 1995;20:458–63.
20. Werner R, Davidoff G, Jackson MD, et al. Factors affecting the sensitivity and specificity of the three-phase technetium bone scan in the diagnosis of reflex sympathetic dystrophy syndrome in the upper extremity. J Hand Surg Am. 1989;14:520–3.

21. Zyluk A. The usefulness of quantitative evaluation of three-phase scintigraphy in the diagnosis of post-traumatic reflex sympathetic dystrophy. J Hand Surg Br. 1999;24(1):16–21.

22. O'Donoghue JP, Powe JE, Mattar AG, et al. Three-phase bone scintigraphy. Asymmetric patterns in the upper extremities of asymptomatic normals and reflex sympathetic dystrophy patients. Clin Nucl Med. 1993;18:829–36.

23. Marsland D, Konyves A, Cooper R, Suvarna SK. Type I complex regional pain syndrome: MRI may be misleading. Injury Extra. 2008;39:102–5.

24. Champak Vas L, Pai R. Ultrasound appearance of forearm muscles in 18 patients with complex regional pain syndrome 1 of the upper extremity. Pain Pract. 2013;13(1):76–88.

25. Pekiindil G, Pekindil Y. Doppler sonographic assessment of post-traumatic reflex sympathetic dystrophy. J Ultrasound Med. 2003; 22:395–402.

26. Harden RN. A clinical approach to complex regional pain syndrome. Clin J Pain. 2000;16(2 Suppl):S26–32.

27. Tran DQH, Duong S. Treatment of complex regional pain syndrome: a review of the evidence. Can J Anesth. 2010;57:149–66.

28. Lichtman DM, Bindra RR, Boyer MI, Putnam MD, Ring D, Slutsky DJ, et al. Treatment of distal radius fractures. J Am Acad Orthop Surg. 2010;18:180–9.

29. Zollinger PE, Tuinebreijer WE, Breederveld RS, Kreis RW. Can vitamin C prevent complex regional pain syndrome in patients with wrist fractures? a randomized, controlled, multicenter dose-response study. J Bone Joint Surg Am. 2007;89(7):1424–31.

30. Zollinger PE, Tuinebreijer WE, Kreis RW, Breederveld RS. Effect of vitamin C on frequency of reflex sympathetic dystrophy in wrist fractures: a randomised trial. Lancet. 1999;354(9195):2025–8.

31. Cazeneuve JF, Leborgne JM, Kermad K, Hassan Y. Vitamin C and prevention of reflex sympathetic dystrophy following surgical management of distal radius fractures. Acta Orthop Belg. 2002;68: 481–4.

32. Shibuya N, Humphers JM, Agarwal MR, Jupiter DC. Efficacy and safety of high-dose vitamin C on complex regional pain syndrome in extremity trauma and surgery—systemic review and meta-analysis. J Foot Ankle Surg. 2013;52(1):62–6.

33. Besse JL, Gadeyne S, Galand-Desme S, Lerat JL, Moyen B. Effect of vitamin C on prevention of complex regional pain syndrome type I in foot and ankle surgery. Foot Ankle Surg. 2009;15(4):179–82.

34. Dommerholt J. Complex regional pain syndrome—2: physical therapy management. J Bodyw Mov Ther. 2004;8:241–8.

35. Perez RS, Zollinger RE, Dijkstra PU, et al. Evidence based guidelines for complex regional pain syndrome type 1. BMC Neurol. 2010;10:20.

36. Kishner S. Complex regional pain syndrome part 2: management and treatment [Internet]. 2012 [updated 11/9/12]. http://now.aapmr.org/pain-neuro/pain-medicine/Pages/CRPS-Part-2.aspx.

37. Kalita J, Vajpayee A, Misra UK. Comparison of prednisolone with piroxicam in complex regional pain syndrome following stroke: a randomized controlled trial. Q J Med. 2006;99:89–95.

38. Grundberg AB. Reflex sympathetic dystrophy: treatment with long acting intramuscular corticosteroids. J Hand Surg Am. 1996;21: 667–70.

39. Christensen K, Jensen EM, Noer I. The reflex dystrophy syndrome response to treatment with systemic corticosteroids. Acta Chir Scand. 1982;148(8):653–5.

40. Braus DF, Krauss JK, Strobel J. The shoulder-hand syndrome after stroke: a prospective clinical trial. Ann Neurol. 1994;36(5):728–33.

41. Kozin F, Ryan LM, Carerra GF, Soin JS, Wortmann RL. The reflex sympathetic dystrophy syndrome (RSDS). III. Scintigraphic studies, further evidence for the therapeutic efficacy of systemic corticosteroids, and proposed diagnostic criteria. Am J Med. 1981; 70:23–30.

42. Grundberg AB. Reflex sympathetic dystrophy: treatment with long acting intramuscular corticosteroids. J Hand Surg Am. 1996;21: 667–70.

43. van de Vusse AC, Stomp-van den Berg SG, Kessels AH, Weber WE. Randomised controlled trial of gabapentin in Complex Regional Pain Syndrome type 1 [ISRCTN84121379]. BMC Neurol. 2004;4:13.

44. Harke H, Gretenkort P, Ladleif HU, Rahman S, Harke O. The response of neuropathic pain and pain in complex regional pain syndrome I to carbamazepine and sustained-release morphine in patients pretreated with spinal cord stimulation: a double-blinded randomized study. Anesth Analg. 2001;92:488–95.

45. Rowbotham MC. Pharmacologic management of complex regional pain syndrome. Clin J Pain. 2006;22:425–9.

46. Brunner F, Bachmann LM, Weber U, et al. Complex regional pain syndrome 1—the Swiss cohort study. BMC Musculoskelet Disord. 2008;9:92.

47. Adami S, Fossaluzza V, Gatti D, Fracassi E, Braga V. Bisphosphonate therapy of reflex sympathetic dystrophy syndrome. Ann Rheum Dis. 1997;56:201–4.

48. Manicourt DH, Brasseur JP, Boutsen Y, Depreseux G, Devogelaer JP. Role of alendronate in therapy for posttraumatic complex regional pain syndrome type 1 of the lower extremity. Arthritis Rheum. 2004;50:3690–7.

49. Varenna M, Zucchi F, Ghiringhelli D, et al. Intravenous clodronate in the treatment of reflex sympathetic dystrophy syndrome. A randomized, double blind, placebo controlled study. J Rheumatol. 2000;27:1477–83.

50. Robinson JN, Sandom J, Chapman PT. Efficacy of pamidronate in complex regional pain syndrome type I. Pain Med. 2004;5: 276–80.

51. Connelly NR, Reuben S, Brull SJ. Intravenous regional anesthesia with ketorolac-lidocaine for the management of sympathetically-mediated pain. Yale J Biol Med. 1995;68:95–9.

52. Namaka M, Gramlich CR, Ruhlen D, Melanson M, Sutton I, Major J. A treatment algorithm for neuropathic pain. Clin Ther. 2004;26:951–79.

53. Azari P, et al. Efficacy and safety of ketamine in patients with complex regional pain syndrome: a systematic review. CNS Drugs. 2012;26(3):215–28.

54. Goldberg ME, et al. Multi-day low dose ketamine infusion for the treatment of complex regional pain syndrome. Pain Physician. 2005;8(2):175–9.

55. Goebel A, Baranowski A, Maurer K, Ghiai A, McCabe C, Ambler G. Intravenous immunoglobulin treatment of the complex regional pain syndrome: a randomized trial. Ann Intern Med. 2010;152(3): 152–8.

56. Fonoff ET, Hamani C, de Ciampi AD, et al. Pain relief and functional recovery in patients with complex regional pain syndrome after motor cortex stimulation. Stereotact Funct Neurosurg. 2011; 89(3):167–72.

57. Low AK, Ward K, Wines AP. Pediatric complex regional pain syndrome. J Pediatr Orthop. 2007;27(2):567–72.

58. Wilder RT. Management of pediatric patients with complex regional pain syndrome. Clin J Pain. 2006;22(5):443–8.

59. Bialocerkowski AE, Daly A. Is physiotherapy effective for children with complex regional pain syndrome type 1? Clin J Pain. 2012; 28(1):81–91.

60. Brooke V, Janselewitz S. Outcomes of children with complex regional pain syndrome after intensive inpatient rehabilitation. PM R. 2012;4(5):349–54.

Fibromyalgia

Levan Atanelov

Abbreviations

ACR	American College of Rheumatology
ANA	Antinuclear antibodies, ANA antinuclear antibody
CAPP	Central amplification of pain perception
CBC	Complete blood count
CBT	Cognitive behavioral therapy
CFIDS	Chronic fatigue immune dysfunction syndrome
CMP	Complete metabolic panel
CPK	Creatine phosphokinase
CRP	C reactive protein
ESR	Erythrocyte sedimentation rate
FDA	Food and drug administration
FIQ	Fibromyalgia impact questionnaire
FIQR	Fibromyalgia impact questionnaire revised
FM	Fibromyalgia
GABA	Gamma-aminobutyric acid
GI	Gastrointestinal
GU	Genitourinary
HEENT	Head, eyes, ears, neck, throat
HIV	Human immunodeficiency virus
HLA	Human leukocyte antigen
HTLV	Human T-lymphotropic virus
MSK	Musculoskeletal
mVASFIQ	Fibromyalgia impact questionnaire
NSAIDs	Nonsteroidal anti-inflammatory drugs
OA	Osteoarthritis
OSA	Obstructive sleep apnea
OT	Occupational therapy
PT	Physical therapy
RA	Rheumatoid arthritis
RF	Rheumatoid factor
SNRIs	Serotonin-norepinephrine reuptake inhibitors
SSI	Symptom severity index
SSRI	Selective serotonin reuptake inhibitors
TCA	Tricyclic antidepressant/s
TMJ	Temporomandibular disorder
TSH	Thyroid-stimulating hormone
WPI	Widespread pain index

- **Definition:** Chronic widespread pain without organic disease sufficient to explain observed symptoms and meeting the diagnostic criteria

Clinical Diagnostic Criteria (Table 25.1 and Fig. 25.1) [1–4]

Epidemiology

Five million Americans (2–5 % of the adult population) are affected [5]

Pathophysiology [6, 7]

- Incompletely understood, neurogenic origin, central (most evidence) and peripheral etiology
- Pain with *allodynia* (pain to non-painful stimuli) and *hyperalgesia* (increased pain response) due to **central amplification of pain perception (CAPP)**
- CAPP due to increased signaling in *ascending* (pro-nociceptive) and decreased signaling in *descending* (anti-nociceptive) pathways
  - *Ascending pathway*: elevated substance P, nerve growth factor, brain-derived neurotrophic factor and glutamate
  - *Descending pathway*: decreased serotonin, norepinephrine and dopamine; increased endogenous opioids and decreased opioid receptor binding
- **Peripheral sensitization**: reduction in the threshold of nociceptive afferent receptors caused by a local change in the sensitivity of sensory fibers initiated by tissue damage.

L. Atanelov, M.D., M.S., B.S. (✉)
Department of Physical Medicine and Rehabilitation, Johns Hopkins Hospital, Baltimore, MD, USA
e-mail: latanel1@jhmi.edu

K.A. Sackheim, *Pain Management and Palliative Care: A Comprehensive Guide*,
DOI 10.1007/978-1-4939-2462-2_25, © Springer Science+Business Media New York 2015

Table 25.1 Current and old diagnostic criteria for fibromyalgia

Old Criteria: 1990 American College of Rheumatology Criteria [1, 2]

  1. Pain is considered widespread when *all* of the following are present (**see** Fig. 25.1):
  – Pain in the *left* side of the body
  – Pain in the *right* side of the body
  – Pain *above* the waist
  – Pain *below* the waist
  – In addition, *axial skeletal pain* (cervical spine or anterior chest or thoracic spine or low back) *must be present*. In this definition, shoulder and buttock pain is considered as pain for each involved side. "Low back" pain is considered lower segment pain
  – Pain > 3 months

  2. Pain in *11 of 18 tender point* sites on digital palpation with approximately 4 kg force. Patient must rate these points as "painful," not "tender"

  18 Points to Examine:
  – Left/right suboccipital muscle insertions
  – Left/right anterior aspects of the intertransverse spaces at C5–C7
  – Left/right trapezius at the midpoint of the upper border
  – Left/right supraspinatus above the scapula spine near the medial border
  – Left/right upper lateral to the second costochondral junction
  – Left/right 2 cm distal to the epicondyles
  – Left/right upper outer quadrants of buttocks in anterior fold of muscle
  – Left/right posterior to the trochanteric prominence
  – Left/right medial fat pad proximal to the joint line

Current Criteria: 2010 American College of Rheumatology Criteria [3]

  1. Widespread Pain Index (WPI) ≥ 7 and Symptom Severity Score (SSS) ≥ 5 *or* WPI between 3 and 6 and SSS ≥ 9

  2. Symptoms present at a similar level for > 3 months

  3. Patient with no disorder that would otherwise explain the pain

  4. WPI—assign a point (0–19) for presence of pain during the *last week* to each of the **following regions**:
  – Left/right shoulder girdle
  – Left/right upper arm
  – Left/right lower arm
  – Left/right upper leg
  – Left/right lower leg
  – Left/right hip (buttock, trochanter)
  – Left/right jaw
  – Chest, neck
  – Abdomen
  – Upper back
  – Lower back

  5. SSS-sum the *severity + extent* of the somatic symptoms (0–12)
  – Rate the *severity* of *fatigue, waking un-refreshed, and cognitive symptoms* on the scale of 0–3 for each
     • Use "0" for no symptoms, "1" for generally mild or intermittent symptoms, "2" for considerable problems, often present and/or at a moderate level, "3" for pervasive, continuous, life-disturbing problems
  – Rate *extent* of somatic symptoms present on the scale of 0–3
     • Use "0" for no, "1" for few, "2" for a moderate number, and "3" for a great deal of symptoms
  – *Some somatic symptoms*: muscle pain, irritable bowel syndrome, fatigue/tiredness, problems thinking or remembering, muscle weakness, headache, pain/cramps in abdomen, numbness/tingling, dizziness, insomnia, depression, constipation, pain in upper abdomen, nausea, nervousness, chest pain, blurred vision, fever, diarrhea, dry mouth, itching, wheezing, Raynaud's, hives/welts, ringing in ears, vomiting, heartburn, oral ulcers, loss/change in taste, seizures, dry eyes, shortness of breath, loss of appetite, rash, sun sensitivity, hearing difficulties, easy bruising, hair loss, frequent urination, painful urination, and bladder spasms [4]

Nociceptor systems in the skin and muscle undergo changes in fibromyalgia patients by yet unknown mechanisms, possibly due to release of algesic substances after muscle or other soft tissue injury [8].
• Imbalances in neurotransmitters associated with mood, fatigue, and sleep dysfunction
• Other abnormalities in: autonomic function, hypothalamic–pituitary–adrenal axis, neurogenic inflammation, gray matter loss, oxidative stress

Risk Factors

• *Genetic*: first-degree relatives of affected patients are affected ×8 compared to relatives of patients affected with rheumatoid arthritis [9], HLA A, B, and DRB1, S/S genotype in the seritonergic transporter promoter region, decrease in the T/T polymorphism in the 5-HT2A receptor

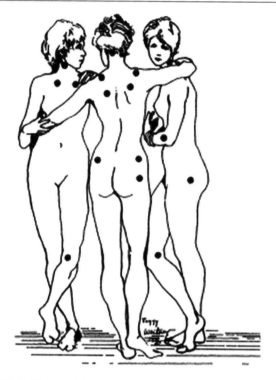

Fig. 25.1 Fibromyalgia "Old" Diagnostic Criteria. *With permission from Johnson JL, Collo MB, Finch WR, Felicetta JV. Fibromyalgia Syndrome. Journal of the American Academy of Nurse Practitioners 1990 Apr–Jun;2(2):47–53. © Wiley and Sons 1990* [43]

gene, D4 dopamine gene, which showed a significant decrease in a specific 7-repeat allele [7]
- *Environmental*: physical trauma or injury, infections (e.g., Lyme disease, hepatitis B/C, HIV, HTLV-1), work/family stress, life-changing events, and abuse history, low job satisfaction [7, 10]
- *Other*: Female sex, Ages 30–50 y/o

Symptoms [11]

- Most commonly: pain bilaterally, above/below waist and axial over 3 months, with fatigue and sleep disturbance (may present with either of these as a predominant complaint)
- May also have tenderness, stiffness, mood, and cognitive symptoms
- Symptoms wax and wane throughout the day and vary in intensity
- Impaired function, most commonly physical function
- Symptoms may vary from mild to severe from patient to patient

Prognosis

Chronic condition, relapsing remitting

History

- *Medical History/Common Comorbidities*: irritable bowel syndrome, tension-type headache/migraine, interstitial cystitis or painful bladder syndrome, chronic prostatitis or prostadynia, temporomandibular disorder (TMJ), chronic pelvic pain, and vulvodynia [12, 13]
- *Psychiatric History/Comorbidities*: anxiety 35–62 %, depression 58–86 %, bipolar 11 % [14, 15]
- *Family History*: first-degree relatives with fibromyalgia [9]
- *Social History/Common Comorbidities*: increased stress, history of sexual abuse, trauma and/or injury are common comorbidities [10]

Differential Diagnoses

- *Drug-induced*: statin-induced myalgia, opioid-induced hyperalgesia
- *Hematologic*: anemia
- *Endocrine*: hypothyroidism, thyroid disease in general
- *Autoimmune/Inflammatory*: inflammatory rheumatic diseases, RA, osteoarthritis, systemic lupus erythematosus, polymyalgia rheumatica, connective tissue disease, spondyloarthropathies
- *Mechanical/Neurological*: myofascial pain, spinal stenosis, neuropathies, sleep disorders (e.g., Obstructive sleep apnea (OSA)), referred discogenic spine pain, localized tendonitis
- *Psychiatric*: mood and anxiety disorders [16]

Please note: myofascial pain syndrome and fibromyalgia have different diagnostic and management criteria (though there is debate over this). *Fibromyalgia* presents with symptoms of *generalized pain without referred pain* and clinical finding of *multiple tender points*. Myofascial pain syndrome presents with *regional (local) referred pain* and clinical finding of *taut bands* of skeletal muscle with characteristic "nodular" texture upon palpation in regional distribution (also known as trigger points). Please note that trigger points may also be present in fibromyalgia, though less commonly. Sleep disturbance, fatigue, parasthesias, irritable bowel, sensation of swelling and headache often co-morbid with *fibromyalgia* are less commonly found with *myofascial pain syndrome*. One difference in clinical treatment is that tender points in fibromyalgia are less likely to improve with local injections than taut bands in myofascial pain syndrome [17, 18].

Physical Exam [11–13, 16]

Diffuse allodynia/hyperalgesia, but otherwise negative, assess for these to narrow the differential

Evaluate for the following to rule out differential and establish clinical diagnosis

- General: alertness, orientation, somnolence (to evaluate for psychiatric, endocrine, and neurological disorders on the differential diagnosis and common comorbidities)
- HEENT: thyroid size (for thyroid disorder on the differential diagnosis), oral ulcers (for autoimmune disorders on the differential diagnosis), TMJ tenderness (a common comorbidity)
- Cardio/Pulm: mitral valve prolapse (may be associated with anxiety, an etiology on the differential diagnosis as well as a common comorbidity)
- Abd: obesity (which may be associated with OSA, a condition on the differential diagnosis)
- GU/GI: vulvodynia/ prostadynia, pregnancy, sexual trauma signs (to evaluate for common comorbidities)
- Extremities: edema, swelling (may be associated with thyroid dysfunction and may help rule it out)
- Musculoskeletal: joint swelling/erythema, tenderness, range of motion, crepitus (to rule out rheumatologic etiologies on the differential diagnosis), **examine all appropriate tender points**, assess for taut bands of skeletal muscle with characteristic "nodular" texture upon palpation (to rule out myofascial pain syndrome)
- Lumbar: range of motion, paraspinal/spinal tenderness, pain on spinal loading (to rule out spine pathologies on the differential diagnosis)
- Neuro: weakness, numbness (to rule out neuropathies on the differential diagnosis)
- Skin: rash, alopecia, ulcers (to rule out autoimmune conditions on the differential diagnosis)
- Psych: anxious, depressed, or manic mood (to assess for psychiatric comorbidities)

Diagnostic studies

- **Labs**:
  - Work-up is negative as this is a diagnosis of exclusion
  - *Screen for to rule in or out other differential diagnoses*: ESR, CRP, CBC, CMP, CPK, TSH, free T3/T4; Levels for vitamin B12, vitamin D, ferritin, iron-binding capacity, and percentage of saturation [16]
  - RF and ANA if suspect autoimmune condition
  - Urinalysis and pregnancy test as needed per history
- **Imaging**: consider joint X-ray to examine for OA/RA, spinal X-ray/MRI to rule out spinal etiology

Treatment

Set treatment goals, use multidisciplinary approach, track symptoms over time, explain the chronic nature of the condition and that there is no specific cure, patient-centered care, start low and go slow with any interventions. Can use medications for symptomatic management.

Symptom-Tracking Tools:
- Validated: Fibromyalgia Impact Questionnaire (FIQ), Fibromyalgia Impact Questionnaire Revised (FIQR), mVASFIQ [19]
- *Not yet* validated: SSI and WPI used in the 2010 ACR diagnosis criteria [3, 19]

Non-pharmacological [19]
- *Education*: provide information about fibromyalgia diagnosis, risk factors, pathology, treatment and prognosis, importance of exercise and sleep. Manage expectations.
- *Physical activity*: walk 10 min/day, build to 30–60 min of low or moderate activity up to 2–3 times/wk, encourage frequent stretching and aerobic activities especially swimming
- *Cognitive Behavioral Therapy (CBT)*: face to face and/or publically available CBT. Web-based resources include: CFIDS and Fibromyalgia Self-Help (www.cfidsselfhelp.org; www.treatcfsfm.org). Arthritis Foundation's Fibromyalgia Self-Help Course
- *Proper sleep hygiene*: create a sleep routine, relaxing environment, TV off, use bed only for sleeping, avoid night-time coffee, exercise during the day, hide clock, etc.
- *Therapy*: PT/OT evaluation and treatment
- *Modalities*: Ultrasound and interferential current often employed by physical and occupational therapists have also proven benefit [20–22].
- *Other*: yoga, massage, acupuncture

Pharmacological:
1. **Antidepressants**:
   - **SNRIs**:
     - *Duloxetine*—Start at 30 mg daily and up-titrate to 60 mg daily, increases activity in pain inhibitory pathways
       Common side effects: nausea, dry mouth, somnolence, fatigue, constipation, decreased appetite, hyperhidrosis. **FDA-approved** [19, 23, 24]
     - *Milnacipran*—12.5 mg daily and up-titrate to 50 mg BID, *increases activity in pain inhibitory pathways*
       Common side effects: nausea, headache, constipation, dizziness, insomnia, hot flush, hyperhidrosis, vomiting, palpitations, increased heart rate, dry mouth, hypertension. **FDA-approved** [19, 23, 24]
     - *Venlafaxine* 75 mg daily (can start at this dose as per study, but many practitioners start at 37.5 mg and titrate up for best tolerance), conflicting results [25]
   - **SSRIs**: inferior to Tricyclic antidepressants (TCAs), inconsistent outcomes
     - *Fluoxetine* 20–80 mg daily, Paroxetine CR 12.5–62.5 mg daily, Citalopram 20–40 mg daily [24]
       Common side effects: nausea, diarrhea, sexual side effects, weight gain, insomnia, may or may not be better than placebo [24]

- **TCAs**: improve sleep, inconsistent improvement of pain *Common side effects*: sedation, constipation, and cardiovascular issues. *Amytriptilyne better than nortriptyline, equal to cyclobenzaprine* [23, 24]
  - E.g. amitriptyline 20–25 mg po qhs [23, 24]
- **MAO inhibitors:**
  - Insufficient data to support use [25]

2. **Antiepileptics**:
   - **Ca-channel blockers**
     - *Pregabalin*: Start at 75 mg BID and up-titrate to 150–225 mg BID, inhibits excitatory pathways (e.g., glutamate)
       Common side effects: dizziness, somnolence, dry mouth, edema, blurred vision, weight gain, difficulty with concentration/attention. **FDA-approved** [19]
     - *Gabapentin*: 300 mg daily up-titrate to 900 mg TID or higher if needed
       Common side effects: dizziness, somnolence, edema, and gait disturbance [26]
   - **Na-channel blocker**
     - *Lacosamide*: little evidence, 400 mg po daily
       Common side effects: nausea, tremor [27]
   - **Unknown**
     - *Phenytoin*: insufficient evidence to support its use [28]
   - **Benzodiazapine**
     - *Clonazepam*: insufficient evidence to support its use [29]
   - **Na-channel, GABA**
     - *Valproic acid*: insufficient evidence to support its use [30]

3. **Analgesics/Opioids**
   - *Nonsteroidal anti-inflammatory drugs (NSAIDs) and opioids*: efficiency NOT demonstrated in trials [19, 23, 24]
   - *Tramadol*: 37.5 mg tramadol/325 mg acetaminophen q4–6 h, *mild opioid with SSRI properties,*
     - *Common side effects*: nausea, headache, pruritis, dizziness, constipation [31] other analgesic agents can be considered, please see specific chapter on analgesic agents

4. **Dopamine Agonists**
   - *Pramipexole* 4.5 mg qhs, possibly affects hypothalamic–pituitary–adrenal axis and hippocampus by modulating adrenergic arousal
     - *Common side effects*: transient anxiety and weight loss [32]

5. **Muscle Relaxants**
   - *Cyclobenzaprine* 10–40 mg qhs or tid of needed and tolerated [23, 24]

6. **Sedative-Hypnotics**
   - Sodium Oxybate 4.5 and 6 g versus placebo, in two divided doses at bedtime and 2.5–4 h later, GSH-Na

salt, *precursor to GABA*, affects both ascending, descending and sleep pathways
  - *Common side effects*: nausea/dizziness [23, 24] other muscle relaxers can be considered, please see specific chapter on muscle relaxers

Tailored Pharmaco-therapy [23]:

- *Pain+sleep disturbance+fatigue*: amitriptyline superior to duloxetine and milnacipran
- *Pain+sleep disturbances*: duloxetine and pregabalin superior to milnacipran
- *Health-related quality of life*: amitriptyline inferior to duloxetine and milnacipran
- *Depressed mood*: duloxetine superior to milnacipran and pregabalin
- *Fatigue*: milnacipran and pregabalin superior to duloxetine
- *Minimize GI side effects*: pregabalin preferred over milnacipran and duloxetine
- *Minimize dry mouth and insomnia side effects*: milnacipran preferred over duloxetine
- *Minimize tachycardia side effect*: avoid milnacipran
- *Minimize weight gain and peripheral edema side effect*: avoid pregabalin
- *Minimize cognitive disturbance side effect*: duloxetine and milnacipran preferred over pregabalin
- *History of depression*: predicts response to venlafaxine

Interventional Treatment Options:

- Trigger point injections have been debated in the literature [33], yet injections improve symptoms to some extent [34]
- Injections appear to be independent of the pharmacological agent used, effective even without any pharmacological agent (aka dry needling) [35, 36]. Therefore, the agent used and the dosing may not change outcomes.
- Combined with stretching exercises, ultrasound treatment and muscle injections are equally effective [37].
- *Toxin*:
  - *Botulism toxin* injection Type A: 50 units versus 1 % lidocaine with statistically significant improvement of pain at 2 and 4 weeks in a small study of 20 patients [38]. One dosing option 50 units in 2 mL NS [39]
- *Analgesic*:
  - Na channel blocker: *Lidocaine* one dosing option: 1 % 1.5 mL [40], may chose over dry-needling to reduce immediate post-injection pain [40, 41]
  - Steroid: *Prednisolone* one dosing option: 25 mg in 1 mL plus saline 0.9 % 1 mL [36]
  - NSAID: *Diclofenac* one dosing option: 50 mg in 2 mL [36]
- *Dry-needling*: One method option is to use 27-gauge hypodermic needle [41]
- Class IV laser therapy: may improve pain and range of motion [42]

Educational Materials:

- Managing Pain Before It Manages You by Caudill (third edition, 2009), The Fibromyalgia Help Book by Fransen and Russell (1996)
- www.knowfibro.com www.fibrotogether.com
- Patient advocacy: www.painfoundation.org, www.healthywomen.org, www.fmcpaware.org

References

1. Barsky AJ, Borus JF. Functional somatic syndromes. Ann Intern Med. 1999;130:910–21.
2. Wolfe F, Smythe HA, Yunus MB, Bennett RM, Bombardier C, Goldenberg DL, et al. The American College of Rheumatology 1990 criteria for the classification of fibromyalgia. Report of the Multicenter Criteria Committee. Arthritis Rheum. 1990;33: 160–72.
3. Wolfe F, Clauw D, Fitzcharles MA, Goldenberg D, Katz RS, Mease P, et al. The American College of Rheumatology preliminary diagnostic criteria for fibromyalgia and measurement of symptom severity. Arthritis Care Res. 2010;62:600–10.
4. Wolfe F, Häuser W. Fibromyalgia diagnosis and diagnostic criteria. Ann Med. 2011;43(7):495–502.
5. Lawrence RC, Felson DT, Helmick CG, et al. Estimates of the prevalence of arthritis and other rheumatic conditions in the United States: part II. Arthritis Rheum. 2008;58(1):26–35.
6. Clauw DJ, Arnold LM, McCarberg BH, FibroCollaborative. The science of fibromyalgia. Mayo Clin Proc. 2011;86(9):907–11.
7. Saxena A, Solitar BM. Fibromyalgia knowns, unknowns, and current treatment. Bull NYU Hosp Jt Dis. 2010;68(3):157–61.
8. Staud R. Are tender point injections beneficial: the role of tonic nociception in fibromyalgia. Curr Pharm Des. 2006;12(1):23–7.
9. Arnold LM, Hudson JI, Hess EV, et al. Family study of fibromyalgia. Arthritis Rheum. 2004;50(3):944–52.
10. Mease PJ, Clauw DJ, Arnold LM, et al. Fibromyalgia syndrome. J Rheumatol. 2005;32(11):2270–7.
11. Arnold LM, Clauw DJ, McCarberg BH, FibroCollaborative. Improving the recognition and diagnosis of fibromyalgia. Mayo Clin Proc. 2011;86(5):457–64.
12. Williams DA, Clauw DJ. Understanding fibromyalgia: lessons from the broader pain research community. J Pain. 2009;10(8):777–91.
13. Ablin K, Clauw DJ. From fibrositis to functional somatic syndromes to a bell-shaped curve of pain and sensory sensitivity: evolution of a clinical construct. Rheum Dis Clin North Am. 2009;35(2):233–51.
14. Arnold LM, Hudson JI, Keck PE, Auchenbach MB, Javaras KN, Hess EV. Comorbidity of fibromyalgia and psychiatric disorders. J Clin Psychiatry. 2006;67(8):1219–25.
15. Thieme K, Turk DC, Flor H. Comorbid depression and anxiety in fibromyalgia syndrome: relationship to somatic and psychosocial variables. Psychosom Med. 2004;66(6):837–44.
16. Yunus MB. A comprehensive medical evaluation of patients with fibromyalgia syndrome. Rheum Dis Clin North Am. 2002;28(2): 201–17, v–vi.
17. Schneider MJ. Tender points/fibromyalgia vs. trigger points/myofascial pain syndrome: a need for clarity in terminology and differential diagnosis. J Manipulative Physiol Ther. 1995;18(6):398–406.
18. Hans SC, Harrison P. Myofascial pain syndrome and trigger point management. Reg Anesth. 1999;22:89–101.
19. Arnold LM, Clauw DJ, Dunegan LJ, Turk DC, FibroCollaborative. A framework for fibromyalgia management for primary care providers. Mayo Clin Proc. 2012;87(5):488–96.
20. Lee SJ, Kim DY, Chun MH, Kim YG. The effect of repetitive transcranial magnetic stimulation on fibromyalgia: a randomized sham-controlled trial with 1-mo follow-up. Am J Phys Med Rehabil. 2012;91(12):1077–85.
21. Moretti FA, Marcondes FB, Provenza JR, Fukuda TY, de Vasconcelos RA, Roizenblatt S. Combined therapy (ultrasound and interferential current) in patients with fibromyalgia: once or twice in a week? Physiother Res Int. 2012;17(3):142–9.
22. Gur A. Physical therapy modalities in management of fibromyalgia. Curr Pharm Des. 2006;12(1):29–35.
23. Han C, Lee SJ, Lee SY, Seo HJ, Wang SM, Park MH, Patkar AA, Koh J, Masand PS, Pae CU. Available therapies and current management of fibromyalgia: focusing on pharmacological agents. Drugs Today (Barc). 2011;47(7):539–57.
24. Mease PJ, Dundon K, Sarzi-Puttini P. Pharmacotherapy of fibromyalgia. Best Pract Res Clin Rheumatol. 2011;25(2):285–97.
25. Tort S, Urrútia G, Nishishinya MB, Walitt B. Monoamine oxidase inhibitors (MAOIs) for fibromyalgia syndrome. Cochrane Database Syst Rev. 2012;(4):CD009807.
26. Moore RA, Wiffen PJ, Derry S, McQuay HJ. Gabapentin for chronic neuropathic pain and fibromyalgia in adults. Cochrane Database Syst Rev. 2011;(3):CD007938.
27. Hearn L, Derry S, Moore RA. Lacosamide for neuropathic pain and fibromyalgia in adults. Cochrane Database Syst Rev. 2012;(2):CD009318.
28. Birse F, Derry S, Moore RA. Phenytoin for neuropathic pain and fibromyalgia in adults. Cochrane Database Syst Rev. 2012;(5):CD009485.
29. Corrigan R, Derry S, Wiffen PJ, Moore RA. Clonazepam for neuropathic pain and fibromyalgia in adults. Cochrane Database Syst Rev. 2012;(5):CD009486.
30. Gill D, Derry S, Wiffen PJ, Moore RA. Valproic acid and sodium valproate for neuropathic pain and fibromyalgia in adults. Cochrane Database Syst Rev. 2011;(10):CD009183.
31. Bennett RM, Kamin M, Karim R, Rosenthal N. Tramadol and acetaminophen combination tablets in the treatment of fibromyalgia pain: a double-blind, randomized, placebo-controlled study. Am J Med. 2003;114(7):537–45.
32. Holman AJ, Myers RR. A randomized, double-blind, placebo-controlled trial of pramipexole, a dopamine agonist, in patients with fibromyalgia receiving concomitant medications. Arthritis Rheum. 2005;52(8):2495–505.
33. Henningsen P, Zipfel S, Herzog W. Management of functional somatic syndromes. Lancet. 2007;369(9565):946–55.
34. Giamberardino MA, Affaitati G, Fabrizio A, Costantini R. Effects of treatment of myofascial trigger points on the pain of fibromyalgia. Curr Pain Headache Rep. 2011;15(5):393–9.
35. Lewit K. The needle effect in the relief of myofascial pain. Pain. 1979;6(1):83–90.
36. Cummings TM, White AR. Needling therapies in the management of myofascial trigger point pain: a systematic review. Arch Phys Med Rehabil. 2001;82(7):986–92.
37. Esenyel M, Caglar N, Aldemir T. Treatment of myofascial pain. Am J Phys Med Rehabil. 2000;79(1):48–52.
38. Smith HS, Audette J, Royal MA. Botulinum toxin in pain management of soft tissue syndromes. Clin J Pain. 2002;18(6):S147–54.
39. Wheeler AH, Goolkasian P, Gretz SS. A randomized, doubleblind, prospective pilot study of botulinum toxin injection for refractory, unilateral, cervicothoracic, paraspinal, myofascial pain syndrome. Spine. 1998;23:1662–6.
40. Garvey TA, Marks MR, Wiesel SW. A prospective, randomized, double-blind evaluation of trigger-point injection therapy for low-back pain. Spine. 1989;14:962–4.
41. Hong CZ. Lidocaine injection versus dry needling to myofascial trigger point. The importance of the local twitch response. Am J Phys Med Rehabil. 1994;73:256–63.
42. Panton L, Simonavice E, Williams K, Mojock C, Kim JS, Kingsley JD, McMillan V, Mathis R. Effects of class IV laser therapy on fibromyalgia impact and function in women with fibromyalgia. J Altern Complement Med. 2012;18:1–8.
43. Johnson JL, Collo MB, Finch WR, Felicetta JV. Fibromyalgia syndrome. J Am Acad Nurse Pract. 1990;2(2):47–53.

Sickle Cell Disease

Leena Mathew

Abbreviations

ASS	Acute splenic sequestration
IV PCA	Intravenous patient controlled analgesia
RBC	Red blood count
SCA	Sickle cell anemia
SCD	Sickle cell disease
WBC	White blood count

Epidemiology [1]

- SCD is a common genetic disorder and major public health concern because of associated morbidity and mortality.
- Affects approximately 30 million persons worldwide
- Pain is the most common symptom for which patient with sickle cell disease (SCD) present to the emergency room.
- Painful episodes may start as early as in the first year of life.
- Acute exacerbations may last from hours to weeks followed by a return to baseline.
- Though stressors such as dehydration, infection, stress, cold temperatures, and fatigue can precipitate painful episodes, most episodes are idiopathic.
- Until recently, pain in SCD was considered an acute pain syndrome, but it is now well accepted that pain associated with SCD should be considered to be a chronic condition and managed as such.
- Painful episodes are often termed "crises." There is an attempt to replace the word crises with a more appropriate term to take out the perception of catastrophe associated with the word.
- 5.2 % of patients with SCD have 3–10 episodes of severe pain every year [2].

L. Mathew, M.D. (✉)
Department of Anesthesiology, Division of Pain Medicine,
New York Presbyterian Hospital, Columbia University,
New York, NY, USA
e-mail: Lm370@cumc.columbia.edu

- During assessment of pain, it is important to get a sense for the strength, resilience, and vulnerability of each patient, as reflected in coping skills, mood, social life, and function.
- Median survival for people with SCD was generally reported to be in the fourth decade.

Pathophysiology [3]

- SCD is a highly phenotypically variable disease.
- A single nucleotide substitution in the beta-globin gene results in a single amino acid substitution of Valine for glutamic acid leading to HbS formation.
- With de-oxygenation, HbS undergoes polymerization and leads to the sickle cell associated with increased erythrocyte density and membrane damage.
- Distorted rigid sickle cells contribute to vaso-occlusion and premature red cell destruction.
- Vaso-occlusion is driven by inflammatory mediators and involves a complex interaction between blood cells, platelets, and endothelial cells.
- Leukocyte adhesion in small postcapillary venules may be one of the key factors contributing to vaso-occlusion. This may offer an attractive therapeutic target for SCD.
- Pulmonary complications and strokes also contribute significantly to premature death.
- Factors that contribute to decreasing disease severity include α-thalassemia and β-thalassemia traits.
- *The most common causes of morbidity are pain and acute chest syndrome episodes.*

Symptoms [4]

Key clinical manifestations are attributed to two major subphenotypes, one attributed to vaso-occlusion and another to hemolysis.

Manifestations of vaso-occlusive subtype

- Pain crises—somatic, visceral, and neuropathic pain
- Acute chest syndrome
- Joint necrosis—dactylitis
- Stroke
- Acute splenic sequestration (ASS)
- Hepatic sequestration and renal failure
- Asplenia

Manifestations of the hemolytic subtype

- Anemia
- Pulmonary hypertension
- Stroke

Crises (vaso-occlusive etiology)

- *Pain*
  - Obstruction of the microcirculation by sickled RBCs
  - Abdominal, bone and joint, as well as soft tissue pain
  - Repeated ischemic injury to spleen causes splenic infarctions and auto-splenectomy and predisposes to sepsis.
  - Other end organ damage including liver and kidney disease may occur.
  - Renal vaso-occlusion leads to papillary necrosis, which may present as an inability to concentrate urine.
- *Acute chest syndrome*
  - Affects 40 % of all people with sickle cell anemia (SCA) and is secondary to vaso-occlusive crises involving the lungs
  - Presents as an infiltrate on chest radiograph with fever and respiratory symptoms
  - Develops after multiple crises and rib or bone marrow or pulmonary infarction
  - Each episode increases likelihood of repeat pulmonary events leading up chronically to pulmonary hypertension.
  - Mortality from acute chest syndrome is 2 % in children and almost 8 % in adults.
  - Death is due to sepsis and Pulmonary embolic events.

Laboratory Studies to Obtain in SCD Patients [5]

Crisis correlates to the presentation and no lab values can signify crisis.

- Anemia: Hemoglobin <10 g/day; Hematocrit <29 % to assess for anemia
- Leukocytosis: WBC count 12,000–20,000 cells/mm^3 (12–20 × 10^9/L), with a predominance of neutrophils >50 %
- Elevated reticulocyte count (normal range in adults is 0.5–1.5 %)
- Peripheral blood smears show sickle erythrocytes
- Presence of Howell–Jolly bodies (RBC) indicates asplenia

General Treatment [6]

- Adequate hydration: (hydration guided by other comorbidities such as renal failure and heart disease)
- Treatment of infections
  - Fever in any sickle cell patient should be considered an indication of infection.
  - Pneumonia, meningitis, influenza, hepatitis, and osteomyelitis are fairly common.
  - Patients should be treated with appropriate intravenous antibiotics.
  - It is also important for patients to prophylactically receive the influenza, hepatitis, and meningitis vaccines.
- Pulmonary toilet
- Oxygen
- Blood transfusions if anemic
- Folic acid and iron supplementation should be provided if these levels are noted to be low.
- Hydroxyurea
  - Only well-studied disease modifying drug
  - Patients who have experienced at least three hospitalizations/year for crisis are good candidates for hydroxyurea therapy.
  - Hydroxyurea can be started at a dose of 10 mg/kg orally, on a daily basis. This can be incrementally increased every 12 weeks to a maximum of 35 mg/kg.
  - The patient's hematologic status should be monitored to rule-out falls in the neutrophil count <2,500 per mm^3 or platelet count <80,000 per mm^3.

Pain Therapy [7, 8]

- Psychosocial support: coping skills, behavioral therapy to treat anxiety and if needed counseling for appropriate opioid usage and education regarding the disease process
- Treatment of pain crises is essential to improving the patient's quality of life [6, 7].
  - *Mild-to-moderate pain*: Acetaminophen with Codeine or a Non-Steroidal Anti-inflammatory agent (Toradol, Ibuprofen, Naproxen, Diclofenac, Meloxicam, Celebrex) (these agents may have an opioid sparing effect or work synergistically with other analgesics)
  - *Moderate-to-severe pain*: Consider long acting opioids at fixed intervals with breakthrough dosing using immediate release agents. Need to ensure appropriate candidates for opioid therapy and frequent assessment to confirm the absence of any aberrant usage or diversion. Long acting medications to consider: Methadone, Oxycodone, Morphine, and Fentanyl
    Severe exacerbations: May need IV PCA as an inpatient

IV bisphosphonates may be a trialled as an adjuvant for pain control in patients presenting with osteonecrosis when standard management fails. Though there are case reports, there are no randomized controlled trials to support their use in the acute setting. Care must be taken to ensure no renal insufficiency prior to instituting bisphosphonate therapy (an intravenous infusion of pamidronate at 1 mg/kg can be infused over 5–10 h and repeated in 3 days if pain continues). The risk of developing osteonecrosis of the jaw is reported with bisphosphonate use.

Key points to remember during administration of analgesia in the acute setting:
- Assess pain with validated pain assessment tools
- Monitor for aberrant behaviors for opioid misuse using saliva or urine drug screens
- Start with parenteral opioids
- Rescue doses may be administered along with a baseline infusion depending on the degree of pain and other comorbidities.
- Avoid a basal infusion in patients with sleep apnea or respiratory insufficiency
- Non-PCA, parenteral administration of opioid analgesics may be given on fixed schedule depending on the opioid half-life and type of medication administered in addition to rescue doses
- Generally speaking, sole regimens of "prn" administration should be avoided.
- PCA is very advantageous since it diminishes the high and low fluctuation in blood levels and thus decreases risk of toxicity.

- Reassess daily opioid use and readjust the dose accordingly
- Monitor for respiratory depression and sedation
- If more than four breakthrough doses are needed by PCA in an hour, readjust the continuous infusion by increasing 25–50 % to allow better analgesia (only if no side effects are noted).
- Medications are tapered to baseline regimen over a week after termination of the crisis.

References

1. Olujohungbe A, Howard J. The clinical care of adult patients with sickle cell disease. Br J Hosp Med (Lond). 2008;69(11):616–9.
2. Platt OS, Thorington BD, Brambilla DJ, Milner PF, Rosse WF, Vichinsky E, et al. Pain in sickle cell disease. Rates and risk factors. N Engl J Med. 1991;325:11–6.
3. Stuart MJ, Nagel RL. Sickle cell disease. Lancet. 2004;364: 1343–60.
4. Platt OS, Brambilla DJ, Rosse WF, Milner PF, Castro O, Steinberg MH, et al. Mortality in sickle cell disease. Life expectancy and risk factors for early death. N Engl J Med. 1994;330(23):1639–44.
5. Bernard AW, Venkat A, Lyons MS. Best evidence topic report. Full blood count and reticulocyte count in painful sickle crisis. Emerg Med J. 2006;23(4):302–3.
6. Brawley OW, Cornelius LJ, Edwards LR, Gamble VN, Green BL, Inturrisi C, et al. National Institutes of Health Consensus Development Conference statement: hydroxyurea treatment for sickle cell disease. Ann Intern Med. 2008;148(12):932–8.
7. Benjamin LJ. The nature and management of acute painful episode in sickle cell disease. In: Forget BG, Higgs D, Nagel RL, Steinberg MH, editors. Disorders of hemoglobin. Cambridge, UK: Cambridge University Press; 2001. p. 671–710.
8. Benjamin LJ, Dampier CD, Jacob AK, et al. Guideline for the management of acute and chronic pain in sickle-cell disease. Glenview: APS Clinical Practice Guidelines Series No 1.

Shan Babeendran and Ariel C. Soucie

Abbreviations

ADR	Adverse reaction
CT	Computed tomography
EtOH	Ethanol
IV	Intravenous
MRI	Magnetic resonance imaging
NSAIDs	Nonsteroidal immunosuppressive drugs
PET	Positron emission tomography
PO	Per os
PRN	Pro Re Nata (as needed)
TENS	Transcutaneous electrical nerve stimulation

Introduction

Assessent and treatment of cancer pain can be very complex and challenging. Unrelieved pain can impact many various aspects of a patient's quality of life. It can significantly impact a patient's ability to endure treatment, return to health as a cancer survivor, or even achieve a peaceful death [1].

Prevalence of Cancer Pain [1]

- 25 % of those newly diagnosed
- 33 % of those undergoing active treatment
- 75 % of those with advanced disease
- Chronic pain in cancer survivors post-treatment is esti-mated to be 75 %

S. Babeendran, D.O. (✉)
Department of Rehabilitation Medicine, New York University
Langone Medical Center, New York, NY, USA
e-mail: ShanBabeendran@gmail.com

A.C. Soucie, D.P.T.
Aureus Medical Group, Portsmouth, NH, USA
e-mail: ariel.soucie@gmail.com

Metastasis to Bone

- *Most common cancers to metastasize to bone are* [2]:
  - Bladder
  - Breast
  - Kidney
  - Lung
  - Melanoma
  - Prostate
  - Thyroid
  - Uterine
- *Imaging modalities to aid in workup for bony metastasis:*
  - Bone Scan—may miss lateral tumors which grow into intervertebral foramens
  - Magnetic resonance imaging (MRI) with contrast
  - PET scan
  - Bone scintigraphy
  - Sacral Imaging
    - MRI may miss lesions that are not midline
    - Scintigraphy may miss lesions if bladder is full
  - Epidural space can be evaluated via CT Myelogram, Plain Myelography, or MRI with and without contrast

Gathering Pertinent History

- Pain should be assessed via self-report when possible
  - In advanced stages, these patients may be suffering from decreased mental status and possible inability to properly communicate

    Vocalizations/grunting, gestures, blinking, and yes/no responses or pointing to yes/no on a paper may be used if the patient is non-verbal or decreased cognition or arousal [3]

    Behavioral pain assessment tools may be helpful in the assessment of non-verbal patients [3].
  - Tumor type and any known spread patterns should be consistent with the reported pain location and type of pain
  - New pain or pain that is inconsistent with the known etiology should be reviewed to determine any new etiology [4]

K.A. Sackheim, *Pain Management and Palliative Care: A Comprehensive Guide*,
DOI 10.1007/978-1-4939-2462-2_27, © Springer Science+Business Media New York 2015

– When a self-reported pain assessment is not feasible, the patient should be thoroughly assessed for potential causes of pain, behavior or lack of behavior, reports of pain/input from the patients' caregivers, and analgesic trials [3]

• Reassess frequently, monitor for changes, document, and communicate with all health care providers involved in the patient's care

• *Pain reports may be affected by factors including*:
  – Patient's mental health, social interactions and/or presence of family or friends at the time of assessment
  – Failing to preserve the patient's modesty as a result of inadequate privacy and/or draping
  – Excess personnel present at the time of assessment
  – Cultural preferences such as the gender and/or mannerisms of the assessor

Selecting an Appropriate Analgesic

• *Mild pain*: patients who are not currently taking opioids can be started on non-opioid analgesics. Pain refractory to non-opioid analgesia, an opioid can be added

• *Moderate to severe pain*: if already on opioid therapy with continued pain, dose or frequency may be increased or change in opioid and/or change in route of administration may be required. Some commonly used opioids include Oxycodone, Fentanyl, Morphine, and Methadone. Some benefits to Methadone include the lack of neuroactive metabolites, clearance is independent of renal function, excellent oral bioavailability, low cost profile, and long half life. It is also important to note that Methadone adverse effects include constipation, fatigue, sweating, and prolonged QTc.

Caveats to Non-Opioid Analgesia

• May have limited value due to low potency and fixed dose ceilings [5–7]

• Aspirin should be avoided for treatment of pain due to high incidence of gastropathy and its irreversible inhibition of platelet agglutination [8]

• IV ketorolac 10 mg q4–6 h to a maximum of 40 mg/day can be administered for up to 5 days to manage postoperative pain in opioid naïve patients
  – Caution should be used in renal patients
  – Several case reports have demonstrated acute renal insufficiency following administration

• Acetaminophen is commonly used as an analgesic
  – Case reports have discussed interactions between anticancer agents and acetaminophen leading to hepatic toxicity [9]
  – Reduced doses of 2,000 mg/day or avoidance of the drug all together is recommended in patients with renal insufficiency, hepatic failure, or strong history of EtOH use [10]

Caveats to Opioid Analgesia

• Mainstay of drug therapy for cancer pain
  – *Symptoms of toxicity can include*:
    Nausea and/or vomiting
    Pruritus
    Drowsiness/dizziness
    Spasticity
    Respiratory compromise
    Seizure

• Codeine is a pro-drug that must undergo metabolism via action of CYP2D6 enzyme. Patients with CYP2D6 enzymes may not be able to convert codeine into morphine
  – Polymorphism of this enzyme varies between ethnic groups, thus altering the level of analgesia achieved 3 % of Asians and African Americans and 10 % of Caucasians are poor metabolizers, leading to reduced analgesic effect [11]
    Other individuals may be ultra-rapid metabolizers and thus may achieve increased serum levels and adverse effects [12]

• Combination medications are commonly used to effectively control moderate pain
  – Oxycodone in conjunction with acetaminophen or ibuprofen
  – Hydrocodone in conjunction with acetaminophen or ibuprofen

• Morphine and oxycodone are commonly used due to availability of immediate and extended release formulations [5–7, 13]

• Oxycodone-administered q4h has been shown to effectively relieve cancer pain and may be less toxic than morphine in patients with narrow therapeutic windows [14, 15]

• Transdermal Fentanyl is most useful in chronic cancer pain patients who are unable to take PO medications and have demonstrated unmanageable toxicity from morphine, oxycodone, or hydromorphone [16, 17]
  – A comparative study of normal vs. low weight cancer patients (defined as 16 kg/m²) who were receiving transdermal fentanyl obtained decreased plasma levels at 48 and 72 h in cachectic patients [18]

Prescribing the Appropriate Opioid Dose

• No set optimal or maximal dose of opioid analgesics when treating cancer pain [5–7, 13, 19, 20]

• Appropriate dose of opioid is identified by its ability to provide pain relief throughout its dosing interval without causing unmanageable toxicity
  – Majority of patients will receive adequate pain control with <morphine 240 mg po per/day [21]
  – Severe cancer pain may require morphine 1,200–1,800 mg po per/day [22]

Table 27.1 Dosing recommendations for acetaminophen and NSAIDs[a]

Drug	Usual dose for adults and children ≥50 kg body weight	Usual dose for adults and children[b] <50 kg body weight
Orally administered acetaminophen and over-the-counter NSAIDs		
Acetaminophen[c]	650 mg q4h	10–15 mg/kg q4h
	975 mg q6h	15–20 mg/kg q4h (rectal)
Aspirin[d]	650 mg q4h	10–15 mg/kg q4h
	975 mg q6h	15–20 mg/kg q4h (rectal)
Ibuprofen (Motrin, Advil)	400–600 mg q6h	5–10 mg/kg q4–6 h
Magnesium salicylate (Doan's, Magan, Mobidin, others)	650 mg q4h	
Naproxen (Naprosyn, Aleve)	250–275 mg q6–8 h	5 mg/kg q8h
Naproxen sodium (Anaprox)	275 mg q6–8 h	
Prescription NSAIDs		
Carprofen (Rimadyl)	100 mg tid	
Choline magnesium trisalicylate[c] (Trilisate)	1,000–1,500 mg q6–8 h	25 mg/kg q6–8 h
Choline salicylate[c] (Arthropan)	870 mg q3–4 h	
Diclofenac (oral) (Voltaren—1 % topical; Pennsaid—1.5 % topical)	50 mg bid–tid oral; 32 g/day topical	Flector (patch): 1 patch bid
Diflunisal[f] (Dolobid)	500 mg q12h	
Etodolac (Lodine)	200–400 mg q6–8 h	
Fenoprofen calcium (Nalfon)	300–600 mg q6h	
Ketoprofen (Orudis)	25–60 mg q6–8 h	
Ketorolac tromethamine[g] (Toradol)	10 mg q4–6 h to a maximum of 40 mg/d	
	IV administration should not exceed 5 days	
Meclofenamate sodium[h] (Meclomen)	50–100 mg q6h	
Mefenamic acid (Ponstel)	250 mg q6h	
Sodium salicylate (Anacin, Bufferin)	325–650 mg q3–4 h	
Parenteral NSAIDs		
Acetaminophen injection	1,000 mg q6h (adults)	15 mg/kg max, 75 mg/kg in 24 h (children aged <13 y)
Ketorolac tromethamine[g–i] (Toradol)	60 mg initially, then 30 mg q6h	
	IV administration should not exceed 5 days	

From the National Cancer Institute http://www.cancer.gov [2]

[a]Only the nonsteroidal anti-inflammatory drugs (NSAIDs) listed here have FDA approval for use as simple analgesics, but clinical experience has also been gained with other drugs

[b]Acetaminophen and NSAID dosages for adults weighing less than 50 kg should be adjusted for weight

[c]Acetaminophen lacks the peripheral anti-inflammatory and antiplatelet activities of the other NSAIDs

[d]The standard against which other NSAIDs are compared. May inhibit platelet aggregation for longer than 1 week and may cause bleeding. Aspirin is not recommended for pain in children

[e]May have minimal antiplatelet activity

[f]Administration with antacids may decrease absorption

[g]Use limited to 5 days or fewer

[h]Coombs-positive autoimmune hemolytic anemia has been associated with prolonged use

[i]Has the same gastrointestinal toxic effects as oral NSAIDs

- – A small population of patients with refractory cancer pain may require particularly high doses of parenteral morphine (Table 27.1) [23]

Route of Medication Administration

- Selection of appropriate route should be guided by using the least invasive
  - – Oral-extended release formulations of opioids add to patient quality of life and independence
  - – Liquid concentrates can be used in patients who cannot swallow pills

- – Rectal formulations of medications can be used but it is important to keep in mind that limitations may include lower bioavailability, varying pharmacokinetic and pharmacological results, and poor predictability of clinical effect.
- – Transdermal fentanyl is an excellent alternative for chronic pain in patients who cannot swallow pills
- – SQ or IV administration of morphine or hydromorphone is preferred over transdermal fentanyl in patients who have only brief periods of inability to use the PO route or in patients with frequent breakthrough pain [5–7, 13]

- Intrathecal administration of opioids should be reserved for patients in whom the combination of systemic analgesics and co analgesics has failed to adequately relieve pain or is accompanied by unmanageable toxicity [6, 7, 24–27]

Schedule Appropriate Dosing Intervals

- Dosing should be given in a manner that minimizes the number of daily doses while consistently preventing end of dose failure with recurrence of pain [5–7, 13]
- If pain returns prior to the end of the expected dosing interval, the dose should be increased in order to maintain the level of analgesia within the patient's therapeutic window of relief without toxicity

Prevent Persistent Pain and Relieve Breakthrough Pain

- Goal of analgesic therapy in cancer patients is to decrease persistent pain as much as possible without toxicity.
  - At the very least, patients' pain levels should be decreased to <5/10
- Pain prevention is also an appropriate goal in the treatment of acute moderate to severe pain [5]
  - Initial therapy of acute pain which is not expected to last >24 h and should consist of PRN dosing for those first 24 h [28]
  - Resolution of the source of acute pain should be anticipated with regular downward dose titration if pain is well-controlled without the need of PRN medication [28]

Titration of Opioid Dose

- Dose titration should be aggressive to expedite the delivery of optimal pain management [5–7, 13]
- Frequent usage of breakthrough analgesics for persistent pain without unmanageable adverse reaction (ADR's) indicates the need for a significant increase in the around-the-clock dosing
  - If a patient is using > two PRN morphine doses per day, the dose of the around-the-clock morphine should be increased by at least the amount of PRN supplements taken with a concordant increase in the PRN dose [28]
  - *Severe pain*: increase dose of oral around-the-clock morphine increased by 50–100 % daily until relief or unacceptable side effects present [28]
  - *Moderate pain*: increase dose by 25–50 % daily
  - *Pain Improvement*: dose tapering is also important in patients whose pain is effectively reduced [5–7, 13]
    - Decrease dose of opioids by 25–50 % each day in such patients as long as there is absence of pain, PRN doses, and presence of ADR's
    - Following a period of regular use of opioid analgesic use, patients who are pain-free should be given

at least 25 % of their previous daily dose in order to prevent a physical withdrawal syndrome [5]

- Prevent and Manage Adverse Reactions of Specific Pharmacotherapy: ADR's of analgesic therapy are often unavoidable and may be effectively managed
- Switching from one opioid to another can eliminate many of the unmanageable ADR's in patients [32–38]
- *Symptoms of hypercalcemia, sepsis, hepatic dysfunction, renal impairment, and brain metastasis can mimic those of opioid toxicity and require aggressive therapy* [13, 29–31]
- Patients on around-the-clock opioids should be on bowel medications to prevent constipation to prevent constipation
- In patients who have achieved good pain control, the initial dose of the new opioid should be 25–50 % less than the calculated equi-analgesic dose to allow for incomplete tolerance (Table 27.2) [5, 13]
- Co-analgesic or adjuvant drugs will enhance the analgesic efficacy of opioids, treat concurrent symptoms that exacerbate pain, and produce independent analgesia for specific types of pain
- Goal of early usage of co-analgesic drugs is to optimize patient's comfort and function by preventing or controlling opioid-induced toxicities [28]
- *Cancer-related pain syndromes which are most amenable to co-analgesic therapy are those related to bony metastasis, nerve compression or damage, and visceral distention* [6, 7, 20, 39, 40]
- Co-analgesics most commonly used in the treatment of cancer pain are nonsteroidal immunosuppressive drugs (NSAID's), corticosteroids, TCA, and anti-convulsants [6, 7, 20, 38, 40] see Table 27.2 (refer to http://www.cancer.gov *for detailed information*)
  - *NSAID's*—shown to be beneficial in the treatment of prostaglandin-mediated pain, inflammatory pain from bone metastases, soft tissue infiltration, arthritis, serositis, and recent surgery [8, 41–43]
  - *Corticosteroids*—found to be helpful in pain caused or exacerbated by mass effect, inflammatory edema such as pain due to acute nerve compression, visceral distention, increased ICP, and soft tissue infiltration [44–46]
  - *TCA's*—used as a first-line co-analgesic therapy of neuropathic pain and also may treat underlying depression [5–7, 13, 47–51]
    - Lower doses than those needed to treat depression may be used in treatment of neuropathic pain
  - *Anticonvulsants*—shown to be helpful in treatment of neuropathic, lancinating, or tic-like pains [5, 7, 13, 44]
    - Usually added to TCA therapy that has not provided adequate relief for neuropathic pain.

Table 27.2 Adjuvant medications with analgesic activity

Class	Drug	Daily dose range[a]	Studies conducted in Cancer patients	Noncancer patients
Antidepressants	Amitriptyline (Elavil)	10–25 mg every day	*Level of evidence: I* [58] *level of evidence: I* [59]	*Level of evidence: I* [60]
	Desipramine (Norpramin)	10–150 mg every day	*Level of evidence: II* [61]	*Level of evidence: II* [62]
	Maprotiline (Ludiomil)	25 mg bid–50 mg tid		*Level of evidence: I* [63]
	Duloxetine (Cymbalta)	20 mg bid–30 mg bid		*Level of evidence: I* [64]
	Nortriptyline (Pamelor, Aventyl)	10–100 mg every day		*Level of evidence: I* [65]
	Venlafaxine (Effexor)	37.5–225 mg every day	*Level of evidence: I* [66] *level of evidence: II* [67]	*Level of evidence: I* [68]
Anticonvulsants	Carbamazepine (Tegretol)	100 mg tid–400 mg tid		*Level of evidence: I* [68]
	Valproate (Depacon)	500 mg tid–1,000 mg tid		*Level of evidence: I* [69]
	Gabapentin (Neurontin)	100 mg tid–1,000 mg tid	*Level of evidence: I* [70] *level of evidence: II* [71]	*Level of evidence: II* [72]
	Clonazepam (Klonopin)	0.5 mg bid–4 mg bid	*Level of evidence: II* [72]	
	Lamotrigine (Lamictal)	25 mg bid–100 mg bid		*Level of evidence: I* [73]
	Pregabalin (Lyrica)	150 mg divided into 2 or 3 doses; increase to 300 mg starting at day 3–7; if needed, increase to 600 mg 7 days later		*Level of evidence: I* [74]
Local anesthetics	Mexiletine (Mexitil)	100 mg bid–300 mg tid		*Level of evidence: I* [75]
	Lidocaine patch (Lidoderm)	5 % patch contains 700 mg; one patch, 12 h on, 12 h off		*Level of evidence: II* [76]
Corticosteroids	Dexamethasone (Decadron)	See text		
	Prednisone	See text		
Bisphosphonates	Clodronate	See text		
	Pamidronate (Aredia)	See text		
	Zoledronic acid (Zometa)	See text	*Level of evidence: II* [77]	
NSAIDs	Refer to Table 27.1 for more information			
Miscellaneous	Baclofen (Lioresal)	5 mg tid–20 mg tid		*Level of evidence: I* [78]
	Calcitonin (Calcimar)	100–200 IU (subcutaneous or intranasal)		
	Clonidine (Catapres)	0.1 mg bid–0.3 mg bid		[79]
	Methylphenidate (Ritalin)	2.5 mg bid–20 mg bid	*Level of evidence: I* [80]	*Level of evidence: II* [81]
	Ketamine (Ketalar)	Refer to the NMDA receptor antagonists section of this summary for more information		

From the National Cancer Institute http://www.cancer.gov [2]

[a]Starting doses should incorporate the lowest possible dose

- May be used alone in patients who cannot tolerate anti-depressant therapy, and those with myoclonic jerks from opioid
  - *Bisphosphonates*:
    - *Skeletal pain is the most common cause of cancer-related pain and can be debilitating for up to two thirds of patients* [2]
    - Effective pain management due to bone metastasis should be integrated with the long-term goal of preventing fractures [2]
    - Patients with metastatic bone pain may benefit from co-analgesic therapy with anti-osteoclast agents such as pamidronate, zolendronic acid, and calcitonin [52–57]
    - Possible dosing schedules:
      Pamidronate 90 mg IV every 3–4 weeks
      Zolendronic Acid 4 mg IV every 3–4 weeks
      (Table 27.3)

Other Modalities to Consider:

- Peripheral Nerve Injection—common are the trigeminal, occipital, sphenopalatine ganglion, intercostals, ilioinguinal and iliohypogastric, pudendal
- Sympathetic Blockade

Table 27.3 Drugs to be avoided for treatment of cancer pain

Class	Drug	Rationale for NOT recommending
Opioids	Meperidine (Demerol)	Short duration (2–3 h) of analgesia
		Repeated administration may lead to CNS toxicity (tremor, confusion, or seizures)
Opioid agonist–antagonists	Pentazocine (Talwin), butorphanol (Stadol), nalbuphine (Nubain)	Risk of precipitating withdrawal in opioid-dependent patients
		Analgesic ceiling
		Possible production of unpleasant psychotomimetic effects (e.g., dysphoria, delusions, hallucinations)
Partial agonist	Buprenorphine (Buprenex)	Analgesic ceiling
		May precipitate withdrawal if administered with full opioid agonist
Antagonists	Naloxone (Narcan), naltrexone (ReVia)	May precipitate withdrawal
		Limit use to treatment of life-threatening respiratory depression. Give in diluted form to opioid-tolerant patients
Combination preparations	Brompton's cocktail[a]	No evidence of analgesic benefit in using Brompton's cocktail over single-opioid analgesics
	DPT (meperidine, promethazine, and chlorpromazine)[b]	Efficacy is poor compared with that of other analgesics
		High incidence of adverse effects
Anxiolytics alone	Benzodiazepines (e.g., alprazolam [Xanax]; clonazepam [Ceberclon]; diazepam [Valium]; lorazepam [Ativan])	Analgesic properties not demonstrated except for some instances of neuropathic pain
		Added sedation from anxiolytics may compromise neurologic assessment in patients receiving opioids by facilitating the development of delirium
Sedative/hypnotic drugs alone	Barbiturates, benzodiazepines	Analgesic properties not demonstrated
		Added sedation from sedative/hypnotic drugs limits opioid dosing and may facilitate the development of delirium

From the National Cancer Institute http://www.cancer.gov [2]

- Neuromodulation:
  - TENS
  - Spinal Cord Stimulator
- Radiofrequency Ablation
- Cryoablation
- High Intensity Focused Ultrasound
- Intrathecal Drug Delivery—for regional pain uncontrolled with oral or IV medications, or for those experiencing significant side effects with oral/IV. Indicated for >3 month life expectancy otherwise should consider tunneled epidural

Consultations to Consider:
- Psychology
- Radiation oncology
- Neurology
- Palliative care

Although very challenging, the treatment and appropriate management of cancer pain can be achieved. Of utmost importance is frequent communication with patients and modification of pain treatment plans as needed.

References

1. Serafini AN. Therapy of metastatic bone pain. J Nucl Med. 2001;42:895–906.
2. Kalso E, Tasmuth T, Neuvonen PJ. Amitriptyline effectively relieves neuropathic pain following treatment of breast cancer. Pain. 1996;64(2):293–302.
3. Coyne PJ, Herr K, Manworren R, et al. Pain assessment in the nonverbal patient: position statement with clinical practice recommendations. Pain Manag Nurs. 2006;7(2):44–52.
4. Du Pen AR, Du Pen SL, Everly R, et al. Implementing guidelines for cancer pain management: results of a randomized controlled clinical trial. J Clin Oncol. 1999;17(1):361–70.
5. Jacox A, Carr DB, Payne R, et al. Management of cancer pain: clinical practice guideline. No. 9 (AHCPR publication no. 94-0592). Rockville: Agency for Health Care Policy and Research; 1994.
6. Miaskowski C, Cleary J, Burney R, et al. Guideline for the management of cancer pain in adults and children, APS clinical practice guidelines series, no. 3. Glenview: American Pain Society; 2005.
7. McNicol E, Strassels S, Goudas L, et al. Nonsteroidal anti-inflammatory drugs, alone or combined with opioids, for cancer pain: a systematic review. J Clin Oncol. 2004;22:1975–92.
8. Kalso E, Vainio A. Morphine and oxycodone hydrochloride in the management of cancer pain. Clin Pharmacol Ther. 1990;47:639–46.
9. Swarm R, Abernethy AP, Anghelescu DL, et al. Adult cancer pain. J Natl Compr Canc Netw. 2010;8:1046–86.

10. Kirchheiner J, Schmidt H, Tzvetkov M, et al. Pharmacokinetics of codeine and its metabolite morphine in ultra rapid metabolizers due to CYP2D6 duplication. Pharmacogenomics J. 2007;7:257–65.

11. Gasche Y, Daali Y, Fathi M, et al. Codeine intoxication associated with ultra rapid CYP2D6 metabolism. N Engl J Med. 2004;351: 2827–31.

12. Body JJ, Bartl R, Burckhardt P, et al. Current use of bisphosphonates in oncology. International Bone and Cancer Study Group. J Clin Oncol. 1998;16:3890–9.

13. American Pain Society. Principles of analgesic use in the treatment of acute pain and chronic cancer pain. 5th ed. Glenview: American Pain Society; 2003.

14. Glare PA, Walsh TD. Dose-ranging study of oxycodone for chronic pain in advanced cancer. J Clin Oncol. 1993;11:973–8.

15. Donner B, Zenz M, Tryba M, et al. Direct conversion from oral morphine to transdermal fentanyl: a multicenter study in patients with cancer pain. Pain. 1996;64:527–34.

16. Kornick CA, Santiago-Palma J, Khojainova N, et al. A safe and effective method for converting cancer patients from intravenous to transdermal fentanyl. Cancer. 2001;92:3056–61.

17. Doyle D, Hanks GWC, MacDonald N, editors. Oxford textbook of palliative medicine. 3rd ed. Oxford: Oxford University Press; 2003.

18. www.cancer.gov

19. Berger A, Portenoy RP, Weisman D, editors. Principles and practice of palliative care and supportive oncology. Philadelphia: Lippincott-Raven; 2002.

20. Coyle N, Adelhardt J, Foley KM, et al. Character of terminal illness in the advanced cancer patient: pain and other symptoms during the last four weeks of life. J Pain Symptom Manage. 1990;5:83–93.

21. Brescia FJ, Portenoy RK, Ryan M, et al. Pain, opioid use, and survival in hospitalized patients with advanced cancer. J Clin Oncol. 1992;10:149–55.

22. Foley KM. Changing concepts of tolerance to opioids: what the cancer patient has taught us. In: Chapman CR, Foley K, editors. Current and emerging issues in cancer pain: research and practice. New York: Raven; 1993. p. 331–50.

23. Kim P. Interventional cancer pain therapies. Semin Oncol. 2005;32:194–9.

24. Bennett G, Burchiel K, Buchser E, et al. Clinical guidelines for intraspinal infusion: report of an expert panel. PolyAnalgesic Consensus Conference. J Pain Symptom Manage. 2000;20:S37–43.

25. Smith TJ, Staats PS, Deer T, et al. Randomized clinical trial of an implantable drug delivery system compared with comprehensive medical management for refractory cancer pain: impact on pain, drug-related toxicity, and survival. J Clin Oncol. 2002;20:4040–9.

26. Sykes N, Fallon M, Patt R, editors. Clinical pain management: cancer pain. New York, NY: Oxford University Press; 2003.

27. Levy H, Samuel T. Management of cancer pain. Semin Oncol. 2005;32:179–93.

28. Cherny N, Ripamonti C, Pereira J, et al. Strategies to manage the adverse effects of oral morphine: an evidence-based report. J Clin Oncol. 2001;19:2542–54.

29. Levy MH. Management of opioid-induced bowel dysfunction. J Natl Compr Canc Netw. 2003;1 Suppl 3:S22–6.

30. McNicol E, Horowicz-Mehler N, Fisk RA, et al. Management of opioid side-effects in cancer-related and chronic non-cancer pain: a systematic review. J Pain. 2003;4:231–56.

31. Galer BS, Coyle N, Pasternak GW, et al. Individual variability in the response to different opioids: report of five cases. Pain. 1992;49:87–91.

32. MacDonald N, Der L, Allan S, Champion P. Opioid hyperexcitability: the application of alternate opioid therapy. Pain. 1993;53:353–5.

33. De Stoutz ND, Bruera E, Suarez-Almazor M. Opioid rotation for toxicity reduction in terminal cancer patients. J Pain Symptom Manage. 1995;10:378–84.

34. Davis MP, Walsh D. Methadone for relief of cancer pain: a review of pharmacokinetics, pharmacodynamics, drug interactions, and protocols of administration. Support Care Cancer. 2001;9:73–83.

35. Bruera E, Pereira J, Watanbe S, et al. Opioid rotation in patients with cancer pain. A retrospective comparison of dose ratios between methadone, hydromorphone, and morphine. Cancer. 1996;78: 852–7.

36. Bruera E, Palmer JL, Bosniak S, et al. Methadone versus morphine as a first-line strong opioid for cancer pain: a randomized, double-blind study. J Clin Oncol. 2004;22:185–92.

37. Bartusch SL, Sanders BJ, D'Alessio JG, et al. Clonazepam for the treatment of lancinating phantom limb pain. Clin J Pain. 1996;12: 59–62.

38. Janjan N. Bone metastases: approaches to management. Semin Oncol. 2001;28(4 Suppl 11):28–34.

39. Cherny NI. The pharmacologic management of cancer pain. Oncology. 2004;18:1499–515.

40. Levy MH. Pharmacologic treatment of cancer pain. N Engl J Med. 1996;335:1124–32.

41. Johnson JR, Miller AJ. The efficacy of choline magnesium trisalicylate (CMT) in the management of metastatic bone pain: a pilot study. Palliat Med. 1994;8:129–35.

42. Simon L, Jacox A, Caudill-Slosberg M, et al. Guideline for the management of pain in osteoarthritis, rheumatoid arthritis, and juvenile chronic arthritis. Glenview: American Pain Society; 2002.

43. Lussier D, Huskey AG, Portenoy RK. Adjuvant analgesics in cancer pain management. Oncologist. 2004;9:571–91.

44. Watanabe S, Bruera E. Corticosteroids as adjuvant analgesics. J Pain Symptom Manage. 1994;9:442–5.

45. Mercadante S, Fulfaro F, Casuccio A. The use of corticosteroids in home palliative care. Support Care Cancer. 2001;9:386–9.

46. Watson CP. The treatment of neuropathic pain: antidepressants and opioids. Clin J Pain. 2000;16(2 Suppl):S49S–55.

47. McQuay HJ, Tramer M, Nye BA, et al. A systematic review of antidepressants in neuropathic pain. Pain. 1996;68:217–27.

48. Dworkin RH, Backonja M, Rowbotham MC, et al. Advances in neuropathic pain: diagnosis, mechanisms, and treatment recommendations. Arch Neurol. 2003;60:1524–34.

49. Rasmussen PV, Jensen TS, Sindrup SH, et al. TDM-based imipramine treatment in neuropathic pain. Ther Drug Monit. 2004;26:352–60.

50. Max MB, Lynch SA, Muir J, et al. Effects of desipramine, amitriptyline, and fluoxetine on pain in diabetic neuropathy. N Engl J Med. 1992;326:1250–6.

51. Eisele Jr JH, Grigsby EJ, Dea G. Clonazepam treatment of myoclonic contractions associated with high-dose opioids: Case report. Pain. 1992;49:231–2.

52. Davis AM, Inturrisi CE. d-Methadone blocks morphine tolerance and N-methyl-D-aspartate-induced hyperalgesia. J Pharmacol Exp Ther. 1999;289:1048–53.

53. DeConno F, Groff L, Brunelli D, et al. Clinical experience with oral methadone administration in the treatment of pain in 196 advanced cancer patients. J Clin Oncol. 1996;14:2836–42.

54. Paice J, Ferrell B. The management of cancer pain. CA Cancer J Clin. 2011;61:157–82.

55. Gralow J, Tripathy D. Managing metastatic bone pain: the role of bisphosphonates. J Pain Symptom Manage. 2007;33:462–72.

56. Ridruejo E, Cacchione R, Villamil AG, et al. Imatinib induced fatal acute liver failure. World J Gastroenterol. 2007;13:6608–11.

57. Heiskanen T, Matzke S, Haakana S, et al. Transdermal fentanyl in cachectic cancer patients. Pain. 2009;144:218–22.

58. Leijon G, Boivie J. Central post-stroke pain—a controlled trial of amitriptyline and carbamazepine. Pain. 1989;36(1):27–36.

59. Holland JC, Romano SJ, Heiligenstein JH, et al. A controlled trial of fluoxetine and desipramine in depressed women with advanced cancer. Psychooncology. 1998;7(4):291–300.

60. Max MB, Kishore-Kumar R, Schafer SC, et al. Efficacy of desipramine in painful diabetic neuropathy: a placebo-controlled trial. Pain. 1991;45(1):3–9; discussion 1–2.

61. Vrethem M, Boivie J, Arnqvist H, et al. A comparison a amitriptyline and maprotiline in the treatment of painful polyneuropathy in diabetics and nondiabetics. Clin J Pain. 1997;13(4):313–23.

62. Raskin J, Pritchett YL, Wang F, et al. A double-blind, randomized multicenter trial comparing duloxetine with placebo in the management of diabetic peripheral neuropathic pain. Pain Med. 2005; 6(5):346–56.

63. Raja SN, Haythornthwaite JA, Pappagallo M, et al. Opioids versus antidepressants in postherpetic neuralgia: a randomized, placebo-controlled trial. Neurology. 2002;59(7):1015–21.

64. Tasmuth T, Härtel B, Kalso E. Venlafaxine in neuropathic pain following treatment of breast cancer. Eur J Pain. 2002;6(1):17–24.

65. Reuben SS, Makari-Judson G, Lurie SD. Evaluation of efficacy of the perioperative administration of venlafaxine XR in the prevention of postmastectomy pain syndrome. J Pain Symptom Manage. 2004;27(2):133–9.

66. Rowbotham MC, Goli V, Kunz NR, et al. Venlafaxine extended release in the treatment of painful diabetic neuropathy: a double-blind, placebo-controlled study. Pain. 2004;110(3):697–706.

67. Harke H, Gretenkort P, Ladleif HU, et al. The response of neuropathic pain and pain in complex regional pain syndrome I to carbamazepine and sustained-release morphine in patients pretreated with spinal cord stimulation: a double-blinded randomized study. Anesth Analg. 2001;92(2):488–95.

68. Kochar DK, Garg P, Bumb RA, et al. Divalproex sodium in the management of post-herpetic neuralgia: a randomized double-blind placebo-controlled study. QJM. 2005;98(1):29–34.

69. Caraceni A, Zecca E, Bonezzi C, et al. Gabapentin for neuropathic cancer pain: a randomized controlled trial from the Gabapentin Cancer Pain Study Group. J Clin Oncol. 2004;22(14):2909–17.

70. Ross JR, Goller K, Hardy J, et al. Gabapentin is effective in the treatment of cancer-related neuropathic pain: a prospective, open-label study. J Palliat Med. 2005;8(6):1118–26.

71. Levendoglu F, Ogün CO, Ozerbil O, et al. Gabapentin is a first line drug for the treatment of neuropathic pain in spinal cord injury. Spine. 2004;29(7):743–51.

72. Hugel H, Ellershaw JE, Dickman A. Clonazepam as an adjuvant analgesic in patients with cancer-related neuropathic pain. J Pain Symptom Manage. 2003;26(6):1073–4.

73. Simpson DM, McArthur JC, Olney R, et al. Lamotrigine for HIV-associated painful sensory neuropathies: a placebo-controlled trial. Neurology. 2003;60(9):1508–14.

74. Lesser H, Sharma U, LaMoreaux L, et al. Pregabalin relieves symptoms of painful diabetic neuropathy: a randomized controlled trial. Neurology. 2004;63(11):2104–10.

75. Oskarsson P, Ljunggren JG, Lins PE. Efficacy and safety of mexiletine in the treatment of painful diabetic neuropathy. The Mexiletine Study Group. Diabetes Care. 1997;20(10):1594–7.

76. Meier T, Wasner G, Faust M, et al. Efficacy of lidocaine patch 5% in the treatment of focal peripheral neuropathic pain syndromes: a randomized, double-blind, placebo-controlled study. Pain. 2003;106(1–2):151–8.

77. Polascik TJ, Given RW, Metzger C, et al. Open-label trial evaluating the safety and efficacy of zoledronic acid in preventing bone loss in patients with hormone-sensitive prostate cancer and bone metastases. Urology. 2005;66(5):1054–9.

78. Dapas F, Hartman SF, Martinez L, et al. Baclofen for the treatment of acute low-back syndrome. A double-blind comparison with placebo. Spine. 1985;10(4):345–9.

79. Lavand'homme PM, Eisenach JC. Perioperative administration of the alpha2-adrenoceptor agonist clonidine at the site of nerve injury reduces the development of mechanical hypersensitivity and modulates local cytokine expression. Pain. 2003;105(1–2):247–54.

80. Bruera E, Chadwick S, Brenneis C, et al. Methylphenidate associated with narcotics for the treatment of cancer pain. Cancer Treat Rep. 1987;71(1):67–70.

81. Cantello R, Aguggia M, Gilli M, et al. Analgesic action of methylphenidate on parkinsonian sensory symptoms: Mechanisms and pathophysiological implications. Arch Neurol. 1988;45(9):973–6.

Palliative Care

Danna Ogden

Abbreviations

BIPAP	Bi-level positive air pressure
BPH	Benign prostatic hyperplasia
CHF	Congestive heart failure
COPD	Chronic obstructive pulmonary disease
EPS	Extrapyramidal symptoms
FDA	Food and drug administration
GI	Gastrointestinal
IM	Intramuscular
IV	Intravenous
MI	Myocardial infarction
MMSE	Mini mental state examination
PO	Per os
PPS	Palliative performance scale
PRN	As needed
QD	One per day
SQ	Subcutaneous

Introduction

Palliative care is specialty level, interdisciplinary care that includes "Active, total care of patients whose disease is not responsive to curative treatment. Control of pain, of other symptoms and of psychological, social, and spiritual problems, is paramount. The goal is the best possible quality of life for patients and their families" [1]. Evidence is showing that patients with early palliative care can have a better quality of life, less depressive symptoms, less aggressive treatment at end-of-life, and longer survival by months [2].

D. Ogden, D.O. (✉)
Hospice and Palliative Medicine,
Kaiser Permanente, Portland, OR, USA
e-mail: danna.j.ogden@kp.org

This therapeutic approach:
- Recognizes the family as the unit of care and is patient-centered
- Uses an interdisciplinary model to address physical, psychological, social, and spiritual needs. Team usually consists of clinical staff, social worker, and chaplain.
- Includes a broad range of interventions and expert symptom management
- Addresses advanced directives, identifies, and coordinates with healthcare proxy or surrogate decision makers
- Identifies caregiver responsibilities and assists with coordination of benefits

Palliative Care vs. Hospice

Palliative care *and* hospice:
- Do not seek to cure, but provide pain relief, symptom management, and address the emotional and spiritual needs of patients and families.
- *Both* stress comprehensive care for the patient and family, need for communication, and value of a clinical team.

Palliative care:
- Aims to relieve suffering in all stages of disease
- Not limited to end-of-life care
- Many patients receive palliative care while they're still pursuing disease modifying therapy

Hospice is a type of palliative care, but differs in important ways, which are addressed in the next chapter. Specifically, patients accepted to hospice have a prognosis of less than 6 months if disease progresses as expected.

Referrals to a palliative care service can include patients with:
- Frequent hospital readmissions for chronic conditions
- Declining functional status, failure to thrive
- Poor symptom management in chronic illness
- Need for goals of care or advanced directive discussions

K.A. Sackheim, *Pain Management and Palliative Care: A Comprehensive Guide*,
DOI 10.1007/978-1-4939-2462-2_28, © Springer Science+Business Media New York 2015

Palliative Performance Scale [3]

Palliative performance scale (PPS) uses five objective domains to *assess functional status*, specifically for patients receiving palliative care. Results correlate with actual survival and median survival time in cancer patients. *Lower scores are indicative of poor performance and poor prognosis.* **PPS of ≤70% is required for hospice eligibility** (Table 28.1).

Symptom Management

Symptom management always takes the patient's prognosis and goals of care into consideration. For each concern, identify potential triggers and treat the underlying cause whenever possible. Treatment of subjective symptoms in palliative care is patient-centered; treatments are offered as a trial and continued when the patient perceives a benefit.

Dyspnea

- Subjective, multidimensional symptom commonly encountered in chronically ill patients including; CHF, COPD, lung cancer
  - Oxygen saturation or respiratory rate may not reflect patient's perception of symptom severity
  - When possible, treat any reversible causes.

General Treatment
- Sit patient upright in bed or chair, as tolerated, to facilitate chest expansion
- Increase air circulation using a bedside fan or open window, reduces the sensation of breathlessness. A gentle breeze from a bedside fan directed at the patient's face can help alleviate dyspnea [4]. This effect is thought to be mediated by stimulation of the thermal and mechanical receptors of the trigeminal nerve in the cheek and nasopharynx [5]
- Play calming music, teach relaxation techniques, minimize the need for patient exertion
- Avoid strong odors, such as smoke, adjust humidity level
- Ensure caregiver understands how to use equipment, nebulizers, BIPAP (bi-level positive air pressure), etc.
- Oxygen therapy: When pulse oximetry is <90 %, start with 2 L/min via nasal cannula and titrate rate to correction of hypoxemia. While supplemental oxygen is usually helpful in patients with low oxygen saturation it may not be for patients with normal oxygen saturation. A perceived benefit in terminally ill patients extends beyond reversing hypoxemia. It is not routinely indicated in all patients.

Specific etiologies and treatments of dyspnea:
- ***Bronchospasm***: Treat with albuterol and/or ipratropium bromide inhaled every 2–4 h as needed. For severe symptoms dexamethasone 4–8 mg/day until improved.
- ***Airway edema***: Consider short trial of steroids (prednisone 5–20 mg daily for 5 days)
- ***Clogged tracheostomy/airway obstruction, copious mucous secretions***: Clean tracheostomy thoroughly by taking out the inner cannula, soaking in hydrogen peroxide

Table 28.1 Palliative Performance Scale (PPS)

%	Ambulation	Activity level evidence of disease	Self care	Intake	Level of consciousness	Estimated median survival (days)		
						a	b	c
100	Full	Normal / *No disease*	Full	Normal	Full	NA	NA	108
90	Full	Normal / *Some disease*	Full	Normal	Full			
80	Full	Normal with effort / *Some disease*	Full	Normal or reduced	Full			
70	Reduced	Can't do normal job or work / *Some disease*	Full	As above	Full	45		
60	Reduced	Can't do hobbies or housework / *Significant disease*	Occasional assistance needed	As above	Full or confusion	29	4	
50	Mainly sit/lie	Can't do any work / *Extensive disease*	Considerable assistance needed	As above	Full or confusion	30	11	41
40	Mainly in bed	As above	Mainly assistance	As above	Full or drowsy or confusion	18	8	
30	Bed bound	As above	Total care	Reduced	As above	8	5	
20	Bed bound	As above	As above	Minimal	As above	4	2	6
10	Bed bound	As above	As above	Mouth care only	Drowsy or coma	1	1	
0	Death	As above						

for at least one minute. Swab out the cannula with cotton swabs or pipe cleaners. Rinse the cannula inside and out, remove any excess water. Reinsert the cannula. Intermittent suction as needed, patient and family education regarding feeding techniques, monitor for signs of aspiration. For atelectasis caused by mucus obstruction, pulmonary complications of cystic fibrosis; consider Mucomyst [6]. Prior to treatment, a bronchodilator by nebulization should be given. *Note: Volume of liquefied bronchial secretions may increase following oral inhalation or intratracheal instillation; potential for airway occlusion*

- **Effusion**: Malignant fluid collections in the chest and abdomen are amenable to percutaneous management with either intermittent thoracentesis or paracentesis or by placement of temporary or permanent drainage catheters. Thoracentesis is a simple way to achieve acute relief of symptoms as well as to assess the degree of symptomatic improvement experienced by the patient. Unfortunately, MPE recurs in 98–100 % of patients within 30 days of thoracentesis and is only controlled for 4 days on average, frequent thoracentesis is likely to be required for palliation of symptoms. The risks of the procedure, including bleeding, infection, pneumothorax, fluid loculation, increase with repeat thoracentesis. For these reasons, treatment of MPE with thoracentesis alone is usually reserved for patients who are likely to respond quickly to systemic therapy or for those with a very short life expectancy [7]. Depending on goals of care, may be appropriate for pleurodesis or permanent indwelling catheter.
- **Volume overload**: Discontinue IV fluids and any artificial feedings, consider trial of diuretic. Add furosemide 20–40 mg orally daily or double dose of current diuretic.
- **Anxiety**: Benzodiazepines are frequently used to alleviate dyspnea in patients with advanced illness when the dyspnea has been optimally treated and the patient is anxious secondary to dyspnea. Consider a trial of low-dose short-acting benzodiazepines, lorazepam 0.5–1 mg every 4–6 h as needed. Combined with medication should be counseling and psychological support. It is important to help the patient anticipate and plan response to breathlessness.
- **Anemia**: Blood transfusion in patients with hemoglobin values of approximately 8 g/dL have been shown to improve anemia-related symptoms on a short-term basis. This benefit is independent of the stage of disease and survival. However, the effects on dyspnea and fatigue tend to decrease within 15 days, despite the maintenance of hemoglobin values attained after transfusions [8]. Policies on blood transfusion are institution-dependent and decisions to transfuse should be based on the patient's medical condition and goals of care. Transfusions can be used to palliate symptoms, and are not offered based on hemoglobin levels alone.

Use of opioids to treat symptoms of dyspnea:

- Opioids relieve symptoms of dyspnea by altering the perception of dyspnea [9], decreasing ventilator drive to both hypoxia and hypercapnia, and reducing oxygen consumption. Although respiratory depression is a commonly cited concern of clinicians, sedation occurs prior to respiratory depression. Dosing of opioids is patient specific and should be ordered PRN, hold for sedation.
- Acute and Severe Dyspnea: In the inpatient setting, or when available, parenteral is the route of choice: 2–5 mg morphine IV every 1 h until relief (first line if no severe renal dysfunction). A continuous opioid infusion with a demand dose that patients or nurses can administer, will provide the timeliest relief. When symptom is improved, continue morphine infusion at 2 mg/h with 5 mg Q1h PRN

Mild-to-Moderate Dyspnea

Opioid naïve: 2–5 mg IV/SQ or 10–15 mg PO morphine every 3–4 h as tolerated, hold for sedation.

Opioid naïve and elderly: Decrease dose to 2 mg PO equivalent morphine initially.

Actively dying 2–5 mg IV morphine every 5–10 min, titrate to effect.

Opioid tolerant: 25–50 % increase above standing dose

While there is no evidence that proper symptom management for terminal dyspnea hastens death, the course and management should be fully discussed with family members, nurses, and others participating in care to avoid confusion about symptom relief vs. fears of euthanasia or assisted suicide [10]. Reassure family and staff, the primary goal of treating symptoms is to relieve suffering, not hasten death.

Nausea and Vomiting

- Protracted nausea and vomiting can effect appetite, pain management, interaction with family and significantly contributes to decreased quality of life.
- Underlying mechanism usually can be categorized as either gastrointestinal, vestibular, cortical, or chemoreceptor trigger zone.
- Evaluate for and treat any reversible causes including medications, constipation, hypercalcemia, gastroenteritis, infection.

General Treatment
- Clear liquid diet, advance as tolerated
- Avoid eating/drinking 1–2 h after vomiting, start with small sips

- Small, frequent feedings. Avoid gas forming foods
- Good oral hygiene. Eliminate offensive food, smells

Specific Etiologies and Treatment

1. **Impaired gastric emptying**: Can present as intermittent nausea, *relieved by vomiting*
   - Prokinetic antiemetic: **Metoclopramide** (10 mg PO, 5 mg SC, 5–10 mg IM Central and peripheral actions. Prokinetic action in GI tract; blocked by anticholinergics. Possible extrapyramidal side effects).
   - For extrinsic compression/obstruction from tumor, diffuse gastric tumor: **Dexamethasone** (4–16 mg PO/IV/SQ Adjuvant antiemetic. Best given in the morning to maintain diurnal rhythm. Monitor for side effects. Review and reduce to lowest effective dose or stop).
   - For patients with gastric irritation or reflux: Proton pump inhibitor
2. **Chemical/metabolic**: Can present as recurrent nausea, *little relief from vomiting*
   - **Haloperidol** 0.5–2 mg I.M., I.V.: Also used off label for postoperative nausea/vomiting [11]. Note: Should not be given to patients with Parkinson's disease, prolonged QTc
   - **Metoclopramide** 10 mg PO/IV Q4h PRN
3. **Cerebellar disease**: (Compression/ irritation by tumor, raised intracranial pressure)
   - **Cyclizine** (histamine H_1 antagonist: 50 mg PO, may repeat in 4–6 h if needed, up to 200 mg/day)
   - **Dexamethasone** Up to 16 mg/day. Doses greater than 4 mg daily are likely to cause side effects after several weeks. Dose should be reviewed at least on a weekly basis. Taper after 2 weeks. Consider use of proton pump inhibitor in patients on high doses of dexamethasone.
4. **Vestibular System**: (motion sickness, base of skull, brainstem disease)
   - **Prochlorperazine**: 5–10 mg PO 3–4 times/day; 5–10 mg IM, 2.5–10 mg IV; may repeat dose every 3–4 h as needed, max 40 mg/day. *Rectal*: 25 mg twice daily. (Caution may cause EPS, anticholinergic effects (constipation, xerostomia, blurred vision, urinary retention); use with caution in patients with decreased gastrointestinal motility, paralytic ileus, urinary retention, BPH (benign prostatic hyperplasia), xerostomia, or visual problems.)
   - **Cyclizine** 50 mg PO Q4–6 h PRN, max 200 mg/day

Avoid combining drugs with a similar mode of action or side effect profile
Do not combine prokinetics with anticholinergics
If patient is vomiting or if oral absorption is questionable, use subcutaneous or rectal route. Prescribe the antiemetic regularly and as required starting with the lowest dose. Review the treatment and response every 24 h until symptoms are controlled.

Constipation

- May be secondary to a complex interaction of physiologic and iatrogenic factors including; decreased activity and oral intake, rectal pain, bowel obstruction or induced by medications.
- Prevention is the single best treatment.

General Treatment
(nonpharmacologic interventions should be implemented):
- Increase dietary fiber
- Increase fluid intake
- Increasing patient mobility
- Removing barriers to get to a bathroom and increase patient privacy
  - Patients on chronic opioid therapy should be on standing senokot and docusate sodium.

Once constipation occurs, it should be aggressively managed in a stepwise approach.
- Begin with:
  - Stool softener—docusate sodium 100–300 mg PO daily
  - Laxative—senokot one to three tabs daily
- *If no bowel movement within 48 h*, consider:
  - Milk of magnesia 30–60 mL PO daily
  - Lactulose 30–45 mL PO daily
- *If no bowel movement after 72 h*, consider:
  - Bisacodyl suppository or enema
  - Perform rectal exam, looking for hemorrhoids, fissures, stool
  - If impacted stool felt on exam, manually disimpact if soft
  - May pretreat patient with sedative, and soften stool with glycerin suppository or oil enema
  - After disimpaction, followup with tap water enema and start patient on standing bowel regimen.
  - Bulk forming fiber and osmotic agents (such as miralax or golytely) are only appropriate for patients who can maintain adequate fluid intake.

Bowel Obstruction

- Mechanical obstruction (partial or complete) of the bowel lumen and/or peristaltic failure
- Assess each patient on the basis of their clinical condition, likely benefits/ risks and patient preferences.
- Some patients with a localized obstruction may benefit from surgery.
- Therapeutic goal is to minimize associated symptoms such as pain, cramping, nausea, and vomiting.

– Start by excluding fecal impaction from history, rectal examination, abdominal X-ray
– Discontinue laxatives and prokinetics (reglan, erythromycin)
– Consider reducing or changing opioids or other medications that may be contributing
– If the patient is dehydrated, IV rehydration may be appropriate initially. Hydration of 1–1.5 L/24 h may reduce nausea but more fluid than this can result in increased bowel secretions and worsen vomiting.
– If obstruction is secondary to a mass, consider trial of steroids to decrease size. Example: Dexamethasone 4–8 mg PO bid
  If no relief in 5 days—discontinue
  If improvement noted—start taper by 1 mg daily after 5 days
- Consider starting anticholinergic (scopolamine one to two patches every 3 days)
- Nausea: Antidopaminergic (Haldol 5–15 mg SQ daily in divided doses). Nausea can usually be fully controlled; vomiting about once a day may be acceptable in bowel obstruction.
- For persistent vomiting: Octreotide 0.1–0.6 mg SQ daily. Inhibits GI secretions and motility.
- Pain relief from colic or tumor pain: Opioid such as fentanyl (reported to have less effect on GI tract), titrate to efficacy, monitor for worsening of symptoms as opioids themselves can be a cause.
- Nasogastric tube: Decompresses stomach in case of intractable vomiting, however can cause aspiration by interfering with coughing. Short-term use only

Anorexia, Cachexia

Decreased appetite and weight loss are predictors of an expected physiological decline seen with the progression of chronic illness.
- Cachexia—significant wasting of adipose tissue and skeletal muscle
  – It reduces quality of life, impairs response to therapy, and is an indicator of poor prognosis. It may occur in up to 80 % of patients with advanced cancer [12]. Most commonly in GI, pancreatic, lung, and prostate cancers.

General Treatment
Nonpharmacological treatments should be recommended which include:
  – Eating frequent, small, high-calorie or high-protein meals, or energy-dense snacks
  – Encourage family to bring in favorite foods from home as tolerated
  – Avoid liquid intake with food to prevent early satiety

– Check oral cavity, for candidiasis or mucositis
– Start routine oral hygiene, remove bad tastes from mouth
– Exercise or physical therapy to maintain muscle mass, decrease fatigue, and improve mood
– Speech and swallow evaluation should be done if dysphagia or a concern for aspiration is present
– Nutrition consultation
- *Pharmacological treatments* evaluated in cancer-related anorexia or cachexia are corticosteroids, progesterone analogs, and serotonin antagonists. Improving appetite or weight gain may be beneficial in some patients, but does not improve survival.
  – **Megestrol**: Starting Dose is 400 mg/day; titrate up to 800 mg QD
    At least two months of continuous therapy is necessary to see benefit. Duration of treatment: No more than 12 weeks at a time
    Post-marketing/case reports have shown duration-dependent increase in thromboembolic phenomena (deep vein thrombosis, pulmonary embolism, thrombophlebitis) [13]
  – **Dronabinol**: 2.5 mg PO twice daily (max: 20 mg/day)
  – **Dexamethasone**: Starting dose is 4 mg PO daily (can also improve pain). Consider benefit vs known side effects of steroids with ongoing use.
    Hyperglycemia, Immunosuppression, Adrenal suppression if taking more than 2 weeks, Psychiatric disturbances, oral candidiasis, myopathy, gastric upset.
  – **Mirtazapine**: 15–30 mg PO at bedtime, onset 1–2 weeks (also beneficial for depression, nausea, and insomnia)

Delirium

Disturbed consciousness, change in cognition, which fluctuates. Develops over a short period.
- Key question for family, "Do you feel he/she has been more confused lately?"
- MMSE<20
  Hyperactive: Increased motor agitation
  Hypoactive: Paucity of speech, slowing or lack of movement, inattentiveness, unaware of environment

Establishing Etiology:
- *Rule out*-infection, electrolyte imbalances, uncontrolled pain, urinary, or fecal retention
- Review all medications being taken for potential side effects.
- Social isolation, emotional distress, and new environments can be contributing factors as well.

- Behavioral modifications—consistent staff, reorient patient to environment
- In end-stage disease, delirium can be caused by brain metastases, seizures, stroke, renal failure, or hepatic failure and is more challenging to treat.

First Line Delirium Treatment: Antipsychotics

Haldol

- First generation. Selectively antagonizes dopamine D2 receptors, metabolized hepatically
- Dosing: 0.5–1 mg Q1h for acute agitation, (can be given IM, IV, PO, SQ) titrate to effect. Maintenance dosing
- Side effects: Dystonia, extrapyramidal symptoms
- Contraindicated in Parkinson's disease. Avoid in patients with prolonged QT. Not approved for dementia-related psychosis.

Risperidone

- Dosing: 0.25–0.5 mg, Q8–12 h, titrate up to effect (max 6 mg/day).
- Preferred for Parkinson's disease, vascular dementia. Less risk of EPS.
- Side effects: Hypotension, EPS, paradoxical insomnia

Quetiapine

- Second generation. Antagonizes dopamine D2 receptors, serotonin 5-HT2 receptors, metabolized hepatically
- Dosing: 12.5–200 mg per day in single or divided doses. Good for sedation at night.
- Side effects: Sedation, headache
- Preferred for Parkinson's disease, vascular dementia
- Note FDA (Food and Drug Administration) black box warning for increased risk of stroke, MI in elderly and weigh risk/benefit ratio of symptom relief in patients with limited prognosis.

Olanzapine

- Promotes weight gain, less EPS (extrapyramidal symptoms), good for long-term use
- Dosing: 1.25–5 mg once daily (wafer available)
- Side effects: Orthostatic hypotension, sedation, hyperglycemia
- Avoid in Parkinson's disease and seizure disorders

Benzodiazepines

Can use as short-term adjunct for acute agitation, can cause paradoxical worsening of delirium. Indicated in alcohol or substance withdrawal.

Lorazepam

- Dosing: 0.5–1 mg PO/IV/SQ q2h as needed, until calm. Most commonly used medication for mild sedation at home.

- Side effects: Sedation, paradoxical agitation

Dry Mouth

Xerostomia:

- Common symptom in palliative care
- Etiologies—dehydration, erosion of mucous membrane lining in the mouth (post chemotherapy or radiation), and a side effect of many medications
- Presentation-dry lips, lips stuck to teeth, difficulty swallowing, sore mouth, foul odorous breath
- Symptom management—includes both saliva substitutes and saliva stimulants.
  - Saliva stimulants include mints, chewing gum, malic acid, and pilocarpine [14].

Simple measures to relieve the dry mouth sensation:

- Good oral hygiene, swab and moisten patient's mouth every hour. Coat lips with ointment liberally
- Drinking liquids
- Humidified air or oxygen
- Sucking on ice, hard candies, or vitamin C tablets, chewing sugarless gum. Pineapple is a natural saliva stimulant and can be enjoyed in frozen form.
- Artificial salvia, products such as biotene, can be found over the counter
- **Pilocarpine** stimulates muscarinic cholinergic receptors and can be used to treat xerostomia at doses of 5–10 mg PO three times daily.

Goals of Care: Overview to Communicating and Negotiating with Families

1. Prepare and plan
   - Establish setting and participants. Find space which allows privacy and minimizes interruptions. Introduce everyone in the room.
   - Review records and discuss with team. Be prepared to answer questions about prognosis, treatments being offered.
2. Explore what the patient and family know, and how much they want to know
   - Actively listen
3. Share medical information in small amounts at a time
   - Pause frequently to check for understanding and to allow questions
   - Discuss prognosis and benefits vs. burdens of treatment options
4. Show empathy as patient and family respond
   - Use silence effectively
5. Identify and resolve conflicts

6. Elicit values and preferences to set goals
   – "What is most important to you?"
7. Summarize and provide support
   – Explain next steps clearly

References

1. World Health Organization. 1993.
2. Temel JS. Early palliative care for patients with metastatic non small cell lung cancer. N Engl J Med. 2010;363:733–42.
3. Anderson F, Downing GM, Hill J. Palliative performance scale (PPS): a new tool. J Palliat Care. 1996;12(1):5–11.
4. Rousseau PC. Nonpain symptom management in terminal care. Clin Geriatric Med. 1996;12:313–27.
5. Dudgeon DJ, Rosenthal S. Management of dyspnea and cough in patients with cancer. Hematol Oncol Clin North Am. 1996;10:157–71.
6. Dynamed. Acetylcysteine: uses. Accessed 2 Oct 2013.
7. Stokes LS. Palliative Interventions in Interventional Radiology. Guest Editor Kent T. Sato M.D. Percutaneous Management of Malignant Fluid Collections. Semin Intervent Radiol. 2007;24(4):398–408.
8. Mercadante S, Ferrera P, Villari P, David F, Giarratano A, Riina S. Effects of red blood cell transfusion on anemia-related symptoms in patients with cancer. J Palliat Med. 2009;12(1):60–3.
9. Bruera E, Macmillan K, Pither J, et al. The effects of morphine on dyspnea of terminal cancer patients. J Pain Symptom Manage. 1990;5:341–4.
10. Von Gunten CF. Morphine and hastened death. 2nd ed. Fast facts and concepts. 2005;8.
11. Gan TJ, Meyer TA, Apfel CC, Chung F, Davis PJ, Habib AS, Hooper VD, Kovac AL, Kranke P, Myles P, Philip BK, Samsa G, Sessler DI, Temo J, Tramèr MR, Vander Kolk C, Watcha M, Society for ambulatory anesthesia. Society for ambulatory anesthesia guidelines for the management of postoperative nausea and vomiting. Anesth Analg. 2007;105(6):1615–28.
12. Holmes S. Understanding cachexia in patients with cancer. Nurs Stand. 2011;25(21):47–56.
13. Loprinzi CL, Ellison NM, Schaid DJ. Controlled trial of megastrol acetate for the treatment of anorexia and cachexia. J Natl Cancer Inst. 1990;82(13):1127–32.
14. Davies AN. The management of xerostomia: a review. Eur J Cancer Care. 1997;6:209–14.

Hospice Medicine

Danna Ogden

Abbreviations

AIDS	Acquired immunodeficiency syndrome
ALS	Amyotrophic lateral sclerosis
BMI	Body mass index
BUN	Blood urea nitrogen
CHF	Congestive heart failure
CNS	Central nervous system
CT	Computed tomography
CVA	Cerebral vascular accident
FAST	Functional Assessment Staging Test
FEV1	Forced expiratory volume
HBsAg	Hepatitis B
INR	International normalized ratio
IV	Intravenous
KPS	Karnofsky Performance Scale
MAC	*Mycobacterium avium* complex
MS	Multiple sclerosis
NYHA	New York Heart Association
PPS	Palliative Performance Scale
PR	Per rectum
PRN	As needed
PT	Prothrombin
RHF	Right heart failure
SQ	Subcutaneous

Introduction

Hospice offers care and support for people who are terminally ill. The focus is on comfort, not on curing an illness. A specially trained team of professionals and caregivers provide care for the "whole person" including his or her physical, emotional, social, and spiritual needs.
- Services may include physical care, counseling, medication, equipment, and supplies related to the terminal illness.
- Care usually takes place in the home
- Family caregivers can also get support
- Hospice is a benefit provided by Medicare but also many private insurances, HMOs and other managed care organizations.

Medicare Hospice Benefits [1]

Patients are eligible for Medicare hospice benefits when all of the following conditions are met:
- Patient is eligible for Medicare Part A (Hospital Insurance, usually age >65 years or receives Medicare disability payments)
- Primary physician and the hospice medical director certify that patient is terminally ill and have ≤6 months to live if the illness runs its normal course
- Informed consent: patient or healthcare proxy signs a statement choosing hospice care instead of other Medicare-covered benefits to treat the terminal illness. (Medicare will still pay for covered benefits for health problems that aren't related)
- Care is provided by a Medicare-certified hospice program

Hospice Myths

Myth: Patient must die within 6 months
Truth: As long as the hospice medical director or other hospice doctor recertifies that patient is terminally ill, they can continue to receive hospice care. Documentation of clinical factors supporting a <6 month life expectancy is always required for certifying initial and continuing eligibility.

D. Ogden, D.O. (✉)
Hospice and Palliative Medicine, Kaiser Permanente,
Portland, OR, USA
e-mail: danna.j.ogden@kp.org

K.A. Sackheim, *Pain Management and Palliative Care: A Comprehensive Guide*,
DOI 10.1007/978-1-4939-2462-2_29, © Springer Science+Business Media New York 2015

Myth: Enrolling in hospice means giving up or withdrawing care.

Truth: Receiving hospice care does not mean giving up hope or that death is imminent. The earlier an individual receives hospice care, the more opportunity there is to stabilize a patient's medical condition and address other needs. Hospice care can improve symptom control and reduce patient/family distress. It is important to clarify this misconception—a hospice referral can mean increasing intensity of home services and available resources.

Myth: You can't keep your primary care doctor

Truth: Hospice reinforces the patient–primary physician relationship by advocating either office or home visits, according to the physician preference. Hospices work closely with the primary physician and consider the continuation of the patient–physician relationship to be a high priority.

Myth: Hospice is a place you go to die

Truth: Hospice care usually takes place in an individual's home, but can be provided in any environment in which a person lives, including a nursing home, assisted living facility, or residential care facility. It is a medical benefit which provides care; it is not a physical place.

Guidelines for Qualifying Hospice Diagnoses [2]

Prognostication can be challenging for providers. Simply, if your answer to the question "Would you be surprised if this patient died within the year?" is "No," a hospice referral may be indicated. Your patient could likely benefit from hospice services if they've been admitted to the hospital several times within the last year with the same symptoms. Also if they wish to remain at home, rather than spend time in the hospital and/or they are no longer receiving treatments intended to cure their disease.

Functional status plays a large role in prognostication and determining eligibility for hospice benefits. The most commonly used and validated tools are the Karnofsky Performance Scale (KPS) (Table 29.1) [3] and the Palliative Performance Scale (PPS).

A patient should have a KPS < 70 % (see below) to be considered for hospice. Progressive clinical decline within the previous year, with documented medical complications, support the prediction of life expectancy < 6 months.

Indications of worsening status for any illness may include:

- Recurrent or intractable fevers, infections such as pneumonia, sepsis, or upper urinary tract, stage III–IV decubitus ulcers after treatment.
- Weight loss not due to reversible causes, decreasing serum albumin or cholesterol
- Dysphagia leading to recurrent aspiration and/or inadequate oral intake
- Increasing frequency of emergency room visits, hospitalizations, or provider visits.

Co-morbidities

When one or more of the following is present, in addition to the terminal diagnosis, it should be taken into account as likely to predict poorer survival:

- Chronic obstructive pulmonary disease
- Congestive heart failure
- Ischemic heart disease
- Diabetes mellitus
- Neurologic disease (CVA, ALS, MS, Parkinson's)
- Renal failure
- Liver disease
- Neoplasia
- AIDS
- Dementia

Disease-Specific Guidelines for Hospice Qualification: used in conjunction with the foregoing general guidelines on clinical decline, if the terminal diagnosis is specific. Note: not all signs are required but support eligibility when present.

Table 29.1 Karnofsky Performance Scale [3]

General category	%	Specific criteria
Able to carry on normal activity	100	Normal general status—no complaint—no evidence of disease
No specific are needed	90	Able to carry on normal activity—minor sign of symptoms of disease
	80	Normal activity with effort, some signs of symptoms of disease
Unable to work	70	Able to care for self, unable to carry on normal activity or do work
Able to live at home and care for most personal needs	60	Requires occasional assistance from others, frequent medical care
Various amount of assistance needed	50	Requires considerable assistance from others, frequent medical care
Unable to care for self	40	Disabled, requires special care and assistance
Requires institutional or hospital care or equivalent	30	Severely disables, hospitalization indicated, death not imminent
Disease may be rapidly progressing	20	Very sick, hospitalization necessary, active supportive treatment necessary
Terminal states	10	Moribund
	0	Dead

End Stage Renal Disease

Clinical Signs

- Uremia: confusion, obtunded, generalized pruritus
- Intractable nausea and vomiting
- Oliguria: urine output of less than 400 cm³/24 h
- Intractable hyperkalemia: persistent serum potassium more than 7.0 not responsive to medical treatment
- Uremic pericarditis
- Hepatorenal syndrome
- Intractable fluid overload, not planning hemodialysis
- Discontinuation of dialysis

Laboratory Criteria

- BUN >100; creatinine clearance of less than 10 cm³/min
- Serum creatinine of more than 8.0 mg/dL, or creatinine >6.0 mg/dL with congestive heart failure or diabetes

End Stage Pulmonary Disease

Clinical Signs

- Dyspnea on exertion or at rest
- Homebound/chair bound
- Increased hospitalizations for pulmonary infections
- Copious/purulent sputum
- Cyanosis: fingertips, lips
- Barrel chested
- Poor response to bronchodilators
- Right heart failure (RHF) secondary to pulmonary disease (Cor pulmonale) (e.g., not secondary to left heart disease or valvulopathy)
- Unintentional weight loss in the past 6 months
- Resting tachycardia

Laboratory Criteria

- Decrease in FEV1 on serial testing of greater than 40 mL/ year (objective evidence of disease progression)
- FEV1 less than 30 % of predicted (objective evidence for disabling dyspnea)
- Hypercapnia; $pCO_2 > 50$ mmHg
- Oxygen dependent; O_2 sat <88 % on room air

End Stage Liver Disease

Clinical Signs

- Cirrhosis/hepatic failure—not a candidate for liver transplant
- Ascites refractory to medical management
- Muscle wasting with reduced strength and endurance
- Hepatic encephalopathy refractory to medical management
- Progressive malnutrition
- Recurrent variceal bleeding/spontaneous bacterial peritonitis
- Hepatorenal syndrome; oliguria, urine Na <10 mEq/L, elevated BUN/creatinine

Laboratory Criteria

- INR >1.5, PT >5 s over control
- Serum albumin <2.5 g/dL

These factors also support an estimated life expectancy of 6 months or less in patients with liver disease:

- Continued active alcoholism (>80 g ethanol/day)
- Hepatocellular carcinoma
- HBsAg (Hepatitis B) positivity or Hepatitis C refractory to interferon treatment

End Stage Cardiac Disease

Clinical Signs

- Symptoms of CHF at rest—NYHA Class IV
- Optimal dose of diuretic and vasodilator therapy
- SVT or ventricular arrhythmia resistant to therapy
- History of cardiac arrest, syncope, cardiogenic brain embolism
- Ejection fraction of 20 % or less (not required but supports eligibility)
- Patient declines or is ineligible for surgical intervention

Cancer/Malignancy

Certain cancers with especially poor prognoses (e.g., small cell lung cancer, brain cancer, and pancreatic cancer) may represent hospice eligibility without use of the below brief guidelines.

- Disease with distant metastases at presentation *or* progression from an earlier stage of disease to metastatic disease with;
- A continued decline in spite of therapy or patient declines further treatment

End-Stage Stroke and Coma

Eligibility guidelines for **end-stage stroke** patients include the following:

- KPS <40 % and inability to maintain hydration and caloric intake with one of the following:
- Weight loss >10 % in the last 6 months or >7.5 % in the last 3 months
- Serum albumin <2.5 g/dL
- Current history of pulmonary aspiration
- Sequential calorie counts documenting inadequate caloric/fluid intake
- Dysphagia severe enough to prevent patient from continuing fluids/foods necessary to sustain life and patient does not receive artificial nutrition and hydration

Diagnostic imaging factors which support poor prognosis after stroke include:

For Non-traumatic Hemorrhagic Stroke

- Large-volume hemorrhage on CT (Infratentorial = 20 mL; Supratentorial = 50 mL)

- Ventricular extension of hemorrhage, surface area of involvement of hemorrhage = 30 % of cerebrum, midline shift = 1.5 cm.
- Obstructive hydrocephalus in patient who declines, or is not a candidate for, ventriculoperitoneal shunt

For Thrombotic/Embolic Stroke

- Large anterior infarcts with both cortical and subcortical involvement, large bihemispheric infarcts, basilar artery occlusion, bilateral vertebral artery occlusion

Eligibility guidelines for **end-stage coma**:

Patients are hospice-eligible if they have any three of the following *on day 3* of coma:

- Abnormal brain stem response
- Absent verbal response
- Absent withdrawal response to pain
- Serum creatinine >1.5 mg/dL

End Stage Alzheimer's

To qualify for hospice a patient needs a FAST score of at least 7 (see below) and must also have one of the following in the past 12 months:

- Recurrent aspiration pneumonia, sepsis
- Pyelonephritis or upper urinary tract infection
- Recurrent fever after antibiotic therapy
- Decubitus ulcers, multiple, stage 3–4
- Inability to maintain sufficient fluid and calorie intake with 10 % weight loss during the previous 6 months or serum albumin <2.5 g/dL.

The FAST score was developed by Barry Reisberg, MD, at New York University Medical Center's Aging and Dementia Research Center. The FAST score measures the stages of Alzheimer's disease. In the absence of a definitive Alzheimer's diagnosis, the FAST score is also used to assess dementia.

Functional Assessment Staging (FAST) [4]

1. **No difficulty**, either subjectively or objectively.
2. Complains of forgetting location of objects. **Subjective work difficulties**.
3. Decreased job functioning evident to co-workers. Difficulty in traveling to new locations. **Decreased organizational capacity**.
4. **Decreased ability to perform complex tasks**, e.g., planning dinner for guests, handling personal finances (such as forgetting to pay bills), difficulty marketing, etc.
5. **Requires assistance in choosing proper clothing** to wear for the day, season, or occasion, e.g., patient may wear the same clothing repeatedly, unless supervised.
6a. **Improperly putting on clothes without assistance or cuing** (e.g. may put street clothes on over night clothes, or put shoes on wrong feet, or have difficulty buttoning

clothing) occasionally or more frequently over the past weeks.
6b. Unable to bathe (shower) properly (e.g., **difficulty adjusting bath-water (shower) temperature**) occasionally or more frequently over the past weeks.
6c. **Inability to handle mechanics of toileting** (e.g., forgets to flush the toilet, does not wipe properly or properly dispose of toilet tissue) occasionally or more frequently over the past weeks.
6d. **Urinary incontinence** (occasionally or more frequently over the past weeks).
6e. **Fecal incontinence** (occasionally or more frequently over the past weeks).
7a. Ability to speak limited to approximately **a half a dozen intelligible different words or fewer**, in the course of an average day or **in the course of an intensive interview**.
7b. Speech ability limited to the use of **a single intelligible word** in an average day or **in the course of an interview** (the person may repeat the word over and over).
7c. Ambulatory ability lost (**cannot walk without personal assistance**).
7d. **Cannot sit up without assistance (e.g., the individual will fall over if there are no lateral rests [arms] on the chair)**.
7e. **Loss of ability to smile.**
7f. **Loss of ability to hold up head independently.**

Adult Failure to Thrive

Both features must be present:
1. Nutritional impairment
   (a) BMI < 22
   (b) Serum albumin <2.5 g/dL
   (c) Unexplained weight loss despite adequate caloric intake
   (d) Refusal of oral/parenteral support
2. PPS or Karnofsky score 40 % or less

Debility Unspecified

Progressive decline of clinical status and function caused by contributing disease processes and co-morbidities, as evidence by:
- Decline of PPS or KPS
- Increasing symptoms of illness, recurrent hospitalizations, emergency visits.
- Dysphagia leading to inadequate nutritional intake or recurrent aspiration
- Nonreversible weight loss, cachexia
- Progressive pressure ulcers in spite of optimal care

- Decline in cognitive level, FAST score 7a or greater.
- Dependence with feeding, ambulation, continence, transfers, bathing, and dressing.

End Stage AIDS

- CD4 count <25 cells/μL; viral load >100,000 copies/mL, KPS<50 %
- CNS lymphoma; untreated, or persistent despite treatment
- Wasting (loss of at least 10 % lean body mass)
- History of successive opportunist infections: *Mycobacterium avium* complex (MAC) bacteremia, progressive multifocal leukoencephalopathy, cryptosporidium infection, toxoplasmosis.
- Visceral Kaposi's sarcoma, unresponsive to therapy

These factors also support an estimated life expectancy of 6 months or less in AIDS patients: chronic persistent diarrhea for 1 year, persistent serum albumin <2.5 g/dL, active substance abuse, age >50 years, absence of or resistance to effective antiretroviral, chemotherapeutic, and prophylactic drug therapy.

Inpatient Hospice Care

Although hospice services are usually provided at home, some patients develop acutely worsening symptoms that require inpatient care for a period of time. Admission to an inpatient unit can also be used as respite for the family and caregivers.

Common problems to anticipate in the inpatient unit include symptoms such as pain, agitation, dyspnea, insomnia, as well as psychosocial issues and preparation for death.

Orders to Consider

- Ativan 0.5 mg Q8h IV/SQ PRN anxiety
- Haldol 0.5 mg IV/SQ PRN agitation/restlessness
- Morphine 2 mg Q4h IV/SQ PRN pain or dyspnea
- Acetaminophen 650 mg PR PRN fever
- Bisacodyl suppository PRN constipation
- Scopolamine patch 1.5 mg Q72h for increased respiratory secretions
- Glycopyrrolate 0.2–0.4 mg SQ Q4h PRN increased respiratory secretions
- Reglan 10 mg IV Q6h PRN nausea/vomiting, or prochlorperazine 25 mg PR Q12h PRN
- Do not resuscitate
- Oral hygiene every 4 h

- Diet; per patient's ability and swallow evaluation. If eating, monitor for aspiration.

Psychosocial Considerations

Religion/Spirituality

Clinicians must address and work to alleviate suffering from all domains. There is a high prevalence of existential distress in terminally ill patients, a spiritual history should be included in the social history for every patient. Patients whose spiritual needs are not met report lower ratings of quality and satisfaction with care.

Spiritual Screening Questions [5]:

- Is religion/spirituality important to you as you cope with your illness?
- How much strength/comfort do you get from your religion/spirituality right now?
- Has there ever been a time when religion/spirituality was important to you?

Exploration of religious or spiritual beliefs, including hope, values, and meaning, demonstrates compassion and caring. Be willing to listen, explore, and empathize without attempting an explanation. This kind of interaction can open up an opportunity to involve professionals, such as hospital chaplains.

Family Dynamics and Addressing Goals of Care

At the end of life, the burden of treatments can outweigh the benefits. A treatment may be withheld if it is seen to be medically futile or withdrawn if there is no demonstrated value [6]. Decisions of how aggressively to treat acute problems, such as malignant bowel obstruction and aspiration pneumonia, can be guided by patient's previous wishes, advanced directives and always include shared medical decision making with patient and family.

Imminently Dying and End of Life Care

When recognized that a patient is imminently dying, this should be communicated in a calm and caring way to the family members to allow for preparation. Notify members of the team and increase emotional support. Provide reassurance to family that the patient's comfort will be prioritized. When handled properly, the family can have realistic expectations which will ease their suffering.

Preparing the family, what to expect;

- **Decreased alertness**
- Patient is expected to be bedbound, sleeping more, have increased weakness and fatigue, can progress to coma.

Fluctuating levels of consciousness may be final phase of terminal delirium. Although patients will often be barely communicative and nonverbal, encourage family, their presence is likely heard and felt.

- **Potential for pressure ulcer formation increases**.
- Gentle turning or repositioning—premedicate with opioid if needed.
- **Decreased appetite**, **anorexia**, **inability to swallow**.
- Teach families that forcing food can actually cause discomfort. Food may be nauseating, or unappealing, patient may express refusal of food by clenching teeth. If not feeding is distressing to the family, offer thing they can do like massaging hands and feet, providing oral hygiene and ice chips.
- **Dehydration**; is a natural part of dying, not associated with thirst or discomfort. Oral intake can lead to choking, aspiration, edema, ascites and does not contribute to comfort or longevity [7]. For comfort maintain oral hygiene and moisture to mouth, nose and eyes. Observe for thrush, coat lips with petroleum jelly, use artificial tears liberally.
- **Decreased ability to swallow and cough**
- Dying process impairs the gag reflex, ability to clear secretions and protect the airway from aspiration. Pooling of saliva in the posterior oropharynx and retention of secretions in the tracheobronchial tree can lead to noisy respirations including gurgling, crackling, and rattling ("death rattle") [8]. Management: suctioning can cause discomfort, instead, reposition to assist postural drainage. Medications: glycopyrrolate 0.2–0.4 mg SQ, atropine drops under tongue, or transdermal scopolamine patches.
- **Changes in circulation**; cyanotic hand or feet, mottling, hypotension, tachycardia, dependent edema in extremities, oliguria/anuria, uremia. Administration of fluids will not reverse circulatory shut down at this stage. Elevating affected extremities against gravity, shifting positions, and massage can be helpful.
- **Changes in breathing**; long periods of apnea, shallow breaths, Cheyne Stokes pattern of irregular respirations. Reassure family, patient is not choking or suffocating. Oxygen is unlikely to help, but may have psychological benefit for patient and/or family [9]. Opioids or benzodiazepines are appropriate to manage sensation of breathlessness.
- **Agitation**; Very distressful symptom for families. When not improved with alteration of modifiable factors, constipation, urinary retention, pain, etc., it can be secondary to terminal delirium. Terminal delirium requires standing medication for patient comfort and safety. Start with ativan 1 mg IV/SC Q8h and adjust as needed.

Pronouncing a Patient

Maintain a quiet, respectful attitude. Introduce yourself and role, determine relationships of persons present. Inform family of purpose; invite to them to remain.

Empathize simply: "I am sorry for your loss."

Death Pronouncement Note

"Patient seen and examined. Absence of spontaneous breathing. Nonresponsive to verbal, tactile, or painful stimulation. Pupils fixed and dilated, absent corneal reflex. Absent heart sounds, no palpable pulse. Make a brief statement of cause of death. Date and time of death. Routine post mortem care." Note: if family present or informed. Note notification of SW, pastoral care, attending physician, as appropriate.

Bereavement is the period after a loss during which grief is experienced and mourning occurs. Allow time and space for grief reaction, even when death is expected. The hospice benefit covers counseling and support from the interdisciplinary team for the family after death. Social workers can assist the family with funeral arrangements, financial concerns.

References

1. http://www.medicare.gov. Accessed 7 Jan 2013.
2. Center for Medicare and Medicaid Services. Indications and limitations of coverage and/or medical necessity.
3. Karnofsky DA, Burchenal JH. The clinical evaluation of chemotherapeutic agents in cancer. In: MacLeod CM, editor. Evaluation of chemotherapeutic agents. New York: Columbia University Press; 1949. 196 p.
4. Reisberg B. Functional assessment staging (FAST). Psychopharmacol Bull. 1988;24:653–9. Copyright © 1984 by Barry Reisberg, MD.
5. Fitchett G, Risk JL. Screening for spiritual struggle. J Pastoral Care Counsel. 2009;62((1, 2)):1–11.
6. Lesage P, Portenoy RK. Ch 30—Pain in medical illness: ethical and legal foundations. In: Bruera ED, Portenoy RK, editors. Cancer pain: assessment and management. Cambridge: Cambridge University Press; 2009. p. 553–60.
7. Bruera E, Hui D, Dalal S, Torres-Vigil I, Trumble J, Roosth J, Krauter S, Strickland C, Unger K, Palmer JL, Allo J, Frisbee-Hume S, Tarleton K. Parenteral hydration in patients with advanced cancer: a multicenter, double-blind, placebo-controlled randomized trial. J Clin Oncol. 2013;31(1):111–8. doi:10.1200/JCO.2012.44.6518. Epub 2012 Nov 19.
8. Quill T, Holloway R, Shah M, Caprio T, Olden A, Storey CP. Primer of palliative care. 5th ed. Chicago: American Academy of Hospice and Palliative Medicine Press; 2010.
9. Abernathy AP, et al. Effect of palliative oxygen versus room air in relief of breathlessness in patients with refractory dyspnoea: a double blind, randomised controlled trial. Lancet. 2010;376:784–93.

Part IV

Pain Management in Patients with Renal Impairment

30

Holly M. Koncicki

Abbreviations

ADH	Antidiuretic hormone
CHF	Congestive heart failure
C_{max}	Concentration max/peak concentration
CNS	Central nervous system
CrCl	Creatinine clearance
CSF	Cerebral spinal fluid
ESRD	End stage renal disease
GFR	Glomerular filtration rate
HD	Hemodialysis
IBW	Ideal body weight
M6G	Morphine-6-glucuronide
NSAID	Nonsteroidal anti-inflammatory drugs
PD	Peritoneal dialysis
SIADH	Syndrome of inappropriate antidiuretic hormone secretion
SNRI	Serotonin–norepinephrine reuptake inhibitors
SSRIs	Selective serotonin reuptake inhibitors
$t_{1/2}$	Half-life
TCA	Tricyclic antidepressants
Vd	Volume of distribution

Introduction [1]

- Pain affects at least 50 % of dialysis patients
- Pain in patients with end stage renal disease (ESRD) on maintenance dialysis has been reported to decrease quality of life, and be under treated.

H.M. Koncicki, M.D., M.S. (✉)
Department of Medicine, Division of Kidney Diseases and Hypertension, Hofstra North Shore-LIJ School of Medicine, Great Neck, NY, USA
e-mail: hollykoncicki@gmail.com

- WHO analgesic ladder has been validated in this population
- Etiology of pain in ESRD patients varies and often there are multiple causes.
  - One study showed the majority (63 %) suffered from "musculoskeletal pain," 13.6 % described recurrent pain related to the dialysis procedure (such as cramping, headaches, and pain related to access), and 12.6 % described pain from "peripheral neuropathy" [2].

Pharmacokinetics

- Evaluation of pharmacokinetics in renal insufficiency may be beneficial if [3]:
  - Drug or active metabolites exhibit a narrow therapeutic index
  - Excretion or metabolism is mostly through the renal system
  - Active metabolites are highly protein bound leading to elevated levels in renal failure
- To achieve therapeutic concentrations a loading dose can be given, or it takes 3–4 $t_{1/2}$ to achieve a steady state [4].
- In renal failure, medication dosing can be altered by decreasing the dose, increasing the dosing interval, or both.
  - A medication can be given at the same frequency if the $t_{1/2}$ is short, and there is a narrow therapeutic range [4].
  - Dosing interval may be increased if there is a broad therapeutic range, long $t_{1/2}$, or for dialysis patients [4].
- *Clearance during dialysis*
  - Properties of drugs that are removed by dialysis:
    Small molecular weight (<500 Da), low protein binding (<90 %), and small volume of distribution (Vd) [4]
  - Drugs cleared by dialysis are usually dosed once daily, and should be dosed after dialysis [4].

K.A. Sackheim, *Pain Management and Palliative Care: A Comprehensive Guide*,
DOI 10.1007/978-1-4939-2462-2_30, © Springer Science+Business Media New York 2015

Estimates of Renal Function

- The FDA recommends use of creatinine clearance (CrCl) calculated by the Cockcroft–Gault formula as measure of glomerular filtration rate (GFR) or renal function when dosing medications [3].
- Based on serum creatinine [3, 5]
  - CrCl = [(140 – age) × IBW (ideal body weight) (in kg)]/ [72 × serum Cr (in mg/dL)]
    In women × 0.85 IBW
  - IBW (Men) = 50.0 kg + 2.3 kg/in over 5 ft
  - IBW (Women) = 45.5 kg + 2.3 kg/in over 5 ft

Definitions of Renal Function [3]

- *Normal renal function*: CrCl > 80 mL/min
- *Chronic kidney disease* (CKD)
  - Mild impairment: CrCl 50–80 mL/min
  - Moderate impairment: CrCl 30–50 mL/min
  - Severe impairment: CrCl < 30 mL/min
  - End stage renal disease (ESRD): patients requiring dialysis

Pain Medication Classifications

Acetaminophen (Tylenol)

National Kidney Foundation recommended as nonnarcotic analgesic for mild–moderate pain in patients with CKD [6].
- **Metabolism**
  - Metabolized in the liver
- **Side effects**
  - Hepatotoxicity
  - Some studies suggest use of 500 mg–1 g/kg for an extended time can cause papillary necrosis.
    Insufficient evidence of acetaminophen causing kidney disease [6]
- **Dosing recommendation** [4, 5]
  - No dose adjustment needed; increase dosing interval:
    - CrCl 10–50 mL/min to every 6 h
    - CrCl < 10 mL/min to every 8 h
    - HD/PD dose as CrCl < 10 mL/min

Nonsteroidal Anti-inflammatory Drugs

- Ex: Celebrex, Naprosyn, Advil, Voltaren
- **Mechanism**
  - Works through inhibition of prostaglandin production by COX-1 and COX-2 enzymes
  - COX-2 selective agents are suggested to have decreased GI and hematological effects, but patients with CKD were excluded from these trials [7].

- Prostaglandins I2 and E2 increase renal perfusion by decreasing vascular resistance through dilation of vasculature [8].
  - Reduction of these prostaglandins may compromise renal blood flow and lead to acute kidney injury
- **Side effects**
  - Increase risk of bleeding
    - Patients with uremia are already predisposed to platelet dysfunction [7].
  - Increased cardiovascular risks with use of COX-2 inhibitors
    - CKD and ESRD patients have higher rates of cardiovascular death at baseline compared to the general population [7].
  - Hypertension
    - Increase systolic blood pressure by 5 mmHg in patients with hypertension [7–10]
    - Use of nonsteroidal anti-inflammatory drugs (NSAIDs) will decrease the antihypertensive effects of diuretics, beta-blockers, and ACE inhibitors [8, 9].
  - Edema
    - Reported in 3–5 % of NSAID users with weight gain of 1–2 kg [7, 8]
    - Effects distal sodium and water reabsorption by inhibiting ADH [8]
  - Electrolyte abnormalities (hyponatremia, hyperkalemia) [7, 8]
    - Risk of hyperkalemia is severe in CKD
    - Increased risk with comorbidities such as diabetes and congestive heart failure (CHF)
    - Increased risk if on medications that may increase potassium including ACE-I, ARB, B blockers, potassium sparing diuretics [7].
      - Indomethacin decreases cellular potassium reuptake [8].
    - Usually resolves with stopping the NSAID [8]
  - Reduction in GFR
    - Important even in patients with ESRD
      - Residual renal function may have benefit in overall morbidity and mortality [7]
      - Increased risk in patients with underlying CKD, the elderly and low perfusion states including CHF and cirrhosis, and those prone to dehydration (e.g., on diuretics) [6, 8]
    - Renal papillary necrosis may be acute or chronic, and cause permanent renal damage
      - Acute damage is associated with NSAID overdose in patients who are dehydrated [8]
      - Chronic is a form of analgesic nephropathy and occurs after prolonged use (5–20 years) [8]
    - Risk of interstitial nephritis and nephrotic syndrome
- **Dosing recommendation**
  - Used with caution for time-limited treatments in ESRD and under the supervision of a physician [6, 7]
  - Not recommended in patients with CKD

Topical Medications

Lidocaine Patch (Lidoderm Patch) [11]
- **Metabolism** [11]
  - Hepatic metabolism to metabolites, some of which are active
  - Excreted by renal system with less than 10 % of parent drug excreted unchanged in urine
  - Dialysis is not useful in treating overdose
    Approximately 70 % protein bound; volume of distribution 0.7–2.7 L/kg
- **Dosing**
  - Not defined

Diclofenac Epolamine Topical Patch (Flector Patch) [12, 13]
- **Metabolism**
  - Topical NSAIDs [12]
    Case reports have described use of topical NSAIDs and development of acute renal failure, suggesting that systemic absorption occurs.
- **Dosing** [13]
  - Not recommended in patients with advanced renal disease
  - If used, monitoring of renal function is recommended

Tricyclic Antidepressants (TCA)

Amitriptyline (Elavil), Nortriptyline (Pamelor), Desipramine (Norpramin)
- **Metabolism**
  - Mostly through hepatic routes
  - ESRD patients may have elevated levels of glucuronidated metabolites, which may increase sensitivity to side effects.
    - Desipramine—metabolized by liver, 70 % excreted in urine [14]
- **Side Effects** [7, 15]
  - *Anticholinergic effects:*
    - Sedation, dry mouth, orthostatic hypotension, constipation, urinary retention, delirium, blurred vision
    - **Desipramine** and **Nortriptyline** have fewer anticholinergic effects and may be better tolerated [15].
    - Dry mouth can worsen thirst and ESRD patients are typically fluid restricted to avoid weight gain between dialysis treatments.
  - Conduction abnormalities including prolonged QTc
    - In ESRD patients, intradialytic hypokalemia, hypocalcemia, and alkalosis may occur, all which may transiently increase QTc [7].
    - Patients maintained on diuretic therapy are also at increased risk of electrolyte abnormalities.

- **Dosing Recommendations** [4, 15, 16]
  - Start at the lowest dose with slow titration every 1–2 weeks
    - Drug level monitoring in hemodialysis patients being treated for depression showed that most were below the lower limit of the therapeutic range of amitriptyline, suggesting inadequate dosing in this population.
    - One study showed a significant decrease in amitriptyline concentrations (26 %) after dialysis, thought to be due to conversion to nortriptyline.
  - **Amitriptyline** [15]
    - CKD dosing ranges from 10 to 150 mg daily
      - No dosing changes for HD/PD [4]
  - **Nortriptyline** [15]
    - CKD dosing ranges from 25 to 150 mg daily
    - No dosing changes for HD/PD [4]

Desipramine [15]
- CKD dosing ranges from 25 to 100 mg daily

Serotonin–Norepinephrine Reuptake Inhibitors (SNRIs)

Venlafaxine (Effexor)
- **Metabolism** [17]
  - Metabolized through hepatic routes into an active metabolite, *O*-desmethylvenlafaxine
  - Primary mode of excretion is through the renal system
    - Elimination $t_{1/2}$ increased by 50 % in renal failure
    - Excretion reduced by 24 % in CrCl < 70 mL/min [17]
    - In ESRD patients clearance is reduced by 57 % and $t_{1/2}$ increased by 180 % [17].
- **Side effects**
  - Fewer side effects than TCAs
  - Nausea, dry mouth
  - Dose-dependent elevations in blood pressure
  - Withdrawal symptoms if discontinuation is abrupt
- **Dosing Recommendations** [4, 17]
  - Dose reduction for CKD
  - Dosing for normal renal function: 75–225 mg daily
    - CrCl 10–50 mL/min: Decrease by 50 % [4]
    - CrCl < 10 mL/min or ESRD: Decrease by 50 %
      - Recommended to dose postdialysis

Duloxetine (Cymbalta)
- **Metabolism**
  - Hepatic metabolism into inactive metabolites [18]
  - 72 % of administered dose is excreted in urine as parent drug or metabolites [18]

- Large Vd and between 95 and 96 % are protein bound [18]
- Peak concentration (C_{max}) and bioavailability (or area under the curve—AUC) for duloxetine exposure were approximately two times higher in ESRD patients [18] In ESRD and non-ESRD patients, $t_{1/2}$ was similar.
- Inactive metabolites had higher C_{max} and AUC in ESRD compared to non-ESRD patients by two- to ninefold
- $t_{1/2}$ of metabolites were 27 h vs. 12 h or 2.1 × longer in ESRD patients [18]
- Mild and moderate renal impairment does not have an important clinical effect on duloxetine levels [18]
- **Side Effects** [18]
  - ESRD patients
    - Nausea, vomiting, and diarrhea were more common
    - Increase in mean supine systolic blood pressure by 10 mmHg
    - Increased orthostasis (decrease in SBP > 15 mmHg) 6 to 12 h after drug administration, though clinically asymptomatic
    - No significant changes in QTc
- **Dosing** [18]
  - Normal dosing for diabetic neuropathy/fibromyalgia is 60 mg daily
  - Dose adjustments not recommended for mild or moderate renal insufficiency (CrCl > 30 mL/min)
  - Not recommended for use in patients with ESRD or severe renal impairment (CrCl < 30 mL/min)

Milnacipran (Savella)
- **Metabolism** [19, 20]
  - Mainly eliminated in urine
    - 80 % of single dose is recovered in urine as parent drug or metabolites in 24 h, 90 % at 5 days [19].
    - Less than 2 % eliminated in the feces
    - 50–60 % of dose excreted unchanged, 20–30 % as conjugated, rest as inactive metabolites
  - Elimination $t_{1/2}$ increased 3 × in patients with severe renal insufficiency [19]
  - Average $t_{1/2}$ 8.3 h, with mean of 15 h for patients with renal insufficiency ranging from 8.6 to 24.6 h [19]
  - Others estimate increase in elimination $t_{1/2}$ by 38, 41, and 122 % in patients with mild, moderate, and severe renal insufficiency [20].
  - Renal insufficiency causes a slower elimination and increase in plasma concentrations, proportional to degree of renal failure [19].
    - Higher and more variable plasma concentrations with AUC increased by 16, 52, and 199 % in mild, moderate, and severe renal insufficiency [19].
    - Low protein binding (13 %) but high volume of distribution, suggestive of poor clearance with dialysis [20].

- **Side Effects** [19, 20]
  - Nausea and vomiting suggested to be more severe in patients with severe renal insufficiency (CrCl < 18 mL/min) [16].
  - Elevation in blood pressure in patients with and without hypertension [20]
  - Hyponatremia due to syndrome of antidiuretic hormone secretion (SIADH).
    Patients at increased risk are elderly, are on diuretics, or are volume depleted [20].
  - Dysuria, urinary retention also described [20]
- **Dosing Recommendations** [20]
  - Recommended to use with caution in patients with moderate renal insufficiency [20]
  - CrCl < 29 mL/min
    - Decrease dose by 50 % to 25 mg twice a day [20]
    - Can increase to 50 mg twice daily based on tolerance
  - Not recommended for use in patients with ESRD [20]

Anticonvulsants

Gabapentin (Neurontin)
- **Metabolism** [7]
  - Elimination correlated to renal function as excreted unchanged in urine
  - Prolonged $t_{1/2}$ in renal failure, from 5–7 h to 52–132 h
  - Dialysis has been estimated to remove approximately 35 % of drug
- **Side Effects** [21, 22]
  - Central nervous system (CNS) effects: asterixis, myoclonus, tremor, confusion, coma, ataxia, somnolence, lethargy, dizziness
  - Increased risk of edema
  - Suggested that patients with renal insufficiency may be at increased risks
- **Dosing Recommendations**
  - *Dose adjustment in CKD:* [5, 23]
    - CrCl > 30–59 mL/min: 400–1400 mg/day
    - CrCl > 15–29 mL/min 200–700 mg/day
    - CrCl 10–50 mL/min some sources recommend increasing dosing interval every 12–24 h [4]
    - CrCl < 15 mL/min: 100–300 mg/day or every 48 h [4]
  - *Hemodialysis:*
    - 300 mg loading dose followed by 200 or 300 mg postdialysis [7]
    - Recommended not to exceed 300 mg/day [7]
  - *Peritoneal Dialysis:*
    - Recommend up to 300 mg every other day [5]

Pregabalin (Lyrica)
- **Metabolism**
  - Mostly excreted in urine

– Dialysis has been estimated to remove 50–60 % of drug [24]
- **Side effects**
  – Dizziness, somnolence, ataxia, and peripheral edema
  – Case reports of decompensated heart failure requiring increased diuretic therapy [25–27]
    ▪ Theorized to be due to the drugs effect on calcium channels in the myocardium
    ▪ Case report of myoclonus in a hemodialysis patient [24]
- **Dosing Recommendations** [28]
  – *Dose adjustment and increased dosing interval for CKD:*
    ▪ CrCl 30–60 mL/min — 50 % of normal dose
      ◆ 75–300 mg/day; dose frequency of two to three times a day
    ▪ CrCl 15–30 mL/min
      ◆ 25–150 mg/day; dose frequency of two times a day or daily
    ▪ CrCl < 15 mL/min
      ◆ 25–75 mg/day; dose frequency daily
  – *Hemodialysis*: supplemental dose given after treatment
    ▪ If on 25 mg qD, supplemental dose of 25–50 mg
    ▪ If on 25–50 mg qD, supplemental dose of 50–75 mg
    ▪ If on 50–75 mg qD, supplemental dose of 75–100 mg
    ▪ If on 75 mg qD, supplemental dose 100 or 150 mg

Topiramate (Topamax)

- **Metabolism** [29]
  – Approximately 70 % is eliminated unchanged in urine
    ▪ Clearance decreased by
      ◆ 42 % in moderate renal impairment (CrCl 30–69 mL/ min/1.72 m^2)
      ◆ 54 % in severe renal impairment (CrCl < 30 mL/ min/1.73 m^2)
  – Cleared 4–6 x greater during greater during dialysis as compared to general population
- **Side Effects**
  – Nonanion gap acidosis [29–33]
    ▪ Described to cause renal tubular acidosis and may have hypokalemia
    ▪ Inhibition of carbonic anhydrase leads to renal loss of bicarbonate [29]
      ◆ For migraine: incidence of persistent decrease in bicarbonate 44 % at doses of 200 mg/day, 39 % for 100 mg/day, 23 % for 50 mg/day [29]
      ◆ Incidence of bicarbonate <17 and >5 mEq/L decrease from pretreatment was 11 % for 200 mg/day, 9 % for 100 mg/day and 2 % for 50 mg/day [29]

    ▪ Untreated acidosis may increase risk of kidney stones, nephrocalcinosis, osteomalacia
  – CKD patients may be at increased risk of acidosis [29]
    ▪ May have increased risk when used with carbonic anhydrase inhibitors
      ◆ Recommend to follow bicarbonate levels during treatment [29, 33]
      ◆ If persistent acidosis can dose reduce, consider switching to a different medication or supplement with alkali (bicarbonate) [29, 33]
  – Kidney stones [29, 34]
    ▪ Of patients being treated with topiramate for seizures, 1.3–1.5 % developed kidney stones [29]
    ▪ Patients with stones had decreased urinary acidification and low urinary citrate [34]
    ▪ Patients should be encouraged to increase water intake to decrease risk of stone formation [33].
- **Dose Adjustments**
  – Moderate to severe renal impairment (CrCl 10–50 mL/min) [5, 29]
    ▪ Dose reduce by 50 %
  – CrCl < 10 [5]
    ▪ Dose reduce by 75 %
      ◆ For migraine dosing in normal renal function — start at 25 mg/day with titration to 100 mg/day divided into BID dosing [29]
  – ESRD on dialysis [29]
    ▪ Dose after dialysis
    ▪ Seizure prophylaxis may require supplemental dosing on dialysis days

Carbamazepine (Tegretol)

- **Metabolism**
  – Hepatic metabolism
  – Renal excretion accounts for 1–3 % of unchanged parent drug and approximately 69 % of metabolites [35, 36].
  – Molecular weight is 236 Da, volume of distribution 0.8–1.8 L/kg, and 75–78 % protein bound [35, 37]
    In cases of overdose, clearance during 4 h, low efficiency hemodialysis has been shown to be approximately 24–25 % [35].
- **Side Effects**:
  – Somnolence, dizzy, ataxia, agranulocytosis, constipation, nausea, CHF, edema, acute renal failure, hepatotoxicity
  – Hyponatremia [36]
- **Dose Adjustment**
  No dose adjustment for ESRD or CKD [4]

Muscle Relaxants

Metaxalone (Skelaxin)
- **Metabolism** [38]
  - Hepatic metabolism
  - Metabolites are excreted in urine
  - Large volume of distribution and is lipophilic
    Suggestive that drug is poorly dialyzable
  - Impact of renal disease on pharmacokinetics have not been determined
- **Side effects** [38]
  - Drowsiness, dizziness, headache, nervousness, nausea, vomiting
- **Dosing** [38]
  - Recommended to use with caution in patients with renal dysfunction
  - Significant impairment is considered a contraindication

Tizanidine (Zanaflex)
- **Metabolism**
  - 70 % is excreted through the renal system
    Compared to patients with normal renal function, clearance is estimated to be reduced by greater than 50 % in elderly patients with CrCl < 25 mL/min [39].
  - AUC in patients with renal failure is seven times that of a patient without renal failure so effect may be prolonged [39]
  - Unclear removal by dialysis [40]
- **Side Effects**
  - Weakness, fatigue, tiredness, somnolence, dry mouth, increased spasm, and dizziness [39]
  - Hypotension and bradycardia [39]
    Case report of bradycardia in a hemodialysis patient [40]
  - Prolonged QT in animal studies of chronic toxicity [39]
- **Dosing Recommendations** [39]
  - *Normal dosing*
    Start at 4 mg and up titrate
    Dosing frequency: every 6–8 h
    Max of 3 doses per day, and maximum dose of 36 mg/day.
  - *Renal dosing*—not well defined
    Recommended to use with caution, and dose reductions should be made
    During titration the dose should be increased rather than the frequency
    Close follow up for symptoms of toxicity

Methocarbamol (Robaxin)
- **Metabolism** [41, 42]
  - Hepatic metabolism to inactive metabolites
  - Decreased clearance in dialysis patients compared to patients with normal renal function
    Similar $t_{1/2}$ in dialysis patients
- **Side Effects**
  - Drowsiness described in hemodialysis patients [41]

- **Dosing**
  - Not defined in renal insufficiency
    Given similar $t_{1/2}$, dosing frequency likely does not need to be adjusted [41]

Chlorzoxazone (Lorzone; Parafon Forte DSC)
- **Metabolism** [43]
  - Hepatic metabolism and excretion in the urine as conjugated form
  - Less than 1 % of unchanged parent drug is excreted in urine in 24 h
- **Dosing**
  - Renal dosing not defined

Cyclobenzaprine (Amrix, Flexeril, Fexmid)
- **Metabolism**
  - Hepatic metabolism and excreted as glucuronides by the renal system [44]
  - Highly protein bound
- **Side Effects**
  - Closely related to TCAs in structure and side effects
  - Unclear data on frequency of QT prolongation though is a reported adverse effect [44, 45]
  - Common adverse effects include dry mouth and drowsiness [44]
    Anticholinergic effects, disorientation, hallucination, coma also seen
  - In overdose: Lethargy, tachycardia, combative behavior are most commonly seen [45]
- **Dosing**
  - Not defined in renal disease

Baclofen (Liorisel)
- **Metabolism**
  - Of the administered drug, 85 % is eliminated through renal system
    Hepatic metabolism of 15 % [46]
  - Clearance is related to renal function [46, 47]
    $t_{1/2}$ is increased in renal insufficiency
  - Low volume of distribution, low protein biding
    Baclofen is cleared by dialysis [47]
    Hemodialysis and peritoneal dialysis have been used to reverse toxicity with improvement in mental status noted after one session [46, 48].
- **Side Effect**
  - Neurotoxicity occurs at increased doses of baclofen [47]
  - Acute intoxications: neurotoxicity, altered mental status, coma, respiratory depression, hypotonia, hyporeflexia, seizures [46, 48, 49]
  - Neurotoxicity in renal insufficiency has been described with daily doses from 5 to 60 mg, with mean dose of 20 mg [47].
    Chronic toxicity: hallucinations, impaired memory, catatonia, mania [48]
    Increased toxicity reported in elderly patients [47]

- **Dosing** [47]
  - No clear guidelines
  - Some recommend avoiding use in patients with an eGFR <30 mL/min/1.73 m^3
  - In patients with eGFR 30–60 mL/min/1.73 m^3 recommended starting at very low doses and long intervals with close monitoring.

Orphenadrine (Norflex)
- **Metabolism**
  - 50 % of dose is excreted in the urine [50, 51]
  - Unlikely to be cleared by dialysis [50, 52]
    - Highly lipid soluble
    - Not detected in dialysis fluid [50]
- **Side effects** [53]
  - Central and peripheral effects seen in overdose due to antihistaminic and anticholinergic properties:
    - Central effects include confusion, seizures, hallucinations, coma
      - ◆ Peripheral effects include mydriasis, anhidrosis, urinary retention, constipation
- **Dosing**
  - No alterations in dosing [5]

Carisoprodol (Soma, Soprodal, Vanadom)
- **Metabolism**
  - Hepatic metabolism
  - Excreted through renal and nonrenal systems [54]
  - Removed by hemodialysis and peritoneal dialysis [54]
- **Side Effects**
  - Most common include drowsiness, dizziness, headache, and nausea [55]
- **Dosing** [54]
  - As drug is excreted by renal system, increased exposure in patients with decreased renal function is expected.
  - Pharmacokinetics have not been evaluated
  - Advised to use with caution

Opioids

Tramadol (Ultram)
- **Metabolism**
  - Metabolized by liver to an active metabolites
  - 30 % of parent drug excreted in the urine; 60 % excreted as metabolites [56]
  - $t_{1/2}$ is doubled in patients with reduced renal function [7]
  - Dialysis has been described to clear <7 % of administered dose [57]
- **Side Effects**
  - Nausea, CNS depression, constipation
  - Epileptogenic in patients with lowered seizure thresholds.

CKD patients may be at increased risk as uremia decreases seizure threshold [7, 57]
  - Case reports of respiratory depression in patients with CKD [7, 58, 59]
- **Dosing Recommendations**
  - Extended release tramadol has not been studied in renal impairment and is contraindicated for use in patients with a CrCl <30 mL/min [60]
  - Requires dose reduction and increase in dosing interval in CKD or ESRD patients with varying recommendations
    - GFR 10–50 mL/min
      Decrease dose: 50–100 mg every 8 h [4]
    - CrCl <30 mL/min to ESRD
      Increase dosing interval to 12 h
      Maximum dose 200 mg daily [56]
    - ESRD on dialysis—maximum dose of 50 mg every 12 h [7]

Codeine
- **Metabolism** [61]
  - Hepatic metabolism into active metabolites
  - Reduced clearance of parent drug and metabolites in renal insufficiency [61]
  - Higher plasma levels of codeine in hemodialysis patients
  - $t_{1/2}$ is increased in hemodialysis patients following one dose
    Accumulation of drug to toxic levels following repeated dosing is suggested [61].
    Normal $t_{1/2}$ 4.04±0.6 h in ESRD 18.69±9.03 h
- **Side Effects**
  - Nausea and vomiting in dialysis patients [61]
  - Cases reports have described CNS depression, hypotension, respiratory arrest, and narcolepsy in patients with renal failure [7, 62, 63].
- **Dosing recommendations** [4, 5, 62, 64]
  - Avoid use in CKD and ESRD
  - If must be used should reduce dose and monitor closely for side effects.
    - GFR 10–50 mL/min—reduce dose by 25 %
    - GFR 10 mL/min—reduce dose by 50 %
    - HD/PD—dose as GFR 10 mL/min

Morphine
- **Metabolism** [63–65]
  - Hepatic metabolism
  - Excreted by renal system [64]
    Of parent compound, <10 % is excreted in urine [62]
  - Metabolites accumulate in renal failure in serum and CSF
  - Morphine-6-glucuronide (M6G) has been suggested to be active and have analgesic properties
  - M6G concentration is 15 times higher in CSF in patients on hemodialysis compared to those with normal renal function [65].

- **Side Effects**
  - Case reports of respiratory and CNS depression in renal insufficiency [66, 67]
  - Case reports of lethal intoxication of morphine in patients with renal insufficiency [68]

    Though hydrophilic molecules are removed during dialysis, there is equilibration of lipophilic molecules so the CNS effects can continue after dialysis [64]
  - Myoclonus
- **Dosing recommendations** [4, 5, 64, 69]
  - Not recommended for use
  - If morphine is used, should only be used for a short time and patient should be transitioned to preferred opioids quickly.
  - Dosing recommendations:
    - GFR 20–50 mL/min—75 % of normal dose
    - GFR 10–20 mL/min—50 % of normal dose
    - GFR <10 mL/min—25–50 % of normal dose
    - HD/PD—recommend 50 % of normal dose

Hydrocodone (Vicodin, Norco)
- Combination with acetaminophen
- **Metabolism**
  - Similar actions to codeine
  - Metabolized by O-demethylation and N-demethylation to hydromorphone and norhydrocodone [62]
  - Parent compound and metabolites are excreted by kidneys [62]

    Within 24 h, 85 % of oral dose is within the urine as metabolites and parent compound [70]
  - Limited data in renal failure

    Data only on hydromorphone and codeine [62]
- **Side Effects**
  - Risk of adverse effects may be increased in patients with renal insufficiency secondary to accumulation of parent medication and metabolites [70]
- **Dosing Recommendations**
  - No data regarding pharmacokinetics in CKD
  - Use is not recommended CrCl < 15 mL/min [62]

Tapentadol (Nucynta)
- **Metabolism**
  - First pass metabolism—96 % is metabolized into inactive metabolites [71]
  - Rapid excretion—50 % excreted after 4 h, 95 % excreted after 24 h [71]
  - In the urine 99 % is excreted as conjugates and 3 % as the unchanged parent compound [71].
  - No change in AUC or C_{max} of parent compound in patients with severe renal insufficiency [72].

    Metabolite tapentadol-O-glycuronide has increased AUC by 1.5, 2.5, and 5.5-fold for mild, moderate, and severe renal insufficiency, respectively [72].

- Large volume of distribution and low protein binding (estimated 20 %) [73]
- **Side effects**
  - Lower GI side effect profile (nausea, vomiting, constipation) compared to oxycodone in elderly patients [74].
  - A study excluding patients with renal insufficiency showed common side effects of nausea, drowsiness, dry mouth, confusion, and constipation, most of which improved over time [75].
- **Dosing Recommendations**
  - No adjustment is recommended in patients with mild or moderate renal impairment [73].
  - Not recommended for use in severe renal insufficiency [72]

Oxycodone
- **Metabolism**
  - Hepatic metabolism [76]

    Nineteen percent of parent drug is excreted in the urine.
  - In patients with renal dysfunction (CrCl < 60 mL/min) $t_{1/2}$ and peak levels of oxycodone and metabolites are increased [76].
  - Extent of clearance during dialysis is unknown [76]

    Large volume of distribution (2.5 ± 0.8 L/kg) and 45 % is protein bound [76]
- **Side effects**
  - Case report of CNS toxicity and respiratory depression in a hemodialysis patient [77]
- **Dosing recommendations**
  - Recommendations
    - Normal adult dosing: 10–30 mg every 4–6 h [76]
    - CrCl 10–50 mL/min—75 % of normal dose [62, 78]
    - CrCl < 15 mL/min not on dialysis: start dose 2.5 mg every 8–12 h [62]

Hydromorphone (Dilaudid)
- Preferred opiod in renal failure
- **Metabolism**
  - Hepatic metabolism to hydromorphone-3-glucuronide and other metabolites, which are excreted by renal system.
  - Longer $t_{1/2}$, of 40 h, in patients with severe renal insufficiency (CrCl < 30 mL/min) as compared to 15 h in patients with normal renal function [79]

    AUC is doubled in patients with moderate insufficiency and increased four times in patients with severe renal insufficiency [80]
  - Clearance during dialysis has been reported to be 40 % of pre-dialysis levels [64, 80].
- **Side effects**
  - Metabolite hydromorphone-3-glucuronide is reported to be neuro-excitatory in animal studies and accumulates in patients with renal failure [64]

- Tremor, myoclonus, agitation, and cognitive dysfunction have been described in CKD patients on parental infusions of hydromorphone [81]
- Reported better tolerance as compared to morphine [82]
- **Dosing Recommendations**
  - Start at lower doses in moderate renal insufficiency [79, 80]
  - Increase dosing interval in severe renal insufficiency [80]

Methadone
- **Metabolism**
  - Hepatic metabolism into inactive metabolite
  - Excreted in urine and stool
    Increased excretion in stool, in patients with decreased renal function [64, 83]
  - Plasma levels of methadone in patients with CKD and ESRD are within normal range [83]
  - Removal during dialysis
    Qualities such as high protein binding and high volume of distribution suggest that it is poorly cleared by dialysis [64]
    Case reports showed poor removal of methadone during dialysis, though inactive metabolite was cleared without clinical effect [83, 84].
- **Side Effects**
  - Anecdotal reports a good safety profile
  - Prolongs QT interval
    Recommended to administer with caution in patients at risk for QT prolongation
    Patients with electrolyte abnormalities may be at increased risk.
    Ex: Diuretic use, transient electrolyte disturbances during dialysis
- **Dosing Recommendations**
  - Dose for normal renal function
    2.5–10 mg q6–8 h [5]
  - No dose adjustment for CrCl > 10 mL/min
  - CrCl < 10 mL/min: 50–75 % of normal dose [5, 62]
  - HD dose as CrCl < 10 mL/min: 50–75 % of normal dose [4]
    No supplemental dosing needed after dialysis

Fentanyl (Duragesic)
- **Preferred opioid in renal failure** as metabolites are inactive and appears to be well tolerated [62]
- **Metabolism**
  - Hepatic metabolism into inactive metabolites that are mostly excreted in urine
  - Clearance may be reduced in CKD
  - Increased $t_{1/2}$ to 25 h, when given as a continuous infusion [62]
  - Removal during dialysis is likely poor given high protein binding, low solubility, high molecular weight, and high volume of distribution [64]

- **Side effects**
  - Case reports that fentanyl is well tolerated in renal failure [85]
  - Some reports of prolonged sedation, and respiratory depression in patients on a continuous infusion or with use of a transdermal patch [62].
- **Dosing Recommendations**
  - Slow titration and careful monitoring for accumulation or toxicity
  - Dose reduction recommended [4, 5, 62]
    - CrCl is 10–50 mL/min—75 % of normal dose
    - CrCl < 10 mL/min—50 % of normal dose
    - HD/PD—dose as CrCl < 10 mL/min—50 % of normal dose
      No supplemental doses are needed

Meperidine (Demerol)
- **Metabolism** [86, 87]
  - Hepatic metabolism to active normeperidine and inactive metabolites.
    Normeperidine has analgesic properties but also carries increased seizure risk compared to Meperidine.
  - Elimination is dependent on renal function and urinary pH
    $t_{1/2}$ of normeperidine is increased in renal insufficiency, which can lead to accumulation [86].
  - Normeperidine levels and normeperidine/meperidine ratio was higher in renal insufficiency than in patients with normal renal function [86, 87]
- **Side effects**
  - Higher incidence in parental compared to oral administration [88]
  - CNS effects
    Hallucinations, psychosis, disorientation, respiratory depression, and tremor [87, 88]
  - Cardiovascular effects
    Hypotension and tachycardia [88]
  - Case reports of seizures, myoclonus, and altered mental status in CKD or ESRD patients [86, 87, 89, 90].
- **Dosing Recommendations**
  - Normal dose 50–100 mg q3–4 h [5]
  - CrCl 10–50 mL/min—75 % of normal dose [4]
  - CrCl < 10 mL/min—50 % of normal dose [4]
  - Avoid in HD/PD [4, 7]
    Case report of hemodialysis use in overdose or for adverse reactions [89].

Buprenorphine Transdermal (Butrans Patch) [91]
- **Metabolism** [91]
  - Hepatic metabolism into one active metabolite, norbuprenorphine.
    Metabolite is excreted by biliary and renal systems.
  - Studies evaluating intravenous buprenorphine found similar concentrations in patients with normal renal function and renal insufficiency.

Table 30.1 Dosing (not defined in renal insufficiency)

Medication	Cautions for use in renal disease	Renal dosing guidelines
Buprenorphine Transdermal [91]	Metabolite excreted by renal system. Plasma levels similar regardless of renal function. Likely poor clearance with dialysis	Studies in renal impairment not done
Tizanidine [39, 40]	Excreted mostly through renal system. Clearance reduced and increased bioavailability in renal insufficiency	Not well defined
		Start with caution
		Dose reduction rather than frequency reduction
Methocarbamol [41, 42]	Similar $t_{1/2}$ in ESRD patients	Not defined. Dosing frequency likely does not need to be adjusted
Carisoprodol [54, 55]	Pharmacokinetics not evaluated, though patients with renal insufficiency likely have increased exposure	Not defined
		Use with caution
Cyclobenzaprine [44, 45]	Metabolites undergo renal excretion	Not defined
Chlorzoxazone [43]	Metabolites undergo renal excretion	Not defined
Lidocaine Patch [11]	Metabolites undergo renal excretion	Not defined

Table 30.2 Recommended medications to AVOID in renal patients

Medication	Cautions for use in renal disease	Renal dosing guidelines
Duloxetine [18]	Increased peak concentration and bioavailability of parent drug and metabolites in renal insufficiency	*CrCl < 30 mL/min or ESRD*: Not recommended
		CrCl > 30 mL/min: No dose adjustment
Milnacipran [16, 19, 20]	$t_{1/2}$ increased three times and bioavailability increased in severe renal insufficiency. Likely poor clearance with dialysis	*ESRD*: Not recommended
		Moderate CKD: Use with caution
		CrCl < 29 mL/min: Decrease dose by 50 % for max dose of 50 mg twice a day
NSAIDs [6–10]	Increased risk of bleeding, hypertension, edema, electrolyte abnormalities, and reduction in GFR	*CKD*: Not recommended
		ESRD: Time-limited trial under physician supervision
Diclofenac transdermal [12, 13]	Possible systemic absorption	*CKD*: Not recommended
Tramadol (Extended release) [4, 7, 56–60]	Extended release tramadol has not been studied in renal impairment	*CrCl < 30 mL/min*: Contraindicated
Codeine [4, 5, 7, 61–64]	Reduced clearance and increased plasma concentrations of the drug in renal insufficiency	*CKD or ESRD*: Not recommended
Morphine [4, 5, 62–68]	Active metabolites accumulate in serum and CSF in patients with renal insufficiency. Side effects including CNS and respiratory depression, as well as myoclonus	*CKD or ESRD*: Not recommended
Meperidine [4, 5, 7, 86–90]	$t_{1/2}$ and plasma levels of active metabolite are increased in renal insufficiency. Side effects include seizures, myoclonus, and altered mental status	*ESRD*: Not recommended
		CrCl 10–50 mL/min: 75 % of normal dose
		CrCl < 10 mL/min: 50 % of normal dose
Tapentadol [71–75]	Increased bioavailability of metabolite in renal insufficiency	*Severe renal insufficiency*: Not recommended
Hydrocodone [62, 70]	Risk of adverse effects may be increased in renal insufficiency due to accumulation of parent medication and metabolites	*CrCl < 15 mL/min*: Not recommended
Baclofen [46–49]	$t_{1/2}$ increased in renal insufficiency. Neurotoxicity in renal insufficiency reported	*eGFR < 30 mL/min/1.73 m3*: Not recommended
Metaxalone [38]	Impact of renal insufficiency on pharmacokinetics not defined	*Significant renal impairment*: Contraindicated

– No significant difference in plasma concentrations before or after dialysis in patients on transdermal buprenorphine. Large volume of distribution and highly protein bound (96 %)

- **Side Effects** [91]
  – Reduction in blood pressure

– Prolonged QTc by 9.2 ms when dose of 40 μg/h used

- **Dosing Recommendations** [91]
  – Studies in patients with renal impairment not done Tables 30.1, 30.2, and 30.3 list dosing, medications to avoid, and preferred medications in renal patients, respectively.

Table 30.3 Preferred medications in renal patients

Medication	Cautions for use in renal disease	Renal dosing guidelines
Tricyclic antidepressants [4, 7, 14–16]	Side effects include anticholinergic effects and conduction abnormalities including prolonged QTc	Start low and titrate slowly
		Amitriptyline—CKD 10–150 mg daily; no changes for HD/PD
		Nortriptyline—CKD 25–150 mg daily; no changes for HD/PD
		Desipramine—CKD 25–100 mg daily
Venlafaxine [4, 17]	Fewer side effects than tricyclic antidepressants. Dose-dependent elevations in blood pressure	Normal renal function: 75–225 mg daily
		CrCl 10–50 mL/min, ESRD on HD/PD: reduce dose by 50 %; Dose after hemodialysis
Gabapentin [4, 5, 7, 21–23]	Increased $t_{1/2}$ in renal insufficiency. Patients with renal insufficiency may be at increased risk of side effects including CNS effects	Start low and titrate slowly *CrCl > 30–59 mL/min*: 400–1400 mg/day
		CrCl > 15–29 mL/min: 200–700 mg/day, Consider increasing dosing interval from every 12 to every 24 h
		Hemodialysis: 300 mg loading dose; 200–300 mg postdialysis; do not exceed 300 mg/day
		Peritoneal Dialysis: 300 mg every other day
Pregabalin [24–28]	Mostly excreted through urine. Side effects including myoclonus, decompensated heart failure, edema, dizziness, ataxia, and somnolence	*CrCl 30–60 mL/min*: 50 % dose reduction; 75–300 mg/day; dose frequency two or three times a day
		CrCl 1 > 5–30 mL/min: 25–150 mg/day; decrease frequency to twice a day or daily
		CrCl < 15 mL/min 25–75/day; dose daily
		Dialysis: supplemental doses based on daily dose; see text
Carbamazepine [4, 35–37]		No adjustment needed for ESRD or CKD
Acetaminophen [4–6]	**National Kidney Foundation recommends** as nonnarcotic analgesic for mild–moderate pain in patients with CKD	*Increase dosing interval for CKD*
		CrCl 10–50 mL/min: every 6 h
		CrCl < 10 mL/min/ HD or PD: every 8 h
Tramadol [4, 7, 56–60] (Immediate release)	$t_{1/2}$ increased in renal insufficiency. Side effects Described in CKD includes respiratory depression. Also may be epileptogenic and patients with CKD have may have a lowered seizure threshold	Requires dose reduction and increase in dosing intervals
		CrCl 10–50 mL/min: 50–100 mg every 8 h
		CrCl < 30 to ESRD: increase dosing interval to every 12 h; max dose of 200 mg/day
		Dialysis: max dose 50 mg every 12 h
Hydromorphone [64, 79–82]	**Preferred opiod in renal failure.** $t_{1/2}$ and bioavailability increased in renal insufficiency. Neuro-excitatory metabolites accumulate in renal insufficiency. Better tolerance than morphine	Start at lower doses in moderate renal insufficiency
		Increase dosing interval in severe renal insufficiency
Oxycodone [62, 76–78]	Peak levels and $t_{1/2}$ increased in renal insufficiency. Case reports of CNS toxicity and respiratory depression in a dialysis patient	Normal adult dosing: 10–30 mg every 4–6 h
		CrCl 10–50 mL/min: 75 % of normal dose
		CrCl < 15 mL/min not on dialysis: starting dose 2.5 mg every 8–12 h
Methadone [4, 5, 62, 64, 83, 84]	Plasma levels in CKD and ESRD within normal range. Anecdotal reports good safety profile. Prolongs QT	Dose for normal renal function
		2.5–10 mg q6–8 h [4]
		CrCl > 10 mL/min: No dose adjustment
		CrCl < 10 mL/min: 50–75 % of normal dose [4, 36]
		HD dose as CrCl < 10 mL/min: 50–75 % of normal dose; no supplemental dose
Fentanyl [4, 5, 62, 64, 85]	**Preferred opioid in renal failure.** Increased $t_{1/2}$ in renal insufficiency. Likely poor removal during dialysis. Some reports of sedation and respiratory depression	Slow titration and careful monitoring for accumulation or toxicity
		CrCl is 10–50 mL/min: 75 % of normal dose
		CrCl < 10 mL/min: 50 % of normal dose
		HD/PD—dose as CrCl < 10 mL/min: 50 % of normal dose; No supplemental doses
Orphenadrine [5, 50–53]	Unlikely cleared by dialysis. Antihistaminic and anticholinergic side effects	No alterations in dosing

References

1. Barakzoy AS, Moss AH. Efficacy of the world health organization analgesic ladder to treat pain in end-stage renal disease. J Am Soc Nephrol. 2003;17:3198–203.

2. Davison SN. Pain in hemodialysis patients: prevalence, cause, severity, and management. Am J Kidney Dis. 2003;42:1239–47.

3. Food and Drug Administration. Guidance for Industry: Pharmacokinetics in patients with impaired renal function—study design, data analysis and impact on dosing and labeling. Rockville: Department of Health and Human Services; 1998.

4. Taal M, Chertow G, Marsden P, Skorecki K, Yu A, Brenner B. Brenner & Rector's The kidney. 9th ed. Elsevier Inc: Philadelphia; 2012.

5. Aronoff GR, Bennett WM, Berns JS, Brier ME, Kasbekar N, Mueller BA, Pasko DA, Smoyer WE. Drug prescribing in renal failure: dosing guidelines for adults and children. 5th ed. Philadelphia: American College of Physicians; 2007.

6. Henrich WL, Agodoa LE, Barrett B, Bennett WM, Blantz RC, Buckalew VM, D'Agati VD, DeBroe ME, Duggin GG, Eknoyan G, Elseviers MM, Gomez A, Matzke GR, Porter GA, Sabatini S, Stoff JS, Striker GE, Winchester JF. Analgesics and the kidney: summary and recommendations to the scientific advisory board of the National Kidney Foundation from an ad hoc committee of the National Kidney Foundation. Am J Kidney Dis. 1996;27:162–5.

7. Kurella M, Bennet WM, Chertow GM. Analgesia in patients with ESRD: a review of available evidence. Am J Kidney Dis. 2003;42:217–28.

8. Whelton A. Nephrotoxicity of nonsteroidal anti-inflammatory drugs: physiologic foundations and clinical implications. Am J Med. 1999;106:S13–24.

9. Johnson AG, Nguyen TV, Day RO. Do nonsteroidal anti-inflammatory drugs affect blood pressure? A meta-analysis. Ann Intern Med. 1994;121:289–300.

10. Pope JE, Anderson JJ, Felson DT. A meta-analysis of the effects of nonsteroidal anti-inflammatory drugs on blood pressure. Arch Intern Med. 1993;153:477–84.

11. Lidoderm [package insert]. Endo Pharmaceuticals Inc., Chadds Ford. 2010. http://dailymed.nlm.nih.gov/dailymed/drugInfo.cfm?id=18476. Accessed 2 Jan 2013.

12. Andrews PA, Sampson SA. Topical non-steroid drugs are systemically absorbed and may cause renal disease. Nephrol Dial Transplant. 1999;14:187–9.

13. Flector [package insert]. Teikoku Seiyaku Co. Ltd., Sanbonmatsu. 2004. http://www.accessdata.fda.gov/drugsatfda_docs/label/2007/021234lbl.pdf. Accessed 2 Jan 2013.

14. Desipramine HCl [package insert]. Sandoz Inc, Princeton. 2011. http://dailymed.nlm.nih.gov/dailymed/lookup.cfm?setid=7ec5f73f-32b6-48c3-b16e-891d06edf6eb. Accessed 30 Oct 2012.

15. Naylor HK, Raymond CB. Treatment of neuropathic pain in patients with chronic kidney disease. CAANT J. 2011;21:34–9.

16. Unterecker S, Müller P, Jacob C, Riederer P, Pfuhlmann B. Therapeutic drug monitoring of antidepressants in haemodialysis patients. Clin Drug Investig. 2012;32:539–45.

17. Venlafaxine [package insert]. Wyeth, Philadelphia. 2004. http://www.accessdata.fda.gov/drugsatfda_docs/label/2004/20151slr028,030,032,20699slr041,048,052_effexor_lbl.pdf. Accessed 24 Sept 2012.

18. Lobo ED, Heathman M, Kuan HY, Reddy S, O'Brien L, Gonzales C, Skinner M, Knadler MP. Effects of varying degrees of renal insufficiency on the pharmacokinetics of duloxetine. Analysis of a single-dose phase I study and pooled steady state data from phase II/III trials. Clin Pharmacokinet. 2010;49:311–21.

19. Puozzo C, Pozet N, Deprez D, Baille P, Ung HL, Zech P. Pharmacokinetics of milnacipran in renal impairment. Eur J Drug Metab Pharmacokinet. 1998;23:280–6.

20. Savella (milnacipran HCl) [package insert]. Forest Pharmaceuticals Inc. 2009. http://www.frx.com/products/savella.aspx. Accessed 30 Oct 2012.

21. Dogukan A, Aygen B, Berilgen MS, Dag S. Gabapentin-induced coma in a patient with renal failure. Hemodial Int. 2006;10:168–9.

22. Bookwalter T, Gitlin M. Gabapentin-induced neurologic toxicities. Pharmacotherapy. 2005;25:1817–9.

23. Neurontin [US physician prescribing information]. Pfizer distributed by Parke-Davis, New York. 2012. http://labeling.pfizer.com/ShowLabeling.aspx?id=630. Accessed 17 Sept 2012.

24. Yoo L, Matalon D, Hoffman RS, Goldfarb DS. Treatment of pregabalin toxicity by hemodialysis in a patient with kidney failure. Am J Kidney Dis. 2009;54:1127–30.

25. Murphy N, Mockler M, Ryder M, Ledwidge M, McDonald K. Decompensation of chronic heart failure associated with pregabalin in patients with neuropathic pain. J Card Fail. 2007;13:227–9.

26. Page II RL, Cantu M, Lindenfeld J, Hergott LJ, Lowes BD. Possible heart failure exacerbation associated with pregabalin: case discussion and literature review. J Cardiovasc Med. 2008;9:922–5.

27. De Smedt RH, Jaarsma T, van der Broek SA, Haaijer-Ruskamp FM. Decompensation of chronic heart failure associated with pregabalin in a 73-year-old patient with postherpetic neuralgia: a case report. Br J Clin Pharmacol. 2008;66:327–8.

28. Lyrica [full prescribing information]. Pfizer distributed by Parke-Davis, New York. 2012. http://labeling.pfizer.com/ShowLabeling.aspx?id=561. Accessed 17 Sept 2012.

29. Topamax [Prescribing Information]. Janseen Ortho LLC, Curabo. 2009. http://www.topamax.com/sites/default/files/topamax.pdf. Accessed 3 Mar 2013.

30. Izzedine H, Launay-Vacher V, Deray G. Topiramate-induced renal tubular acidosis. Am J Med. 2004;116:281–2.

31. Fernández-de OL, Esteban-Fernández J, Aichner HF, Casillas-Villamor Á, Rodriguez-Álvarez S. Topiramate-induced metabolic acidosis: a case study. Nefrologia. 2013;32:403–4.

32. Sacré A, Jouret F, Manicourt D, Devuyst O. Topiramate induces type 3 renal tubular acidosis by inhibiting renal carbonic anhydrase. Nephrol Dial Transplant. 2006;21:2995–6.

33. Mirza N, Marson A, Pirmohamed M. Effect of topiramate on acid-base balance: extent, mechanism and effects. Br J Clin Pharmacol. 2009;68:655–61.

34. Lamb EJ, Stevens PE, Nashef L. Topiramate increased biochemical risk of nephrolithiasis. Ann Clin Biochem. 2004;41:166–9.

35. Prabahar MR, Karthik KR, Sing M, Singh RB, Singh S, Dhamodharan J. Successful treatment of carbamezapine poisoning with hemodialysis: a case report and review of the literature. Hemodial Int. 2011;15:407–11.

36. Carbamazepine [package insert]. Distributed by Novartis Pharmaceuticals Corporation, East Hanover. 2012. http://www.pharma.us.novartis.com/product/pi/pdf/tegretol.pdf. Accessed 2 Nov 2012.

37. Pilapil M, Petersen J. Efficacy of hemodialysis and charcoal hemoperfusion in carbamazepine overdose. Clin Toxicol. 2008;46:342–3.

38. Skelaxin [package insert]. Corepharma LLC, Middlesex. 2011. http://dailymed.nlm.nih.gov/dailymed/drugInfo.cfm?id=51427. Accessed 26 Sept 2012.

39. Tizanidine [package insert]. Dr. Reddy's Laboratories Limited, Bachepalli. http://dailymed.nlm.nih.gov/dailymed/drugInfo.cfm?id=16397. Accessed 25 Sept 2012.

40. Kitabata Y, Orita H, Kamimura M, Shiizaki K, Narukawa N, Abe T, Kobata H, Akizawa T. Symptomatic bradycardia probably due to tizanidine hydrochloride in a chronic hemodialysis patient. Ther Apher Dial. 2005;9:74–7.

41. Sica DA, Comstock TJ, Davis J, Manning L, Powell R, Melikian A, Wright G. Pharmacokinetics and protein binding of methocarbamol in renal insufficiency and normals. Eur J Clin Pharmacol. 1990;39:193–4.

42. Robaxin [package insert]. Schwarz Pharma LLC, Smynra. 2009. http://dailymed.nlm.nih.gov/dailymed/drugInfo.cfm?id=38053#nlm34068-7. Accessed 25 Sept 2012.

43. Chlorzoxazone [package insert]. Watson Pharma Private Limited, Verna, Salcette Goa. 2010. http://dailymed.nlm.nih.gov/dailymed/drugInfo.cfm?id=52547#nlm34068-7. Accessed 2 Jan 2013.

44. Flexeril [product insert]. Merck & Co. Inc, West Point. 2001. http://www.accessdata.fda.gov/drugsatfda_docs/label/2003/017821s045lbl.pdf. Accessed 25 Sept 2012.

45. Spiller HA, Winter ML, Mann KV, Borys DJ, Muir S, Krenzelok EP. Five-year multicenter retrospective review of cyclobenzaprine toxicity. J Emerg Med. 1995;13:781–5.

46. Brvar M, Vrtovec M, Kovač D, Pezdir T, Bunc M. Haemodialysis clearance of baclofen. Eur J Clin Pharmacol. 2007;63:1143–6.

47. El-Husseini A, Sabucedo A, Lamarche J, Courville C, Peguero A. Baclofen toxicity in patients with advanced nephropathy: proposal for new labeling. Am J Nephrol. 2011;34:491–5.

48. Chen YC, Chang CT, Fang JT, Huang CC. Baclofen neurotoxicity in uremic patients: is continuous ambulatory peritoneal dialysis less effective than intermittent hemodialysis? Ren Fail. 2003;25:297–305.

49. Chou CL, Chen CA, Lin SH, Huang HH. Baclofen-induced neurotoxicity in chronic renal failure patients with intractable hiccups. South Med J. 2006;99:1308–9.

50. Stoddart JC, Parkin JM, Wynee NA. Orphenadrine poisoning. A case report. Brit J Anaesth. 1968;40:789–90.

51. Hespe W, de Roos AM, Nauta WT. Investigation into the metabolic fate of orphenadrine hydrochloride after oral administration to male rats. Arch Int Pharmacodyn Ther. 1965;156:180–200.

52. Mao YC, Hung DZ, Yang CC, Wang JD. Full recovery from a potentially lethal dose of orphenadrine ingestion using conservative treatment: a case report. Hum Exp Toxicol. 2010;29:961–3.

53. Garza MB, Osterhoudt KC, Rutstein R. Central anticholinergic syndrome from orphenadrine in a 3 year old. Pediatr Emerg Care. 2000;16:97–8.

54. Carisoprodol [package insert]. Vintage Pharmaceuticals Inc, Charlotte. 2010. http://dailymed.nlm.nih.gov/dailymed/drugInfo.cfm?id=22442. Accessed 25 Sept 2012.

55. Serfer GT, Wheeler WJ, Sacks HJ. Randomized, double-blind trial of carisoprodol 250 mg compared with placebo and carisoprodol 350 mg for the treatment of low back spasm. Curr Med Res Opin. 2010;26:91–9.

56. Ultram (tramadol hydrochloride) [full prescribing information]. Janssen Ortho LLC, Guarabo. 2008. http://www.accessdata.fda.gov/drugsatfda_docs/label/2009/020281s032s033lbl.pdf. Accessed 24 Sept 2012.

57. Gardner JS, Blough D, Drinkard CR, Shantin D, Anderson G, Graham D, Alderfer R. Tramadol and seizures: a surveillance study in a managed care population. Pharmacotherapy. 2000;20:1423–31.

58. Barnung SK, Treschow M, Borgbjerg FM. Respiratory depression following oral tramadol in a patient with impaired renal function. Pain. 1997;71:111–2.

59. Stamer UM, Stüber F, Muders T, Musshoff F. Respiratory depression with tramadol in a patient with renal impairment and CYP2D6 gene duplication. Anesth Analg. 2008;107:926–9.

60. Durotram XR [product information]. iNova Pharmaceuticals, Thornleigh. 2008. http://www.medsafe.govt.nz/profs/datasheet/d/durotramxrtab.pdf. Accessed 17 Sept 2012.

61. Guay DR, Awni WM, Findlay JW, Halstenson CE, Abraham PA, Opsahl JA, Jones EC, Matzke GR. Pharmacokinetics and pharmacodynamics of codeine in end-stage renal disease. Clin Pharmacol Ther. 1988;43:63–71.

62. Murtagh FE, Chai MO, Donohoe P, Edmonds PM, Higginson IJ. The use of opioid analgesia in end-stage renal disease patients managed without dialysis: recommendations for practice. J Pain Palliat Care Pharmacother. 2007;21:5–16.

63. Talbott GA, Lynn AM, Levy FH, Zelikovic I. Respiratory arrest precipitated by codeine in a child with chronic renal failure. Clin Pediatr. 1997;36:171–3.

64. Dean M. Opioids in renal failure and dialysis patients. J Pain Symptom Manage. 2004;28:497–504.

65. D'Honneur G, Gilton A, Sandouk P, Scherrmann JM, Duvaldestin P. Plasma and cerebrospinal fluid concentrations of morphine and morphine glucuronides after oral morphine. The influence of renal failure. Anesthesiology. 1994;81:87–93.

66. Bodd E, Jacobsen D, Lund E, Ripel Å, Mørland J, Wiik-Larsen E. Morphine-6-glucuronide might mediate the prolonged opioid effect of morphine in acute renal failure. Hum Exp Toxicol. 1990;9:317–21.

67. Angst MS, Bührer M, Lötsch J. Insidious intoxication after morphine treatment in renal failure: delayed onset of morphine-6-glucuronide action. Anesthesiology. 2000;92:1473–6.

68. Lagas JS, Wagenaar JF, Huitema AD, Hillebrand MJ, Koks CH, Gerdes VE, Brandjes DP, Beijnen JH. Lethal morphine intoxication in a patient with sickle cell crisis and renal impairment: case report and a review of the literature. Hum Exp Toxicol. 2011;30:1399–403.

69. Bunn R, Ashley C. The renal drug handbook. Oxford: Radcliffe Medical Press; 1999.

70. Vicodin (Hydrocodone Bitartrate and Acetaminophen) [package insert]. Abott Laboratories, North Chicago. 2011. http://www.rxabbott.com/pdf/vicodin.pdf. Accessed 30 Oct 2012.

71. Terlinden R, Ossig J, Fliegert F, Lange C, Göhler K. Absorption, metabolism, and excretion of ¹⁴C-labeled tapentadol HCl in healthy male subjects. Eur J Drug Metab Pharmacokinet. 2007;32:163–9.

72. Hartick C. Tapentadol immediate-release for acute pain. Expert Rev Neurother. 2010;10:861–9.

73. Nucynta (tapentadol) [package insert]. Ortho-McNeil-Janssen Pharmaceuticals Inc, Raritan. 2010. http://dailymed.nlm.nih.gov/dailymed/lookup.cfm?setid=07c33315-90c9-4a73-bf1d-bca70c7e0ff5. Accessed 30 Oct 2012.

74. Vorsanger G, Xiang J, Biondi D, Upmalis D, Delfgaauw J, Allard R, Moskovitz B. Post hoc analyses of data from a 90-day clinical trial evaluating the tolerability and efficacy of tapentadol immediate release and oxycodone immediate release for the relief of moderate to severe pain in elderly and nonelderly patients. Pain Res Manag. 2011;16:245–51.

75. Mercadante S, Porzio G, Ferrera P, Aielli F, Adile C, Ficorella C, Giarratano A, Casuccio A. Tapentadol in cancer pain management: a prospective open-label study. Curr Med Res Opin. 2012;28:1–5.

76. Lugo RA, Kern SE. The pharmacokinetics of oxycodone. J Pain Palliat Care Pharmacother. 2004;18:17–30.

77. Foral PA, Ineck JR, Nystrom KK. Oxycodone accumulation in a hemodialysis patient. South Med J. 2007;100:212–4.

78. Broadbent A, Khor K, Heaney A. Palliation and chronic renal failure: opioid and other palliative medications—dosage guidelines. Prog in Palliat Care. 2003;11:183–90.

79. Dilaudid [Package Insert]. Abbott Laboratories, North Chicago. 2007. http://medlibrary.org/lib/rx/meds/dilaudid/. Accessed 18 Sept 2012.

80. Durnin C, Hind ID, Wickens MM, Yates DB, Molz KH. Pharmacokinetics of oral immediate-release hydromorphone (Dilaudid® IR) in subjects with renal impairment. Proc West Pharmacol Soc. 2001;44:81–2.

81. Paramanandam G, Prommer E, Schwenke DC. Adverse effects in hospice patients with chronic kidney disease receiving hydromorphone. J Palliat Med. 2011;14:1029–33.

82. Lee MA, Leng ME, Tiernan EJ. Retrospective study of the use of hydromorphone in palliative care patients with normal and abnormal urea and creatinine. Palliat Med. 2001;15:26–34.

83. Kreek MJ, Schecter AJ, Gutjahr CL, Hect M. Methadone use in patients with chronic renal disease. Drug Alcohol Depend. 1980;5:197–205.

84. Furlan V, Hafi A, Dessalles MC, Bouchez J, Charpentier B, Taburet AM. Methadone is poorly removed by haemodialysis. Nephrol Dial Transplant. 1999;14:254.

85. Karanikolas M, Aretha D, Kiekkas P, Monantera G, Tsolakis I, Filos KS. Intravenous fentanyl patient-controlled analgesia for perioperative treatment of neuropathic/ischaemic pain in haemodialysis patients: a case series. J Clin Pharm Ther. 2010;35:603–8.

86. Szeto HH, Inturrisi CE, Houde R, Saal S, Cheigh J, Reidenberg MM. Accumulation of normeperidine, an active metabolite of meperidine, in patients with renal failure or cancer. Ann Intern Med. 1977;86:738–41.

87. Kaiko RF, Foley KM, Gabinski PY, Heidrich G, Rogers AG, Inturrisi CE, Reidenberg MM. Central nervous system excitatory effects of meperidine in cancer patients. Ann Neurol. 1983;13:180–5.

88. Miller RR, Jick H. Clinical effects of meperidine in hospitalized medical patients. J Clin Pharmacol. 1978;18:180–9.

89. Hassan H, Bastani B, Gellens M. Successful treatment of normeperidine neurotoxicity by hemodialysis. Am J Kidney Dis. 2000;35:146–9.

90. Hochman MS. Meperidine-associated myoclonus and seizures in long-term hemodialysis patients. Ann Neurol. 1983;14:593.

91. Butrans patch [package insert]. LTS Lohmann Therapie-Systeme AG, Andernach. 2010. http://dailymed.nlm.nih.gov/dailymed/drugInfo.cfm?id=65886. Accessed 2 Jan 2013.

Pain Management in Patients with Hepatic Impairment

Adam C. Ehrlich and Amir Soumekh

Abbreviations

AUC	Area under the curve
Cmax	Maximum concentration
CNS	Central nervous system
COX	Cyclooxygenase
CYP	Cytochrome P450
FDA	Food and Drug Administration
INR	International normalized ratio
LFTs	Liver function tests
NAPQI	N-Acetyl-p-benzoquinone imine
NMDA	N-Methyl-D-aspartate
NSAIDs	Non-steroidal anti-inflammatory drugs
SNRIs	Serotonin-norepinephrine reuptake inhibitors

Introduction

Liver disease/cirrhosis affects an estimated 4.5–9.5 % of the overall population [1]. As a pain management physician, it is very important to treat patients with medications that will not cause exacerbation or progression of their liver pathology.

A.C. Ehrlich, M.D., M.P.H. (✉)
Department of Medicine, Section of Gastroenterology,
Temple University Hospital, Philadelphia, PA, USA
e-mail: adam.ehrlich@tuhs.temple.edu

A. Soumekh, M.D.
Department of Medicine, Division of Gastroenterology
and Hepatology, Weill Cornell Medical College,
New York, NY, USA
e-mail: ams2041@med.cornell.edu

Pharmacokinetics

Drug metabolism occurs in the liver by a combination of three different mechanisms:
1. Conjugation of drug molecule to glucuronic acid, sulfate, glycine, glutathione, acetate, or a methyl group
2. Oxidation/reduction/hydrolysis reactions by the cytochrome P450 (CYP) enzyme system
3. Biliary excretion [2]

Adjusting dosing/medications for hepatic patients:
- Drug choice and dosages do not necessarily need to be modified in patients with asymptomatic chronic liver disease without cirrhosis. Approval from their treating physician is recommended.
- In patients post-liver transplant without cirrhosis, medication choice should be dictated by drug interactions with immunosuppressive medications and not necessarily on liver disease

Cirrhosis Effects on Drug Metabolism

- Liver disease appears to have varying and complex effects on drug metabolism
- As the severity of liver dysfunction increases → metabolism of drugs is more highly impaired [3]
- Due to increased intestinal permeability, drug absorption may be increased in cirrhotics, which may lead to toxicity [4, 5]
- Conversely, drug absorption may be decreased due to gut edema secondary to portal hypertension or from poor motility [6, 7]
- Ascites and peripheral edema increase the volume of distribution of hydrophilic drugs; thus, they may be less effective
- Individuals with chronic liver disease often have unpredictable responses to medications, so expert consensus

K.A. Sackheim, *Pain Management and Palliative Care: A Comprehensive Guide*,
DOI 10.1007/978-1-4939-2462-2_31, © Springer Science+Business Media New York 2015

suggests considering modifying drug-prescribing for all patients with known or suspected cirrhosis

- In patients who have developed cirrhosis, the degree of alteration in drug metabolism is more severe in those patients with decompensated cirrhosis compared to compensated patients

Types of Pain in Cirrhosis

- Cirrhotic patients are susceptible to all of the same pain syndromes and injuries as healthy patients
- Cirrhotic patients are also at risk for abdominal and low back pain related to ascites formation, as well as mastalgia related to gynecomastia
  - When reference is made to mild, moderate, and severe hepatic impairment, we are generally referring to the classification scheme below
  - *Child-Turcotte-Pugh score classifies patients with cirrhosis into Class A, B, or C based on scoring five different clinical and laboratory parameters with Class A being mild and Class C being severe* [8, 9]:
    - ↑ bilirubin
    - ↑ INR
    - ↓ albumin
    - Presence of encephalopathy
    - Presence of ascites

Pain Medication Classifications

Acetaminophen (Tylenol)

- **Metabolism and side effects**
  - Largely hepatic with combination of glucuronidation, sulfation, and hydroxylation
  - NAPQI, produced as an intermediate metabolite prior to conjugation to glutathione, is the toxic metabolite that causes acute liver toxicity
- **Dosing recommendations**
  - Despite common misconception, acetaminophen is not contraindicated in patients with liver disease and is often an excellent first-line drug for chronic pain. It is always recommended to approve this medication use with the patients treating physician.
  - Older studies suggest that acetaminophen is safe at recommended doses. Cirrhotic patients given 4 g/day had no evidence of drug accumulation or hepatotoxicity [10, 11]
  - Cirrhotics who are actively abusing alcohol can have hepatotoxicity, hepatic necrosis, and death at ingestions much less than what is seen with the general population (<4 g vs. 10 g) [12]

- *Acetaminophen administration should be limited to < 2 g/day to ensure drug concentrations well below the potentially toxic levels* [13]

Combination Drugs

- Often include acetaminophen. Ex Percocet (oxycodone–acetaminophen), Vicodin (hydrocodone–acetaminophen), and other over the counter remedies
- Patients with liver diseases should be counseled to carefully read packaging of any medication or consult with their physician to ensure they remain below the 2 g/day guideline for acetaminophen

Non-steroidal Anti-inflammatory Drugs (NSAIDs)

- **Metabolism and side effects**
  - Largely hepatic and mostly protein bound
  - Idiopathic and idiosyncratic hepatotoxicity has been reported [14]
  - Risk of hepatorenal syndrome exists in cirrhotic patients and is thought to be driven by NSAID-related inhibition of prostaglandins, which are necessary to counteract the renin-aldosterone-angiotensin system and the sympathetic stimulation that results in decreased renal perfusion [15]
  - NSAIDs can increase the risk of mucosal bleeding in a patient who already has thrombocytopenia due to effects on cyclooxygenase (COX) [16]
- **Dosage recommendations**
  - *Avoid NSAIDs in patients with cirrhosis*
  - COX-2 inhibitors need further study

Topical medications

- **Metabolism and side effects**
  - Depends on active ingredient (e.g., lidocaine patches have risk of systemic toxicity as lidocaine is metabolized by liver; however, diclofenac patch has risks associated with NSAIDs)
- **Dosage recommendations**
  - *Lidocaine patches or gel should be used with caution*
  - *Diclofenac patches or gel should be avoided*
  - Dosing of other topical medications should be based on risk of active ingredient

Tricyclic antidepressants

- **Metabolism and side effects**
  - Largely by hepatic biotransformation using CYP proteins and then renal excretion

- Known side effects of sedation and intestinal stasis may put cirrhotics at higher risk of ence-phalopathy
- May also be at higher risk of anticholinergic side effects if degradation impaired by liver dysfunction
- **Dosage recommendations**
  - No specific recommendations exist but would start at low doses and titrate slowly. Always proceed with caution and monitor frequently to assess for side effects.
  - *Desipramine and nortriptyline are preferred over older agents as they have fewer sedating properties and a lower likelihood of hypotension* [17]

Serotonin-Norepinephrine Reuptake Inhibitors (SNRIs)—Venlafaxine (Effexor), Desvenlafaxine (Pristiq), Duloxetine (Cymbalta), Milnacipran (Savella)

- **Metabolism and side effects**
  - Varying degrees of hepatic CYP metabolism vs. glucuronidation
  - Common side effects include drowsiness, fatigue, and anorexia
  - Hepatotoxicity has been reported with duloxetine and milnacipran, most notably in patients with preexisting liver disease [18, 19]
- **Dosage recommendations**
  - *Avoid use of duloxetine and milnacipran in any patients with liver disease* [18, 19]
  - Venlafaxine can be used with dose reduction of 50 % in patients with mild-moderate liver disease but should be avoided in those with severe liver disease [20]
  - Desvenlafaxine can be used with starting doses of 50 mg/day and should not be increased >100 mg/day [21]

Anticonvulsants

Gabapentin (Neurontin, Gralise)
- **Metabolism and side effects**
  - Eliminated unchanged via renal excretion [22]
  - *Not metabolized by the liver and minimally bound to proteins, making it a good choice for patients with liver disease*
  - Need to be wary of sedation and dizziness side effects
- **Dosage recommendations**
  - *No adjustment in dosing necessary but suggest starting at low dose and titrating as needed*

Pregabalin (Lyrica)
- **Metabolism and side effects**
  - Similar to gabapentin
  - *No metabolism by liver [23]*
  - *Single case report of likely acute liver failure due to pregabalin [24]*

- **Dosage recommendations**
  - *No adjustment in dosing necessary but suggest starting at low dose and titrating as needed*

Topiramate (Topamax)
- **Metabolism and side effects**
  - *Eliminated largely unchanged via renal excretion*
  - *No metabolism by liver*
  - Plasma levels may be increased in liver disease but mechanism not well understood [25]
- **Dosage recommendations**
  - *No adjustment in dosing necessary but suggest starting at low dose and titrating as needed*

Muscle Relaxants

Metaxalone (Skelaxin)
- **Metabolism and side effects**
  - *Metabolized by hepatic CYP proteins and excreted by renal system as unidentified metabolites [26]*
  - Sedation is major side effect, but this is less than with other muscle relaxants [27]
- **Dosage recommendations**
  - *Should be used with extreme caution in patients with liver disease and should be avoided in patients with advanced cirrhosis*

Tizanidine (Zanaflex)
- **Metabolism and side effects**
  - *Primarily metabolized by CYP1A2*
  - *Can cause liver function test (LFT) abnormalities in patients without liver disease, and patients should have frequent LFTs*
  - *Can cause sedation, hypotension, and psychosis*
- **Dosage recommendations**
  - *Because of significant hepatic metabolism, tizanidine should be avoided or used with extreme caution in patients with established liver disease [28]*

Methocarbamol (Robaxin)
- **Metabolism and side effects**
  - *Unclear metabolism, but likely via dealkylation, hydroxylation, and conjugation in the liver*
  - *Clearance in patients with cirrhosis was decreased by approximately 70 % [29]*
  - Side effects similar to other central nervous system (CNS) depressants, including drowsiness
- **Dosage recommendations**
  - *No specific dosing recommendations available for chronic liver disease so would avoid use in these patients*

Chlorzoxazone (Parafon Forte)

- **Metabolism and side effects**
  - Primarily metabolized hepatically by CYP450 2E1
  - Can cause drowsiness and lightheadedness
  - Case reports of hepatotoxicity, including severe, fulminant liver failure, and death [30]
  - FDA warning for hepatotoxicity exists for this drug [31]
- **Dosing recommendations**
  - *Not well studied in hepatic dysfunction*
  - *No specific dosing recommendations available for chronic liver disease so would avoid use in these patients*

Cyclobenzaprine (Flexeril)

- **Metabolism and side effects**
  - Largely by hepatic biotransformation using CYP proteins and then renal excretion
  - Has similar chemical structure to tricyclic antidepressants and so has similar risks of anticholinergic side effects [27]
  - A study of patients with mild hepatic impairment showed double the pharmacokinetic measurements of AUC and Cmax compared to healthy controls [32].
- **Dosage recommendations**
  - *Be aware of long $t_{1/2}$ and sedating properties*
  - *Start with low dose and only titrate up if absolutely necessary*

Baclofen

- **Metabolism and side effects**
  - Low liver metabolism (15 %), mainly excreted unchanged by the kidneys
  - Can cause drowsiness
  - No cases of encephalopathy or other hepatic side effects noted in a study of patients with alcoholic cirrhosis [33]
- **Dosing recommendations**
  - *No dosage adjustment recommended in patients with liver disease*

Orphenadrine (Norflex)

- **Metabolism and side effects**
  - Extensive hepatic metabolism
  - Derivative of diphenhydramine with unclear mechanism of action
  - Known to have anticholinergic activity, histaminic activity, and NMDA receptor antagonist properties [34]
  - Anticholinergic side effects
- **Dosing recommendations**
  - *Not well studied in hepatic dysfunction*
  - *No specific dosing recommendations available for chronic liver disease so would avoid use in these patients*

Carisoprodol (Soma)

- **Metabolism and side effects**
  - Largely in liver by CYP2C19 into metabolite, meprobamate, which is a schedule III drug and has addictive properties [35]
  - Sedation is major side effect
- **Dosage recommendations**
  - *Because of significant hepatic metabolism, carisoprodol should be used with caution in patients with established liver disease [35]*

Benzodiazepines

- **Metabolism and side effects**
  - Largely hepatic metabolism with drug highly protein bound [36–39]
  - Expect longer $t_{1/2}$ with these medications
  - Major side effects to consider are sedation and hepatic encephalopathy
- **Dosage recommendations**
  - *Slight variation between drugs, but generally recommendations are to use caution in patients with cirrhosis*
  - *Most drugs will likely need dose reduction or widening of dosing interval [40, 41]*

Opioids

Tramadol (Ultram)

- **Metabolism and side effects**
  - Metabolized into several metabolites, including the main active metabolite (O-demethyl-tramadol) via CYP2D6 with excretion by kidneys [42]
  - Unpredictable serum levels of the therapeutic metabolite in setting of hepatic dysfunction, but longer $t_{1/2}$ in patients with cirrhosis
  - Fewer opiate-related side effects because of its multiple modes of analgesic action
  - As with all opiates, may induce or worsen hepatic encephalopathy and cause constipation and ileus
- **Dosing recommendations**
  - *Immediate-release form dose for patients with cirrhosis is 50 mg every 12 h [42]*
  - *Extended-release formulation should not be used in advanced cirrhosis [43]*

Codeine

- **Metabolism and side effects**
  - Metabolized into active metabolite (morphine) by the liver via CYP2D6 [44]
  - Unpredictable serum levels of the therapeutic metabolite in setting of hepatic dysfunction
  - Can cause CNS depression, hypotension, and drowsiness
  - As with all opiates, may induce or worsen hepatic encephalopathy and cause constipation and ileus

- **Dosing recommendations**
  - *Avoid use in hepatic impairment*
  - *If must be administered, use lowest available dose (15 mg) and titrate up slowly while monitoring for side effects* [44]

Morphine
- **Metabolism and side effects**
  - Well absorbed by gastrointestinal tract, but with significant first-pass metabolism by the liver
  - Metabolites are excreted by renal system and reduced glucuronidation of morphine has been shown in cirrhosis [45, 46]
  - However, extrahepatic metabolism of morphine may increase in the setting of cirrhosis, reducing the effect of liver disease on drug metabolism [46]
  - Oral morphine may have much higher bioavailability in patients with cirrhosis compared to controls [47]
  - Intravenous dosing may result in similar drug levels in patients with liver disease compared to healthy controls [48]
  - Toxic metabolites accumulate in the setting of concomitant renal failure with marked increase in side effects like respiratory depression, myoclonus, and seizures
  - As with all opiates, may induce or worsen hepatic encephalopathy and cause constipation and ileus [49]
- **Dosing recommendation**
  - *No specific dosing recommendations available*
  - *Start with lowest recommended dose for healthy patients for given indication and titrate up slowly as tolerated*
  - *Consider widening dosing interval*

Hydrocodone (Component of Vicodin and Norco)
- **Metabolism and side effects**
  - Metabolized to hydromorphone by liver via CYP2D6 [50]
  - Variable metabolism to active compound in setting of liver disease can cause unpredictable serum levels
  - As with all opiates, may induce or worsen hepatic encephalopathy and cause constipation and ileus
- **Dosing recommendations**
  - *Avoid use in hepatic impairment if possible*
  - *Avoid hydrocodone in combination formulations such as Vicodin (hydrocodone combined with acetaminophen), which can have additional hepatic toxicity*

Tapentadol (Nucynta)
- **Metabolism and side effects**
  - Not extensively studied in hepatic impairment
  - Extensive first-pass effect in healthy adults with only 32 % bioavailability and concern for significantly higher bioavailability in severe liver disease [51]
  - Higher maximum plasma concentration in liver disease

  - Thought to have fewer opiate-related side effects because of its multiple modes of analgesic action
  - Can cause CNS depression, hypotension, and drowsiness
  - As with all opiates, may induce or worsen hepatic encephalopathy and cause constipation and ileus (though less frequently than other opiates)
- **Dosing recommendations**
  - *No dosage adjustment necessary in mild liver disease* [52]
  - *In moderate hepatic impairment, use lower doses (starting dose for immediate release form is 50 mg every 8 h, and for extended-release form is 50 mg every 24 h)*
  - *Not studied and not recommended for patients with severe liver disease*

Oxycodone
- **Metabolism and side effects**
  - Metabolized by liver to the primary active metabolite, oxymorphone, via CYP3A4 and excreted renally
  - Serum levels of hepatic metabolites (including the active metabolite) are unpredictable, causing unpredictable analgesic and toxic effects
  - Drug clearance is prolonged in liver disease [53]
  - Can cause increased ventilator depression in patients with end-stage liver disease [54]
  - As with all opiates, may induce or worsen hepatic encephalopathy and cause constipation and ileus
- **Dosing recommendations**
  - *Use reduced initial doses (can decrease dose to one-third or one-half of regular dosing) and lengthen dosage intervals* [55]
  - *Long-acting oxycodone (Oxycontin) use is recommended with caution in end-stage liver disease; avoid if possible*

Oxymorphone (Opana)
- **Metabolism and side effects**
  - Metabolized in liver to oxymorphone-3-glucuronide and other metabolites
  - Bioavailability of oral forms are approximately 10 %, so hepatic function is crucial in limiting active compound; bioavailability in mild hepatic impairment increased 1.6-fold, in moderate impairment 3.7-fold, and in severe hepatic impairment 12.2 fold [56]
  - Can get markedly increased serum levels when given concomitantly with ethanol ingestion [57]
  - Recent possible association between hepatitis C and thrombotic thrombocytopenic purpura in patients who abuse intravenous oxymorphone [58]
  - As with all opiates, may induce or worsen hepatic encephalopathy and cause constipation and ileus

- **Dosing recommendations**
  - *Use with caution in patients with mild hepatic impairment, starting with the lowest available dose (5 mg orally every 4–6 h) and titrating cautiously*
  - *Contraindicated in moderate or severe hepatic impairment*

Hydromorphone (Dilaudid)
- **Metabolism and side effects**
  - Metabolized in liver to hydromorphone-3-glucuronide and other metabolites, which are renally excreted
  - Most metabolites appear nontoxic, making hydromorphone safer to use in liver dysfunction than other opiates
  - Clearance likely prolonged in cirrhosis [59, 60]
  - As with all opiates, may induce or worsen hepatic encephalopathy and cause constipation and ileus
- **Dosing recommendations**
  - *A preferred opiate in cirrhosis* [13]
  - *Reduce dose in liver disease*
  - *Use prolonged dosage intervals in cirrhosis*
  - *Appears to be a safe choice in hepatorenal syndrome due to safety in both hepatic and renal dysfunction*

Methadone
- **Metabolism and side effects**
  - Heavily protein bound (80 % of drug) while circulating, which raised concern that serum levels may be increased in low albumin states such as cirrhosis [50]
  - However, most of the drug is bound to alpha-1-acid glycoprotein, and hypoalbuminemia has not been shown to affect drug distribution [61]
  - High bioavailability due to very low first-pass metabolism and significant absorption from gastrointestinal tract
  - Half-life is increased, but drug clearance does not appear to be significantly altered in severe liver disease [62]
  - Can prolong QT interval and caution advised in patients at risk for QT prolongation, including diuretic use, risk of hypokalemia, or hypomagnesaemia
  - As with all opiates, may induce or worsen hepatic encephalopathy and cause constipation and ileus
- **Dosing recommendations**
  - *No dose adjustment for mild or moderate liver disease* [63]
  - *Avoid if possible in severe liver disease*

Fentanyl (Duragesic)
- **Metabolism and side effects**
  - Metabolized by liver into inactive metabolites via CYP3A4, which are renally excreted
  - Heavily protein bound (approximately 85 %) while circulating, which raised concern that serum levels may be increased in low albumin states such as cirrhosis

  - Less likely to cause hemodynamic changes (hypotension) than other opiates [64]
  - Continuous infusion (intravenous or by a transdermal patch) associated with sedation and respiratory depression
  - As with all opiates, may induce or worsen hepatic encephalopathy and cause constipation and ileus
- **Dosing recommendations**
  - Intravenous bolus form is a preferred short-acting opiate in cirrhosis with no specific dose changes recommended
  - Fentanyl patch is considered less safe due to continuous drug absorption
    - Mild or moderate liver disease: Reduce dose by 50 %
    - Severe liver disease: Use with caution but can use starting dose of 12.5 μg every 72 h [13]
    - *Recommend careful monitoring for accumulation/ toxicity, and slow titration*
  - *Appears to be a safe choice in hepatorenal syndrome due to safety in both hepatic and renal dysfunction* [65]

Buprenorphine (Butrans patch, Suboxone)
- **Metabolism and side effects**
  - Metabolized by the liver (via CYP3A4) into inactive and partially active metabolites, but has not been well studied in liver disease
  - Acute hepatitis has been reported with buprenorphine [66]
  - Has risk of QT prolongation as well as CNS depression, hypotension, drowsiness
  - As with all opiates, may induce or worsen hepatic encephalopathy and cause constipation and ileus (though less frequently than other opiates)
- **Dosing recommendations**
  - *Patients with mild or moderate hepatic impairment should use only the lowest dose (5 μg/h)* [67]
  - *Not studied and not recommended for patients with severe liver disease*

Meperidine (Demerol)
- **Metabolism and side effects**
  - Metabolized in liver to active normeperidine, which has serious CNS toxicity, especially in the setting of concomitant renal dysfunction
  - Heavily protein bound (approximately 70 %) with marked increase in bioavailability in cirrhosis [50, 68]
  - Increased half-life in setting of end-stage liver disease, up to two times that of patients with normal liver function [69]

- Can cause neuromuscular irritability, CNS depression, respiratory depression, psychosis, hyperactivity, and seizures
- Has multiple drug interactions
- **Dosing recommendations**
  - *Avoid use in patients with liver disease* [70]

Summary and Recommendations

- In patients without cirrhosis, pain medication doses usually do not need to be altered; however, in patients with cirrhosis, many medications need lower doses or are contraindicated.
- Patients with cirrhosis should not take any new medications without first discussing with the provider of their liver care.
- Acetaminophen can be used safely at doses *up to 2 g/day*, but providers should caution patients that many over the counter medications contain acetaminophen as well.
- *NSAIDs should be avoided in cirrhotic patients.*
- Neuropathic pain medications and muscle relaxants vary in their use in liver patients. Check the body of this chapter and associated tables for further recommendations about specific drugs.
- **If opioid pain medications are to be used, hydromorphone and fentanyl are the best choices in patients with liver disease.**

References

1. Lim YS, Kim WR. The global impact of hepatic fibrosis and end-stage liver disease. Clin Liver Dis. 2008;12(4):733–46, vii.
2. Elbekai R, Korashy H, El-Kadi A. The effect of liver cirrhosis on the regulation and expression of drug metabolizing enzymes. Curr Drug Metab. 2004;5(2):157–67.
3. Verbeeck RK. Pharmacokinetics and dosage adjustment in patients with hepatic dysfunction. Eur J Clin Pharmacol. 2008;64(12):1147–61.
4. Parlesak A, Schafer C, Schutz T, Bode JC, Bode C. Increased intestinal permeability to macromolecules and endotoxemia in patients with chronic alcohol abuse in different stages of alcohol-induced liver disease. J Hepatol. 2000;32:742–7.
5. Keshavarzian A, Holmes EW, Patel M, Iber F, Fields JZ, Pethkar S. Leaky gut in alcoholic cirrhosis: a possible mechanism for alcohol-induced liver damage. Am J Gastroenterol. 1999;94:200–7.
6. Isobe H, Sakai H, Satoh M, Sakamoto S, Nawata H. Delayed gastric emptying in patients with liver cirrhosis. Dig Dis Sci. 1994;39:983–7.
7. Ishizu H, Shiomi S, Kawamura E, Iwata Y, Nishiguchi S, Kawabe J, Ochi H. Gastric emptying in patients with chronic liver diseases. Ann Nucl Med. 2002;16:177–82.
8. Child CG, Turcotte JG. Surgery and portal hypertension. In: Child CG, editor. The liver and portal hypertension. Philadelphia: Saunders; 1964. p. 50–64.
9. Pugh RN, Murray-Lyon IM, Dawson JL, et al. Transection of the oesophagus for bleeding oesophageal varices. Br J Surg. 1973;60(8):646–9.
10. Benson GD. Acetaminophen in chronic liver disease. Clin Pharmacol Ther. 1983;33:95–101.
11. Zimmerman HJ, Maddrey WC. Acetaminophen (paracetamol) hepatotoxicity with regular intake of alcohol: analysis of instances of therapeutic misadventure. Hepatology. 1995;22:767.
12. Kuffner EK, Dart RC, Bogdan GM, Hill RE, Casper E, Darton L. Effect of maximal daily doses of acetaminophen on the liver of alcoholic patients: a randomized, double-blinded, placebo-controlled trial. Arch Intern Med. 2001;161:2247.
13. Chandok N, Watt KDS. Pain management in the cirrhotic patient: the clinical challenge. Mayo Clin Proc. 2010;85(5):451–8.
14. Rossi S, Assis DN, Awsare M, Brunner M, Skole K, Rai J, Andrel J, Herrine SK, Reddy RK, Navarro VJ. Use of over-the-counter analgesics in patients with chronic liver disease: physicians' recommendations. Drug Saf. 2008;31(3):261–70.
15. Laffi G, La Villa G, Pinzani M, Marra F, Gentilini P. Arachidonic acid derivatives and renal function in liver cirrhosis. Semin Nephrol. 1997;17(6):530–48.
16. Castro-Fernandez M, Sanchez-Munoz D, Galan-Jurado MV, Larraona JL, Suarez E, Lamas E, Rodriguez-Hornillo MC, Pabon M. Influence of nonsteroidal antiinflammatory drugs in gastrointestinal bleeding due to gastroduodenal ulcers or erosions in patients with liver cirrhosis. Gastroenterol Hepatol. 2006;29(1):11–4.
17. Thanacoody HK, Thomas SH. Tricyclic antidepressant poisoning: cardiovascular toxicity. Toxicol Rev. 2005;24(3):205–14.
18. Cymbalta [package insert]. Indianapolis: Eli Lilly and Company; 2012.
19. Savella [package insert]. St. Louis: Forest Pharmaceuticals; 2009.
20. Effexor [package insert]. Philadelphia: Wyeth Pharmaceuticals; 2004.
21. Pristiq [package insert]. Philadelphia: Wyeth Pharmaceuticals; 2012.
22. Neurontin [package insert]. New York: Parke-Davis Division of Pfizer; 2012.
23. yrica [package insert]. New York: Parke-Davis Division of Pfizer; 2012.
24. Einarsdottir S, Bjornsson E. Pregabalin as a probable cause of acute liver injury. Eur J Gastroenterol Hepatol. 2008;20(10):1049.
25. Topamax [package insert]. Titusville: Janssen Pharmaceuticals; 2009.
26. Skelaxin [package insert]. Bristol: King Pharmaceutical Inc.; 2007.
27. See S, Ginzburg R. Skeletal muscle relaxants. Pharmacology. 2008;28(2):207–13.
28. Zanaflex [package insert]. Hawthorne: Acorda Therapeutics Inc.; 2010.
29. Robaxin [package insert]. Smyrna: Schwarz Pharma, LLC; 2009.
30. Jackson J, Anania FA. Chlorzoxazone as a cause of acute liver failure requiring liver transplantation. Dig Dis Sci. 2007;52(12):3389–91.
31. Nightingale SL. Chlorzoxazone warning on hepatotoxicity is strengthened. JAMA. 1995;274:1903.
32. Flexeril [package insert]. Fort Washington: McNeil Consumer Healthcare, Division of McNeil-PPC, Inc.; 2010.
33. Addolorato G, Leggio L, Ferrulli A, Cardone S, Vonghia L, Mirijello A, Abenavoli L, D'Angelo C, Caputo F, Zambon A, Haber PS, Gasbarrini G. Effectiveness and safety of baclofen for maintenance of alcohol abstinence in alcohol-dependent patients with liver cirrhosis: randomised, double-blind controlled study. Lancet. 2007;370(9603):1915–22.
34. Desaphy JF, Dipalma A, De Bellis M, Costanza T, Gaudioso C, Delmas P, George Jr AL, Camerino DC. Involvement of voltage-gated sodium channel blockade in the analgesic effects of orphenadrine. Pain. 2009;142(3):225–35.

35. Soma [package insert]. Somerset: Meda Pharmaceuticals, Inc.; 2011.

36. Xanax [package insert]. New York: Pfizer, Inc.; 2011.

37. Midazolam [package insert]. Minneapolis: Paddock Laboratories, Inc.; 2008.

38. Valium [package insert]. Nutley: Roche Pharmaceuticals; 2008.

39. Restoril [package insert]. St. Louis: Mallinckrodt Inc.; 2006.

40. Trouvin JH, Farinotti R, Haberer JP, Servin F, Chauvin M, Duvaldestin P. Pharmacokinetics of midazolam in anaesthetized cirrhotic patients. Br J Anaesth. 1988;60(7):762–7.

41. Macgilchrist AJ, Birnie GG, Cook A, Scobie G, Murray T, Watkinson G, Brodie MJ. Pharmacokinetics and pharmacodynamics of intravenous midazolam in patients with severe alcoholic cirrhosis. Gut. 1986;27:190–5.

42. Ultram [package insert]. Raritan: Ortho-McNeil Pharmaceutical, Inc.; 2003.

43. Durotram XR [package insert]. Thornleigh: iNova Pharmaceuticals; 2008.

44. Codeine [package insert]. Philadelphia: Lannett Company, Inc.; 2010.

45. Tegeder I, Lotsch J, Geisslinger G. Pharmacokinetics of opioids in liver disease. Clin Pharmacokinet. 1999;37:17–40.

46. Crotty B, Watson KJ, Desmond PV, Mashford ML, Wood LJ, Colman J, Dudley FJ. Hepatic extraction of morphine is impaired in cirrhosis. Eur J Clin Pharmacol. 1989;36:501–6.

47. Hasselstrom J, Eriksson S, Persson A, Rane A, Svensson JO, Säwe J. The metabolism and bioavailability of morphine in patients with severe liver cirrhosis. Br J Clin Pharmacol. 1990;29(3):289–97.

48. Patwardhan RV, Johnson RF, Hoyumpa Jr A, Sheehan JJ, Desmond PV, Wilkinson GR, Branch RA, Schenker S. Normal metabolism of morphine in cirrhosis. Gastroenterology. 1981;81(6):1006–11.

49. Laidlaw J, Read AE, Sherlock S. Morphine tolerance in hepatic cirrhosis. Gastroenterology. 1961;40:389–96.

50. Smith HS. Opioid metabolism. Mayo Clin Proc. 2009;84(7):613–24.

51. Hartrick CT. Tapentadol immediate-release for acute pain. Expert Rev Neurother. 2010;10(6):861–9.

52. Nucynta [package insert]. Raritan: Ortho-McNeil-Janssen Pharmaceuticals; 2010.

53. Kaiko RF. Pharmacokinetics and pharmacodynamics of controlled-release opioids. Acta Anaesthesiol Scand. 1997;41(1 Pt 2):166–74.

54. Tallgren M, Olkkola KT, Seppala T, Höckerstedt K, Lindgren L. Pharmacokinetics and ventilatory effects of oxycodone before and after liver transplantation. Clin Pharmacol Ther. 1997;61(6):655–61.

55. Oxycodone [package insert]. St. Louis: Tyco Healthcare; 2005.

56. Opana ER [package insert]. Chadds Ford: Endo Pharmaceuticals; 2011.

57. Opana (oxymorphone) [package insert]. Chadds Ford: Endo Pharmaceuticals; 2011.

58. Centers for Disease Control and Prevention. MMWR weekly: thrombotic thrombocytopenic purpura (TTP)—like illness associated with Opana ER intravenous abuse. 2013. http://www.cdc.gov/mmwr/preview/mmwrhtml/mm6201a1.htm

59. Durnin C, Hind ID, Ghani SP, Yates DB, Molz KH. Pharmacokinetics of oral immediate-release hydromorphone (Dilaudid IR) in subjects with moderate hepatic impairment. Proc West Pharmacol Soc. 2001;44:83–4.

60. Dilaudid [package insert]. North Chicago: Abbott Laboratories; 2007.

61. Eap CB, Buclin T, Baumann P. Interindividual variability of the clinical pharmacokinetics of methadone: implications for the treatment of opioid dependence. Clin Pharmacokinet. 2002;41(14):1153–93.

62. Novick DM, Kreek MJ, Fanizza AM, Yancovitz SR, Gelb AM, Stenger RJ. Methadone disposition in patients with chronic liver disease. Clin Pharmacol Ther. 1981;30(3):353–62.

63. Dolophine (methadone) [package insert]. Columbus: Roxane Laboratories, Inc., 2006.

64. Jacobi J, Fraser GL, Coursin DB, Riker RR, Fontaine D, Wittbrodt ET, Chalfin DB, Masica MF, Bjerke HS, Coplin WM, Crippen DW, Fuchs BD, Kelleher RM, Marik PE, Nasraway Jr SA, Murray MJ, Peruzzi WT, Lumb PD. Clinical practice guidelines for the sustained use of sedatives and analgesics in the critically ill adult. Crit Care Med. 2002;30(1):119–41.

65. Niscola P, Scaramucci L, Vischini G, Giovannini M, Ferrannini M, Massa P, Tatangelo P, Galletti M, Palumbo R. The use of major analgesics in patients with renal dysfunction. Curr Drug Targets. 2010;11(6):752–8.

66. Hervé S, Riachi G, Noblet C, Guillement N, Tanasescu S, Goria O, Thuillez C, Tranvouez JL, Ducrotte P, Lerebours E. Acute hepatitis due to buprenorphine administration. Eur J Gastroenterol Hepatol. 2004;16:1033–7.

67. Butrans patch [package insert]. Stamford: Purdue Pharma L.P.; 2010.

68. Pond SM, Tong T, Benowitz NL, Jacob P, Rigod J. Presystemic metabolism of meperidine to normeperidine in normal and cirrhotic subjects. Clin Pharmacol Ther. 1981;30(2):183–8.

69. Klotz U, McHorse TS, Wilkinson GR, Schenker S. The effect of cirrhosis on the disposition and elimination of meperidine in man. Clin Pharmacol Ther. 1974;16(4):667–75.

70. Goodman F. Criteria for use of meperidine. Hines (IL): VHA Pharmacy Benefits Management Strategic Healthcare Group and the Medical Advisory Panel (US). 2003. www.vapbm.org

Pain Management During Pregnancy and Breast-Feeding

32

Yolanda Scott

Abbreviations

CNS	Central nervous system
FDA	Food and Drug Administration
GABA	Gamma-aminobutyric acid
LBP	Low back pain
MOA	Mechanism of action
NERI	Norepinephrine reuptake inhibitor
NMDA	N-methyl-D-aspartate
SNRIs	Serotonin-norepinephrine reuptake inhibitors
TCA	Tricyclic antidepressant
TCAs	Tricyclic antidepressants
TENS	Transcutaneous electrical nerve stimulation
TERIS	Teratogen Information System

Introduction

Pregnancy leads to an increased incidence of low back pain (LBP) and other painful conditions [1, 2–4]. Unfortunately, practitioners are limited in their treatment options for these patients. This chapter will discuss safe treatment options that can be used during pregnancy.

Painful Conditions in Pregnancy

In all painful conditions in pregnant patients, an obstetrician should be consulted prior to ensure no surgical or threatening pathology is present. If any severe pain, bleeding, fever, or other ominous signs are noted, patient should be sent to

Y. Scott, M.D. (✉)
Department of Rehabilitation Medicine, Icahn School of Medicine at Mount Sinai, New York, NY, USA

emergency room immediately. After urgent conditions are ruled out, other nonemergent etiologies can be considered.

Back pain: Approximately 50 % pregnant women [5]
- Hormonal changes in pregnancy lead to increased mobility at joints and laxity at ligaments
- *Low back pain*:
  - Increased lordosis contributes pain at this region
- *Upper back pain*:
  - Myofascial/ligamentous laxity
- *Sacroiliac joint pain*
  - Usually due to ligamentous laxity
  - *Symptoms*: Lower back and buttock pain which may radiate to the posterior thigh (less often below the knee, not to foot/ankle), may worsen with weight bearing
- *Sciatica/radiculopathy*
  - *Symptoms*: Lower back and buttock pain which may radiate to the posterior thigh foot/ankle
- *Back pain treatment*: Instruct on proper lifting, body mechanics, pain avoidance activities, physical therapy, aqua therapy, heat/ice, TENs, approved topical medications
  In refractory cases consider acetaminophen, if severe opioids can be considered if cleared with obstetrician

Headache [5]
- Estrogen levels increase during pregnancy which usually decreases headache occurrence
- All headaches in pregnancy should be carefully evaluated/cleared by a neurologist and obstetrician prior to symptomatic treatment from a pain physician
- In severe/refractory cases consider MRI if not done previously
- If no neurological symptoms and threatening conditions (preeclampsia, brain hemorrhage, pseudo-tumor cerebri, etc.) have been ruled out symptomatic treatment can be initiated if needed. Minimizing the risk to the fetus is always considered priority.

K.A. Sackheim, *Pain Management and Palliative Care: A Comprehensive Guide*,
DOI 10.1007/978-1-4939-2462-2_32, © Springer Science+Business Media New York 2015

- *Treatment*: Biofeedback, relaxation techniques, trigger food avoidance, appropriate quantities of caffeine, acetaminophen
  If refractory consider prophylactic treatment with propranolol

Abdominal wall and ligamentous pain [5]

Once threatening etiologies have been ruled out consider the following:

- Round ligament pain
  - Ligament is stretched due to growth of the uterus
  - *Treatment*: Bed rest and local heat
    If refractory, consider approved oral analgesics
- Rectus abdominus hematoma (rare)
  - Muscles/sheath stretch as uterus expands
  - When severe can dehisce
  - *Treatment*: Bed rest, local heat
    If refractory consider approved oral analgesics

Pelvic pain:

- *Symphysiolysis*:
  - Pubic symphysis: Provides 40 % of pelvic stability, during pregnancy several pathophysiological changes occur, to allow laxity of the pelvic region [6]
  - This includes hormonal changes, as well as structural widening of the symphysis, which occurs in the 10th to 12th week [6, 7].
  - If there is physiological separation of the pelvis, than it is termed Pubic Diastasis which can separate up to 1 cm. The disjointing can occur with forceful descent of the fetal head against the pelvic ring, which can result in a spontaneous rupture or separation of the pubic symphysis.
  - *Symptoms*: Pain at suprapubic area, pain can radiate to the medial thighs and increase with movement of the lower extremities, difficulty walking up stairs, carrying heavy objects [8, 9]. Possible audible crack during delivery.
  - *Physical exam*: Tenderness at suprapubic area, palpable gap where the pubic rami intersect, duck-like gait.
  - *Treatment*: Conservative treatment includes 24–48 h of bed rest postpartum, ice, pelvic belt, ambulating with a walker, and/or acetaminophen. A last resort would be a pelvic sling or surgery, which involves an open reduction and internal fixation of the pubic symphysis [8]

Hip pain

- *Osteonecrosis*
  - Commonly at the Femoral Head [10, 11]
  - More frequently during the third trimester

  - As the patient approaches the third trimester of pregnancy, cortisol levels increase almost 3× that of a nonpregnant female [8].
  - *Pathophysiology*: Unknown cause but one theory associates it with an increase in adrenocortical activity compounded by an increase stress from weight gain in addition to an increase in estrogen and progesterone [9, 10].
  - *Symptoms*: Deep pain at the groin that may radiate to the knee and painful range of motion at the hip.
  - *Treatment*: Conservative management includes symptomatic management during pregnancy—limitation of vigorous physical activity, reduction in weight bearing, and physical therapy
    A small number of patients have undergone Total Hip Arthroplasties. One study performed joint aspiration with weight-bearing precautions, which resulted in complete recovery [11].
    Pourbagher et al. was able to achieve 100 % accuracy using the ultrasound-guided injections to remedy osteoarthritis [12].
- *Transient osteoporosis of the hip*
  - Rare, usually during the third trimester, unknown etiology
  - *Symptoms*: Pain in the groin [8]. Pain may be acute or gradual and is mainly appreciated with weight-bearing activities.
  - *Physical examination*: Painful and limited range of motion at the hip
  - *Treatment*: Symptomatic management during pregnancy—limit/avoid weight bearing to avoid fracture. Symptoms are self limiting and can spontaneously resolve between 6 and 8 months [6]. Patients are encouraged to remain non-weight bearing with the use of a walker or crutches, and mild analgesics can be prescribed. If weight-bearing activities are not avoided, then a fracture of the femoral neck may occur, and surgery will be the only treatment option.
- *Meralgia Paresthetica*
  - Sensory mononeuropathy that involves the lateral femoral cutaneous nerve [8, 9]
    - Occurs in pregnancy secondary to entrapment of the nerve as it passes around the anterior superior iliac spine or as it passes through the inguinal ligament (Fig. 32.1) [8, 13, 14].
  - Woman may present with numbness or tingling on the anterior lateral region of the thigh.
  - *Treatment*: Conservative management includes minimizing periods of standing, loose fitting clothing, and the removal of any factor that may increase tension around the anterior superior iliac spine with hip extension, including belts. Most importantly, reassurance to

Fig. 32.1 Pathway of the lateral femoral cutaneous nerve and the area most affected with Meralgia Paresthetica. © Mayo Clinic [14]

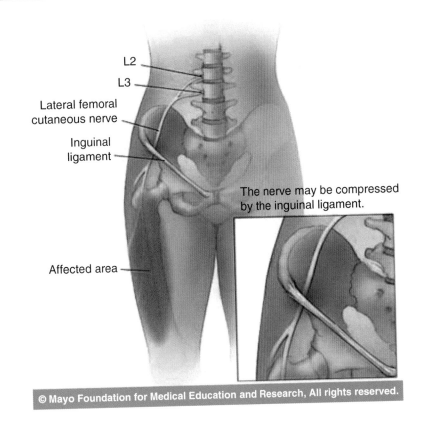

L2

L3

Lateral femoral cutaneous nerve

Inguinal ligament

The nerve may be compressed by the inguinal ligament.

Affected area

Table 32.1 Chart of the FDA pregnancy categories modified from the FDA website [14]

Category A	Category B	Category C	Category D	Category X
Adequate and well-controlled studies have failed to demonstrate a risk to the fetus in the first trimester of pregnancy (and there is no evidence of risk in later trimesters)	Animal reproduction studies have failed to demonstrate a risk to the fetus and there are no adequate and well-controlled studies in pregnant women	Animal reproduction studies have shown an adverse effect on the fetus and there are no adequate and well-controlled studies in humans, but potential benefits may warrant use of the drug in pregnant women despite potential risks	There is positive evidence of human fetal risk based on adverse reaction data from investigational or marketing experience or studies in humans, but potential benefits may warrant use of the drug in pregnant women despite potential risks	Studies in animals or humans have demonstrated fetal abnormalities and/or there is positive evidence of human fetal risk based on adverse reaction data from investigational or marketing experience, and the risks involved in use of the drug in pregnant women clearly outweigh potential benefits

the expecting mother that the condition is self-limiting and not harmful to the infant.

Medications

Medications are divided into categories for use during pregnancy, which denote increased or decreased safety (see Table 32.1). Below we discuss various analgesic medications and possible options for refractory pain during pregnancy. Medications during pregnancy should always be avoided if possible to ensure safety of the fetus. Medication avoidance is most critical during early development.

Factors that decrease medication transfer across placenta and excretion into breast milk: [5]
- High molecular weight (larger molecules)
- Ionized state (polar molecules)
- Increased protein binding
- Lipophobic/hydrophilic
- Increased maternal metabolism
- Early gestation [7, 8] given the fetal hepatic system is not developed

Breast-Feeding [5]
- Neonatal dose during breast-feeding is 1–2 % of the maternal dose.

- This can still be dangerous, as infants have decreased metabolism and potential for allergic reaction.
- If medically necessary, minimize drug transfer by taking medications after breast-feeding or during the longest time period between feedings. Pumping and dumping may be required in certain circumstances.
- Avoid long-acting medications in patients who are breast-feeding

Pain Medication Classifications

Acetaminophen (Tylenol)

- **Mechanism**
  - Not completely understood, it is believed to work by inhibiting the synthesis of prostaglandin in the central nervous system (CNS)
- **Metabolism**
  - Hepatically metabolized
  - *Risk during pregnancy*:
    - Category B
  - *Risk during breast-feeding*
    - Acetaminophen is excreted in breast milk, use with caution [15–17]

Nonsteroidal anti-inflammatory drugs (NSAIDs)

- **Mechanism**
  - Inhibit the synthesis of prostaglandins
- **Metabolism**
  - Hepatically metabolized via CYP450
  - *Risk during pregnancy*:
    - Category B until the third trimester and then it becomes a class D [16]
    - All NSAIDs used near term may cause premature closure of the ductus arteriosus and inhibit labor. More common complications include Oligohydramnios with prolonged use.
  - *Risk during breast-feeding*:
    - Most NSAIDs are excreted in breatmilk so it is not advised due to potential cardiovascular complications to the infant [16].

Topical medications

Lidoderm
- **Mechanism**
  - Topical application produces an analgesic effect by stabilizing neuronal membranes thereby inhibiting ionic impulses.

- **Metabolism**
  - Extensively metabolized through the liver (CYP450), approximately 3 % systemically absorbed
  - *Risk during pregnancy*
    - Category B
    - No adequate studies of the lidocaine patch performed on human subjects
    - Should only be used during pregnancy if clearly indicated
  - *Risk during breast-feeding*
    - Lidocaine is excreted in human milk; caution should be used in breast-feeding women [16]

Tricyclic antidepressants (TCAs)

Amitriptyline
- **Mechanism**
  - By increasing both serotonin and norepinephrine. Onset of therapeutic action works between 2 and 4 weeks
- **Metabolism**
  - Hepatic metabolism via CYP 1A2 and CYP 2D6 isoenzymes
- **Dosing recommendation**
  - Initial dose of 25 mg/day at bedtime, and increase by 25 mg q3–7 days
  - Dosage: 50–100 mg/day
  - *Risk during pregnancy*
    - Category C
    - No link between TCA use and congenital abnormalities
    - Crosses the placenta
  - *Risk during breast-feeding*
    - Drug can be found in breast milk
    - Recommend bottle-feeding or discontinuing the drug [16]

Nortriptyline
- **Mechanism**
  - Increasing norepinephrine and blocks the neurotransmitter's reuptake pump. At high doses it can also increase the level of serotonin.
- **Metabolism**
  - Hepatically metabolized via the CYP450
  - Onset of therapeutic action is between 2 and 4 weeks
- **Dosing Recommendation**
  - Initial dose of 10–25 mg/day at bedtime and increase by 25 mg q3–7 days with a maximum dose of 300 mg/day.
  - Dosage: 75–150 mg/day daily for depression. 50–150 mg/day for chronic pain

– *Risk during pregnancy*:
  - Risk Category D
  - Crosses the Placenta
  - Should only be used if benefits outweigh the risk
– *Risk during breast-feeding*:
  - Drug found in mother's milk
  - Either discontinue the medication or bottle-feed [16]

Desipramine

- **Mechanism**
  – Norepinephrine reuptake inhibitor. Onset of therapeutic action is 2–4 weeks.
- **Metabolism**
  – Hepatically metabolized via the CYP450
- **Dosing Recommendation**
  – Initial dose of 25 mg/day at bedtime, increase by 25 mg q3–7 days
  – Dosage: 100–200 mg/day for depression, 50–150 mg/day for chronic pain
  – *Risk during pregnancy*:
    - Risk Category C
    - Crosses the Placenta
  – *Risk during breast-feeding*:
    - Drug found in mother's milk
    - Either discontinue the medication or bottle-feed [16].

Serotonin-norepinephrine reuptake inhibitors (SNRIs)

Cymbalta

- **Mechanism**
  – Inhibition of the reuptake of serotonin and norepinephrine
- **Metabolism**
  – Hepatic metabolism via CYP 1A2 and CYP 2D6 isoenzymes [16]
- **Dosing recommendation**
  – Start with 30 mg/day and increase to 60 mg daily.
  – Dosage: 60 mg daily
  – *Risk during pregnancy*
    - Category C
    - Limited number of studies available but Duloxetine crosses the placenta [18]
    - One study published in the Arch Womans Ment Health in 2011 showed no malformation or withdrawal symptoms from in utero exposure to Duloxetine, more studies are needed to confirm its safety [19].
  – *Risk during breast-feeding*
    - Drug found in mother's milk with exposure of 0.14–0.25 % of the maternal dose [20]

- Briggs et al. published a case report that showed Duloxetine can be excreted in breast milk, but the concentration is very low [17].
- A Study showed that an infant exclusively breast-fed by a mother on a dose of 60 mg/day did not show signs of toxicity after 32 days [18].

Milnacipran

- **Mechanism**
  – It *blocks serotonin reuptake and increases neurotransmitters*
  – *Weak* NMDA-receptor antagonist
- **Metabolism**
  – Hepatically metabolized via CYP450
- **Dosing Recommendation**
  – Start at 12.5 mg daily and increase by 25 mg/day on Day 2, 50 mg in two divided doses on day 4, 100 mg in two divided doses on day 7 with a max dose of 200 mg/day
  – Dosage: 30–200 mg/day twice a day
  – *Risk during pregnancy*
    - Category C
    - Not recommended for use during pregnancy, especially during the first trimester
  – *Risk during breast-feeding*
    - Unknown if the medication is transmitted into breast milk
    - Should only be used if benefits outweigh the risk [16]

Anticonvulsants

Gabapentin (Neurontin)

- **Mechanism**
  – It is a structural analog of GABA, which binds to a subunit of a calcium-sensitive channel inhibiting calcium influx by changing the channels function. This results in a decrease in the release of neurotransmitters.
- **Metabolism**
  – Renal excreted without being metabolized [16, 21]
- **Dosing Recommendation**
  – Start with 300 mg/day for 1 day and increase by 300 mg every 1–3 days as tolerated.
  – Dosage: For Neuropathic Pain: 300–1800 mg/day up to 3600 mg/day
  – *Risk during pregnancy*
    - Category C
    - There is currently no data available on gabapentin during pregnancy [16, 21]
    - Patients should consider terminating the medication before and during pregnancy.
  – *Risk during breast-feeding*

■ Some drug is found in the mother's breast milk; recommended to discontinue taking the medication or bottle-feed

Pregabalin (Lyrica)
- **Mechanism**
  - Structural analog of GABA, which binds to a subunit of a calcium-sensitive channel inhibiting calcium influx by changing the channels function. This results in a decrease in the release of neurotransmitters.
- **Metabolism**
  - Renal excretion without being metabolized
- **Dosing recommendation**
  - For Fibromyalgia: 30–450 mg/day
  - Neuropathic pain: 100–600 mg/day
  - Risk during pregnancy
    - Category C
    - There are no adequate studies on human subjects
  - Risk during breast-feeding
    - Not known if it is excreted in breast milk
    - Recommended to discontinue taking the medication or bottle-feed
    - If the mother continues to take the medication while breast-feeding, the infant should be monitored for adverse effects [16].

Topiramate (Topamax)
- **Mechanism**
  - GABA (A) receptor augmentation and sodium channel blocker
- **Metabolism**
  - Renally excreted
  - Risk during pregnancy
    - Category C
  - Risk during breast-feeding
    - Highly recommended to discontinue medication prior to breast-feeding or bottle-feed [16]

Carbamazepine
- **Mechanism**
  - It interacts with sodium channels inhibiting the release of glutamate.
- **Metabolism**
  - Hepatically metabolized by Cytochrome P450 CYP3A4 [16, 21]
- **Dosing recommendation**
  - Trigeminal Neuralgia: 100 mg twice a day, increase up to 200 mg/week with a max daily dose of 1,200 mg
  - Risk during pregnancy
    - Category D
    - Studies on mice have shown a significant number of fetuses with congenital defects of the CNS or urogenital system [21]

- Use during pregnancy can cause neural tube defect
  - Risk during breast-feeding
    - The drug has been found in breast milk
    - Recommended to discontinue taking the medication or bottle-feed
    - If the mother continues to take the medication while breast-feeding, the infant should be monitored for adverse effects [17].

Opioids

Tramadol
- **Mechanism**
  - Due to low- and high-affinity binding to the Mu receptor as well as inhibition of the reuptake of serotonin and norepinephrine.
- **Metabolism**
  - Hepatically metabolized via Cytochrome P450 isozymes
  - Maximum daily dose of 400 mg
  - Risk during pregnancy
    - Category C
    - No adequate studies in pregnant woman
  - Risk during breast-feeding
    - Safety has not been studied in nursing mothers [16]

Codeine
- **Mechanism**
  - Codeine acts very similar to Morphine, but its specific MOA is not well defined but it is thought to be selective for the Mu receptor.
- **Metabolism**
  - Hepatically metabolized
  - Risk during pregnancy
    - Category C
    - Only use in pregnancy if the benefits outweigh the risk.
  - Risk during breast-feeding
    - It is excreted in breast milk
    - Maternal use of codeine can lead to severe adverse reactions such as death [16].

Morphine
- **Mechanism**
  - It's a Mu Receptor agonist on the opioid receptor in the CNS and peripheral nervous system.
- **Metabolism**
  - Metabolized in the liver
  - Risk during pregnancy
    - Category C
    - There are no well-controlled studies on chronic in utero exposure with human subjects.

- If there is fetal exposure, they may experience symptoms of withdrawal but this is dependent on the mother's last dose and rate of elimination from the fetus.
- *Risk during breast-feeding*
  - Low amounts of Morphine Sulfate have been detected in breast milk [16]

Hydrocodone
- **Mechanism**
  - Weak Mu receptor within the CNS
- **Metabolism**
  - Hepatically metabolized through the Cytochrome 450 CYP2D6
  - *Risk during pregnancy*
    - Category C
    - There are no adequate studies in pregnant woman.
    - The drug should only be used if the benefits outweigh the risk to the fetus.
  - *Risk during breast-feeding*
    - Unknown if the drug can be excreted in breast milk
    - Mothers should discontinue the drug or bottle-feed [16].

Tapentadol
- **Mechanism**
  - Centrally acting opioid that binds to the Mu receptor.
- **Metabolism**
  - Hepatically metabolized
  - *Risk during pregnancy*
    - Category C
    - No adequate studies in pregnant women
  - *Risk during breast-feeding*
    - Unknown if the drug can be excreted in breast milk
    - Not recommended for use in nursing women [16]

Oxycodone
- **Mechanism**
  - Mu Receptor agonist on the opioid receptor in the CNS and peripheral nervous system
- **Metabolism**
  - Hepatically metabolized
  - *Risk during pregnancy*
    - Category B
    - Chronic use of the medication during pregnancy can cause adverse reaction in the newborn including respiratory depression
  - *Risk during breast-feeding*
    - Low concentrations of oxycodone have been detected in breast milk
    - Nursing should not occur if the mother is taking an opioid.
    - Infants can experience withdrawal symptoms if exposed to the drug through breast milk [16].

Oxymorphone (Opana)
- **Mechanism**
  - Mu agonist that can hyperpolarize channels reducing neuronal excitability
- **Metabolism**
  - Hepatically metabolized
  - *Risk during pregnancy*
    - Category C
    - No adequate studies in pregnant women
    - Opioids do cross the placenta and may cause respiratory depression on the neonate [22]
  - *Risk during breast-feeding*
    - Unknown if it can be found in breast milk, but caution should be exercised [22]
    - Not recommended for use in nursing women [16].

Hydromorphone
- **Mechanism**
  - Mu agonist that can cause hyperpolarizable channels reducing neuronal excitability
- **Metabolism**
  - Hepatically metabolized
  - *Risk during pregnancy*
    - Category C
    - No adequate studies in pregnant women
  - *Risk during breast-feeding*
    - Found in breast milk
    - Not recommended for use in nursing women [16]

Methadone
- **Mechanism**
  - Mu agonist and NMDA-receptor antagonist
- **Metabolism**
  - Hepatically metabolized by Cytochrome P450 enzymes
  - *Risk during pregnancy*
    - Category C
    - No adequate studies in pregnant women but review of the Teratogen Information System (TERIS) stated that a well-monitored and controlled regimen was unlikely to post a substantial teratogenic risk, however the data is insufficient.
  - *Risk during breast-feeding*
    - Methadone has been detected in human breast milk
    - Mothers on Methadone maintenance should be properly counseled to wean the infant from breast-feeding slowly [16].

Fentanyl
- **Mechanism**
  - Mu Receptor agonist on the opioid receptor in the CNS and peripheral nervous system.

- **Metabolism**
  - Hepatically metabolized
  - *Risk during pregnancy*
    - Category C
    - No reports of congenital abnormalities in infants born to mothers on fentanyl
  - *Risk during breast-feeding*
    - Fentanyl is excreted in breast milk
    - Not recommended for use in nursing women [16]

Buprenorphine (Butrans patch, Suboxone)

- **Mechanism**
  - Buprenorphine is a partial agonist at the mu-opioid receptor and an antagonist at the kappa-opioid receptor.
- **Metabolism**
  - Hepatically metabolized.
  - *Risk during pregnancy*
    - Category C
  - *Risk during breast-feeding*
    - Buprenorphine was found to pass into breast milk
    - Breast-feeding is not advised while on Buprenorphine [23].

Meperidine

- **Mechanism**
  - Mu receptor agonist
- **Metabolism**
  - Hepatically metabolized
  - *Risk during pregnancy*
    - Category C
    - No adequate studies in pregnant women
  - *Risk during breast-feeding*
    - It appears in breast milk
    - Mothers should discontinue the drug or bottle-feed [16].

Other Medications

Bisphosphonates (Pamidronate)

- **Mechanism**
  - Bisphosphonates work on bone metabolism by affecting osteoclastogenesis by causing apoptosis of osteoclast and macrophages.
  - Unknown how Pamidronate works but it is believed to cause apoptosis on osteoclast and macrophages
- **Metabolism**
  - Renally excreted
- **Dosing recommendation**
  - Dosage: 60–90 mg IV
    Paget's disease: 30 mg daily for 3 days

Osteolytic bone lesions: 90 mg monthly
Osteolytic bone metastasis: 90 mg every 2–4 weeks
  - *Risk during pregnancy*
    - Category D
  - *Risk during breast-feeding*
    - It is not known if Pamidronate passes into breast milk
    - Mothers should discontinue the drug or bottle-feed [16].

Muscle Relaxants

Metaxalone (Skelaxin)

- **Mechanism**
  - Believed to be due to CNS depression
- **Metabolism**
  - Hepatically metabolized
  - *Risk in pregnancy*
    - Not categorized due to lack of data but likely category B
  - *Risk in breast-feeding*
    - Unknown if it is excreted in breast milk [16]

Tizanidine (Zanaflex)

- **Mechanism**
  - Exact mechanism is unknown but it's a centrally acting muscle relaxant
- **Metabolism**
  - Hepatically metabolized
  - *Risk in pregnancy*
    - Category C
  - *Risk in breast-feeding*
    - Unknown if it is excreted in breast milk [24]

Cyclobenzaprine (Flexeril)

- **Mechanism**
  - Centrally acting muscle relaxant, potentiates norepinephrine and binds to serotonin receptors thereby reducing spasticity
- **Metabolism**
  - Hepatically metabolized
  - *Risk in pregnancy*
    - Category B
  - *Risk in breast-feeding*
    - Unknown if it's excreted in breast milk.
    - Given its close relation to TCA, some of which is excreted in human milk, precaution should be taken [25].

Carisoprodol (Soma)

- **Mechanism**
  - GABA(A) modulator

- **Metabolism**
  - Hepatically metabolized
  - *Risk in pregnancy*
    - Category C
  - *Risk in breast-feeding*
    - Drug is excreted in breast milk
    - Can cause sedation [16]

Methocarbamol (Robaxin)
- **Mechanism**
  - General CNS depression
- **Metabolism**
  - Hepatically metabolized.
  - *Risk in pregnancy*
    - Category C
    - Unknown if the drug can cause harmful affects on fetus [24]
  - *Risk in breast-feeding*
    - Excreted in breast milk [16]

Orphenadrine (Norflex)
- **Mechanism**
  - Centrally acting muscle relaxant by blocking histamine and NMDA receptors.
- **Metabolism**
  - Hepatically metabolized
  - *Risk in pregnancy*
    - Category C
  - *Risk in breast-feeding*
    - Excretion in breast milk is unknown [16]

Baclofen
- **Mechanism**
  - GABA (B) agonist. It inhibits mono and polysynaptic spinal reflexes.
- **Metabolism**
  - Hepatically metabolized.
  - *Risk in pregnancy*
    - Category C
  - *Risk in breast-feeding*
    - Oral baclofen is excreted in breast milk and should not be used [16].

Chlorzoxazone (Parafon Forte)
- **Mechanism**
  - Centrally actiging muscle relaxant; Inhibits polysynaptic spinal reflexes [24]
- **Metabolism**
  - Hepatically metabolized
  - *Risk in pregnancy:*
    - Category C
  - *Risk in breast-feeding*
    - Unknown if excreted in breast milk. Safety advised

Alternative Treatment

- **TENS unit**:
  - TENS unit (Transcutaneous Electrical Nerve Stimulator) device that provides electrical signal lead wires attached to a patients skin used to relieve pain by stimulating nervous system pathways within the spinal cord which blocks the transmission of pain [7].
  - It has been safely used during pregnancy and has even been used during labor pains [7].
  - No adverse effects have been reported in either the fetus or the mother and a recent study showed reduced LBP with TENS in the third trimester of pregnancy compared to treatment with just exercise and acetaminophen [7].
  - *Precautions should be taken with*:
    History of Epilepsy
    Implantation devices (i.e., pacemaker or defibrillator)
    History of miscarriage or abortion
- Placing leads over acupuncture points most likely to induce labor [7]. When using a TENS unit for labor pain relief, one should take several precautions which include the settings and the placement of the electrodes. According to a study by Bundsen et al., the current density should not be greater than 0.5 $\mu A/mm^2$. The electrodes should not be placed surpapubically if the mother is thin. The TENS unit is more likely to be effective if placed over the lumbosacral nerve roots for spinal and pelvic girdle pain [26],
- **Physical therapy**
  - One systematic review of the literature published in 1985 was inconclusive on the benefits of physical therapy for pregnancy-related LBP [27].
  - A 2007 Cochrane review analyzed 8 studies with a total of 1,305 patients and found that physical therapy and acupuncture reduced the amount of sick days by 12 % [28].
  - A Supervised, low-to-moderate intensity strength training program during pregnancy can be safe and efficacious for pregnant women [29, 30].
- **Chiropractic treatment**
  - In a randomized control trial comparing exercise, spinal manipulation, and neuro emotional techniques as a way to treat pregnancy-related back pain, 50 % of patients experienced improvement in symptoms [29].
  - Studies have shown the relative safety and effectiveness of chiropractic treatment for LBP during pregnancy [30, 31]
- **Bracing**
  - **Pelvic and Sacroiliac belts**
    Hypothesis for back pain in pregnancy is the hormonal changes alter the lumbopelvic ligaments, thereby affecting the stability [32].

Table 32.2 A list of commonly used medications and its safety and side effects based on the FDA Pregnancy category

Drug	Category	Safe with lactation	Precautions
Tylenol	B	Safe	
Ibuprofen	B	Safe	Not to be taken during third trimester
Benadryl	B	Probably safe	
Claritin	B	Probably safe	Category B in third trimester
Colace	C	Safety unknown	
Pseudoephedrine	C	Conditional safety	

Please refer to Table 32.1 for FDA category explanation

The effectiveness of a pelvic belt in reducing pelvic pain in pregnancy remains controversial.

The theory behind its benefits is that the belt brings the articular surface of the Sacroiliac joint together [4].

The positioning of the belt is more effective than the tension of the belt with reducing SI joint laxity [4].

A review article that studied published literature on the effectiveness of pelvic belts concluded that there is little evidence that the use of pelvic belt will independently reduce pregnancy-related LBP or pelvic girdle pain [4].

Table 32.2 lists common medications used during pregnancy.

References

1. Morgan IM, Pohjanen AI. Low back pain and pelvic pain during pregnancy: prevalence and risk factors. Spine. 2005;30:983–91.
2. Dowswell T, Bedwell C, Lavender T, Neilson JP. Transcutaneous electrical nerve stimulation (TENS) for pain relief in labour. Cochrane Database Syst Rev 2009: CD007214. doi:10.1002/14651858.CD007214.pub2.
3. Sadr S, et al. The treatment experience of patients with low back pain during pregnancy and their chiropractors: a qualitative study. Chiropr Man Therap. 2012;20(1):32.
4. Ho S, Yu W, et al. Effectiveness of maternity support belts in reducing lower back pain during pregnancy: a review. J Clin Nurs. 2009;18:1523–32.
5. Raj P. Pain medicine: a comprehensive review. 2nd ed. Chapter 8, p. 49–57.
6. Smith M, Marcus P, Wurtz L. Orthopedic issues in pregnancy. Obstet Gynecol Surv. 2008;63(2):103–11.
7. Keskin EA, Onur O, Keskin HL, et al. Transcutaneous electrical nerve stimulation improves low back pain during pregnancy. Gynecol Obstet Invest. 2012;74:76–83.
8. Richie J. Orthopedic considerations during pregnancy. Clin Obstet Gynecol. 2003;46(2):456–66.
9. Lee S, Jeong C, Lee H, Yoon M, Kim W. Ultrasound guided obturator nerve block: a single interfascial injection technique. J Anesth. 2011;25:923–6.
10. Taha A. Ultrasound-guided obturator nerve block: a proximal interfascial technique. Anesth Analg. 2012;114(1):236–9.
11. Myllynen P, Makela A, Kontula K. Aseptic necrosis off the femoral head during pregnancy. Obstet Gynecol. 1988;71:495–8.
12. Pourbagher MA, Ozalay M, Pourbagher A. Accuracy and outcome of sonographically guided intra-articular sodium hyaluronate injections in patients with osteoarthritis of the hip. J Ultrasound Med. 2005;24:1391–5.
13. Ng I, Vaghadia H, Choi PT, Helmy N. Ultrasound imaging accuracy identifies the lateral femoral cutaneous nerve. Anesth Analg. 2008;107:1070–4.
14. http://Mayoclinic.org.
15. Smith H, Pappagello M. Essential pain pharmacology. Cambridge: Cambridge University Press; 2012.
16. Adams K, et al. Safety of pain therapy during pregnancy and lactation in patients with inflammatory arthritis: a systematic literature review. J Rheumatol Suppl. 2012;90:59–61.
17. Briggs G, Ambrose P, Illett K, et al. Use of duloxetine in pregnancy and lactation. Ann Pharmacol. 2009;43(11):1898–902.
18. Boyce P, Hackett L, Illett K. Duloxetine transfers across the placenta during pregnancy and into mild during lactation. Arch Womens Ment Health. 2011;14:169–72.
19. Patil A, Kuller J, Rhee E. Antidepressants in pregancy: a review of commonly prescribed medications. Obstet Gynecol Surv. 2011;66(12):777–87.
20. Wlodarczyk BJ, Palacios AM, George TM, Finnell RH. Antiepileptic drugs and pregnancy outcomes. Am J Med Genet A. 2012;158A:2071–90.
21. Ferreira CW, Alburquerque-Sendı NF. Effectiveness of physical therapy for pregnancy-related low back and/or pelvic pain after delivery: a systematic review. Physiother Theory Pract. 2013;29(6):419–31.
22. http://Opana.org.
23. http://Suboxone.com.
24. http://Rxlist.org
25. http://Amrix.com.
26. Bundsen P, Ericson K. Pain relief in labour by transcutaneous electrical nerve stimulation safety aspects. Acta Obstet Gynaecol Scand. 1982;61(1):1–5.
27. Pennick VE, Young G. Interventions for preventing and treating pelvic and back pain in pregnancy. Cochrane Database Syst Rev. 2007;2, CD001139.
28. Peterson C, Haas M, Gregory T. A pilot randomized controlled trial comparing the efficacy of exercise, spinal manipulation, and neuro emotional technique for the treatment of pregnancy related low back pain. Chiropr Man Therap. 2012;20:18.
29. Braddom RL, Buschbacher RM. Physical medicine and rehabilitation. Philadelphia: Saunders; 2000.
30. O'Conner P, Poudevigne M, Cress M. Safety and efficacy of supervised strength training adopted in pregnancy. J Phys Act Health. 2011;8(3):309–20.
31. Stuber KJ, Smith DL. Chiropractic treatment of pregnancy-related low back pain: a systematic review of the evidence. J Manipulative Physiol Ther. 2008;31:447–54.
32. Damen L, Spoor C, Snijders C, Stam H. Does a pelvic belt influence sacroiliac joint laxity? Clin Biomech. 2002;17:495–8.

Pain Management in Geriatric Patients

33

Earl L. Smith and Tita Castor

Abbreviations

APAP	Acetaminophen
ASA	Aspirin
AV	Arteriovascular
BP	Blood pressure
CABG	Coronary artery bypass grafting
CCB	Calcium channel blockers
COX	Cyclooxygenase
CV	Cerebrovascular
EtOH	Ethanol
GERD	Gastroesophageal reflux disease
GIB	Gastrointestinal bleeding
IV	Intravenous
MSK	Musculoskeletal
NSAIDs	Nonsteroidal anti-inflammatory drugs
OIC	Opioid induced constipation
OT	Occupational therapy
PHN	Postherpetic neuralgia
PO	Per os
PPI	Proton pump inhibitor
prn	As-needed
PT	Physical therapy
PUD	Peptic ulcer disease
QoL	Quality of life
SQ	Subcutaneous
TBI	Traumatic brain injury

E.L. Smith, M.D., Ph.D., FAAPMR (✉)
Department of Rehabilitation Medicine, Emory Palliative
Care Center, Emory University, Atlanta, Georgia, USA
e-mail: earl.smith@emory.edu

T. Castor, M.D., F.A.C.P.
Elmhurst Hospital Center, Elmhurst, NY, USA

Icahn School of Medicine at Mount Sinai, New York, NY, USA
e-mail: castort@nychhc.org

Introduction

- Persistent pain affects 25–50 % of community-dwelling elderly persons and 45–80 % of older residents of long-term care facilities [1].
- Several painful conditions occur more commonly in older than in younger adults and often go unrecognized (see Table 33.1) [1–4].
- Some painful syndromes result from therapies decades earlier, e.g., Radiation therapy, surgeries such as CABG (coronary artery bypass grafting), amputations, etc.
- Untreated pain may lead to a decline of functional status and quality of life, depression, falls, and increased health-care utilization.

Physiologic Changes in Geriatric Population [1, 2, 4]

- Slowed absorption results in delayed onset and delayed time to peak serum concentration.
- Slowed metabolism—decreased renal and hepatic clearance may lead to toxicities, especially with polypharmacy, e.g., sedation, confusion, constipation, and urinary retention in geriatric patients
- Other changes—lower albumin, increased fat mass, decreased muscle and body water affect distribution, i.e., delayed onset, increased free-drug concentration, and increased washout time [4].

Recommendations When Treating Geriatric Patients

- Use least invasive route of administration of pain medications
- **Avoid intramuscular medications**: No specific advantages over IV or PO medications, absorption of

K.A. Sackheim, *Pain Management and Palliative Care: A Comprehensive Guide*,
DOI 10.1007/978-1-4939-2462-2_33, © Springer Science+Business Media New York 2015

Table 33.1 Pain syndromes encountered with higher frequency in the older adult

Athridites (e.g., OA, RA)	Temporal arteritis and other rheumatic disorders
Vertebral body compression fractures	
Amputations	
Cancer pain	Both direct and as a consequence of treatments
Late sequelae of surgery	May occur decades after treatment (i.e., noncardiac chest pain; post-CABG; postthoracotomy
Late sequelae of radiation therapy	May occur decades after treatment (i.e., mucositis, proctitis) often poorly localized
Neuralgias	Postherpetic neuralgia/shingles
	Trigeminal neuralgia
	"Double Crush" after chemotherapy, EtOH use, diabetes, etc.
Peripheral neuropathies	Due to diabetes, atherosclerosis, PVD, ischemic pain, etc.

OA osteoarthritis, *RA* rheumatoid arthritis, *CABG* coronary artery bypass grafting, *PVD* peripheral vascular disease, *EtOH* ethanol

intramuscular medications vs. IV or PO is less predictable in older patients. Some medications, such as APAP (acetaminophen) and opioids, work well as suppositories

- Dosing recommendations are difficult to obtain, as they have not been systematically studied in older adults [1, 4, 5].
- *Caution to avoid cognitive impairment which can lead to falls/fractures, avoid exacerbating constipation, and renal or hepatic worsening of pathology*
  - Widespread differences amongst prescribing practices for older adults [5] due to few quality studies of pain management in the elderly, those with cognitive impairment, and/or the frail
- **"Start low and go slow"**: Analgesics have widespread effects on many systems which may be compromised by diseases and/or by age-related changes, making side effects less predictable [1–4, 6] *Monitor for side effects such as cognitive impairment which can lead to falls/fractures, constipation, and renal or hepatic worsening of pathology*
  - Clinician must be guided by:
    Understanding of pharmacokinetics [7]
    Vigilance for the **quietly crashing patient**, who may show no changes in vital signs, mental status, nor lab values but be critically ill [1–6].

American Geriatrics Society Guidelines

- 2012 Beers Criteria allow most opioids except meperidine (See Table 33.2) [6]
  - Recommend least invasive route of drug administration when possible
  - Around-the-clock dosing for continuous pain treatment
  - Use of short-acting medications for breakthrough pain on an as-needed (prn) basis

Common Geriatric Pain Syndromes

See Table 33.1 for a list of common pain syndromes, which may afflict geriatric patients with higher frequency than younger adults.

Pain Assessment in Older Adults

- More complicated than in younger adults
- Geriatrics may have lower pain threshold [2].
- **Vision and hearing impairment** lead to inaccurate assessments when formal measurement scales are used.
- **Geriatric pain assessment instruments** for older adults should be simple, readily available to patients and staff, and in large print. They should also describe pain in language that patients comprehend. Familiar words such as slight, mild, moderate, severe, or extreme may be preferred over the traditional 1–10 rating scale.
- Ask family members the patient's pain history to elucidate etiology and treatment. Be wary not to "sideline" the patient as that may hinder development of therapeutic rapport and treatment efficacy
- **Nihilism**: Health care workers' cultural or societal beliefs, e.g., pain is inevitable with aging, may present barriers to treatment.
- **Cognitive impairment** (stroke, delirium, or dementia) must differentiate various distressful external vs. internal stimuli, e.g., the moaning patient might be delirious, not in pain.
- **Physical exam** may elicit grimacing, movement, on palpation of a suspected painful region.
- **Medical workup** for reversible causes of Altered Mental Status is required.
- New behavioral problems in dementia patients may reflect a number of uncomfortable situations, including urinary tract infections, constipation, or discomfort from falls or injuries. Treating the patient's underlying disorder may reduce use of pain medication and anxiolytics, antipsychotics prescribed for agitation, or other symptoms of delirium.

Patients with Cognitive Impairment

- Patients with cognitive impairment may not be able to request prn medications and may require standing medications [1, 2, 8]. May necessitate the use of less well-studied routes of administration such as SQ, suppository,

Table 33.2 Dosing and titration of opioid medications for the older adult [1, 2, 4, 5, 7, 8]

Generic name	Brand names	Dosing	Clinical comments
Buprenorphine patch	Butrans	Begin 5 μg/h q7days	Only the patch is approved for pain; SL form is for treatment of withdrawal (significant first-pass metabolism precludes oral)
		Titrate to 10 then 20 μg/h at 3-day intervals	Sublingual tablets approved only for opioid dependence and requires DEA waiver
			Not suitable for patients who require >80 mg PO morphine in 24 h
			Safe in renal impairment because of fecal excretion
			Rarely covered by insurance
Codeine with acetaminophen	Tylenol #3	30 mg/300 mg 1 tab PO q4–6 h PRN	Rarely used due to high risk of adverse events
			Complicated metabolism: Must be metabolized to morphine before good pain relief
			Highest risk of injurious falls (huang)
Fentanyl	Transdermal: Duragesic	Smallest patch is 12.5 μg/h but difficult to obtain. Most common starting dose is 25 μg/h. Do not use before 60 mg PO morphine/24 h	Not for opioid-naïve patients
			Dosing, absorption, and pharmacokinetics difficult to predict
			Geriatric half-life much longer than younger adults: May take days to achieve pain control and steady state, both for starting and stopping
			For severe chronic and malignant pain
			Rarely helpful in cachectic patients
	Actiq, Fentora, Subsys	100 μg troche, spray or lozenge equivalent	Do not use if fever >39 °C (102 °F)
			Little role on the Rehab floor/hospital wards
			SL formulations are approved only for cancer pain; rarely covered by insurance
Hydrocodone	Vicodin, Lortab/ Norco (APAP) Vicoprofen (ibuprofen)	2.5–5 mg every 4–6 h	Recently changed to DEA Schedule II
			Nonopioid medications in combination vary in dose, and may be dose-limiting
Hydromorphone	Dilaudid	1–2 mg PO every 3–4 h	
		0.2 mg IV every every hour PRN	
		Titrate as required	
Meperidine	Demerol		Inappropriate for geriatrics, per 2012 Beers Criteria
Methadone	Dolophin	Doses for pain typically much lower than for substance abuse	**Consult expert before prescribing**
			Not for opioid naïve patients
		2.5–5 mg PO at bedtime	Variable pharmacokinetics
			Risk of QT prolongation/torsades
Morphine	Immediate release: Morphine, Roxonol elixir	2.5–10 mg every 4 h, 2 mg IV	First-line weak opioid but not often used on Rehab floor. Decreased first-pass metabolism results in higher bioavailability
			Decreased renal clearance may result in increased toxicity
	Sustained release: MS-Contin, Avinza, Kadian	15 mg every 8–12 h	Monitor for end-of-dose failure
Oxymorphone	Opana IR	5 mg q6	Significant interactions with food
	Opana ER	5 mg q12	Significant alcohol toxicity
Oxycodone with acetaminophen	Oxycodone, Roxicodone	Elixir: 2–10 mg every 4 h as needed for pain	Highest potential for abuse of legal opioids: Can be activating/euphorigenic
	Combinations: Percocet, Roxicet	Combination: 5 mg/325 mg or 10 mg/325 mg PO. 1 or 2 tabs q4 h PRN pain	Available in elixir or sustained release
			Sustained release forms may be prohibitively expensive, even generic
			Increasing reluctance by third-party payors to cover sustained release, even generic
	Sustained release: OxyContin	Sustained release: 10 mg PO every 12 h	Monitor for end-of-dose failure
Tapentadol	Nucynta	50–100 PO q4–6 h as needed for moderate-to-severe	Short term (postoperative) and chronic pain
			Some studies show less constipation
	Nucynta ER	Sustained release: 50–250 mg PO q12	Nociceptive and neuropathic pain
			Recently on market so often requires preauthorization for coverage
Tramadol	Ultram	25 mg PO q4 or 6 h	Has the usual opioid side effects, including constipation, urinary retention, potential for aberrant use
			Weak opioid with ceiling dose
			Some states are changing to Schedule II

- Consider specialist (Pain Management, Geriatrics, Palliative Care) for nonroutine dosing
- For all opioids, begin bowel regimen immediately; **geriatrics are at high risk for fecal impaction**. At minimum a cathartic
- Extended release formulations are usually started after initial dose determined by effects of immediate release
- Monitor mental status and mood (sedation, delirium) and rotate opioid as required
- May require concomitant dosing of stimulants, e.g., methylphenidate or modafenil
- Synthetic and semisynthetic opioids with "cleaner metabolism" have lower risk of opioid-induced neurotoxicity (see text)

DEA drug enforcement administration

SQ, and the assistance of caregivers to provide optimal management [1, 2, 4–8].

- Opioid-sparing strategies such as **adjuvant pain** medications may provide greater benefit while minimizing side effects when compared to escalating the dose of a single agent [1, 3, 8].
- Geriatrics are more susceptible to **opioid-induced neurotoxicity**: Monitor closely for any one or more of delirium, hyperreflexia, dysesthetic touch, muscle twitching (both subjective and objective reports), widespread pain (total body pain), reports of vivid dreams and/or nightmares.

Pain Medication Classes

Acetaminophen (Tylenol)

First-line treatment to relieve most types of mild-to-moderate pain

- Scheduled (around-the-clock) dosing vs. as-needed dosing of acetaminophen improves efficacy for treatment of chronic pain. Total daily dose should not exceed 3,000–4,000 mg divided every 6–8 h. Elderly patients are more susceptible to liver toxicity and caution should be used when giving max daily doses to these patients.
- *Caution with combination medications* that also may contain acetaminophen such as Percocet, Vicodin/Norco). These must be included in total acetaminophen daily dosage. If combination drugs are necessary, use formulations that contain only 325 mg of acetaminophen.
- *Caution with existing liver pathology (cirrhosis, hepatitis)*

Nonsteroidal anti-inflammatory drugs (NSAIDs)

- **Mechanism of action:**
  - Traditional NSAIDs (Nonselective COX inhibitors) treat inflammation in musculoskeletal tissues through COX 2 inhibition, while also limiting COX-1 protective activity in the gastric mucosal lining.
    - Proton pump inhibitors (PPIs) reduce the risk of developing PUD (peptic ulcer disease)/GIB (gastrointestinal bleeding)/Gastric upset. Remember to stop PPI if NSAIDs are discontinued to reduce polypharmacy as PPIs can cause delirium, osteopenia, and weaken the GI intrinsic immune system.
    - Misoprostol, a synthetic prostaglandin, reduces risk of PUD, though the side effect of diarrhea limits compliance.
  - COX-2 inhibitors and choline magnesium trisalicylate (Trilisate) have reduced gastrointestinal side-effect risk, but still require monitoring for renal toxicity (hypertension and limb edema).

- *Use with caution in patients with history of*:
  - Renal/hepatic pathology
  - PUD/GERD (gastroesophageal reflux disease)
  - Concurrent use of anticoagulant, antiplatelet, or corticosteroid medications
  - Bleeding diatheses
- *Do not use in patients with moderate—severe renal disease*: See more details in Chap. 30.
- NSAIDs are for short-term use only.

Opioids

- Indicated for moderate-to-severe pain refractory to other medications
- Pain severity, medical and cognitive status, and side-effect tolerance may guide selection of this class of medications.
- Episodic moderate-to-severe pain: PRN dosing, e.g., Dosing in arthroplasty patients 20–30 min prior to PT/OT aides in therapy tolerance.
- Scheduled doses of short-acting medications should be titrated for desired effect, and then conversion to long-acting formulas may be performed if needed.
- Continuous pain can be treated with long-acting preparations; risks of overdose and side effects are higher. Given impaired metabolism, short-acting may suffice in the elderly.
- Titrate less often than with younger patients.
- Opioid equivalency tables, SmartPhone apps, and online must be used with **caution**, due to paucity of studies of older adults [5]. Decrease for incomplete cross-tolerance
- **Side effects of opioids**
- Nausea and Constipation are most common. Nausea secondary to opioids and metabolites habituates after 2–3 days. Severe symptoms may require opioid rotation or symptom control with antiemetic medications.
- Laxatives/stool softeners must be initiated with opioids to avoid stool impaction, typically senna and docusate. Magnesium or phosphorous preparations are not first line in elderly as can cause electrolyte abnormalities. If lactulose is used, docusate is not required.
- Methylnaltrexone is approved in the United States for opioid-induced constipation (OIC) as SQ (subcutaneous) injection. Patient should have tried at least two other laxation agents prior. Dosing is weight-based. Advise patient to expect copious bowel movements within 30 min of dosing. Administer only to a patient who will be awake as sleeping patients tend not to defecate. IV and PO studies are in progress. (Prucalopride is not yet approved in the United States). Lubiprostone is now approved for OIC.
- Monitor for sedation, impaired cognition, dizziness, dry mouth, and urinary retention. Respiratory depression is rare if opioids are titrated at the correct rate (see Table 33.3).

Table 33.3 Nonopioid medications for geriatric patients: acetaminophen, NSAIDs, and adjuvants

Generic name	Brand names	Dosing	Clinical comments
Acetaminophen	Tylenol	Maximum daily dose of 4 g per 24 h	Effective in musculoskeletal pain
		Include "hidden sources" from combination pills	Relatively contraindicated in liver failure
		2 g if regular EtOH use	
Nonselective NSAIDs:			
Ibuprofen	Motrin, Advil	200–400 mg PO q6 h	Use with extreme caution if safer therapies have failed
			Do not use in active PUD, CKD, CHF
			Do not take more than one for pain control
			Patients taking ASA for cardiac protection should not take ibuprofen
Naproxen	Aleve, Naprosyn	500–750 mg PO q8 h	Naprosyn has lowest risk of CV events
Diclofenac	Voltaren, Zipsor	50 mg q12, or 25 mg q6 h, or 75 mg extended release daily	Assess regularly for GI and renal toxicity
Choline magnesium salicylate	Trilisate	500–750 mg PO q8	Trilisate may have less antiplatelet action
COX-2 inhibitors			
Celoxicib	Celebrex	100 mg daily	
Tricyclic drugs Amitriptyline Desimpramine Nortriptyline	Elavil Norpramin Pamelor, Aventyl	The typical starting dose of any TCA for treatment of neuropathic pain is 10–25 mg nightly. Increase by 10–25 mg every 3–7 days as tolerated. Older persons rarely tolerate doses greater than 75–100 mg per day. Tertiary tricyclic antidepressants (amitriptyline, imipramine, doxepin) should be avoided because of higher risk for adverse effects. Secondary amine tricyclic antidepressants (desipramine, nortriptyline) may have fewer adverse effects than amitriptyline	Significant risk of adverse effects in elderly: Anticholinergic (visual, urinary, GI), orthostasis and AV block
SNRIs			
Duloxetine	Cymbalta	20 mg daily	Multiple drug–drug interactions
			Avoid when CrCl <30 mL/min
			Can increase BP and HR
Venlafaxine	Effexor	25 or 37.5 mg daily	Caution in renal insufficiency. If CrCl <30 mL/min, decrease by 50%. May cause constipation, nausea, hot flashes, dry mouth, palpitations, HTN, hyperhydrosis
Milnacipran	Savella	Start at 12.5 mg daily and titrate to 50 BID. Discontinuation requires tapering	
Anticonvulsants			
Carbamazepine	Tegretol	100 mg daily	Monitor transaminases, CBC, Cr, BUN, electrolytes, serum levels. Multiple drug–drug interactions
Gabapentin	Neurontin	Start at 100 mg PO qHS titrate PRN	Sedation, ataxia, edema, weight gain
	Gralisse	300 mg PO qHS; titrate PRN	Sedation, ataxia, edema, weight gain
Pregabalin	Lyrica	50 mg PO qHS; titrate PRN	Sedation, ataxia, edema, weight gain rapid onset may cause more delirium
Topicals			
Capsaicin 8 % patch	Quetenza	1–4 patches for 60 min; repeat q3mos PRN	Application site may develop erythema, pain, pruritus, papules, or hyperalgesia. Pretreat with topic anesthetic if required
Capsaicin 0.025–0.1 %		TID or QID as tolerated	Patch is FDA-approved only for PHN, but both patch and lotion are effective in HIV
			Lotion may require application for days/weeks

(continued)

Table 33.3 (continued)

Generic name	Brand names	Dosing	Clinical comments
Corticosteroids			
Prednisone Methylprednisolone	Deltasone Medrol dosepak	e.g., 5–60 mg daily	Use lowest dose possible
			Monitor for fluid retention, glycemic effects, delirium.
			For short-term use, except in end-of-life care
			Taper as rapidly as feasible
			Also give PPI
Dexamethasone	Decadron	4 mg PO/IV q6 then q8 on day 2	

Consider specialist such as Pain Management, Geriatrics, or Palliative Care for nonroutine cases

Monitor mental status and mood (sedation, delirium)

NSAIDs nonsteroidal anti-inflammatory drugs, *PPI* proton pump inhibitor, *PO* per os, *IV* intravenous, *FDA* Food and Drug Administration, *PRN* as-needed, *PHN* postherpetic neuralgia, *HIV* human immunodeficiency virus, *CBC* complete blood count, *Cr* creatinine, *BUN* blood urea nitrogen, *HTN* hypertension, *BP* blood pressure, *HR* heart rate, *GI* gastrointestinal, *PUD* peptic ulcer disease, *CKD* chronic kidney disease, *CHF* congestive heart failure

- **Opioid-induced hyperalgesia (OIH)** is a serious side effect and a sign of Opioid-Induced Neurotoxicity
- **Opioid-induced neurotoxicity (OIN)**: Monitor closely for any one or more of delirium, hyperreflexia, dysesthetic touch, muscle twitching (both subjective and objective reports), widespread pain (total body pain), reports of vivid dreams and/or nightmares
- OIN occurs more often at higher doses and with chronicity. Treatment may include reducing dose or rotation to a different opioid. Avoid polypharmacy; i.e., use same opioid for long-acting and for short-acting PRN dosing
- Histamine release is frequently mislabeled allergy and usually habituates in 2–3 days. Pruritus can be treated with pramoxine lotion; use systemic antihistamines only if absolutely necessary.
- Sedation: Consider stimulants such as methylphenidate or modafinil in cardiac stable patients. Monitor heart rate and BP if these are a concern.

Neuropathic pain medications

- **Neuropathic pain syndromes**
  - Neuropathic pain is often described with a "burning," "squeezing," "like pressure" or "pins and needles," "like insects crawling" or "numb."
  - **Dysesthetic** touch: Light touch, even e.g., bedsheets, perceived as painful.
    - Neuropathic pain may occur with intracranial injuries such as stroke or traumatic brain injury (TBI). Post-stroke pain syndromes are **common** (>50 % of stroke patients)
    - **Peripheral neuropathy** may arise from diabetes, micronutrient deficiencies, and other metabolic disorders, EtOH use, liver pathology, HIV, chemotherapy.
    - HIV neuropathy responds well to topicals such as capsaicin (see Table 33.3) [9, 10].

- **Phantom limb pain** or pain resulting from neuroma formation in the residual limb. **Neuromas** can form in a variety of postoperative sites, resulting in a panoply of **noncardiac chest pain syndromes** such as post-CABG, postmastectomy, postthoracotomy pain syndromes. These may become symptomatic decades after surgery if patient develops "**double crush**" from e.g., diabetes or chemotherapy.

Tricyclic antidepressants

- Commonly used for neuropathic conditions in adults, but rarely used for older adults due to burdensome side-effect profile.
- Significant side effects include QT prolongation and anticholinergic effects which may lead to severe dry mouth, cognitive impairment, bowel, and bladder dysfunction.
- Amitriptyline, nortriptyline, and desipramine, even at low dose, are considered only if refractory to all other medications. Close side effects monitoring is recommended. Nortriptyline has the most side-effect burden.

Anticonvulsants medications

- Used to treat virtually all neuropathic pain syndromes.
- Gabapentin, with its low side-effect profile and slow onset is commonly prescribed. Renal clearance reduces interactions with other medications, and monitoring of drug levels and liver function is not necessary. See Table 33.1 for dosing. Close monitoring for edema and neurological side effects is recommended.
  - Likelihood of peripheral edema increases with dose, age, and decreased renal function.
- Other seizure medications, such as phenytoin, valproate, and carbamazepine, also may be prescribed for

neuropathic pain. These are dosed to lowest dose required to control pain; typically lower than "therapeutic level" for seizure prophylaxis. Periodic monitoring of levels and liver function is required.

Topical analgesic medications

- As well as opioids and adjuvants such as gabapentin, use Lidoderm patch once the vesicles have crusted. There are numerous reports for use in other localized pain syndromes. Lidocaine jelly can be used in e.g., rectal/anal/intertriginous areas.
- Capsaicin cream or lotion, believed to deplete pain fiber nerve terminals of substance P, may be used to treat neuropathic or nociceptive pain. Avoid accidental placement of the medication in mucous membranes and eyes. Careful hand washing and careful movement of clothing, bed linens, or dressings over treated regions reduces this risk.
- Topical Medications Generally Perceived as Safe for the Older Adult: Diclofenac patch (Flector) and gel (Voltaren), ASA (aspirin) gel (SportsCreme, AsperCreme), menthol creams (BenGay), capsaicin, lidocaine patch (Lidoderm)

Nonpharmacological Pain Management Strategies

- Osteopathic manipulation has been demonstrated to improve pain and QoL in many patients, including geriatrics. Techniques include postural examination and palpation using soft tissue techniques designed to increase proprioception and posture [11].
- Massage
- PT/OT/splinting/sling
- Music therapy (nursing home, dementia)
- Recreation therapy (relief of boredom)
- Tai Chi—proprioception, lowers MSK pain

Overall, caution should always be taken when prescribing medications to elderly patients as they are likely more susceptible to side effects and overdose potential.

References

1. American Geriatrics Society Panel on Pharmacological Management of Persistent Pain in Older Persons. Pharmacological management of persistent pain in older persons. J Am Geriatr Soc. 2009;57(8):1331–46.
2. Kaye AD, Baluch A, Scott JT. Pain management in the elderly population: a review. Ochsner J. 2010;10(3):179–87.
3. Siefferman JW. Postamputation pain in the geriatric population: part 1. Top Pain Manag. 2013;28(7):1–9.
4. Huang AR, Mallet L. Prescribing opioids in older people. Maturitas. 2013;74(2):123–9.
5. Bell JS, Klaukka T, Ahonen J, Hartikainen S. National utilization of transdermal fentanyl among community-dwelling older people in Finland. Am J Geriatr Pharmacother. 2009;7(6):355.
6. American Geriatrics Society 2012 Beers Criteria Update Expert Panel. American Geriatrics Society updated Beers Criteria for potentially inappropriate medication use in older adults. J Am Geriatr Soc. 2012;60(4):616–31.
7. McLachlan AJ, Bath S, Naganathan V, Hilmer SN, Le Couteur DG, Gibson SJ, Blyth FM. Clinical pharmacology of analgesic medicines in older people: impact of frailty and cognitive impairment. Br J Clin Pharmacol. 2011;71(3):351–64.
8. Pergolizzi J, Böger RH, Budd K, Dahan A, Erdine S, Hans G, Kress HG, Langford R, Likar R, Raffa RB, Sacerdote P. Opioids and the management of chronic severe pain in the elderly: consensus statement of an International Expert Panel with focus on the six clinically most often used World Health Organization Step III opioids (buprenorphine, fentanyl, hydromorphone, methadone, morphine, oxycodone). Pain Pract. 2008;8(4):287–313.
9. Simpson DM, Brown S, Tobias J, NGX-4010 C107 Study Group. Controlled trial of high-concentration capsaicin patch for treatment of painful HIV neuropathy. Neurology. 2008;70(24):2305–13.
10. American Geriatrics Society Workgroup on Vitamin D Supplementation for Older Adults. Recommendations abstracted from the American Geriatrics Society Consensus Statement on vitamin D for Prevention of Falls and Their Consequences. J Am Geriatr Soc. 2014;62:147–52.
11. Papa L, Mandara A, Bottali M, Gulisano V, Orfei S. A randomized control trial on the effectiveness of osteopathic manipulative treatment in reducing pain and improving the quality of life in elderly patients affected by osteoporosis. Clin Cases Miner Bone Metab. 2012;9(3):179–83.

Acute Postsurgical Pain and PCA Management

34

Christopher A.J. Webb, Paul D. Weyker,
Brandon Esenther, and Leena Mathew

Abbreviations

CNS	Central nervous system
CSF	Cerebrospinal fluid
CT	Computed tomography
FLACC	Face, legs, activity, cry, consolability
IM	Intramuscular
INR	International normalized ratio
IV	Intravenous
LMWH	Low molecular weight heparin
MAOIs	Monoamine oxidase inhibitors
MRI	Magnetic resonance imaging
NA	Not available
NMDA	N-methyl-D-aspartate
NPO	Nil per os
NSAIDs	Nonsteroidal anti-inflammatory drugs
PCA	Patient-controlled analgesia
PO	Per os
PONV	Postoperative nausea and vomiting
TURP	Transurethral resection of the prostate
VAS	Visual analog scale

Introduction

Despite advances in pain medicine, postsurgical pain remains undertreated. It is a subject that has received greater attention over the last two decades [1, 2]. A vast majority of patients will suffer from some degree of discomfort during their postoperative recovery. Adequate evaluation, acknowledgement, and management of postoperative pain are integral to standard of care.

Brief Overview of Acute Pain

- *Acute pain or nociceptive pain*:
    - Related to a precipitating event (acute onset) and lasts <3 months
    - Mediated through the system and developed as an adaptive mechanism to mitigate further tissue damage [3].
- Acute pain can be categorized into somatic or visceral pain
    - **Somatic pain**: A delta fibers
      Superficial somatic pain: Well-localized, sharp, stabbing, or pinprick pain.
      Deep somatic pain: Arises from muscles, bones, joints, is less well localized and often described as dull, aching pain [4, 5].
    - **Visceral pain**: C fibers
      Deep visceral pain: Arises from the visceral organs. Dull, pressure-like pain that is diffused and poorly localized.
      Parietal pain: Localized or referred pain and is sharp/stabbing in nature [6, 7].

Evaluating the Postsurgical Patient with Pain

- Evaluation begins with the preoperative anesthetic assessment
- Comorbidities should be identified
- Patients at risk for significant postoperative pain

C.A.J. Webb, M.D. • P.D. Weyker, M.D.
Department of Anesthesia and Perioperative Care,
University of California San Francisco Medical Center,
University of California San Francisco, San Francisco, CA, USA

B. Esenther, M.D.
Department of Anesthesiology, New York Presbyterian—Columbia,
New York, NY, USA

L. Mathew, M.D. (✉)
Division of Pain Medicine, Department of Anesthesiology,
New York Presbyterian Hospital, Columbia University,
New York, NY, USA
e-mail: Lm370@columbia.edu

K.A. Sackheim, *Pain Management and Palliative Care: A Comprehensive Guide*,
DOI 10.1007/978-1-4939-2462-2_34, © Springer Science+Business Media New York 2015

Focused History of Present Illness

1. Location and radiation of pain
2. Temporal association
3. Quality of pain
4. Pain assessment
   - Visual analog scale (VAS): Reliable tool to quantify acute pain and is used to monitor the effectiveness of analgesic modalities [8, 9].
   - In noncommunicative or unconscious patients, objective measures such as heart rate, blood pressure, respiratory rate (over breathing on ventilator), agitation, and facial expression can also be used to assess pain in nonverbal patients [10].
5. Chronic pain syndromes
   - Imperative to document any previously diagnosed pain syndromes
   - Identify current treatment modalities/medications
   - Past analgesic modalities trialed
     - What treatment modalities have worked?
     - What treatment modalities have not worked and why?
       - Inadequate dose escalation
       - Adverse reactions to medications: Tolerable or intolerable

Post-Surgical Physical Exam

- Physical exam should focus on the neurological, musculoskeletal, and vascular systems with considerations of the surgical site.
- *Examination of the catheter site*:
  - Evaluate location of catheter at the skin and confirm location with intraoperative records. Catheters should be 4–5 cm in the epidural space. Migration either into or out of the epidural space can account for insufficient analgesia or unblocked dermatomal segments (patchy coverage).
  - Evaluate for leakage around the insertion site, bleeding, erythema, or signs of injection. Catheter site should be clean, dry, and intact.
- *Use of neuraxial opioids (epidural)*:
  - Neuraxial opioids
    Neuraxial fentanyl: Mode of intraoperative analgesia as onset and duration are relatively short
    Neuraxial morphine: Mode of postoperative analgesia as onset is several hours and lasts up to 24 h
- *Perioperative analgesics*
  - *Ketorolac*: Used in all surgeries where there are no contraindications (Renal dysfunction, neurosurgery, etc.)
  - *Intravenous paracetamol*:
    Can be given on scheduled basis while patients are NPO

Oral acetaminophen should be given when patients tolerating PO.
May be opioid sparing
- *Gabapentinoids* [11]:
  Gabapentin may be started preoperatively and continued postoperatively especially when neuropathic pain is predominant.
  Evidence to support this is mostly anecdotal
  Avoid gabapentin in gastric bypass patients as these patients have the duodenum "bypassed" from their GI tract, the sole site of gabapentin absorption.
- *Benzodiazepines*:
  Decrease perioperative anxiety
  Anxiety is a significant component of pain perception.
  Muscle relaxant properties effective in treating muscle spasm pain
  Avoid in elderly due to increased risk of contributing to postoperative delirium

Specific Surgery Considerations

- *Orthopedic procedures*: Can be accomplished with peripheral nerve blocks/catheters or Neuraxial techniques
- *NSAIDs*: Avoid in patients with chronic kidney disease or in surgeries with a high risk of bleeding or where bleeding cannot be easily controlled (i.e., neurosurgical procedures)
- *Neuraxial infusions with epidural catheters*: Consider in large abdominal surgeries

Patient Considerations

- *Elderly*: Can have increased sensitivity to medications, use lower doses and longer dosing intervals (see specific chapter for more details)
- *Delirium*: Benzodiazepines should be avoided especially in the elderly
- *Hepatic or renal dysfunction*: Effects metabolism and excretion of drugs or metabolites (see specific chapters for more details)
  - Active metabolites of Morphine in patients with renal dysfunction can lead to neurotoxicity [12]
  - Meperidine in the elderly and those with renal dysfunction can result in seizures due to accumulation of active metabolite Normeperidine [13, 14].

Allergies

- True allergies to opioids are uncommon
- Patients may perceive adverse reactions as allergies and request not to have certain opioids (Table 34.1).
  - Opioid equianalgesic chart with doses (Table 34.2)

Table 34.1 Pharmacokinetics (metabolism, elimination half-life, excretion, active metabolites)

Opioid	Phase 1 metabolism	Phase 2 metabolism	Active metabolites
Morphine	None	Glucuronidation	Morphine-3-G Glucuronide, Morphine-6-G Glucuronide
Codeine	CYP2D6	None	None
Hydrocodone	CYP2D6	None	None
Oxycodone	CYP3A4, CYP2D6	None	Noroxycodone
Methadone	CYP3A4, CYP2B6, CYP2C8, CYP2C19, CYP2D6, CYP2C9	None	None
Tramadol	CYP3A4, CYP2D6		O-desmethyltramadol
Fentanyl	CYP3A4		None
Hydromorphone	None	Glucuronidation	Hydromorphone-3-Glucuronide
Oxymorphone	None	Glucuronidation	6-Hydroxy-oxymorphone

Table 34.2 Opioid equianalgesic chart

Opioid	IV (mg)	PO (mg)	IV:PO ratio	Duration of action (hours)
Morphine	10	30	1:3	3–4
Codeine	130	200	1:1.5	3–4
Hydrocodone	N/A	30	N/A	3–4
Oxycodone	N/A	20–30	N/A	3–4
Methadone	10	3–5	1:2.5	4–12
Fentanyl	0.1	N/A	N/A	1–3
Hydromorphone	1.5	7.5	1:5	3–4
Oxymorphone	1	10	1:10	3–4

Opioid Analgesics

- *Morphine*
  - Prototypical long-acting opioid in the perioperative period
  - Widely available and cost-effective
  - Can be administered IV, IM, or PO
  - PO formulation is available in short-acting and sustained-release preparations
  - Avoid in patients with renal dysfunction
    Clinically active metabolites: Morphine 3 Glucuronide and Morphine 6 Glucuronide. Morphine's use is not recommended in patients with renal dysfunction as morphine-6-glucuronide can accumulate in renal failure leading to respiratory depression, myoclonus, and seizures.
- *Hydromorphone*
  - Roughly five times more potent than morphine
  - Good alternative for morphine intolerant patients
  - Available in IV and PO formulary [15, 16].
  - It is metabolized in the liver to hydromorphone-3-glucoronide (H3G) which itself has no analgesic properties. However, this H3G metabolite is renally cleared. There is some literature to suggest that H3G accumulation in renal failure can lead to neuroexcitation with symptoms such as restlessness, agitation, hallucination, and hyperalgesia. Therefore caution is advised when using hydromorphone in this patient population.
- *Fentanyl*
  - Highly potent analgesic
  - 75–125 times more potent than morphine
  - Relatively short duration of action
  - Being the most commonly used opioid intraoperatively, fentanyl is an excellent choice for the first hours after surgery as a patient's response to the drug may already be known.
  - Safe option in cases of hepatic dysfunction
- *Methadone*
  - Long-acting opioid
  - Highly variable potency and bioavailability
  - The analgesic profile is much shorter than its pharmacokinetic profile (i.e., severe respiratory suppression and somnolence despite inadequate pain control).
  - Acts as a mu receptor agonist and a *N*-methyl-D-aspartate (NMDA) antagonist
  - Can be used to limit tolerance and overall dosage of other opioids postoperatively in patients requiring high-dose opioids.
  - Available in IV and PO formulation
  - At high doses >100 mg, it can cause a prolonged QT syndrome
  - Metabolized in the liver to inactive metabolites

- *Meperidine*
  - Synthetic opioid
  - Limited use due to its active metabolite Normeperidine
  - Toxicity can cause myoclonus and seizures
  - Acts as a mu agonist and has some alpha-2 agonist properties
  - Inhibits the uptake of serotonin and may precipitate serotonin syndrome
  - Used in low dose for the treatment of postoperative rigors
- *Oxycodone*
  - Synthetic oral opioid useful for moderate-to-severe pain
  - Available in short- and long-acting formulations
  - Low-dose combination formulations with NSAIDS useful for mild-to-moderate pain
  - Caution in patients with drug abuse history
- *Oxymorphone*
  - Semisynthetic opioid derivative of morphine
  - Available in IV, short- and long-acting oral and suppository formulation
- *Tramadol*
  - Oral agent only
  - Acts weakly at the mu receptor in addition to inhibition of serotonin and norepinephrine reuptake
  - Caution in patients with a seizure history and those on warfarin therapy
  - Use contraindicated in patients on MAOIs
  - Can precipitate serotonin syndrome
- *Buprenorphine*
  - Mixed opioid agonists–antagonist
  - Mu receptor agonist–antagonist
  - Great affinity for the mu receptor (50 times that of morphine)
  - Associated with respiratory suppression resistant to naloxone treatment (Tables 34.1 and 34.2)

Complications

- *Overdose*:
  - Miosis, stupor, apnea, respiratory suppression
  - Other management can be found in Opioid Overdose chapter

Side-Effect Management

- *Constipation*
  - Bowel regimen with Senna, Docusate and/or Dulcolax
  - For persistent constipation or ileus, Methylnaltrexone subcutaneous dose of 0.15 mg/kg every other day has been used with success in chronic pain populations [17, 18].

- *Sedation*
  - Decreasing demand dose or continuous infusion, changing lock out time
  - In opiate naïve or patient's sensitive to medications, consider no continuous infusion as this can avoid excess sedation
  - Consider opioid rotation
- *Nausea/vomiting*
  - Consider opioid rotation depending on severity of symptoms
  - Antiemetics available as needed [19]
    Ondansetron 4–8 mg every 6–8 h
    Metoclopramide 10 mg every 6–8 h
    Promethazine 12.5–25 mg every 4–6 h
- *Pruritus*
  - Consider opioid rotation in severe cases
  - Diphenhydramine may be beneficial but can cause unwanted sedation.
    Diphenhydramine 12.5–25 mg IV, 25–50 mg PO every 4–6 h
  - Naloxone: At low doses can effectively decrease pruritus without increasing pain scores [20]
  - Nalbuphine: Up to 10 mg may be given in divided doses without reversing analgesia

Opioid Antagonists

- Naloxone:
  - A competitive opioid antagonist
  - Duration of action of 20–90 min
  - If there is respiratory depression opioids should be discontinued and Naloxone should be given
  - Start at 0.04 mg to avoid precipitating severe withdrawal symptoms [21]
  - Naloxone dose can be increased every 2 min up to a maximum of 15 mg [22].
  - Given that the action of naloxone is shorter than the action of many if profound respiratory depression remains following discontinuation of the patient-controlled analgesia (PCA) a naloxone infusion or endotracheal intubation maybe necessary to maintain ventilation [22, 23]

Nonopioid Analgesics

- *NSAIDS*
  - Can decrease opioid requirements and decrease PONV
  - Theoretical concerns of platelet function and bone healing must be considered.
  - NSAIDS must be used with caution in patients with renal dysfunction and those with gastritis.

- *Acetaminophen or Paracetamol* (*intravenous acetaminophen*)
  - Opioid sparing effects
  - Available in injectable, suppository, or oral forms
  - Avoid in liver dysfunction or in allergy states
- *Alpha-2 agonists*: *Clonidine and Dexmedetomidine*
  - Shown to decrease opioid requirements
  - Can be given as a postoperative sedative
  - Can cause hemodynamic changes
- *Anticonvulsants*: *Gabapentin, pregabalin*
  - To treat chronic neuropathic pain
  - A single oral preoperative dose can decrease opioid requirements postoperatively.
  - Can decrease chronic postsurgical pain
- *NMDA-receptor antagonists*: *Ketamine*
  - Given intravenously to decrease postoperative pain
  - Bolus of 0.5 mg/kg followed by a continuous infusion of 2–4 µg/kg/min during surgery and continued post-operatively in a monitored setting.
- *Glucocorticoids*: *Dexamethasone*
  - 0.1–0.2 mg/kg can reduce postoperative pain and opioid consumption

Analgesic Techniques

- *Intravenous PCA* (*Table 34.3, 34.4, 34.5, and 34.6*)
  - Delivery of medications through the dose-metered infusion pumps operated by patient based on their level of pain.
  - Inter-patient variability of opioid requirements and reported pain score response to analgesics make PCA ideal for patients with severe pain [24].
  - Self-titration of opioids to maintain a minimal blood concentration at which pain is alleviated without producing undesirable side effects [25, 26].
  - Titration of a predetermined demand dosage and set time (lock out interval) at which the patient can self-administer an analgesic.
  - PCA use has been associated with increased patient satisfaction and greater pain control.
  - Pain scores, side effects, and daily opioid requirements have to be documented by medical staff.
  - If adequate pain control is not attained due to side effects the PCA settings or the delivered opioid must be changed.

Table 34.3 Common patient-controlled analgesia regimens (opioid naïve patients)

Opioid	Demand dose	Lockout (minutes)	Continuous Basal
Morphine	1–2 mg	6–10	0–2 mg/h
Hydromorphone	0.2–0.4 mg	6–10	0–0.4 mg/h
Fentanyl	20–50 µg	5–10	0–60 µg/h

Table 34.4 PCA troubleshooting

General	Always check vitals and r/o respiratory depression
	Check pump to verify correct usage
	Check catheter depth, connection, and tubing
	Check for CSF prior to any bolus
	For any opioid adverse events consider changing to plain bupivacaine
Patient in pain	Check BP; Bolus; Monitor for comfort and vitals
	Consider increasing dose or decreasing lockout time (15 min)
Sedation	Assess for respiratory distress Naloxone? 02
	Check PCA settings
	IV: Decrease dose; change opioid
	Epi: Change to plain bag
Respiratory depression	Stop Pump!! Check ABGs, Assess, Arouse
	Titrate Naloxone (dilute to 40 µg/mL
Confusion	Change opioid
Pruritus	Decrease dose; change opioid; Benadryl
	Naloxone (20–40) µg
Nausea/ vomiting	Decrease dose; Change opioid; Antiemetic

Table 34.5 Epidural PCA issues

Hypertension	Aspirate catheter and check for CSF
	Decrease rate of stop infusion
Unilateral analgesia	Withdraw catheter 1 cm
	Bolus in lateral position painful side down
Lower extremity weakness	Aspirate catheter and check for CSF
	Decrease rate or stop infusion
	Neuro/NS consult if does not resolve
Blood/fluid around catheter	Change dressing and check catheter depth

Table 34.6 PCA guidelines

IV PCA guidelines starting dose	**Morphine**: (2 mg/mL: 0/14/8
	Fentanyl: (25 µg/mL: 0/18/8
	Hydromorphone: (2 mg/mL): 0/0.2/8
Epidural PCA guidelines (all + 0.1 % Bupivacaine; yellow tubing)	Standard + Fentanyl 5 µg/mL
	Low-dose + Fentanyl 2 µg/mL
	Plain = no Fentanyl
	Common orders: 4/2/20 or 6/2/20
	Peripheral Catheter: Plain @ 8–10 mL/h

08/0.8/7 = 0 basal; 0.8 bolus; 8 min lockout; 7 doses/h

- PCA is contraindicated in patients with altered mental status or those unable to grasp concept of PCA (low education level or mental retardation).
- Opioid/dosing regimens: (Table 34.7)
  - In an opioid naïve patient, a background continuous infusion is associated with a greater occurrence of respiratory suppression in adult patients [26, 27].
  - Once a patient's pain is resolving, PCA usage should be terminated and converted to an as-needed basis (PRN) of IV or PO regimens.

Table 34.7 Common patient-controlled epidural analgesia infusions

Drug combination	Solution (%)	Bolus dose of Bupivacaine (%)	Basal infusion	Demand dose	Basal infusion adjustment for inadequate pain control
Morphine	0.01	0.5–0.25	6–8 mL/h	1–2 mL every 10–15 min	1 mL of solution
Bupivacaine	0.05–0.1				
Fentanyl	0.001	0.5–0.25	0.1–0.15 mL/kg/h	1–2 mL every 10–15 min	1 mL of solution
Bupivacaine	0.05–0.1				
Hydromorphone	0.0025–0.005	0.5–0.25	6–8 mL/h	1–2 mL every 10–15 min	1 mL of solution
Bupivacaine	0.05–0.1				

Neuraxial Analgesia

Brief overview

- Local anesthetics and opioids placed for anesthesia in surgical procedures provide additional postoperative analgesia.
- Randomized controlled trials have yet to demonstrate decreased perioperative morbidity and morality in patients managed with Neuraxial anesthesia as compared to general anesthesia.
- Can decrease incidence of venous and arterial thrombosis and also decrease blood loss in total hip or knee surgery [28, 29]

Indications and contraindications:

- Lower extremity orthopedic procedures, abdominal surgery, and thoracic surgery
- Perioperative regional anesthesia may decrease the incidence of postsurgical chronic pain [30].
- In the presence of anticoagulation therapy, use ASRA guidelines for Neuraxial techniques [31, 32].
- *Absolute and relative contraindications* [33]:
  - Sepsis
  - Site infection
  - Severe hypovolemia or hypotension
  - Coagulopathy
  - Severe valvular disease
  - Patient refusal

Techniques:

- Intrathecal opioids
- Epidural analgesia with local anesthetics

Postoperative management:

- Dosing regimens for postoperative analgesia
  - *Epidural*: Commonly used epidural opioid/ Bupivacaine combination [34]
  - *Continuous spinal analgesia*:
    - Use dilute Bupivacaine 0.0625 %+Fentanyl 2 µg/ mL solution at 2 mL/h
    - No bolus to avoid high spinal
  - *Single bolus intrathecal opioids*:
    - Decrease need for systemic opioids
    - Intrathecal morphine >500 µg produces more side effects [35–38]
    - Analgesia and respiratory depression with hydrophilic opioids peaks within 6 h and persists for 18–24 h [38].
    - Patients should be closely monitored by continuous pulse oximetry for 12 h
- *Low dose* (knee replacement, hip replacement, TURP): 50–200 µg
- *Moderate dose* (Abdominal hysterectomy, colon surgery, spinal surgery) [38, 39]: 200–400 µg
- *High dose* (Major abdominal aortic surgery, cardiac surgery, thoracotomy surgery [38, 39]: 400–500 µg (Table 34.8)

Troubleshooting epidural/spinal catheters

- Check dermatomal distribution by assessing sensation to cold or pinprick
- Check catheter insertion site at skin. Ideally catheters should be 4–5 cm within the epidural space and 2–3 cm within the intrathecal space.
- Check tubing. Look for leakage around the catheter site.
- When dosing through a Neuraxial catheter, always monitor HR, BP, and respiratory status for 15–20 min after bolus dose.

  - *Nonfunctional catheter/no analgesia*:
    - Always aspirate catheter to check to in advertent intravascular or intrathecal migration
      Intrathecal: 1–2 mL of 0.25–0.5 % Bupivacaine
      Epidural: 3–5 mL of 2 % Lidocaine
  - *Inadequate analgesia*:
    - Always aspirate catheter to check to inadvertent intravascular or intrathecal migration and increase infusion by 2 mL/h.
      Intrathecal: 1–2 mL 0.25 % Bupivacaine
      Thoracic epidural: 3–5 mL of 2 % lidocaine, 0.25–0.5 % Bupivacaine
      Lumbar epidural: 5–10 mL of 2 % Lidocaine, 0.25–0.5 % Bupivacaine

- *Migrated catheter*:
  - Aspirate through catheter
  - Repeat test dose with 3 mL 1.5 % lidocaine with Epinephrine 1:200,000
  - If one-sided options are to increase infusion rate or bolus 5–10 mL of 0.25–0.5 % Bupivacaine. If block continues to be one-sided, withdraw catheter 1–2 cm and reassess.
  - If no resolution removes existing catheter and replaces with new catheter at same site or adjacent intervertebral level.
- *Disconnected catheter*:
  - Using a sterile technique, clean catheter with Chlorhexidine or alcohol and cut off 2 in. from the end of catheter with sterile scissors.
  - Reconnect to a new filter and restart infusion
- *Hypotension*:
  - Depending on cardiopulmonary status, fluid bolus 500–1,000 mL of crystalloid.
  - Decrease infusion rate
  - With persistent hypotension, consider stopping infusion and control pain with intravenous analgesics/opioid PCAs.

Complications and Management

- Signs/symptoms of local anesthetic overdose/toxicity
  - *Immediate signs*: Circum-oral numbness, Dysphoria/confusion, tinnitus, restlessness, agitation
  - *CNS depression*: Drowsiness, loss of consciousness, slurred speech, tonic clonic seizures
  - *Respiratory depression or arrest*
  - *Cardiovascular depression*: Myocardial depression, Bradycardia, Ventricular fibrillation

Treatment of Overdose or Toxicity

- Catheter removal: Check American Society of Regional Anesthesia Guidelines for anticoagulation details [31, 32, 40].
- Stop infusion and transition patient to PO analgesics or initiate opioid PCA
- Intra-lipid dosing regimens [41, 42]:
  - 1.5 mL/kg of 20 % Intra-lipid IV bolus followed by an infusion of 0.25 mL/kg/min for 30 min. Increase infusion to 0.5 mL/kg/min for 60 min

Management of Retained Catheter

- There are no consensus guidelines

- Case reports and expert opinions recommend computed tomography (CT) imaging to localize catheter fragment.
- Many catheters are ferromagnetic, so magnetic resonance imaging (MRI) is not recommended
- If patients are asymptomatic, conservative observation is recommended
- For patients with persistent paresthesias, neurosurgical consultation for fragment removal should be considered [43, 44].

Anticoagulation and Neuraxial Catheters

- For catheter removal INR <1.5
  - *Unfractionated heparin*:
    For patients on subcutaneous heparin for >4 days, check platelets to rule out heparin-induced thrombocytopenia.
    Remove catheter 2–4 h after last heparin dose. Wait 1 h after catheter removal before restarting heparin
  - *Low molecular weight heparin (LMWH)*:
    Remove catheter 10–12 h after last dose of LMWH. Wait 2 h after catheter removal before redosing LMWH.

Peripheral Nerve Blocks

- Postoperative peripheral nerve blocks can be excellent analgesia option
- Types:
  - Single-shot peripheral nerve blocks
  - Continuous peripheral [45, 46] nerve blocks
- Benefits
  - Earlier return of bowel function
  - Earlier ambulation
  - Decreased nausea/vomiting
  - Decreased inflammatory stress response
  - Decreased perioperative use of opioids [47, 48]
  - Immunomodulation associated with local anesthetics may decrease cancer recurrence [45, 46]

1. **Interscalene blocks:**
   - *Indications*:
     - Shoulder surgery (total, hemiarthroplasty, rotator cuff repair, arthrodesis)
     - Frozen shoulder syndrome
     - Biceps surgery, proximal humerus fractures
   - *Dosing*:
     - Bolus 20 mL 1.5 % Mepivacaine + 20 mL of 0.5 % Ropivacaine
     - Infusion 0.2 % Ropivacaine at 5–10 mL/h

2. **Clavicular blocks** (**Supraclavicular, infraclavicular**):
   - *Indications*:
     - Elbow surgery/trauma
     - Distal Humerus surgery/trauma
     - Ulnar surgery/trauma
     - Hand surgery/trauma
   - *Dosing*:
     - Bolus: 20 mL 1.5 % Mepivacaine + 20 mL of 0.5 % Ropivacaine
     - Infusion: 0.2 % Ropivacaine at 5–10 mL/h
3. **Thoracic paravertebral blocks**:
   - *Indications*:
     - Breast augmentation/surgery
     - Thoracotomy
     - Rib fractures
     - Abdominal surgery: Laparotomy, nephrectomy, cystectomy
   - *Dosing*:
     - Bolus: Per catheter: 10 mL 1.5 % Mepivacaine + 10 mL 0.5 % Ropivacaine.
     - Infusion: 0.2 % Ropivacaine at 5–10 mL/h
4. **Lumbar plexus blocks**:
   - *Indications*:
     - Hip surgery/trauma
     - Femur surgery/trauma
   - *Dosing*:
     - Bolus: 10 mL 1.5 % Mepivacaine + 10 mL 0.5 % Ropivacaine
     - Infusion: 0.2 % Ropivacaine at 5–10 mL/h
5. **Lower extremity blocks**:
   - *Indications*:
     - Femoral block—Femur surgery/trauma
     - Femoral block/sciatic block—Knee surgery/trauma
     - Popliteal/Femoral—Sciatic—Tibial surgery/trauma
     - Popliteal—Fibula surgery/trauma
     - Ankle block/Popliteal block/Femoral—Sciatic blocks—Ankle surgery/trauma
   - *Dosing*:
     - Femoral nerve + Sciatic/Popliteal
       - Bolus: 10 mL 1.5 % Mepivacaine + 10 mL 0.5 % Ropivacaine
       - Infusion: 0.2 % Ropivacaine at 5–8 mL/h

Guidelines for Anticoagulation

- No specific guidelines exist for performing peripheral nerve blocks in anticoagulated patients
- When performing deep blocks and/or plexus blocks, it may be prudent to follow the guidelines for Neuraxial techniques as defined by the American society of regional anesthesia and pain medicine [31, 32, 40].

Key Points in Managing the Postsurgical Pediatric Patient

Pain assessment:
- Pediatric pain management is a challenging subspecialty of pain medicine
- There are several cognitive, maturational, and communication differences.
- Validated, age-specific pain scales such as the FACES scale or the face, legs, activity, cry, consolability (FLACC) scale attempt to assimilate behavioral changes with severity and intensity of pain.
- Acute pain in the pediatric patient population is under-recognized and undertreated [49].

Respiratory depression:
- Close monitoring with continuous pulse oximetry is imperative
- These patients are particularly sensitive to postoperative respiratory depression
- Children <60 weeks postconceptual age are monitored for 24 h after general anesthesia.
- Nonopioid analgesic regimens/doses:
  To minimize respiratory depression, multimodal analgesia with nonopioid analgesics is commonly used
  - Acetaminophen:
    - Maximum daily amount:
      For patients <60 kg: 75–100 mg/kg or 4,000 mg, whichever is less
      For patients >60 kg: 4,000 mg
      Rectal: 40 mg/kg
      Orally: 10–15 mg/kg
  - Ketorolac:
    - Neonates: Not routinely used
    - Infants >1 month and Children <2 years: 0.5 mg/kg IV every 6–8 h for up to 72 h [50, 51]
    - Children >2 years:
      0.5 mg/kg IV, max 30 mg
  - Ibuprofen:
    - Children <60 kg: Dose 5–10 mg/kg PO every 6–8 h; maximum dose 40 mg/kg/day
    - Children >60 kg: Dose 400–600 mg PO every 6–8 h; maximum dose 2,400 mg per day

Opioid Analgesic Regimens/Doses (Table 34.8 and 34.9)

Perioperative Management of the Chronic Pain/Opioid-Dependent Patient

- Opioid-dependent patients present a formidable challenge to the pain physician during the acute postoperative period.

Table 34.8 Common pediatric opioid analgesic regimens

Opioid	Bolus doses (IV) (<50 kg)	Bolus doses (IV) (>50 kg)	PO:IV ratio	PO dose (immediate release)
			NA	NA
Fentanyl	0.5–1 µg/kg every 1–2 h	25–50 µg every 1–2 h		0.05 mg/kg every 4 h
Hydromorphone	15 µg/kg every 1–2 h	15 µg/kg every 1–2 h	5:1	0.3 mg/kg every 4 h
Morphine	0.05–0.1 mg/kg every 1–2 h	0.05–0.1 mg/kg every 1–2 h	3:1	0.2 mg/kg every 4–8 h
Methadone	0.1 mg/kg every 5–10 h	0.1 mg/kg every 5–10 h	2:1	0.5–1 mg/kg every 4 h
Codeine	NA	NA	NA	0.1 mg/kg every 4 h
Oxycodone	NA	NA	NA	0.1 mg/kg every 4 h
Hydrocodone	NA	NA	NA	

Table 34.9 Common pediatric patient-controlled analgesia regimens

Weight (kg)	Opioid	Demand dose	Continuous infusion	Lock out (minutes)
<50	Morphine	15 µg/kg	10 µg/kg/h	8
	Fentanyl	0.5–1 µg/kg	0.5–1 µg/kg/h	8
	Hydromorphone	2–5 µg/kg	3 µg/kg/h	8
>50	Morphine	0.5–2.5 mg	0.5–1 mg/h	8
	Fentanyl	20–40 µg	20 µg/h	8
	Hydromorphone	0.1–0.4 mg	0.1–0.2 mg/h	8

- These patients are tolerant to many different analgesics and have developed hyperalgesia
- They may be physiologically dependent on opioids or other drugs such as alcohol.
- Polysubstance abuse may be present as well.
- Patient's pain is related to periprocedural over the basal requirements from previously diagnosed pain syndromes.

Strategies

Multimodal analgesia should always be employed when clinically applicable and not contraindicated [52–54].

- *Preoperative*:
  - No published guidelines
  - Continue their scheduled opioid regimens on the morning of surgery with a sip of water [52, 53].
  - Patients on methadone or buprenorphine maintenance regimens should continue their regimens on the day of surgery and restart the regimen once oral intake has resumed [52, 53].
  - For patients who have not received their basal opioid requirements, provide oral equivalent doses in the preoperative holding area or incorporate equivalent doses intravenously during induction of anesthesia [52, 53].
  - Effective communication between the pain physician and the anesthesiologist is crucial to good patient care.
  - Transdermal patch or implantable pumps
    - Continue intrathecal pumps or patches during the perioperative period.
    - For cases during which a warming blanket will be used, there are cases of opioid overdose in the literature due to changes in transdermal opioid absorption from increased blood flow [55].
    - Of note, despite removing the patch, significant doses of opioids will continue to be absorbed from the skin layers for up to 12 h [52].
    - When restarting fentanyl transdermal patches postoperatively, it may take 6–12 h to establish baseline analgesic effects, with peak effects being reached in 20–72 h [53].
    - When restarting transdermal fentanyl patches, short-acting opioids rather than long-acting opioid analgesics should be used in combination with close monitoring by continuous pulse oximetry to avoid respiratory depression [52, 53].
- *Postoperative:*
  - Opioid dose regimens: Incorporate basal opioid requirements in addition to a 20–50 % increase in opioid doses above baseline to account for acute surgical pain.
  - Downtitration to presurgical doses is dependent on the type of surgery and should be done slowly 3–7 days [53].
  - PCA
  - Methadone:
    - Through activation of a different subtype of mu opioid receptors more resistant to morphine tolerance, activation of descending alpha adrenergic receptors and NMDA glutamate receptor antagonism, methadone may mitigate morphine tolerance and opioid-induced hyperalgesia [53].
    - Opioid rotations: In opioid-dependent patients, adequate pain may not be achieved with dose escalations [56–58]. Oftentimes, opioid rotations may allow for improved pain control at lower

Equianalgesic doses [56–58]. Opioid doses should be decreased by 25–75 % to account for incomplete cross tolerance [52, 56–58]

Withdrawal: see specific chapter on this

- Opioid withdrawal syndrome is characterized by increased sympathetic and parasympathetic responses with nausea, vomiting, muscle aches, lacrimation, pupillary dilation, diarrhea, fever, and insomnia being common symptoms.

References

1. Phillips DM. JCAHO pain management standards are unveiled. Joint Commission on Accreditation of Healthcare Organizations. JAMA. 2000;284:428–9.
2. Apfelbaum JL, Chen C, Mehta SS, Gan TJ. Postoperative pain experience: results from a national survey suggest postoperative pain continues to be undermanaged. Anesth Analg. 2003;97:534–40. Table of contents.
3. Woolf CJ. Pain: moving from symptom control toward mechanism-specific pharmacologic management. Ann Intern Med. 2004;140:441–51.
4. Mannion RJ, Woolf CJ. Pain mechanisms and management: a central perspective. Clin J Pain. 2000;16:S144–56.
5. Woolf CJ. Somatic pain—pathogenesis and prevention. Br J Anaesth. 1995;75:169–76.
6. Woolf CJ. Generation of acute pain: central mechanisms. Br Med Bull. 1991;47:523–33.
7. Ladabaum U, Minoshima S, Owyang C. Pathobiology of visceral pain: molecular mechanisms and therapeutic implications V. Central nervous system processing of somatic and visceral sensory signals. Am J Physiol Gastrointest Liver Physiol. 2000;279:G1–6.
8. Paul-Dauphin A, Guillemin F, Virion JM, Briancon S. Bias and precision in visual analogue scales: a randomized controlled trial. Am J Epidemiol. 1999;150:1117–27.
9. Bijur PE, Silver W, Gallagher EJ. Reliability of the visual analog scale for measurement of acute pain. Acad Emerg Med. 2001;8:1153–7.
10. Schnakers C, Chatelle C, Majerus S, Gosseries O, De Val M, Laureys S. Assessment and detection of pain in noncommunicative severely brain-injured patients. Expert Rev Neurother. 2010;10:1725–31.
11. Schmidt PC, Ruchelli G, Mackey SC, Carroll IR. Perioperative gabapentinoids: choice of agent, dose, timing, and effects on chronic postsurgical pain. Anesthesiology. 2013;119:1215–21.
12. Angst MS, Buhrer M, Lotsch J. Insidious intoxication after morphine treatment in renal failure: delayed onset of morphine-6-glucuronide action. Anesthesiology. 2000;92:1473–6.
13. Stone PA, Macintyre PE, Jarvis DA. Norpethidine toxicity and patient controlled analgesia. Br J Anaesth. 1993;71:738–40.
14. McHugh GJ. Norpethidine accumulation and generalized seizure during pethidine patient-controlled analgesia. Anaesth Intensive Care. 1999;27:289–91.
15. Hong D, Flood P, Diaz G. The side effects of morphine and hydromorphone patient-controlled analgesia. Anesth Analg. 2008;107:1384–9.
16. Angst MS, Drover DR, Lotsch J, Ramaswamy B, Naidu S, Wada DR, Stanski DR. Pharmacodynamics of orally administered sustained-release hydromorphone in humans. Anesthesiology. 2001;94:63–73.
17. Thomas J, Karver S, Cooney GA, Chamberlain BH, Watt CK, Slatkin NE, Stambler N, Kremer AB, Israel RJ. Methylnaltrexone for opioid-induced constipation in advanced illness. N Engl J Med. 2008;358:2332–43.
18. Portenoy RK, Thomas J, Moehl Boatwright ML, Tran D, Galasso FL, Stambler N, Von Gunten CF, Israel RJ. Subcutaneous methylnaltrexone for the treatment of opioid-induced constipation in patients with advanced illness: a double-blind, randomized, parallel group, dose-ranging study. J Pain Symptom Manage. 2008;35:458–68.
19. Rawlinson A, Kitchingham N, Hart C, McMahon G, Ong SL, Khanna A. Mechanisms of reducing postoperative pain, nausea and vomiting: a systematic review of current techniques. Evid Based Med. 2012;17:75–80.
20. Murphy JD, Gelfand HJ, Bicket MC, Ouanes JP, Kumar KK, Isaac GR, Wu CL. Analgesic efficacy of intravenous naloxone for the treatment of postoperative pruritus: a meta-analysis. J Opioid Manag. 2011;7:321–7.
21. Inturrisi CE. Clinical pharmacology of opioids for pain. Clin J Pain. 2002;18:S3–13.
22. Boyer EW. Management of opioid analgesic overdose. N Engl J Med. 2012;367:146–55.
23. Evans JM, Hogg MI, Lunn JN, Rosen M. Degree and duration of reversal by naloxone of effects of morphine in conscious subjects. Br Med J. 1974;2:589–91.
24. Woodhouse A, Ward ME, Mather LE. Intra-subject variability in post-operative patient-controlled analgesia (PCA): is the patient equally satisfied with morphine, pethidine and fentanyl? Pain. 1999;80:545–53.
25. Austin KL, Stapleton JV, Mather LE. Relationship between blood meperidine concentrations and analgesic response: a preliminary report. Anesthesiology. 1980;53:460–6.
26. Grass JA. Patient-controlled analgesia. Anesth Analg. 2005;101:S44–61.
27. George JA, Lin EE, Hanna MN, Murphy JD, Kumar K, Ko PS, Wu CL. The effect of intravenous opioid patient-controlled analgesia with and without background infusion on respiratory depression: a meta-analysis. J Opioid Manag. 2010;6:47–54.
28. Tuman KJ, McCarthy RJ, March RJ, DeLaria GA, Patel RV, Ivankovich AD. Effects of epidural anesthesia and analgesia on coagulation and outcome after major vascular surgery. Anesth Analg. 1991;73:696–704.
29. Christopherson R, Beattie C, Frank SM, Norris EJ, Meinert CL, Gottlieb SO, Yates H, Rock P, Parker SD, Perler BA, et al. Perioperative morbidity in patients randomized to epidural or general anesthesia for lower extremity vascular surgery. Perioperative Ischemia Randomized Anesthesia Trial Study Group. Anesthesiology. 1993;79:422–34.
30. Andreae MH, Andreae DA. Local anaesthetics and regional anaesthesia for preventing chronic pain after surgery. Cochrane Database Syst Rev. 2012;10, CD007105.
31. Horlocker TT, Wedel DJ, Rowlingson JC, Enneking FK, Kopp SL, Benzon HT, Brown DL, Heit JA, Mulroy MF, Rosenquist RW, Tryba M, Yuan CS. Regional anesthesia in the patient receiving antithrombotic or thrombolytic therapy: American Society of Regional Anesthesia and Pain Medicine Evidence-Based Guidelines (Third Edition). Reg Anesth Pain Med. 2010;35:64–101.
32. Horlocker TT, Wedel DJ, Rowlingson JC, Enneking FK. Executive summary: regional anesthesia in the patient receiving antithrombotic or thrombolytic therapy: American Society of Regional Anesthesia and Pain Medicine Evidence-Based Guidelines (Third Edition). Reg Anesth Pain Med. 2010;35:102–5.
33. Cwik J. Postoperative considerations of neuraxial anesthesia. Anesthesiol Clin. 2012;30:433–43.

34. de Leon-Casasola OA, Lema MJ. Postoperative epidural opioid analgesia: what are the choices? Anesth Analg. 1996;83:867–75.

35. Meylan N, Elia N, Lysakowski C, Tramer MR. Benefit and risk of intrathecal morphine without local anaesthetic in patients undergoing major surgery: meta-analysis of randomized trials. Br J Anaesth. 2009;102:156–67.

36. Blay M, Orban JC, Rami L, Gindre S, Chambeau R, Batt M, Grimaud D, Ichai C. Efficacy of low-dose intrathecal morphine for postoperative analgesia after abdominal aortic surgery: a double-blind randomized study. Reg Anesth Pain Med. 2006;31:127–33.

37. Palmer CM, Emerson S, Volgoropolous D, Alves D. Dose-response relationship of intrathecal morphine for postcesarean analgesia. Anesthesiology. 1999;90:437–44.

38. Rathmell JP, Lair TR, Nauman B. The role of intrathecal drugs in the treatment of acute pain. Anesth Analg. 2005;101:S30–43.

39. Mugabure Bujedo B. A clinical approach to neuraxial morphine for the treatment of postoperative pain. Pain Res Treat. 2012;2012:612145.

40. Horlocker TT. Regional anaesthesia in the patient receiving antithrombotic and antiplatelet therapy. Br J Anaesth. 2011;107 Suppl 1:i96–106.

41. Corcoran W, Butterworth J, Weller RS, Beck JC, Gerancher JC, Houle TT, Groban L. Local anesthetic-induced cardiac toxicity: a survey of contemporary practice strategies among academic anesthesiology departments. Anesth Analg. 2006;103:1322–6.

42. Rosenblatt MA, Abel M, Fischer GW, Itzkovich CJ, Eisenkraft JB. Successful use of a 20% lipid emulsion to resuscitate a patient after a presumed bupivacaine-related cardiac arrest. Anesthesiology. 2006;105:217–8.

43. Mitra R, Fleischmann K. Management of the sheared epidural catheter: is surgical extraction really necessary? J Clin Anesth. 2007;19:310–4.

44. Forsythe A, Gupta A, Cohen SP. Retained intrathecal catheter fragment after spinal drain insertion. Reg Anesth Pain Med. 2009;34:375–8.

45. Exadaktylos AK, Buggy DJ, Moriarty DC, Mascha E, Sessler DI. Can anesthetic technique for primary breast cancer surgery affect recurrence or metastasis? Anesthesiology. 2006;105:660–4.

46. Kavanagh T, Buggy DJ. Can anaesthetic technique effect postoperative outcome? Curr Opin Anaesthesiol. 2012;25:185–98.

47. Aguirre J, Del Moral A, Cobo I, Borgeat A, Blumenthal S. The role of continuous peripheral nerve blocks. Anesthesiol Res Pract. 2012;2012:560879.

48. Carli F, Kehlet H, Baldini G, Steel A, McRae K, Slinger P, Hemmerling T, Salinas F, Neal JM. Evidence basis for regional anesthesia in multidisciplinary fast-track surgical care pathways. Reg Anesth Pain Med. 2011;36:63–72.

49. Chidambaran V, Sadhasivam S. Pediatric acute and surgical pain management: recent advances and future perspectives. Int Anesthesiol Clin. 2012;50:66–82.

50. Burd RS, Tobias JD. Ketorolac for pain management after abdominal surgical procedures in infants. South Med J. 2002;95:331–3.

51. Moffett BS, Wann TI, Carberry KE, Mott AR. Safety of ketorolac in neonates and infants after cardiac surgery. Paediatr Anaesth. 2006;16:424–8.

52. Mehta V, Langford RM. Acute pain management for opioid dependent patients. Anaesthesia. 2006;61:269–76.

53. Mitra S, Sinatra RS. Perioperative management of acute pain in the opioid-dependent patient. Anesthesiology. 2004;101:212–27.

54. Smith HS. Perioperative intravenous acetaminophen and NSAIDs. Pain Med. 2011;12:961–81.

55. Frolich MA, Giannotti A, Modell JH. Opioid overdose in a patient using a fentanyl patch during treatment with a warming blanket. Anesth Analg. 2001;93:647–8.

56. Nalamachu SR. Opioid rotation in clinical practice. Adv Ther. 2012;29:849–63.

57. Mercadante S. Opioid rotation for cancer pain: rationale and clinical aspects. Cancer. 1999;86:1856–66.

58. Pereira J, Lawlor P, Vigano A, Dorgan M, Bruera E. Equianalgesic dose ratios for opioids: a critical review and proposals for long-term dosing. J Pain Symptom Manage. 2001;22:672–87.

Julia Sackheim, Thomas Riolo, and Jeremy J. Robbins

Abbreviations

aPTT	activated partial thromboplastin time
ASA	Aspirin
ASRA	Anesthesia Society of Regional Anesthesia and Pain Medicine
COX	Cylcooxygenase inhibitor
HIT	Heparin Induced Thrombocytopenia
INR	International normalized ratio
IV	Intravenous
ISIS	International Spine Interventional Society
LMWH	Low molecular weight heparin
NSAIDs	Non-steroidal anti-inflammatory drugs
PLT	Platelet
PT	Prothrombin time
SQ	Subcutaneous
UFH	Ultrafractionated heparin

Introduction

Blood thinning agents should be held prior to spinal injections to avoid bleeding complications in these patients. There is no exact method as to when to hold each hematologic-altering medication. Each physician has his/her own preference and different resources state different information,

J. Sackheim, D.O.
Department of Internal Medicine, Stony Brook University Hospital, Stony Brook, NY, USA
e-mail: julia.sackheim@stonybrookmedicine.edu

T. Riolo, D.O. (✉)
Department of Rehabilitation Medicine, New York University Langone Medical Center, New York, NY, USA
e-mail: Thomas.Riolo@nyumc.org

J.J. Robbins, D.O.
Department of Anesthesiology, University of Missouri Health System, Columbia, MO, USA
e-mail: robbsinsjj@health.missouri.edu

therefore always proceed with caution for the best results and the least amount of risks. It is important to always speak with the prescribing physician to see if it is ok to stop any medication prior to an injection. If the risk is too high to stop the medication, the procedure may not be able to be performed.

Antiplatelet Medications

It is recommended to use other resources when making decisions about when to stop and restart these medications.

- **Aspirin and Salicylate medications**
    - Can continue if strong indication for use [1]
    - Per ISIS, it is not necessary to stop ASA [2]
    - If patient is healthy with no strong indication, ok to discontinue prior
    - Low-dose ASA (81 mg) has higher bleeding risk than high dose [3]
    - In outpatient setting, consider stopping ASA 7 days before lumbar injections and 10 days prior to cervical epidurals [4].
    - *Increased caution when doing cervical and thoracic epidurals while patient is on these medications as the epidural space in these regions is smaller and more functional risk associated with hematoma formation at these locations* [1].
    - Patients with recently implanted coronary stents or unstable coronary syndromes have **increased risk of morbidity and mortality if aspirin is stopped before a procedure** [5–7]
    - Patients with drug eluting stents should only stop taking aspirin before an operation when there is a life-threatening bleeding risk [8].
    - ASA alone does not significantly increase the risk of spinal hematomas, unless there are comorbid factors [1].
- **NSAIDs and COX-2 inhibitors**
    - Include ibuprofen, Naproxen, Mobic, Arthrotec, Voltarin, Relafen, Daypro, Celebrex, and any other NSAIDs)

K.A. Sackheim, *Pain Management and Palliative Care: A Comprehensive Guide*,
DOI 10.1007/978-1-4939-2462-2_35, © Springer Science+Business Media New York 2015

- NSAIDs alone don't significantly increase risk of spinal hematoma [1]
- Not necessary to stop [2]
- Continue if strong indication for use. Discontinue 3 or more days before if patient has no strong indication [1].
- *Increased caution when doing cervical and thoracic due to reasons mentioned prior* [1].
- Spinal injection when the patient is only on ASA or NSAIDS has only shown to cause intraspinal hematomas when complications occurred, such as technical difficulties, concomitant heparin administration, and epidural venous angiomas [1].
- Combination of ASA or NSAIDs with Unfractionated heparin (UFH), LMWH, oral anticoagulants, and thrombolytics, as well as each other increases risk of spontaneous hemorrhaging, bleeding at site of injection, and spinal hematoma [1].
- COX-2 inhibitors have not been found to cause an increase in bleeding alone [1].
  COX-2 inhibitors + Warfarin → increase PT causing an increased risk of hemorrhagic complications [3]
- ASA, NSAIDs, and COX-2 inhibitors are ideal for the perioperative period with spinal injections [1].

- **Clopidogrel (Plavix)**
  - Injection with concurrent Clopidogrel is contraindicated due to high risk of bleeding [7]
  - Discontinue 7 days prior to procedure [1]
  - No incidences of spinal hematomas have been reported with Clopidogrel [1].
  - Many cardiac patients are on Clopidogrel and ASA. This combination has shown to increase the risk of spinal hematomas [1].
    In this situation, discontinue the Clopidogrel 7 days before, and continue the ASA. Restart the Clopidogrel 1-2 days after the procedure.

- **Ticlopidine (Ticlid)**
  - Discontinue 10–14 days prior to procedure [1], 14 days per ISIS [2]
  - Spinal hematomas have been reported with Ticlopidine [1]

- **Ticagrelor**
  - Greatly increase risk of bleeding [9]
  - Discontinue 5 days prior [9]

- **Platelet GP IIb/IIIa receptor antagonists**
  - *Abciximab (Repro)*
    Last dose must be at least 24–48 h prior [1]
  - *Eptifibatide (Integrelin)*
    Last dose must be 4–8 h prior [1]
  - Tirofiban (Aggrastat)
    Last dose must be 4–8 h prior [1]
  - Be aware that platelet GP IIb/IIIa receptor antagonists are typically prescribed in combination with ASA or heparin [3].

- **Cilastozal (Pletal)**
  - Hold 2 days [10]
- **Dipyridamole (Persantine) and Dipyridamole/ASA (Aggrenox)**
  - Hold 7 days [10]

Anticoagulant Medications

Permission should be obtained by prescribing physician before any of these medications are discontinued. Any procedure done on a patient who was on anticoagulants should be single needle a-traumatic placement. All patients on anticoagulant medications should be monitored for neurological issues following any spinal procedure. If the risks outweigh the benefits, you may not be able to proceed with injection.

Do not administer spinal injections if the patient displays signs of excessive anticoagulation, such as petechiae, bruising, bleeding from the IV site, or if the patient displays any pathological process such as sepsis, uremia, meningitis, skin, or soft tissue infections [4].

- **Warfarin (Coumadin)**
  - Contraindication if patient took Warfarin within 5 days prior [2, 3]
  - Check INR day of injection [1]
    - Ok to proceed with injection only if PT and INR are within normal limits [3]
    - INR ≤ 1.5 before spinal injection [1]
- **Heparin**
  - SQ Heparin (5,000 U q12h)
    - Minimal risk of spinal hematoma [3]
    - Perform injection before heparin is given [1]. Next dose of Heparin should be held for at least 1 h [11–15].
    - Risk of Heparin Induced Thrombocytopenia, which would present with decreased Platelets for > 5 days [1]
  - IV Heparin
    - Wait over 6 h after heparin administration to give spinal injection [4].
    - Wait at least 1 h after spinal injection to give heparin [3]
  - ASRA guidelines recommend holding dose prior to injection, restart 1 h after, monitor aPTT, and measure Platelet count prior to procedure if on unfractionated heparin for over 4 days
  - Therapeutic doses of Heparin are associated with a higher risk of bleeding than prophylactic doses.
  - Procedure should only be performed when APTT (or Anti-Xa) has normalized [16, 17]
  - Per ISIS, UFH is not contraindicated if the patient is receiving less than 5,000 U twice daily [2]
  - Concomitant use of Heparin with other anticoagulants/antiplatelets increase the risk of spinal hematomas [3]

- Bloody or difficult neuraxial needle placement may increase risk of bleeding, but no data has been found to support cancellation of procedure [1]
- **Low Molecular Weight Heparin (LMWH)**
  - Lovenox
    - If patient is receiving prophylactic Enoxaparin (Lovenox) at 1.5 mg/kg BID → Administer spinal injection 12 h after last LMWH dose [1]
    - If patient is receiving therapeutic Lovenox at 1 mg/kg BID or Lovenox 1.5 mg/kg QD → Administer spinal injection 24 h after last LMWH dose [1]
  - If patient is receiving Dalteparin (Fragmin) 120 U/kg BID or 200 U/kg QD, and Tinzaparin (Innohep) 175 U/kg QD → Administer spinal injection 24 h after last LMWH dose [1]
  - **Restarting LMWH after injection**
    - *When the patient is on BID dosing*:
      - Wait at least 24 h after spinal injection before restarting LMWH. The second dose of LMWH should be given another 24 h after the first dose [1].
    - *When the patient is on single-daily dosing*:
      - Wait 6–8 h after spinal injection before restarting LMWH. Administer second dose at least 24 h after the first dose [1].
- **Xarelto (Rivaroxaban)**
  - US boxed warning [18]. New medication with limited data
  - Epidural and Spinal Hematomas have occurred with use of spinal injection [18].
  - Discontinue at least 18 h prior to spinal injection [18].
  - Restart medication 6 h after spinal injection, and if traumatic puncture, do not restart until 24 h after [18]
- **Fondaparinux (Arixtra)**
  - US Boxed Warning [18]
  - Use with extreme caution, due to risk of developing spinal and epidural hematomas [19].
  - If prophylactic use, consider holding for 36 h prior to procedure and 12 h after procedure [20].
  - If therapeutic use (5–10 mg), do not perform procedure due to high risk of accumulation of drug [20].
- **Fibrinolytic/Thrombolytic drugs**
  - No definite recommendations
  - Contraindicated in Spinal Anesthesia [21]
  - Avoid these for 10 days after the procedure [22]
  - Reteplase, Alteplase, Anistreplase, Streptokinase, Tenecteplase
  - Follow fibrinogen levels (1.5–3 g/L)
- **Thrombin inhibitors**
  - No reported cases of spinal hematomas with injection, but may still be at risk [1]
  - No definitive recommendations, but thrombin inhibitors increase risk of bleeding.
  - Monitor by aPTT

- Lepirudin (Refludan)
  - Warning/Caution with neuraxial procedures [23]
  - Bleeding is the major adverse affect of the drug alone [23].
- *Desirudin (Revasc)*
  - Boxed warning [24]
  - Consider risk versus benefit [24]
- *Bivalirudin (Angiomax)*
  - Proximal use of spinal/epidural anesthesia is contraindicated [25]
- *Argatroban (Acova)*
  - Need to determine if patient is taking this due to history of HIT or acute HIT type II in which therapeutic anticoagulation is needed.
  - If HIT is acute, neuraxial blockade is not recommended [8]
- *Dabigatron (Pradaxa)*
  - *Discontinue 1–2 days prior if normal kidney function, and 3–5 days prior if kidney impairment [8]*
  - *Start 4 h after [3]*
  - *No reported spinal hematomas, but lack data [3]*
  - *Manufacturer advises AGAINST neuraxial blockade [8]*
- No antidote is available
- Concomitant use of the prior mentioned therapies with other anticoagulants/antiplatelets may increase the risk of bleeding [1]

Vitamins and Supplements

- **Vitamin C**
  - No box warnings or precautions advised with Vitamin C supplementation
- **Vitamin E (greater than 400 IU)**
  - Stop 7 days prior to procedure [10]
- **Hydroxocobalamin (Vitamin B12)**
  - No box warnings or precautions advised with B12 supplementation
- **Folic acid**
  - No box warnings or precautions advised with Folic Acid
- **Fish oil and Omega 3 fatty acids**
  - High doses (3–15 g/day) of fish oil increase bleeding time, but have not been shown to increase clinical bleeding [26].

Herbal Therapy

- Unlikely to cause increased risk of bleeding; not mandated to discontinue them or avoid regional anesthetic techniques [3].
- **Garlic** (standard dose is 4 g (2 cloves) [3]
  - Consider holding 7 days [1]

Table 35.1 Anticoagulants with half-lives, time to discontinue prior and restart after procedure

Drug	Preprocedure hold	Postprocedure restart	Monitoring	Metabolism	Platelet effect
UFH (PPX/TX)	6 h	1 h	aPTT, antifactor Xa	Renal	–
LMWH (PPX/TX)	12/24 h	6–8/24[a]	aPTT, antifactor Xa	Renal	–
ASA	7–10 days[b]	–	–	Liver/gut/plasma	Irreversible
Clopidrogel	7 days	–	–	Liver	Irreversible
Ticlodipine	10–14 days	–	–	Liver	Irreversible
Warfarin	Hold 5 days until INR under 1.4	–	PT/INR	Liver	–
Fondaparinux (PPX/TX)	36 h/contraindication	12 h/contraindication	None	Renal	–
Argatroban	Procedures contraindicated in acute HIT	–	aPTT	Liver	–
Dabigatran	2–5 days, although manufacturer advises against procedures	4 h	None	Liver/renal	–
Rivaroxaban	24 h[c]	6–8 h	None	Liver/renal/gut	–
NSAIDs	3 days	–	–	Renal	Reversible
Glycoprotein IIb/IIIa antagonists	Abciximab: 24–48 h	–	–	–	–
	Eptifibatide: 4–8 h				
	Tirofiban: 4–8 h				
Herbal medications	Variable	–	–	–	–

aPTT activated partial thromboplastin time, *PT* prothrombin time, *INR* international normalized ratio
[a]24 h hold until restart in cases of traumatic procedure
[b]ASA (aspirin) hold ONLY if on dual therapy with heparins
[c]Extreme caution should be used secondary to lack of sufficient literature

- **Ginkgo** (standard dose is 120–240 mg of standardized extract daily) [3]
  - Consider holding 36 h [1]
- **Ginseng** (standard dose of 1–2 g of root or 200 mg daily) [3]
  - Consider waiting 24 h [1]
  - Stop taking 10–14 days before, and restart 7 days after [27]
- **Feverfew**
  - Stop taking 7 days before [10]
- Concomitant use of the prior mentioned herbal therapies with other anticoagulants/antiplatelets may increase the risk of bleeding [3].

Table 35.1 lists anticoagulants with half-lives, the time to discontinue prior to a procedure, and when to restart after a procedure.

References

1. Benzon HT. Anticoagulants and neuraxial anesthesia. In: Benzon HT, Raja SN, Molloy RE, Liu SS, Fishman SM, editors. Essentials of pain medicine and regional anesthesia. 2nd ed. Philadelphia: Elsevier; 2005. p. 708–17.
2. Bogduk N. Practice guidelines for spinal diagnostic and treatment procedures. 2nd ed. San Francisco: International Spine Intervention Society; 2013. p. 9–15.
3. Horlocker TT, Wedel DJ, Rowlingson JC, Enneking FK, Kopp SL, Benzon HT. Regional anesthesia in the patient receiving antithrombotic or thrombolytic therapy. Reg Anesth Pain Med. 2010;35(1):64–101.
4. Fleisher LA, Gaiser R, Placement E. Lumbar epidural placement. Procedures consult. Philadelphia: Elsevier; 2008. http://www.proceduresconsult.com/medical-procedures/lumbar-epidural-placement-AN-016-procedure.aspx.
5. Ferrari E, et al. Coronary syndromes following aspirin withdrawal: a special risk for late stent thrombosis. J Am Coll Cardiol. 2005;45(3):456–9.
6. Collet JP, et al. Impact of prior use or recent withdrawal of oral antiplatelet agents on acute coronary syndromes. Circulation. 2004;110(16):2361–7. Epub 2004 Oct 11.
7. Burger W, et al. Low-dose aspirin for secondary cardiovascular prevention—cardiovascular risks after its perioperative withdrawal versus bleeding risks with its continuation—review and meta-analysis. J Intern Med. 2005;257(5):399–414.
8. Gogarten W, et al. Regional anaesthesia and antithrombotic agents: recommendations of the European Society of Anaesthesiology. Eur J Anaesthesiol. 2010;27(12):999–1015.
9. UpToDate. [Internet]. Lexi-comp Online™. Hudson: Ticagrelor: drug information. c1978-2013. [cited 2013 Feb 13]. http://www.uptodate.com/contents/ticagrelor-drug-information?source=search_result&search=ticagrelor&selectedTitle=1~28
10. Pauza K. Educational guidelines for interventional spinal procedures. American Academy of Physical Medicine and Rehab. 2001. http://www.google.com/url?sa=t&rct=j&q=&esrc=s&source=web&cd=13&ved=0CDwQFjACOAo&url=http%3A%2F%2Fwww.aapmr.org%2Fpractice%2Fguidelines%2FDocuments%2Fedguidelines.pdf&ei=ensIUYH0B5PC9gTLkoGoAw&usg=AFQjCNHkhq9aX8Y8rdMKmAC8L-P6YV01zQ&sig2=eYAzFfbzpp0CEqabZTifYQ&bvm=bv.41642243,d.eWU&cad=rja
11. Liu SS, Mulroy MF. Neuraxial anesthesia and analgesia in the presence of standard heparin. Reg Anesth Pain Med. 1998;23(6 Suppl 2):157–63.
12. Liau Pitarch JV, et al. Hemostasis-altering drugs and techniques for regional anesthesia and analgesia: safety recommendations. Rev Esp Anestesiol Reanim. 2005;52(4):248–50.

13. Gogarten W, et al. The use of concomitant antiplatelet drugs during neuraxial anesthesia is contraindicated in Germany. Reg Anesth Pain Med. 2003;28(6):585–6. author reply 586.

14. Horlocker TT, et al. Regional anesthesia in the anticoagulated patient: defining the risks. Reg Anesth Pain Med. 2003;28(3):172–97.

15. Kozek-Langenecker SA, et al. Locoregional anesthesia and coagulation inhibitors. Recommendations of the Task Force on Perioperative Coagulation of the Austrian Society for Anesthesiology and Intensive Care Medicine. Anaesthesist. 2005;54(5):476–84.

16. Vandermeulen EP, Van Aken H, Vermylen J. Anticoagulants and spinal-epidural anesthesia. Anesth Analg. 1994;79(6):1165–77.

17. Tryba M. European practice guidelines: thromboembolism prophylaxis and regional anesthesia. Reg Anesth Pain Med. 1998;23 (6 Suppl 2):178–82.

18. UpToDate. [Internet]. Lexi-comp Online™. Hudson: Rivaroxaban: drug information. c1978-2013. [cited 2013 Feb 13]. http://www.uptodate.com/contents/rivaroxaban-drug-information?source=search_result&search=rivaroxaban&selectedTitle=1~42

19. UpToDate. [Internet]. Lexi-comp Online™. Hudson: Fondaparinux: drug information. c1978-2013. [cited 2013 Feb 13]. http://www.uptodate.com/contents/fondaparinux-drug-information?source=search_result&search=fondaparinux&selectedTitle=1~47

20. Singelyn FJ, et al. The safety and efficacy of extended thromboprophylaxis with fondaparinux after major orthopedic surgery of the lower limb with or without a neuraxial or deep peripheral nerve catheter: the EXPERT Study. Anesth Analg. 2007;105(6):1540–7.

21. Clinical Pharmacology [Internet]. Elsevier. c2013. [cited 2013 Feb 13]. http://www.clinicalpharmacology-ip.com

22. Layton K, Kallmes D, Horlocker T. Recommendations for anticoagulated patients undergoing image-guided spinal procedures. AJNR Am J Neuroradiol. 2006;27:468–70. http://www.ajnr.org/content/27/3/468.full.

23. UpToDate. [Internet]. Lexi-comp Online™. Hudson: Lepirudin: drug information. c1978-2013. [cited 2013 Feb 13]. http://www.uptodate.com/contents/lepirudin-drug-information?source=search_result&search=lepirudin&selectedTitle=1~15

24. UpToDate. [Internet]. Lexi-comp Online™. Hudson: Desirudin: drug information. c1978-2013. [cited 2013 Feb 13]. http://www.uptodate.com/contents/desirudin-drug-information?source=search_result&search=desirudin&selectedTitle=1~4

25. UpToDate. [Internet]. Lexi-comp Online™. Hudson: Bilvarudin: drug information. c1978-2013. [cited 2013 Feb 13]. http://www.uptodate.com/contents/bilvarudin-drug- information?source=search_result&search=bivalirudin&selectedTitle=1~31

26. Knapp HR, Reilly IA, Alessandrini P, FitzGerald GA. In vivo indexes of platelet and vascular function during fish-oil administration in patients with atherosclerosis. N Engl J Med. 1986;314(15):937.

27. http://www.uwhealth.org/ [Internet]. Wisconsin: University of Wisconsin Hospitals and Clinics Authority. c06/20/2011. http://www.uwhealth.org/healthfacts/B_EXTRANET_HEALTH_INFORMATION-FlexMember-Show_Public_HFFY_112665 1115765.html

Injections in Patients with Bleeding Risks and Comorbid Conditions

36

Thomas Riolo, Brian Richard Forzani, and Aleksandr Levchenko

Abbreviations

aPTT	activated partial thromboplastin time
DDAVP	Desmopressin
GP	Glycoproteins
HELLP	**H** (hemolysis, which is the breaking down of red blood cells) **EL** (elevated liver enzymes) **LP** (low platelet count)
INR	International normalized ratio
LMWHs	Low molecular weight heparins
PLT	Platelet
PT/INR	Prothrombin time/international normalized ratio
U	Factor IX loading dose
VWD	von Willebrand's disease
VWF	von Willebrand factor

Introduction

Assessing bleeding risk for patients who are to undergo spinal/epidural or peripheral joint injections is patient dependent. As a physician, you will encounter patients with varying medical comorbidities that can affect their susceptibility to bleed. It is important to keep an open line of communication with the physicians managing their medical bleeding conditions to determine the safest way to proceed.

T. Riolo, D.O. (✉) • B.R. Forzani, M.D. • A. Levchenko, D.O.
Department of Rehabilitation Medicine, New York University
Langone Medical Center, New York, NY, USA
e-mail: Thomas.Riolo@nyumc.org; Brian.Forzani@nyumc.org;
Aleksandr.Levchenko@nyumc.org

Bleeding Risk of Spinal/Epidural Injections

- Bleeding is an inherent risk with potentially catastrophic effects when located in the small spaces surrounding the spinal cord.
- *Increased bleeding risk* [1–13]:
  - Abnormal acquired coagulation (Renal Failure, Liver Failure, Disseminated Intravascular Coagulation, HELLP, Malignancy)
  - Congenital bleeding disorders
  - Anticoagulant/Antiplatelet/Fibrinolytic medications
  - Thrombocytopenia—Platelet (PLT) count $</\mu$L 100,000
  - Elderly
  - Female
  - Spinal abnormalities (spina bifida/stenosis, spinal tumors, ankylosing spondylitis)
  - Presence of blood in the catheter during insertion/removal
  - Receive immediate pre- or postinjection anticoagulant administration

Risks of Peripheral Joint Injections

- Musculoskeletal and joint injections are regarded as low-risk procedures with papers quoting mild and self-limiting adverse events in only 2.4–12 % of patients [14–18]. Although infrequent, bleeding or hemarthrosis are the most common complications with joint injections [19].
- In patients with bleeding disorders or those taking anticoagulants, joint aspiration, or injection is controversial, however, the risks are low. A study by Bettencourt showed that patients taking warfarin, with international normalized ratios (INR) of 4.5 or greater, did not demonstrate an increased risk of significant bleeding [20].

K.A. Sackheim, *Pain Management and Palliative Care: A Comprehensive Guide*,
DOI 10.1007/978-1-4939-2462-2_36, © Springer Science+Business Media New York 2015

Hemarthrosis

- Accumulation of blood within the joint cavity, which has been shown to produce synovitis and joint destruction [21–24].
- Final result of these changes is referred to as chronic hemophilic arthropathy, which is characterized by pain, stiffness, functional disability, and deformity [25].

Spinal Bleeding

- Epidural hematomas are most common but still infrequent with an overall incidence of 1/150,000–190,000 epidural procedures [21].
- Epidural space is densely packed with vascular structures (epidural venous plexus) is implicated as the likely source of bleeding and puncture may result is devastating consequences.
- Subdural hematomas are far less common but can result in grave consequences [23].

  In a review of 61 reports of epidural or subdural hematomas following neuraxial procedures, a clotting anomaly or use of anticoagulant medication was present in 69 % of the cases [14]. Generally, presenting symptoms are the onset of radicular pain followed by progressive neurologic dysfunction.

Management of Bleeding Disorders Prior to Injections

- There is limited literature and no specific guidelines concerning the appropriate way to approach spinal procedures in patients with bleeding disorders.
- It is crucial to understand the bleeding risks associated and involve a hematologist familiar with bleeding disorders to improve patient safety.
- Bleeding complications from a preexisting hemorrhagic disorder in a patient with no history of excessive bleeding is a rare event [26–30].
- During history and physical it is important to elicit current and prior history of bleeding, easy bruising, renal, hepatic or oncological disease, systemic lupus erythematosus, as well as family history of bleeding can help identify those who need to be screened further [31].

Screening Tests for at Risk Patients

- *Prothrombin time/international normalized ratio (PT/ INR)*
  - Extrinsic pathway (I, II, V, VII, X)
  - Normal range INR: 0.9–1.1 [32]

- *Activated partial thromboplastin time (aPTT)*
  - Intrinsic pathway (VIII, IX, XI, XII)
  - Normal range aPTT: 25–35 s [32]
- *Platelet count*
  - Normal range: 150,000–450,000/μL [32]
  - If known or suspected thrombocytopenia, platelet count <150,000/μL [33]
  - In the absence of platelet dysfunction, most individuals can tolerate invasive procedures with platelet counts >80,000/μL [34]. Caution should be taken when platelet <100,000/μL.
- *Bleeding time*
  - Bleeding time prolongation occurs in patients with platelet disorders
  - If procedure performed on patient with history of spontaneous bleeding and platelet dysfunction, limit to only those patients with a normal platelet count prior to injection [33].
  - There is increasing evidence that the bleeding time is not a very reliable test [35] and does not correlate with risk of bleeding during invasive procedures [34].
  - No current indication before image-guided procedures [32]
- *Most common congenital bleeding disorders include*:
  - von Willebrand's disease
  - Hemophilia A (factor VIII deficiency)
  - Hemophilia B (factor IX deficiency)
  - Factor XI deficiency (Hemophilia C) [27]
- Idiopathic thrombocytopenic purpura is the most common acquired bleeding disorder [28, 29]

Von Willebrand's Disease (VWD)

- Autosomal-dominant transmitted disease with decreased, absent, or defective von Willebrand factor (VWF) that results in impaired platelet adhesion.
- *Three types of VWD*:
  - Type 1—least severe with partial deficiency of VWF and accounts for 70 % of cases [36].
  - Type 2—four subtypes (2A, 2B, 2M, and 2N) that reflect qualitative variants of VWF deficiencies.
  - Type 3—virtually complete deficiency of VWF
- Symptoms: may include bruising and mucosal bleeding
- Routine screening tests may reveal a prolonged aPTT and bleeding time. Platelet function analysis and specialized assays can confirm the diagnosis.
- Treatment prior to injection involves desmopressin (DDAVP), which raises VWF and factor VIII levels [33].
  - Dosing and timing may vary per physician, this should be discussed with a hematologist prior to injection
  - Dosing: 0.3 μg/kg IV in 50 mL saline over 20 min [34]

– Use in most patients with type 1, variable in type 2 (thrombocytopenia may worsen in type 2B patients), not for type 3
- Treatment prior to injection can also involve factor VIII/VWF replacement with concentrates containing all VWF multimers or cryoprecipitate [34]:
  – Dosing: 20–30 U/kg every 12 h for 5–7 days with goal VWF levels of 50 % prior to injection.
  – Use for type 2B and severe type 3
- Antifibrinolytic agents are additional options [34]:
  – E-aminocaproic acid
    Dosing: 50 mg/kg orally for 4–5 days prior to injection
  – Tranexamic acid
    Dosing: 25 mg/kg orally for 3–4 days prior to injection
  – They may be used alone or in combination with other agents and are useful in mucosal bleeding

Hemophilia

- Hemophilia A and B are inherited X-linked recessive disorders with defects in factor VIII and IX, respectively, that primarily afflict men.
- Severe hemophiliacs bleed with an annual average of 20–30 episodes of spontaneous or excessive bleeding, particularly into joints and muscles [26]. Mildly affected patients can bleed significantly after trauma or surgery.
- Hemophilia A and B both have prolonged aPTT; however, PT and bleeding times are normal.
- Prior to injection treatment includes factor VIII replacement [34]:
  – One unit of factor VIII activity per kilogram of body weight will result in an increase of factor VIII in the recipient's plasma of approximately 2 U/day.
  – Factor VIII loading dose (U) = $0.5 \times$ (% desired rise in factor VIII) × (patient weight in kg).
  – To maintain a level at or above the desired factor VIII activity, one half of the loading dose should be repeated every 8 h.
- Factor IX replacement [34]:
  – Factor IX loading dose (U) = $0.75 \times$ (% rise in factor IX desired) × (patient weight in kg).
  – Half-life of factor IX is 12–24 h
- Recombinant factor VIIa, a "universal" hemostatic agent, maybe used as well to control surgical or trauma-associated bleeding in hemophilia [26, 36, 37].
- Monitoring of factor levels is critical to prevent under- and overdosing. For most surgical procedures, the desired factor activity level should be between 80 and 100 % and duration of therapy between 7 and 10 days [34].

Immune Thrombocytopenic Purpura (ITP)

- An acquired autoimmune disorder, which results from antibodies directed against platelet glycoproteins (GP IIb/IIIa) [32].
- Thrombocytopenia may be clinically silent or associated with petechiae, easy bruising, or mucosal bleeding [33].
- Asymptomatic patients with platelet counts >50,000/μL and not receiving drugs that interfere with platelet function do not need medical intervention and can safely undergo minimally invasive procedures [34]. Some clinicians prefer >100,000/μL for safety.
- In patients with platelets count <50,000/μL, medical intervention with steroids, intravenous immune globulin, or platelet transfusions may be required to raise the platelet count [34].
- The management of these patients should be made in conjunction with a hematology specialist since no single algorithm is suitable for all patients [33].

Liver Disease: Coagulation Abnormalities

- Liver disease can lead to thrombocytopenia, platelet dysfunction, reduced production of clotting factors, increased factor consumption, and increased fibrinolysis [38]. All stages of liver disease increase the risk of bleeding [39, 40].
- Pre-procedure screening should include a platelet count, platelet function analysis, hemoglobin, PT, aPTT, and fibrinogen level [38].
- Fresh frozen plasma can be administered to correct markedly prolonged PT/aPTT times [34]. Repetitive infusions of 10–15 mL/kg every 12 h may be needed [33, 39].
- Other management strategies include vitamin K supplementation, platelets, and cryoprecipitate [38].
  – Cryoprecipitate infusions should be used if fibrinogen levels are less than 75 mg/dL [39]. One bag of cryoprecipitate may raise the serum concentration by 5 mg/dL with typically, two bags of cryoprecipitate should be given per 10 kg of body weight, every 12 h and the fibrinogen should be maintained above 125 mg/dL [33, 39].
  – Vitamin K supplementation may be sufficient in patients with biliary tract disorders or sterilization of the gut by broad-spectrum antibiotics with typical doses of 10 mg given subcutaneously on a daily basis and the PT being closely monitored [39].
  – Platelets should be maintained above 70,000–80,000/μL [34].

Renal Disease: Coagulation Abnormalities

- The potential for bleeding during invasive procedures in patients with uremia is significant [34]. Defects in platelets, subendothelial metabolism, platelet vessel interactions, and anemia may occur [41].
- Bleeding in uremic patients is typically mucosal, genito-urinary, subdural, or gastrointestinal [33].
- Renal disease augments the effects of antiplatelet drugs and low molecular weight heparins (LMWHs) [38]. Current LMWH preparations used in renal failure will have an impaired clearance and a prolonged half-life and are not completely reversed with protamine [34].
- A comprehensive coagulation profile must be performed in renal failure patients that are pending an invasive procedure.
  - Screening tests in these individuals include a PT and an aPTT [34].
  - The bleeding time is typically prolonged in uremia and is not predictive of bleeding [30]. Bleeding time, however, is useful in monitoring response to therapy [40].
- The coagulation abnormality may be corrected with pre-procedure dialysis, abstinence from platelet active drugs, correction of anemia, desmopressin, cryoprecipitate infusions, or estrogens [33].
  - A 10 U infusion of cryoprecipitate normalizes bleeding time in 50 % of uremic patients [41].
  - Cryoprecipitate has been largely replaced by desmopressin unless other coagulation factors such as fibrinogen need replacement [40, 41].
  - Intravenous administration of desmopressin (0.3–0.4 μg/kg over 20–30 min) improves bleeding time within 1 h, and this effect is maintained for 4–8 h [41].
  - Conjugated estrogen infusions (0.6/mg/kg/day × 5 days) or oral estrogens (50 mg/kg/day) shorten the bleeding time in uremia [34, 41]. The effect is slower in onset—about 6 h after the initial intravenous dose or 2 days after initiation of oral treatment and lasts for about 2 weeks after completing 5 days of intravenous treatment, but only 4 or 5 days after oral doses are stopped [41].
  - Correction of anemia in renal failure also improves the bleeding time. Blood transfusion or the use of erythropoietin to raise the hematocrit above 30 % appears to restore platelet-vessel wall interactions [34].

In conclusion, as a pain physician, it is always of the utmost importance to understand your patient's full medical history. Patients with any conditions increasing their risk for bleeding should determine if their spinal injection is urgent and communication should always occur with the treating physician.

References

1. Abram S. Complications associated with epidural, facet joint, and sacroiliac joint injections. In: Moore R, editor. Handbook of pain and palliative care. New York: Springer; 2012. p. 247–57.
2. Bush K, Hillier S. A controlled study of caudal epidural injections of triamcinolone plus procaine for the management of intractable sciatica. Spine. 1991;16:572–5.
3. Dilke TF, Burry HC, Grahame R. Extradural corticosteroid injection in management of lumbar nerve root compression. Br Med J. 1973;2:635.
4. Hollander JL, Brown Jr EM, Jessar RA, et al. Hydrocortisone and cortisone injected into arthritic joints; comparative effects of and use of hydrocortisone as a local antiarthritic agent. JAMA. 1951;147(17):1629–35.
5. Snibbe JC, Gambardella RA. Use of injections for osteoarthritis in joints and sports activity. Clin Sports Med. 2005;24(1):83–91.
6. Lavelle W, Lavelle E, Lavelle L. Intra-articular Injections. Anesthesiol Clin. 2007;25:853–62.
7. Derby R, et al. Complications following cervical epidural steroid injections by expert interventionalists in 2003. Pain Physician. 2004;7(4):445–9.
8. McGrath JM, Schaefer MP, Malkamaki DM. Incidence and characteristics of complications from epidural steroid injections. Pain Med. 2011;12(5):726–31.
9. Karaman H, et al. The complications of transforaminal lumbar epidural steroid injections. Spine. 2011;36(13):E819–24.
10. Botwin KP, Baskin M, Rao S. Adverse effects of fluoroscopically guided interlaminar thoracic epidural steroid injections. Am J Phys Med Rehabil. 2006;85(1):14–23.
11. Benny B, Azari P, Briones D. Complications of cervical transforaminal epidural steroid injections. Am J Phys Med Rehabil. 2010;89(7):601–7.
12. Reid D. Complications of low back pain therapies. Tech Reg Anesth Pain Manag. 1998;2(3):147–51.
13. Green L, Machin SJ. Managing anticoagulated patients during neuraxial anaesthesia. Br J Haematol. 2010;149(2):195–208. doi:10.1111/j.1365-2141.2010.08094.x. Epub 2010 Feb 8.
14. Vandermeulen EP, Van Aken H, Vermylen J. Anticoagulants and spinal-epidural anesthesia. Anesth Analg. 1994;79(6):1165–77.
15. Tehranzadeh J, Mossop EP, Golshan-Momeni M. Therapeutic arthrography and bursography. Orthop Clin North Am. 2006;37:393–408.
16. Creamer P. Intra-articular corticosteroid treatment in osteoarthritis. Curr Opin Rheumatol. 1999;11:417–21.
17. Saupe N, Zanetti M, Pfirrmann CWA, Weis T, Schwenke C, Hodler J. Pain and other side effects after MR arthrography: prospective evaluation in 1085 patients. Radiology. 2009;250:830–8.
18. Hugo III PC, Newberg AH, Newman JS, Wetzner SM. Complications of arthrography. Semin Musculoskelet Radiol. 1998;2:345–8.
19. Peterson C, Hodler J. Adverse events from diagnostic and therapeutic joint injections: a literature review. Skeletal Radiol. 2011; 40:5–12.
20. Bettencourt RB, Linder MM. Arthrocentesis and therapeutic joint injection: an overview for the primary care physician. Prim Care. 2010;37:691–702.
21. Horlocker TT, Wedel DJ. Infectious complications of regional anesthesia. Best Pract Res Clin Anaesthesiol. 2008;22(3):451–75.
22. Shanthanna H, Park J. Acute epidural haematoma following epidural steroid injection in a patient with spinal stenosis. Anaesthesia. 2011;66(9):837–9.
23. Reitman CA, Watters III W. Subdural hematoma after cervical epidural steroid injection. Spine. 2002;27(6):E174–6.
24. Jansen NW, Roosendaal G, Wenting MJ, et al. Very rapid clearance after a joint bleed in the canine knee cannot prevent adverse effects

on cartilage and synovial tissue. Osteoarthritis Cartilage. 2009; 17:433–40.

25. Solimeno L, et al. Knee arthropathy: when things go wrong. Haemophilia. 2012;18 Suppl 4:105–11.

26. Mannucci PM, Tuddenham EGD. The hemophilias—from royal genes to gene therapy. N Engl J Med. 2001;344(23):1773–9.

27. Bolton-Maggs PHB. The rare inherited coagulation disorders. Pediatr Blood Cancer. 2013;60(S1):S37–40.

28. Englbrecht JS, Pogatzki-Zahn EM, Zahn P. [Spinal and epidural anesthesia in patients with hemorrhagic diathesis: decisions on the brink of minimum evidence?]. Anaesthesist. 2011;60(12):1126–34. Epub 2011/08/02. Ruckenmarknahe Regionalanasthesie bei Patienten mit hamorrhagischen Diathesen : Entscheidungen am Rande des Evidenzminimums?.

29. Cines DB, Blanchette VS. Immune thrombocytopenic purpura. N Engl J Med. 2002;346(13):995–1008.

30. Peterson P, Hayes TE, Arkin CF, Bovill EG, Fairweather RB, Rock Jr WA, et al. The preoperative bleeding time test lacks clinical benefit: College of American Pathologists' and American Society of Clinical Pathologists' position article. Arch Surg. 1998; 133(2):134–9.

31. Close HL, Kryzer TC, Nowlin JH, Alving BM. Hemostatic assessment of patients before tonsillectomy: a prospective study. Otolaryngol Head Neck Surg. 1994;111(6):733–8. Epub 1994/12/01.

32. Patel IJ, Davidson JC, Nikolic B, Salazar GM, Schwartzberg MS, Walker TG, et al. Consensus guidelines for periprocedural management of coagulation status and hemostasis risk in percutaneous image-guided interventions. J Vasc Interv Radiol. 2012; 23(6):727–36.

33. Raj PP, Shah RV, Kaye AD, Denaro S, Hoover JM. Bleeding risk in interventional pain practice: assessment, management, and review of the literature. Pain Physician. 2004;7(1):3–51. Epub 2006/07/27.

34. Cobos E, Cruz J-C, Day M. Etiology and management of coagulation abnormalities in the pain management patient. Curr Rev Pain. 2000;4(5):413–9.

35. Soliman DE, Broadman LM. Coagulation defects. Anesthesiol Clin North America. 2006;24(3):549–78.

36. Mannucci PM, Federici AB. Management of inherited von Willebrand disease. Best Pract Res Clin Haematol. 2001; 14(2):455–62.

37. Aldouri M. The use of recombinant factor VIIa in controlling surgical bleeding in non-haemophiliac patients. Pathophysiol Haemost Thromb. 2002;32 Suppl 1:41–6.

38. Shah RV, Kaye AD. Bleeding risk and interventional pain management. Curr Opin Anaesthesiol. 2008;21(4):433–8. Epub 2008/07/29.

39. Sallah S, Bobzien W. Bleeding problems in patients with liver disease. Ways to manage the many hepatic effects on coagulation. Postgrad Med. 1999;106(4):187–90. Epub 1999/10/26.

40. DeLoughery TG. Management of bleeding with uremia and liver disease. Curr Opin Hematol. 1999;6(5):329–33. Epub 1999/09/01.

41. Weigert AL, Schafer AI. Uremic bleeding: pathogenesis and therapy. Am J Med Sci. 1998;316(2):94–104.

SriKrishna Chandran and Phong Kieu

Abbreviations

AP   Action potential
GABA   Gamma aminobutyric acid

Introduction

This chapter focuses on injectable medications used in the field of pain management. As a clinician, it is always important to understand the risks associated with each medication being used in the procedure and to choose the safest option.

Local Anesthetics

Mechanism of Action

- Block action potential (AP) conduction via inhibition of ion channels
  - Principally inhibit sodium channels of neuronal cell membranes [1]
- Resulting decreased permeability prevents AP propagation
  - *Smaller nerve fibers*: require a shorter length of fiber to be exposed to local anesthetics for blockade to occur
  - *Larger nerve fibers*: have larger internodal distances (distance between Nodes of Ranvier) which makes them increasingly resistant to local anesthetic blocks [2].

- Block peripheral nerve action by degrading transmitted electrical patterns such as after potentials and after oscillations [3].
- When administered to the intrathecal space, these medications diffuse within the spinal cord interacting with a variety of ion channels.
  - *This results in*:
    Altered excitation and depolarization of presynaptic terminals
    Altered release of neurotransmitters with both pre- and postsynaptic receptor sites [4]
- Local anesthetics also act centrally to prevent the release/binding of certain nociceptive neurotransmitters (such as Substance P) and promote other neurotransmitters (such as gamma aminobutyric acid [GABA] and acetylcholine) [2].

Chemical Structure

- Local anesthetics are classified as amides or esters based on their chemical structure.
  - *Amide type*: bupivacaine, dibucaine, etidocaine, lidocaine, mepivacaine, prilocaine, ropivacaine. Most commonly used are bupivacaine and lidocaine. Widely used in diagnostic and therapeutic injections and may be associated fewer true allergic reactions [5–8].
  - *Ester type*: benzocaine, chloroprocaine, cocaine, procaine, and tetracaine. Associated with a risk of severe allergic reactions stemming from their metabolite para-aminobenzoic acid [7].

Clinical Effect

- Certain physiochemical properties of local anesthetics are known to influence their activity
  - Lipid solubility
  - pKa
  - Protein binding
- Each of these factors contributes to a local anesthetic's potency, speed of onset, and duration of action.

S. Chandran, M.D. (✉)
Department of Physical Medicine and Rehabilitation,
Johns Hopkins Hospital, Baltimore, MD, USA
e-mail: schand13@jhmi.edu

P. Kieu, M.D.
Department of Orthopedics and Sports Medicine, John Peter Smith Hospital, Arlington, TX, USA
e-mail: pkieu@rocketmail.com

K.A. Sackheim, *Pain Management and Palliative Care: A Comprehensive Guide*,
DOI 10.1007/978-1-4939-2462-2_37, © Springer Science+Business Media New York 2015

Table 37.1 Local anesthetic dosage ranges

	Procedure	Concentration (location dependent) (%)	Volume (location dependent)	Maximal single dose (location dependent) (mg)
Lidocaine hydrochloride (Xylocaine© APP pharmaceuticals, Shamburg IL, USA)	Peripheral nerve	1–2	1–20 mL	20–300
	Percutaneous infiltration	0.5–1	1–60 mL	5–300
Bupivacaine hydrochloride (Sensorcaine© APP pharmaceuticals, Shamburg IL, USA)	Peripheral nerve	0.25–0.5	12.5–max mL	175
	Local infiltration	0.25	Up to max dose	175

Note: Information obtained from specific product insert. Concentrations, volumes, suggested and max doses vary significantly depending on the location and purpose of injection. Please refer to specific product insert prior to use

- *Potency is related to a local anesthetic's lipid solubility.*
  - Increasing lipid solubility→easier nerve membrane penetration→greater Na channel affinity
  - Bupivacaine is more potent and more lipophilic than lidocaine [5, 6].
- Onset of action is associated with a local anesthetic's pKa. pKa is defined as the pH at which a specific drug is half ionized and half in its neutral, unionized form.
  - The unionized form is more able to diffuse across the nerve membrane.
  - Local anesthetics that have a pKa closer to the injection site's physiologic pH have a faster onset of action [5].
  - Onset of action is not changed by the amount of local anesthetics administered.
- Duration of action is associated with protein binding, location of administration, administered dose, and lipid solubility (Table 37.1).

Tachyphylaxis

- Clinical phenomenon of decreasing efficacy is noted with repeated administration of the same dose of local anesthetics.
  - Short dosing intervals that prevent pain from occurring may prevent the appearance of tachyphylaxis [2].

Adverse Reactions/Toxicity

- *Caution is advised in administering amide type local anesthetics in those with liver dysfunction.*
  - Metabolized via the cytochrome P450 system and are thus dependent upon hepatic blood flow, extraction, and enzyme function [5].
- *CNS toxicity*
  - Bupivacaine≫Ropivacaine≫Lidocaine [9–13]
  - Symptoms include: Shivering, muscle twitching, tremor, hypoventilation, respiratory arrest, generalized convulsions [10]. Hiccups have also been noted following epidural administration of bupivacaine [11].

- In animal models, bupivacaine had a markedly lower threshold dose to induce generalized convulsions than either lidocaine or ropivacaine [12].
- *Cardiac toxicity*
  - Bupivacaine≫Lidocaine or Ropivacaine [14, 15]
  - Symptoms include: sympathetic activation, arrhythmias, cardiovascular depression, cardiovascular collapse [10, 14].
- *Skeletal muscle toxicity*
  - Bupivacaine is characterized with a high rate of myotoxicity, when compared to lidocaine and ropivacaine [16–20].
  - All local anesthetics in experimental settings are noted to be myotoxic in clinical concentrations with a dose dependent rate of toxicity [16–18].
  - The clinical effect of local anesthetic myotoxicity remains controversial.
  - Clinical evidence of myotoxicity is rare and may be due to rapid recovery and tissue regeneration [10].
- *Articular cartilage toxicity*
  - Several studies have shown that local anesthetics are cytotoxic to chondrocytes in large volumes [21–23].
  - Addition of epinephrine to lidocaine and bupivacaine in intra-articular injections has been shown in some studies to lead to increased chondrocyte toxicity.
    - Postulated to be the result of the lower pH in these combinations [23].
    - Addition of epinephrine to local anesthetics in intra-articular injections is not advised [10].
  - There are few cases of clinically significant chondrocyte toxicity after a single dose of local anesthestics and the use of local anesthetics for joint pain has been successfully employed for decades.
  - This may be because the concentrations used for in vitro experiments may not be seen in vivo, due to the dilutional effects of joint fluid and active synovial absorption [21].

– Therefore, further clinical studies are needed to fully assess the implications of these findings in cases of single dose administration.

Select Contraindications

- Symptoms include: history of hypersensitivity or allergy to a local anesthetic of the same class (amide, ester), history of anaphylaxis [10].
- *Absolute contraindications*: unstable joint, uncontrolled diabetes mellitus, charcot joint, bacteremia/sepsis, septic arthritis, osteomyelitis, or osteochondral fracture of adjacent bone, local infection, coagulopathy [24].
- *Relative contraindication for combination local anesthetics*: epinephrine/norepinephrine is concurrent use of a monoamine oxidase inhibitor/tricyclic antidepressant due to the risk of severe, persistent hypertension (a result of possible systemic agent absorption) [25, 26].

Corticosteroids

Background

- Corticosteroids are synthetic analogues of the adrenal glucocorticoid hormone cortisol, secreted from the adrenal cortex and involved in protein and glucose metabolism [27, 28]. It was later discovered that they have important anti-inflammatory properties.
- Due to their anti-inflammatory properties, they are a commonly used medication for office-based joint and soft tissue injections in combination with local anesthetics for a wide variety of disorders:
  - Joints, bursae, tendon sheaths, tendon insertion sites, muscular trigger points, epidural, transforaminal, perineural, interdigital neuroma, cyst and ganglion conditions.
  - Often used in patients who cannot tolerate systemic nonsteroidal anti-inflammatory drugs due to their local administration [29].

Mechanism of Action

- Precise pharmacological effects are unclear.
  - *Anti-inflammatory*:
    - At the cellular level, corticosteroids affect immune and inflammatory responses possibly by modulation of transcription [27].
    - Inhibits production of local inflammatory mediators such as arachidonic acid, prostaglandins, leukotrienes, cytokines, and other acute phase reactants [28].
  - *Direct neural membrane stabilization*:
    - Studies have shown that corticosteroids may reduce spontaneous ectopic discharge rates seen after nerve injuries [29].

- Reversible inhibition of nociceptive C-fiber transmission has been studied [28].
- Modulation of peripheral nociceptor neurons and spinal cord dorsal horn cells has been demonstrated [29].
  - *Excretion*:
    - Corticosteroids bind to albumin or globulins after absorption [28].
    - They then undergo sequential oxidative reduction to form inactive compounds [28].
    - This is followed by hepatic-mediated conjugation resulting in water-soluble metabolites that are excreted in the urine [28].

Chemical Structure

- Common synthetic corticosteroids are derivatives of prednisolone [10]:
  - *Methyl derivative*: Methylprednisolone acetate (Depo-Medrol, Solu-Medrol, Duralone, Medralone)
  - *Fluorinated derivative*: Betamethasone (Celestone Soluspan, Betaject), Dexamethasone (Decadron phosphate, Adrenocot, Decaject), Triamcinolone (Kenalog)
  - *Particulate/ester preparations*:
    "Acetates"—highly lipophilic—highly insoluble
    - Efficacy and duration are greater than non-esters in joints as they require hydrolysis prior to activation [10].
    - They form microcrystalline suspensions which may result in flocculations with preservatives in some local anesthetics, ultimately creating particulates
    - Risk for damage to soft tissue, neural, and vascular structures (i.e., Artery of Adamkiewicz)
  - *Non-particulate/non-ester preparations*:
    Salt, "sodium phosphate"—water soluble
    - Dexamethasone is the non-ester and non-particulate formulation most commonly used.
    - It is water soluble, and therefore has a much faster onset of action, but reduced duration of action [10].
    - Celestone Soluspan is a combination ester and salt with theoretical short- and long-term action duration, although not clinically significant [10].

Clinical Effect (Table 37.2)
Adverse Effects/Toxicity

- Mostly described from systemic usage [30, 31]:
  - Fluid retention, elevated blood pressure, elevated blood glucose levels, generalized erythema, facial flushing, allergic reaction, menstrual irregularities, gastritis—peptic ulcer disease, hypothalamic–pituitary–adrenal-axis suppression, Cushing syndrome, bone demineralization, steroid myopathy, brief euphoric or manic reactions

Table 37.2 Equivalent potencies of select corticosteroids [2, 4–6]

Medication	Half-life (h)	Equivalent potency (mg)	Solubility (percent weight/volume)	Particle aggregation
Hydrocortisone	8–12	1	Freely soluble	Not studied
Methylprednisolone acetate	12–36	5	0.001	Few
Triamcinolone acetonide	12–36	5	0.0002	Extensive
Betamethasone acetate/sodium phosphate	36–72	25	Acetate—highly insoluble	Some
			Sodium phosphate—freely soluble	
Dexamethasone sodium phosphate	36–72	25	Freely soluble	None

Table 37.3 Medication codes

Medication code	1 U equivalent
J1030	Depo-Medrol 40 mg
J1040	Depo-Medrol 80 mg
J1100	Dexamethasone 1 mg
J3301	Kenalog 10 mg
J0702	Celestone 3 mg
J3490	Lidocaine/Marcaine (1 U only)
J1885	Toradol 15 mg
Q9965	Omnipaque (1 U only)

- More specific to injections—theoretical risk of weakened ligaments, possible increased risk of infection, postinjection pain, skin hypopigmentation, sterile meningitis, and arachnoiditis [32].
- Special considerations
  - Methylprednisolone acetate (Depo-Medrone) is noted to cause more postinjection pain and carries an increased risk of a rare anaphylactoid reaction due to succinate salts [10, 28, 31].
  - Diabetes Mellitus—injected steroids do increase the frequency of hyperglycemia, but its clinical significance is uncertain. Long-term effects have not been found, but caution should be used in brittle diabetics.
  - Artery of Adamkiewicz—thoracic and upper-lumbar level to L2-3. Caution when performing transforaminal epidural steroid injection or selective nerve root block with particulate steroids as this could result in spinal cord ischemia or infarction [10, 31, 32].

Select Contraindications

- Absolute contraindications: local infection, intra-articular infection, and systemic infection, joint fractures, joint instability, coagulopathy [10].
- Relative contraindications: Osteoporosis
- No more than three injections/year in the same joint and no sooner than 6 weeks apart

Table 37.3 lists medication codes and Table 37.4 shows properties of steroids used in spinal injections.

Table 37.4 Properties of steroids used in spinal injections

Agent	Biological half-life (h)	Anti-inflammatory potency	Salt-retaining potency	Particulate size (aggregation)
Hydrocortisone (hydrocortone)	8–12	1	1	
Triamcinolone (Kenalog 40)	12–36	5	0	RBC size to 133 (extensive, densely packed)
Methylprednisolone (Depo-Medrol)	12–36	5	0.5	RBC size (few, densely packed)
Dexamethasone (Decadron)	36–72	25	0	RBC size (none)
Betamethasone (Celestone Soluspan)	36–72	25	0	Varied size (extensive, densely packed)

Information adapted and modified from *Essentials of Pain Management*, *Benzon*

References

1. Nau C, Wang GK. Interactions of local anesthetics with voltage-gated Na⁺ channels. J Membr Biol. 2004;201(1):1–8.
2. Liu SS. Local anesthetics: clinical aspects. In: Benzon H, Raja S, Molloy R, Liu S, Fishman S, editors. Essentials of pain medicine and regional anesthesia. 2nd ed. Philadelphia: Elsevier Science; 2005. p. 558–65.
3. Raymond SA. Subblocking concentrations of local anesthetics: effects on impulse generation and conduction in single myelinated sciatic nerve axons in frog. Anesth Analg. 1992;75(6):906–21.
4. Gokin A, Strichartz G. Local anesthetics acting on the spinal cord. Access, distribution, pharmacology and toxicology. In: Yaksh TL, editor. Spinal drug delivery: anatomy, kinetics and toxicology. 1st ed. New York: Elsevier; 1999. p. 477–501.
5. Sitzman B, Chen Y, Clemans R, Fishman S, Benzon H. Pharmacology for the interventional pain physician. In: Benzon H, Raja S, Molloy R, Liu S, Fishman S, editors. Essentials of pain medicine and regional anesthesia. 2nd ed. Philadelphia: Elsevier; 2005. p. 166–80.
6. Butterworth IV JF, Strichartz GR. Molecular mechanisms of local anesthesia: a review. Anesthesiology. 1990;72:711–34.
7. Cox B, Durieux ME, Marcus MA. Toxicity of local anaesthetics. Best Pract Res Clin Anaesthesiol. 2003;17(1):111–36.

8. Holmdahl MH. Xylocain (lidocaine, lignocaine), its discovery and Gordh's contribution to its clinical use. Acta Anaesthesiol Scand Suppl. 1998;113:8–12.

9. Krunic AL, Wang LC, Soltani K, Weitzul S, Taylor RS. Digital anesthesia with epinephrine: an old myth revisited. J Am Acad Dermatol. 2004;51(5):755–9.

10. MacMahon P, Eustace S, Kavanagh E. Injectable corticosteroid and local anesthetic preparations: a review for radiologists. Radiology. 2009;25(3):647–67.

11. McAllister R, McDavid A, Meyer T, Bittenbinder T. Recurrent persistent hiccups after epidural steroid injection and analgesia with bupivacaine. Anesth Analg. 2013;116(2):1834–6.

12. Liu PL, Feldman HS, Giasi R, Patterson MK, Covino BG. Comparative CNS toxicity of lidocaine, bupivacaine, and tetracaine in awake dogs following rapid intravenous administration. Anesth Analg. 1983;62(4):375–9.

13. Groban L. Central nervous system and cardiac effects from long-acting amide local anesthetic toxicity in the intact animal model. Reg Anesth Pain Med. 2003;28(1):3–11.

14. Gristwood RW. Cardiac and CNS toxicity of levobupivacaine: strengths of evidence for advantage over bupivacaine. Drug Saf. 2002;25(3):153–63.

15. Leone S, Di Cianni S, Casati A, Fanelli G. Pharmacology, toxicology, and clinical use of new long acting local anesthetics, ropivacaine and levobupivacaine. Acta Biomed. 2008;79(2):92–105.

16. Brun A. Effect of procaine, carbocain and xylocaine on cutaneous muscle in rabbits and mice. Acta Anaesthesiol Scand. 1959;3(2):59–73.

17. Hogan Q, Dotson R, Erickson S, Kettler R, Hogan K. Local anesthetic myotoxicity: a case and review. Anesthesiology. 1994;80(4):942–7.

18. Foster AH, Carlson BM. Myotoxicity of local anesthetics and regeneration of the damaged muscle fibers. Anesth Analg. 1980;59(10):727–36.

19. Benoit PW, Belt WD. Destruction and regeneration of skeletal muscle after treatment with a local anaesthetic, bupivacaine (Marcaine). J Anat. 1970;107(Pt 3):547–56.

20. Yagiela JA, Benoit PW, Buoncristiani RD, Peters MP, Fort NF. Comparison of myotoxic effects of lidocaine with epinephrine in rats and humans. Anesth Analg. 1981;60(7):471–80.

21. Chu CR, Izzo NJ, Coyle CH, Papas NE, Logar A. The in vitro effects of bupivacaine on articular chondrocytes. J Bone Joint Surg Br. 2008;90(6):814–20.

22. Piper SL, Kim HT. Comparison of ropivacaine and bupivacaine toxicity in human articular chondrocytes. J Bone Joint Surg Am. 2008;90(5):986–91.

23. Dragoo JL, Korotkova T, Kanwar R, Wood B. The effect of local anesthetics administered via pain pump on chondrocyte viability. Am J Sports Med. 2008;36(8):1484–8.

24. Thumboo J, O'Duffy JD. A prospective study of the safety of joint and soft tissue aspirations and injections in patients taking warfarin sodium. Arthritis Rheum. 1998;41(4):736–9.

25. Goulet JP, Pérusse R, Turcotte JY. Contraindications to vasoconstrictors in dentistry: Part III. Pharmacologic interactions. Oral Surg Oral Med Oral Pathol. 1992;74(5):692–7.

26. Karaoglu S, Dogru K, Kabak S, Inan M, Halici M. Effects of epinephrine in local anesthetic mixtures on hemodynamics and view quality during knee arthroscopy. Knee Surg Sports Traumatol Arthrosc. 2002;10(4):226–8.

27. Saunders S, Longworth S. The drugs. In: *Injection techniques in orthopaedic and sports medicine: a practical manual for doctors and physiotherapists*. 3rd ed. Philadelphia: Churchhill Livingstone/Elsevier; 2006.

28. Sitzman BT. Pharmacology for the spine injectionist. In: Fenton D, Czervionke L, editors. Image-guided spine intervention. Philadelphia: Saunders Elsevier; 2003.

29. Devor M, Govrin-Lippman R, Raber P. Corticosteroids suppress ectopic neural discharge originating in experimental neuromas. Pain. 1985;22:127–37.

30. Stitik T, Kumar A, Kim J, Tran J, Lee C. Chapter 2: pharmacotherapy of joint and soft tissue injections. In: Stitik P, editor. Injection procedures: osteoarthritis and related conditions. New York: Springer; 2010.

31. Collighan N, Gupta S. Epidural steroids. Cont Educ Anaesth Crit Care Pain. 2010;10(1):1–5.

32. Catalano III LW, Glickel SZ, Barron OA, Harrison R, Marshall A, Purcelli-Lafer M. Effect of local corticosteroid injection of the hand and wrist on blood glucose in patients with diabetes mellitus. Orthopedics. 2012;35(12):e1754–8.

Radiation Safety and Monitoring

Anuj Malhotra

Abbreviations

ABC   Automatic brightness control
CT   Computed tomography

Introduction

Fluoroscopic guidance: used for pain procedures to identify bony landmarks located near target joints and nerves. Views are two dimensional, necessitating a mobile unit that can be rotated (C-arm) to provide different angles to determine appropriate needle localization

X-rays: part of electromagnetic spectrum of radiation, produce ionizing radiation in the body which can cause damage via direct DNA damage or free radical production

Radiation Units

Exposure: Roentgen or Coulomb/kg (1 R $= 2.5 \times 10^{-4}$ C/kg)

Radiation absorbed dose: rad or Gray (100 rad $=$ 1 Gy)

Radiation equivalent in man: rem or Sievert (100 rem $=$ 1 Sv)

X-ray equivalency: 1 R $\approx$ 1 rad $\approx$ 1 rem

C-arm Components (See Fig. 38.1)

X-ray tube (*source*): position under table to limit radiation exposure to room personnel, should be positioned as far as possible from patient to minimize exposure

Image intensifier (*detector*): position above table captures X-rays that pass through patient to produce an image based on penetrability of tissues

Camera: captures image from detector

Display monitors: displays image from camera, can be rotated or saved as needed for reference and medical record keeping

Collimators: can adjust the X-ray beam to minimize area exposed to radiation and to improve image contrast (Iris—circular shutters, Linear—side shutters), increased use of collimators also decreases scatter

Fluoroscopy Settings

Current: Increased current increases number of X-rays produced, darkens image

Exposure time: Increased exposure time darkens image

Voltage: Increased voltage increases X-ray penetration

Automatic brightness control (*ABC*): adjusts voltage and current to optimize image, generally increases voltage to increase penetration while minimizing current to limit dose

New vs. old machines: generally decreased exposure with newer machines due to optimization of current and voltage settings

A. Malhotra, M.D. (✉)
Division of Pain Medicine, Department of Anesthesiology,
Icahn School of Medicine at Mount Sinai, New York, NY, USA
e-mail: anuj.malhotra@mountsinai.org

K.A. Sackheim, *Pain Management and Palliative Care: A Comprehensive Guide*,
DOI 10.1007/978-1-4939-2462-2_38, © Springer Science+Business Media New York 2015

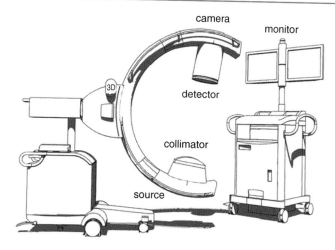

Fig. 38.1 C-arm components

Fluoroscopy Modes

Intermittent mode: individual, spot images, low dose, exposure based on number of images

Continuous mode: increased dose time to allow for live evaluation, real-time spread of injected contrast

Pulsed mode: intermittent images at a set time interval to decrease exposure of continuous mode

Digital subtraction: high-dose fluoroscopy used to remove static structures from a live image, better evaluates for intravascular injection

Occupational Exposure

Inverse-square law: radiation is inversely proportional to the square of the distance from the X-ray source

Scatter: majority of occupational exposure occurs from scattered radiation off the table on the side of the X-ray source. Larger patients and increased distance from the X-ray source to the table will increase scatter.

Common Radiation Exposures per Procedure [1]

- Chest X-ray: 10 mrem
- Head CT: 200 mrem
- Fluoroscopy, intermittent: 0.7–3 mrem
- Fluoroscopy, boost: 2–20 mrem
- Fluoroscopy, continuous: 200–1,000 mrem/min
- Fluoroscopy, digital subtraction: 2,000–4,000 mrem/min

Annual Maximal Permissible Radiation Dose [2]

- Total body: 5 rem
- Thyroid: 50 rem
- Lens of eye: 15 rem
- Fetus: 0.5 rem

Minimum Organ Radiation Dose Exposure to Produce Damage [3]

- Lens of the eye, cataracts: 200 rad (8 years latency)
- Skin, dermatitis: 500 rad (1–2 days latency)
- Body, hematopoietic crisis: 200–700 rad (4–6 weeks latency)

Lead Shielding

Fixed shielding: walls, doors, and windows should have a lead equivalence of 1–3 mm

Mobile shielding: barriers or screens can be placed between the X-ray source and personnel and can produce the largest decrease in radiation exposure; however, these should generally be used in addition to personal shielding as they can be difficult to reliably position between operator and X-ray source at all times

Effective personal shielding includes lead aprons, thyroid shields, and leaded glasses

It is recommended not to use lead gloves as most fluoroscopy units will compensate for the increased radiodensity by increasing voltage, thereby increasing exposure and scatter.

Lead Thickness Protection Under Commonly Used Fluoroscopy Settings [4]

- **1 mm**: blocks 99 %+ of radiation
- **0.72 mm**: blocks 98–99 %+ of radiation
- **0.5 mm**: blocks 95–99 %+ of radiation
- **0.22 mm**: blocks 87–95 % of radiation

Most aprons are 0.25–0.5 mm lead equivalence for reasons of weight:
- One-sided aprons 0.35 mm is appropriate
- Wrap-around aprons, 0.25 mm is sufficient so long as the apron is oriented correctly with the overlap in front to yield 0.5 mm with 0.25 mm in the back

Monitoring

- *Radiation badge*: Should be used by all personnel who work with a C-arm, required for personnel who may receive exposure to >25 % of the annual limit, consists of film that darkens with exposure to beta and gamma radiation
  - Over the collar: approximates exposure to lens of the eye
  - Under the apron: approximates exposure to shielded organs

Minimizing Radiation Exposure [5]

- *Training*: Proper radiation training
- *Inspections*: Maintain regular quality control of fluoroscopy equipment to prevent overexposure
- *Protection*: Use proper lead protection including leaded glasses, apron, thyroid shield, and/or standing shield: Ensure lead shielding is positioned between personnel and the X-ray source at all times (e.g., facing the C-arm if using single-sided lead aprons)
- *Patient positioning*: Properly position the patient on the table, remove belt buckles or buttons that might obscure view (this can help minimize reimaging and dose)
- *C-arm positioning*:
  - Position C-arm over area to be imaged prior to beginning fluoroscopy to minimize number of "finder" images (increased amount of images → increased radiation exposure)
  - Keep X-ray source below table in AP views to decrease scatter
  - If only lateral imaging is required, consider positioning the patient lateral on the table to keep the X-ray source below the table
  - If lateral imaging is required only part of the time, ensure the operator is opposite the X-ray source and on the side of the image detector
- *Collimating*: Utilize ABC settings and collimation to optimize voltage and current settings and limit exposure area for the patient (collimated views → less radiation exposure)
- *Increase distance*: Increase operator distance from X-ray source by use of foot pedals, fixed standing shields, and extensions/connectors during live injection of contrast
- *Use pulse*: Use intermittent/pulse as opposed to live fluoroscopy when possible

References

1. Rathmell J. Atlas of image-guided intervention in regional anesthesia and pain medicine. 2nd ed. Philadelphia: Lippincott Williams & Wilkins; 2011. p. 8–15.
2. Benzon H, Raja SN, Fishman SM, Liu S, Cohen SP. Essentials of pain medicine. 3rd ed. Philadelphia: Saunders; 2011. p. 502–10.
3. International Commission on Radiological Protection. Recommendations of the ICRP, Publication 103. Oxford: Pergamon Press; 2007.
4. Singer G. Occupational radiation exposure to the surgeon. J Am Acad Orthop Surg. 2005;13:69–76.
5. Fishman SM, Smith H, Meleger A, Sievert JA. Radiation safety in pain medicine. Reg Anesth Pain Med. 2002;27:296–305.

Benjamin P. Lowry and Adam M. Savage

Abbreviations

AP	Anteroposterior
CMBB	Cervical Medial Branch Blocks
CPT	Current Procedural Terminology
CSF	Cerebrospinal fluid
IL-CESI	Interlaminar cervical epidural steroid injection
RFA	Radiofrequency ablation
UTI	Urinary tract infection

Introduction

Cervical spine pathology may contribute to a variety of pain symptoms including headache, facial pain, neck pain, shoulder pain, and paresthesias within the upper extremities. A thorough evaluation is essential for a correct diagnosis as well as determining appropriate treatment options. Interventions in or around the cervical spine have the potential for a multitude of complications including intravascular injection or neuronal injury. The utilization of fluoroscopy, as well as the more recent use of sonography, has allowed for an improvement in needle placement, safety, and procedural efficacy [1, 3].

Cervical Injection Contraindications

- *Absolute contraindications*
  - Patient refusal
  - Local infection at the site

B.P. Lowry, M.D. (✉)
Department of Anesthesiology, Baylor Scott & White
Health/Texas A&M College of Medicine, Temple, TX, USA
e-mail: blowry@sw.org

A.M. Savage, M.D.
Department of Anesthesiology—Pain Management, Scott & White
Hospital, Temple, TX, USA

  - Systemic infection (UTI, pneumonia, etc.)
  - Bleeding disorder
  - Full anticoagulation
  - Allergic reaction to injectants
  - Local malignancy
  - Acute cord compression
- *Relative contraindications*
  - Pregnancy
  - Poorly controlled diabetes
  - Poorly controlled hypertension
  - Immunosuppression
  - Previous surgery altering the targeted anatomy
  - Intraspinal vascular dilation or anomalies near target site
  - Congestive heart failure [1–3]

Patient Positioning for Cervical Procedures

- Patient is placed prone with arms at their side. Two pillows are placed under their chest and a small towel/sheet beneath the forehead to facilitate cervical spine flexion. Arms are best tucked under the anterior thighs to prevent patient movement and to assure the shoulders are not inhibiting the lateral view. Cervical pillow can be used as a substitute to the above positioning.

Interlaminar Cervical Epidural Steroid Injection (IL-CESI)

- **Indications**
  - Most common indication: nerve root inflammation resulting in *cervical neuritis* or *radicular symptoms* Both diagnostic and therapeutic
  - Radiculopathy or Radiculitis
  - Neck/arm Pain
  - Central canal stenosis
  - Neuroforaminal stenosis
  - Herniated Disc [1–3]

K.A. Sackheim, *Pain Management and Palliative Care: A Comprehensive Guide*,
DOI 10.1007/978-1-4939-2462-2_39, © Springer Science+Business Media New York 2015

- – Discogenic pain
- – Degenerative Disc Disease
- – Cervicogenic headache
- *Interlaminar approach*: Most common approach to the epidural space
  - – Epidural space is accessed between the vertebral laminae using a posterior approach near midline most commonly at the C7-T1 interspace.
  - – Entry at higher levels is not advisable because of the noncontinuity of the ligamentum flavum at these levels.
- *Transforaminal approach* (*selective nerve root block*): poses an increased risk of intravascular injection and is discouraged by many pain physicians. Due to the increased danger, this approach will not be discussed.
- **Anatomy**
  - – *Borders of the epidural space:* laminae posteriorly, pedicles laterally, and vertebral bodies anteriorly
  - – The ligamentum flavum defines the posterior border of the epidural space, but its thickness and completeness is less reliable at the cervical region than in the thoracic and lumbar spine.
  - – Epidural space contains a thin layer of adipose to cushion the thecal sac, a robust venous plexus and loose areolar tissue.
- **Fluoroscopy**
  - – Obtain an AP view of the targeted interspace. Locate a good opening between the lamina. If needed, the C-arm can be moved caudally to maximize the interlaminar opening at C7-T1 (Fig. 39.1)
- **Procedure**
  - – Posterior neck is prepped and draped in a sterile manner

- – *Entry point*: at or slightly to the side of midline at the interlaminar opening
- – Skin and subcutaneous tissue overlying the target site are anesthetized with 1 % lidocaine
- – A Tuohy needle is inserted through the anesthetized skin and advanced using a coaxial technique and intermittent fluoroscopy to assure midline or close to midline needle positioning (Fig. 39.2).
- – Prior to or once the interspinous ligament is engaged, obtain a lateral view to assure proper depth. (*Depth can be assessed at anytime during this procedure with lateral view to ensure safety.*)
- – Once the ligament is approached, LOR syringe containing a small amount of air or sterile preservative-free saline is attached to the needle. The loss of resistance technique is used cautiously while slowly advancing the needle in the same trajectory. During this process, intermittent lateral fluoroscopy is used until the epidural space is identified. *Remember the ligamentum at this region is very thin.*
- – Once a loss is obtained, aspirate for the presence of blood or cerebrospinal fluid (CSF) (Fig. 39.3)
  - ▪ *If aspiration is positive for blood*: reposition the needle within the same interlaminar space or at a different level to avoid intravascular needle placement
  - ▪ *If aspiration is positive for CSF*: consider reaccessing the epidural space at an adjacent or different level to avoid intrathecal medication injection. Procedure discontinuation can also be considered depending on the circumstances.

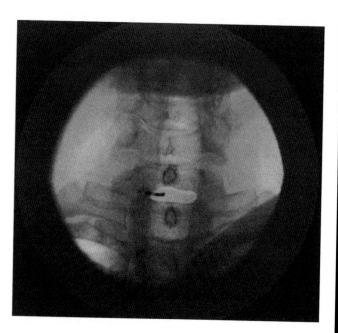

Fig. 39.1 AP view of the cervical spine. C7-T1 intralaminar interspace maximized with cephalocaudal tilt. Allows for needle placement utilizing a midline or paramedian approach

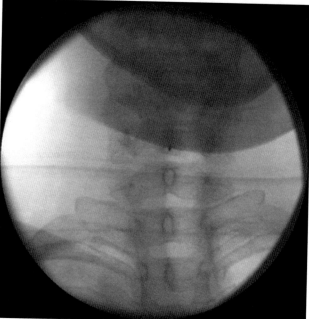

Fig. 39.2 Note needle tip placement is aligned in a midline position between the spinous processes of C6-C7

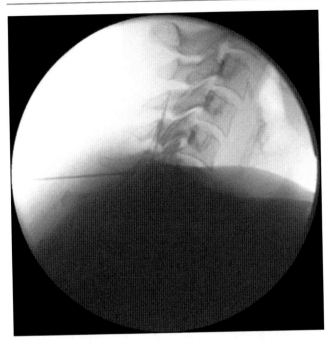

Fig. 39.3 Needle tip is located in the posterior epidural space just anterior to the spinous processes of C7 and T1. Contrast confirms spread within the posterior epidural space without anterior or posterior vascular uptake or intrathecal contrast spread

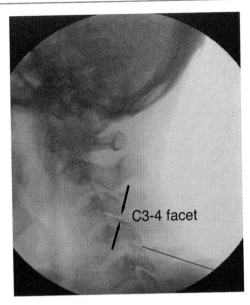

Fig. 39.4 The C3-4 cervical facet joint in a lateral view is illustrated between the *arrows*. Entry point (cervical facet joint injection)—Entry point should be directly overlying the posterior joint space once the joint is coaxially aligned anterior to posterior

- ▪ *If aspiration is negative:* needle placement can be verified by injecting 1–3 mL of contrast and confirming spread in the epidural space in both the AP and lateral views while also excluding vascular or intrathecal spread.
- ▪ Once needle placement is confirmed, medications are injected [1–3]
- • **Contraindications**: See contraindication section at the beginning of the chapter.
- • **Medications injected**
  - – *Mixture of*:
    - ▪ Steroid diluted in 1–2 mL of sterile preservative-free normal saline
    - ▪ Safest steroids to inject in the cervical region are non-particulate or low-particulate. Dexamethasone is most commonly used.
  - – *Total volume*: 2–4 mL
  - – Smaller volumes may be indicated in stenotic patients or patients in excruciating radicular pain as increased pressure from the medications can cause brief heightened pain [3, 4].

Cervical Facet Joint Injections

- • **Indications**
  - – Diagnostic and therapeutic treatment of facetogenic axial neck pain

  - – Cervical Spondylosis/Facet arthropathy
  - – Facetogenic headache
- • **Contraindications**
  - – Similar to contraindications for epidural steroid injections, although thought to have less risk of bleeding, intrathecal injection, or nerve trauma.
  - – See contraindication section at the beginning of the chapter.
- • **Anatomy**
  - – Facet joints are formed from the superior articular process of the inferior vertebra and the inferior articular process of the superior vertebra (Fig. 39.4).
  - – *C1-2 joint*: Injection to the atlantoaxial joint is discouraged because of close proximity to the vertebral artery
  - – *C2-3 joint*: the most frequent cervical facet pain generator is aligned 70° from the sagittal plane and 45° from the axial plane, which minimizes cervical rotation.
  - – *C5-6 joint*: the second most affected cervical joint is where the cervical facets transition to their posterolateral position.
  - – *Each facet joint is innervated by two medial branch nerves.*
  - – The facet joint is a true synovial joint with a limited volume of 0.5–1.0 mL in the cervical region [5–8].
- • **Fluoroscopy**
  - – Obtain and AP view of the targeted level. C-arm can be rotated caudally 25–35° in order to bring the axis of the X-rays in line with the axis of the facet joints.

Fig. 39.5 Lateral image of needle tip within the facet joint. Needle tip noted within the posterior aspect of the cervical facet joint. Contrast confirms intra-articular spread. Needle tip should not be advanced past posterior joint line to avoid possible vertebral artery puncture

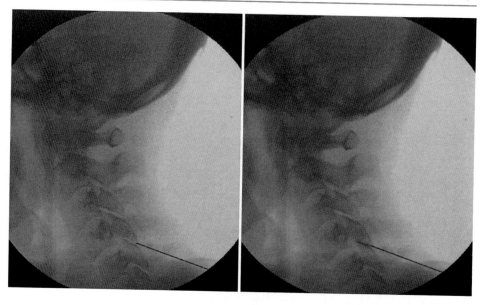

- **Procedure**
  - The skin and subcutaneous tissue are anesthetized overlying the facet joint with lidocaine 1 %.
  - A 25 gauge, curved 3.5 in. spinal needle is advanced in a coaxial orientation until the surface of the joint space is contacted. A lateral view is obtained to assure proper needle depth and the needle slightly advanced to penetrate the posterior joint capsule, but not between the articular surfaces (Fig. 39.5).
- **Medications injected**
  - *Mixture of*:
    Can be diagnostic with just anesthetic or steroid can be added for longer therapeutic response.
    Dexamethasone is most commonly used in the cervical region.
    Bupivacaine 0.25 % or lidocaine 1–2 %
  - *Each Level*: 0.5–1 mL per level of total volume [5–8]

Cervical Medial Branch Blocks (CMBB)

- **Indications**
  - Diagnostic and therapeutic treatment of facetogenic neck pain
    - Therapeutic blockade with steroid may provide several months of pain relief. Typically, if the patient has two successful blocks with >50 % symptomatic relief lasting <2 months, radiofrequency ablation is considered. If pain relief if long lasting, therapeutic medial branch block can be considered instead of radiofrequency.
  - Cervical Spondylosis/Facet arthropathy
  - Facetogenic headache

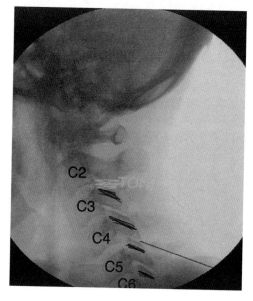

Fig. 39.6 Lateral image of the cervical spine shows the variable locations of the medial branch nerves coursing along the articular pillars

- **Contraindications**
  - Similar to contraindications for epidural steroid injections, although thought to have less risk of bleeding, intrathecal injection, or nerve trauma.
  - See contraindication section at the beginning of the chapter.
- **Anatomy**
  - The medial branch is the terminal division of the posterior ramus that provides sensory innervations to the facet joint (Fig. 39.6).
  - *Innervation*:
    - The innervation of the cervical facets is more varied and complicated than that of the thoracic and lumbar spine.

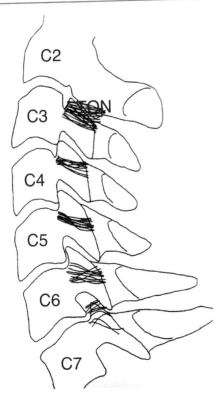

Fig. 39.7 Skeletal portrayal of the cervical medial branch nerves coursing around the articular pillars

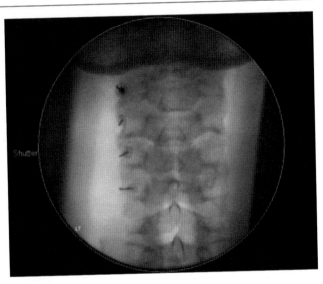

Fig. 39.8 Needles placed in near coaxial plane with tips at the waist of the articular pillars of C3-6 on the patient's left

- *C2-3 facet joint innervation*: stems from the greater occipital nerve (C2) and the third occipital nerve (C3)
- *C3-4 through C7-T1 facet joints*: receive innervation from the medial branches at the same level and the level above. Both nerves must be blocked in order to treat/diagnose pain emanating from affected level.

– The medial branch nerves for the cervical spine are targeted as they curve around the waist of the articular pillar (Fig. 39.7) [5–8].

• **Fluoroscopy** (Fig. 39.8)

– The medial branch nerves in the cervical spine may be approached posteriorly or laterally. However, when doing lateral approach, the needle is directed toward the spinal cord. Since the posterior approach avoids this risk and is the conventional approach for radiofrequency treatment, we will describe this below.

– Obtain an AP view to identify the appropriate level. C-arm can be caudally tilted 25–35° in order to maximize visualization of the articular pillars and square up the end plates.

• **Procedure**

– *Entry point*: Anesthetize the skin and subcutaneous tissue overlying the middle of the articular pillar with lidocaine 1 % (Fig. 39.9).

– Advance a 25-gauge, curved 3.5-in. spinal needle in a coaxial plane toward the invagination or "waist" of the articular pillar. Needle approach is best done with the needle curve facing medially. Once bone is approached the tip can be turned laterally to advance to desired location.

– *Target*: The needle is gently seated on the lateral margin of the facet column.

– A lateral view should confirm needle depth and proper placement to be in the middle of the facet column, seen as the center of the trapezoid (Fig. 39.10).

– Always aspirate prior to injection to ensure negative for heme, CSF, or air.

– Once needle position is confirmed and aspiration is negative, medications are injected.

• **Medications injected**

– Diagnostic block may be done with 0.5–1.0 mL of local anesthetic at each level

- Usually, a series of two injections are performed with differing local anesthetics to monitor the amount of time with pain relief

  ♦ Lidocaine 1 % should diminish pain for 1–3 h

  ♦ Bupivacaine 0.25 % should diminish pain for 4–8 h

– Some clinicians also use steroid for added and prolonged therapeutic affect [5–8]

- Dexamethasone is safest in the cervical region

– *Each level*: 0.5–1.0 mL of total volume [5, 8]

Fig. 39.9 Needle entry site should be directly over the waist of the articular pillars of target medial branch nerve sites or 1–3 mm lateral to target site depicted by *white dots*

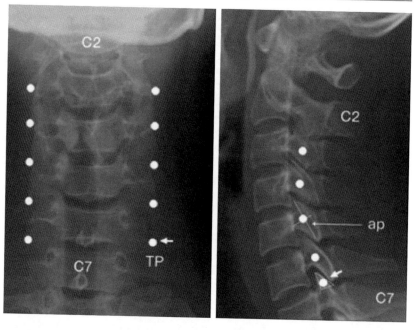

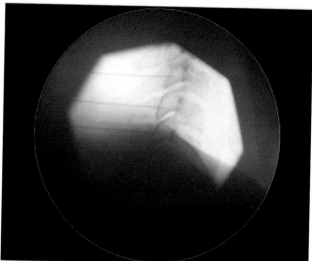

Fig. 39.10 Needle tips at the mid aspect of the trapezoid

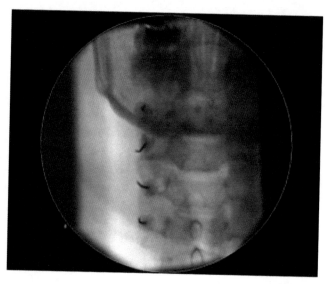

Fig. 39.11 Entry site directly overlying waist of target articular pillar. Image best obtained with slight caudal tilt of image intensifier. Needles should be advanced in a coaxial plane with the needle tip overlying the "trapezoid" of the cervical articular pillar

Cervical Radiofrequency Ablation (RFA)

- **Indications**
  - Facet-mediated pain that responds with at least 50 % relief with two medial branch blocks. Radiofrequency is usually considered if pain relief from blocks is <2 months. If pain relief with blocks is longer lasting, therapeutic blocks can be done instead of radiofrequency depending on patient needs.
- **Contraindications**: See contraindication section at the beginning of the chapter.
  - *Caution with pacemakers and defibrillators*
- **Anatomy**: See medial branch blocks section [5–8]

- **Fluoroscopy**: See medial branch blocks section
- **Procedure**
  - *Entry point*: Anesthetize the skin and subcutaneous tissue overlying the middle of the articular pillar with lidocaine 1 % (Fig. 39.11).
  - Obtain an AP view to identify the appropriate level. C-arm can be caudally tilted 25–35° in order to maximize visualization of the articular pillars and square up the end plates.
  - Once the lateral margin of the facet column is contacted, the needle is walked laterally off the facet and advanced 2–3 mm beyond the facet joint in the lateral view.

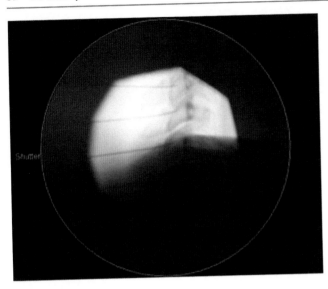

Fig. 39.12 Needle tips at mid aspect of the cervical articular pillars

- Obtain a lateral view to confirm that the needle does not extend into the neural foramen (Fig. 39.12).
- *Sensory stimulation*: performed eliciting pain, pressure, or tingling at <0.5 V at 50 Hz.
- *Motor stimulation*: up to 2.0 V should cause no motor stimulation into the affected myotome. *If muscle activity is noted in the upper extremity, needle must be repositioned.*
- Once proper needle placement is confirmed by fluoroscopy view and nerve stimulation, each level is then anesthetized with 0.5 mL of lidocaine 1–2% and subsequently treated with thermocoagulation, typically at 80 °C for 60–90 s.

- **Medications injected**
  - *Mixture of*: Bupivacaine 0.25 % and dexamethasone
  - *Each level*: 0.5–1.0 mL total volume [5–8]

Cervical Injection Complications (Please See Complication Chapter for More Details)

- *Procedure Complications*
  - Localized bleeding, bruising, and/or soreness at needle entry site
  - Dural puncture
  - Headache
  - Transient vagal episode
  - Paresthesias
  - Increased radicular pain

  - Direct trauma to spinal cord or spinal nerves
  - Infection such as epidural abscess
  - Hemorrhage such as epidural hematoma
  - Intravascular injection
  - Nerve root or spinal cord infarction
  - Paralysis
  - Joint damage or articular surface abrasion
  - Exacerbation of pain
- *Pharmacologic complications*
  - Seizure
  - Bradycardia
  - Hypotension
  - Allergic reaction
  - Neurotoxicity
  - Weight gain
  - Fluid retention
  - Hypertension
  - Congestive heart failure
  - Cushing's syndrome [1–8]

References

1. Rathmell JP. Chapter 5: Interlaminar epidural injection. In: Atlas of image-guided intervention in regional anesthesia and pain medicine. 2nd ed. Philadelphia: Lippincott Williams & Wilkins; 2012. p. 34–63.
2. Stizman BT. Epidural injections. In: Fenton DS, Czervionke LF, editors. Image-guided spine intervention. Philadelphia: Saunders; 2003.
3. Molloy RE, Benzon HT. Interlaminar epidural steroid injections for cervical radiculopathy. In: Benzon HT, Raja SN, Molloy RE, Liu SS, Fishman SM, editors. Essentials of pain medicine and regional anesthesia. 2nd ed. Philadelphia: Elsevier; 2005.
4. Rathmell JP. Chapter 6: Transforaminal and selective spinal nerve injection. In: Atlas of image-guided intervention in regional anesthesia and pain medicine. 2nd ed. Philadelphia: Lippincott Williams & Wilkins; 2012. p. 64–79.
5. Rathmell JP. Chapter 7: Facet injection: intra-articular injection, medial branch block, and radiofrequency treatment. In: Atlas of image-guided intervention in regional anesthesia and pain medicine. 2nd ed. Philadelphia: Lippincott Williams & Wilkins; 2012. p. 80–117.
6. Czervionke LF, Fenton DS. Facet joint injection and medial branch block. In: Fenton DS, Czervionke LF, editors. Image-guided spine intervention. Philadelphia: Saunders; 2003.
7. Raj PP, Lou L, Erdine S, Staats PS, Waldman SD. Chapter 30: Cervical facet block and median branch blocks. In: Radiographic imaging for regional anesthesia and pain management. Philadelphia: Churchill Livingstone; 2003. p. 185–96.
8. Clemons RR, Benzon HT. Facet syndrome: facet joint injections and facet nerve blocks. In: Benzon HT, Raja SN, Molloy RE, Liu SS, Fishman SM, editors. Essentials of pain medicine and regional anesthesia. 2nd ed. Philadelphia: Elsevier; 2005.

Thoracic Injections

40

Benjamin P. Lowry

Abbreviations

AP   Anteroposterior
CSF   Cerebrospinal fluid
IL-TESI   Interlaminar thoracic epidural steroid injection
LOR   Loss of resistance
RF   Radiofrequency
UTI   Urinary tract infection

Introduction

Thoracic back pain may be caused by trauma, spinal degenerative changes, neuropathic etiologies, or issues involving intrathoracic viscera. A thorough evaluation is essential for a correct diagnosis as well as determining appropriate treatment options. Interventions in or around the thoracic spine has the potential for a multitude of complications including pneumothorax, intravascular injection, or neuronal injury. The utilization of fluoroscopy, as well as the more recent use of sonography, has allowed for an improvement in needle placement, safety, and procedural efficacy.

Thoracic Injection Complications

- *Absolute contraindications*
  - Patient refusal
  - Local infection at the site
  - Systemic infection (UTI, pneumonia, etc.)

B.P. Lowry, M.D. (✉)
Department of Anesthesiology, Baylor Scott & White
Health/Texas A&M College of Medicine, Temple, TX, USA
e-mail: blowry@sw.org

  - Bleeding disorder
  - Full anticoagulation
  - Severe allergic reaction to injectants
  - Acute cord compression
- *Relative contraindications*
  - Pregnancy
  - Poorly controlled diabetes
  - Poorly controlled hypertension
  - Immunosuppression
  - Previous surgery altering the targeted anatomy
  - Intraspinal vascular dilation or anomalies near target site
  - Congestive heart failure [1–3]

Patient Positioning for Thoracic Procedures

- Patient is placed prone with 1–2 pillows or chest rolls underneath the anterior thorax to exaggerate thoracic kyphosis and improve access to the targeted interlaminar interspace. Additional pillows can be placed under their feet for comfort.

Interlaminar Thoracic Epidural Steroid Injection (IL-TESI)

- **Indications**
  - Most common indication is nerve root inflammation resulting in *thoracic neuritis* or *radicular symptoms*
    - Both diagnostic and therapeutic
  - Discogenic pain
  - Neuroforaminal stenosis
  - Central canal stenosis
  - Herpes zoster or zoster sin herpete
  - Postherpetic neuralgia

K.A. Sackheim, *Pain Management and Palliative Care: A Comprehensive Guide*,
DOI 10.1007/978-1-4939-2462-2_40, © Springer Science+Business Media New York 2015

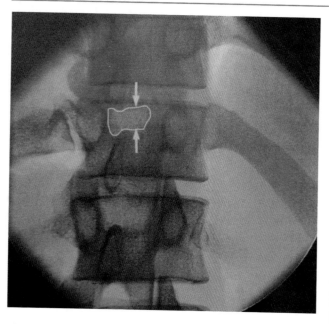

Fig. 40.1 Interlaminar interspace of T10-11 is outlined in *white*. The two *arrows* depict the superior and inferior aspects of the interspace

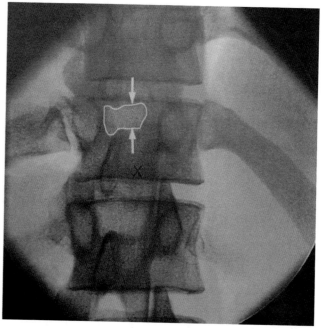

Fig. 40.2 The initial starting point is depicted by the *red X*. The superior and inferior end plates are squared utilizing cranial–caudal tilt of the fluoroscopy tube. The C-arm is then obliqued right or left 5–15° to maximize the view of the interlaminar interspace. The initial starting point typically overlies the inferior endplate of the vertebral body directly below the target interspace

- Posttraumatic neuralgia
- Vertebral fractures [1–3]
- *Interlaminar approach*—Most common approach to the epidural space
- Epidural space is accessed between the vertebral laminae using a posterior approach near midline in upper (T1-2 and T2-3) and lower thoracic levels (T11–12 and T12-L1)
- Paramedian approach is typically used in the mid thoracic spine (T4-10) due to the wider lamina and increased angulation of the spinous processes.
- *Transforaminal approach* (*selective nerve root block*)— poses an increased risk of intravascular injection and is discouraged by many pain physicians. Due to the increased danger, this approach will not be discussed.
- **Anatomy**
  - Borders of the epidural space are the laminae posteriorly, pedicles laterally, and vertebral bodies anteriorly (Fig. 40.1).
  - The ligamentum flavum defines the posterior border of the epidural space and is shaped like a hemicylinder with the most midline portion being the apex of the hemicylinder.
  - The epidural space contains a thin layer of adipose to cushion the thecal sac, a venous plexus, and loose areolar tissue.
- **Fluoroscopy**
  - Obtain an A-P image of the desired interlaminar space with slight caudal/cranial tilt to "square off" the vertebral endplate (view the superior endplate in a parallel

fluoroscopic plane) to improve visualization of the targeted interspace [5–10] degrees of oblique tilt may provide improved visualization of desired intralaminar interspace [1–3].

- **Procedure**
  - Anesthetize the skin and subcutaneous tissues 1 cm lateral and 2–3 cm inferior to the desired space with 1 % lidocaine (Fig. 40.2)
  - Tuohy needle is then inserted through the anesthetized skin
  - Needle is advanced until the lamina and base of the spinous process of the inferior level is contacted. The needle is slightly redirected cephalad until the needle tip has cleared the superior laminar edge is cleared.
  - Once the needle tip has cleared the superior laminar edge, change to lateral view, and use the loss of resistance (LOR) technique to locate the epidural space.
  - Once a loss is obtained, aspirate for the presence of blood or cerebrospinal fluid (CSF)
    - *If aspiration is positive for blood:* reposition the needle within the same interlaminar space or access at a different level
    - *If aspiration is positive for CSF:* consider re-accessing the epidural space at an adjacent level, or procedure can be discontinued depending on circumstances.

- *If aspiration is negative:* needle placement can be verified by injecting 1–3 mL of contrast and confirming spread in the epidural space in both the AP and lateral views while also excluding vascular or intrathecal spread (Fig. 40.3 and 40.4).
  – Once needle placement is confirmed, medications can be injected

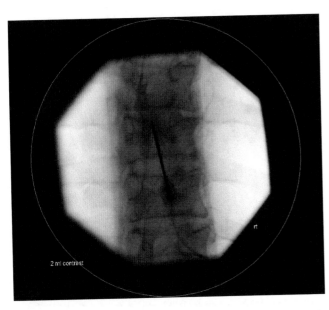

Fig. 40.3 Contrast spread noted in AP view within the thoracic epidural space

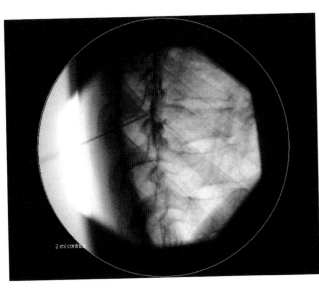

Fig. 40.4 Contrast spread noted in lateral view within the posterior thoracic epidural space

- **Medications injected**
  – *Mixture of:*
    - Non-particulate steroid diluted in 1–2 mL of sterile preservative-free normal saline
    - Some clinicians choose to add of 0.25 % Bupivacaine as well
    - Caution with injection of a high volume of anesthetic as it may cause the patient to feel temporary weakness and/or numbness at the lower extremities
  – *Total volume:* 3–5 mL
  – Smaller volumes may be indicated in stenotic patients or patients in excruciating radicular pain as increased pressure from the medications can cause brief heightened pain [1–3].

Thoracic Facet Joint Injections

- **Indications**
  – Diagnostic and therapeutic treatment of facetogenic mid-back pain
  – Thoracic spondylosis/Facet arthropathy
- **Contraindications**
  – Similar to contraindications for epidural steroid injections, although thought to have less risk of bleeding, intrathecal injection, or nerve trauma.
  – See contraindication section at the beginning of chapter.
- **Anatomy**
  – Facet joints are formed from the superior articular process of the inferior vertebra and the inferior articular process of the superior vertebra.
  – Joint orientation is nearly vertical and uniformly angled 110° from midline posterior sagittal plane
  – Each facet joint is innervated by two medial branch nerves originating at the level of the joint and the level directly above.
  – The facet joint is a true synovial joint with a limited volume of 0.4–0.6 mL in the thoracic region [4–7].
- **Fluoroscopy**
  – AP view is used to identify level. The joint is situated directly posterior to the unilateral pedicle. A lateral view is required to appreciate the joint line and confirm final needle placement [4–7].
- **Procedure**
  – The skin and subcutaneous tissue are anesthetized overlying the pedicle one level **below** target joint.
  – A 22 or 25 gauge spinal needle is advanced in a cephalad orientation toward the inferior aspect of the pedicle underlying target joint.

- The needle is walked superiorly until the joint capsule is penetrated.
- A lateral view is utilized to confirm needle tip is within the joint [4–7].
- **Medications injected**
  - *Mixture of:*
    Non-particulate steroid (if therapeutic)
    Bupivacaine 0.25–0.5 % or lidocaine 1–2 % (0.5 cc per level)

Thoracic Medial Branch Blocks (TMBB)

- **Indications**
  - Diagnostic and therapeutic treatment of facetogenic axial pain. Therapeutic blockade with steroid may provide several months of pain relief. Typically, if the patient has two successful blocks with >50 % symptomatic relief lasting <2 months, radiofrequency ablation is considered [4–7]
- **Anatomy**
  - *In the upper thoracic region (T1-T8)* the medial branch nerves course from the superolateral aspect of the transverse process inferomedially toward the facet joint. *In the lower thoracic region,* the medial branch nerves take a more medial course over the transverse process traversing inferomedially near the superior articular process (Fig. 40.5).
  - Thoracic facet joints are innervated by the medial branch at the same level and the level above. Both of these nerves must be blocked in order to diagnose/treat pain emanating from affected level.
    - Each joint is innervated by two medial branch nerves. For example, the T7-T8 facet joint is innervated by the T6 and T7 medial branch nerves [4–7].
- **Fluoroscopy**
  - Obtain an AP view to identify the appropriate level and the superior endplate is squared.
  - The transverse process of affected level is identified.
  - The target depends on the level to be blocked
    - T1-7 target is superolateral aspect of transverse process
    - T8-10 target is mid aspect of transverse process
    - T11-12 target is at the junction of the transverse process and the superior articular process [4–7]
- **Procedure**
  - Anesthetize the skin and subcutaneous tissue at the entry point with Lidocaine 1 % (Fig. 40.6).
  - Advance a 22 g spinal needle in a coaxial plane toward the superior aspect of the transverse process until os is

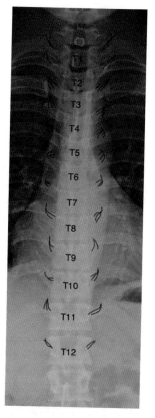

Fig. 40.5 The variable course of the thoracic medial branch nerves is illustrated above. In the superior and mid aspect of the thoracic spine the medial branch nerves typically course medially along the superior lateral aspect of the transverse process. The inferior thoracic spine medial branch nerves course over the transverse process near the junction of the superior articular process

contacted. The target will depend on the thoracic level to be blocked.
  - Check a lateral view to confirm needle placement (Fig. 40.7)
  - Always aspirate prior to injection to ensure negative for heme, CSF, or air.
  - Once needle position is confirmed, medications are injected [4–7].
- **Medications injected**
  - Diagnostic block may be done with 0.5–1.0 mL of local anesthetic at each level
    - Usually a series of two injections are performed with differing local anesthetics to monitor the amount of time with pain relief
      - Lidocaine should diminish pain for 1–3 h
      - Bupivacaine should diminish pain for 4–8 h
  - Some clinicians also use non-particulate steroid for added therapeutic affect [4–7]
  - *Each level:* 1.0 mL

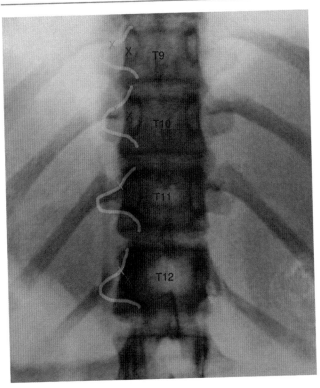

Fig. 40.6 Transverse processes outlined in *green*. The *red X* represents the starting point directly over the thoracic pedicle. The *orange X* represents the final needle tip target for block of the left T8-11 medial branch nerves

Thoracic Radiofrequency Ablation (RF)

- **Indications**
  - Facet-mediated pain that responds well to medial branch blocks for a short duration
- **Contraindications**: Same as for medial branch blocks Caution with pacemakers and defibrillators [4–7]
- **Anatomy**: See medial branch blocks (Fig. 40.7 and 40.8)
- **Fluoroscopy**: Same as medial branch blocks except with 25–30° caudal angulation [4–7]
- **Procedure**
  - Skin anesthesia same as medial branch blocks
  - Needle placement is typically started inferior to the target and advanced until the non-insulated portion of the needle lies parallel to the medial branch nerve.
  - Once the needle contacts bone at the superior margin of the transverse process it can be walked off the superior margin and advanced 2–3 mm beyond the facet joint in the lateral view. Confirm in the lateral radiographic view that the needle does not extend into the neural foramen or intrathoracic cavity.
  - *Sensory stimulation* is performed eliciting pain, pressure, or tingling at <0.5 V at 50 Hz
  - *Motor stimulation* up to 2.0 V should cause no motor stimulation into the abdominal or thoracic wall. *If muscle activity is noted the needle must be repositioned*

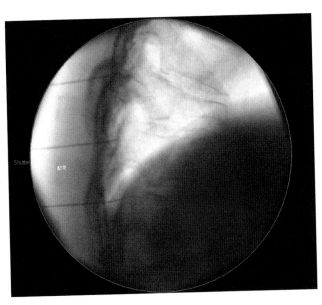

Fig. 40.7 Lateral view of radiofrequency ablation needle tips noted to be posterior to the thoracic neuroforamen

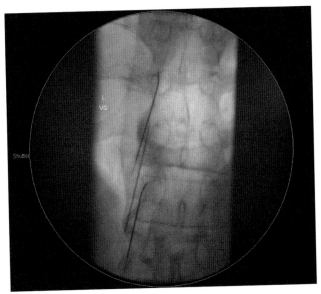

Fig. 40.8 Radiofrequency needles depicted with the active tips overlying thoracic medial branch nerves

– Each level is then anesthetized with 1 mL of lidocaine and subsequently treated with thermocoagulation, typically at 80 °C for 60–90 s [4–7].
• **Medications injected**
– Mixture of Bupivacaine 0.25 % and non-particulate steroid
– *Each level:* 0.5–1.0 mL

Intercostal Nerve Block

• **Indications**
– May be used as diagnostic procedure or to alleviate acute pain emergencies
– Thoracic neuritis
– Postherpetic neuralgia
– Postthoracotomy pain
– Rib pain (Traumatic or metastatic process)
– Pleuritic pain secondary to metastatic process
• **Contraindications**:
– Same as above
– Caution with coagulopathy, contralateral phrenic palsy, contralateral pneumonectomy, or end-stage pulmonary disease [6–11]
• **Anatomy**:
– Arises from anterior division of thoracic paravertebral nerve
– Neurovascular bundle courses along inferior border of rib.
– Situated only 2–10 mm posterior to pleura
• **Fluoroscopy**:
– Identify target level in AP view
– Fluoroscope is obliqued to ipsilateral side to enhance posterior rib [6, 9]
• **Procedure**
– Skin entry site is directly over inferior half of target rib.
– Entry site is anesthetized with 1 % lidocaine
– A 22–25 g spinal needle is advanced in a coaxial plane toward rib until os is contacted.
– Needle depth is noted
– The needle is walked off inferior border of rib and slowly advanced 2–3 mm
– Aspirate carefully looking for heme, CSF, or air.
– Contrast may be injected looking for spread along neurovascular bundle
– 3–5 mL of local anesthetic may be injected per level. If multiple levels are to be blocked, ensure total injectate below recommended toxicity dose
– For chronic pain conditions, intercostal nerves may be ablated utilizing cryoablation, thermal radiofrequency ablation, or neurolytic agents

• **Medications injected**
– Bupivacaine 0.25 %
– Steroid may be added for inflammatory etiologies
– *Each level:* 3–5 mL
• **Procedure Complications**
– Headache from accidental dural puncture (most common)
– Back pain
– Increased radicular pain
– Direct trauma to spinal cord or spinal nerves
– Infection such as epidural abscess
– Hemorrhage such as epidural hematoma
– Pneumothorax
– Intravascular injection
– Nerve root or spinal cord infarction
• *Pharmacologic complications*
– Seizure
– Bradycardia (anesthestizing cardiac accelerators)
– Hypotension
– Allergic reaction
– Neurotoxicity
– Weight gain
– Fluid retention
– Hypertension
– Congestive heart failure
– Cushing's syndrome

References

1. Rathmell JP. Chapter 5: interlaminar epidural injection. In: Atlas of image-guided intervention in regional anesthesia and pain medicine. 2nd ed. Philadelphia: Lippincott Williams & Wilkins; 2012. p. 34–63.
2. Stizman BT. Epidural injections. In: Fenton DS, Czervionke LF, editors. Image-guided spine intervention. Philadelphia: Saunders; 2003.
3. Raj PP, Lou L, Erdine S, Staats PS, Waldman SD. Chapter 13: spinal neuroaxial blocks. In: Interventional pain management—image guided procedures. Philadelphia: Saunders Elsevier; 2008. p. 267–78.
4. Rathmell JP. Chapter 7: Facet injection: intra-articular injection, medial branch block, and radiofrequency treatment. In: Atlas of image-guided intervention in regional anesthesia and pain medicine. 2nd ed. Philadelphia: Lippincott Williams & Wilkins; 2012. p. 80–117.
5. Czervionke LF, Fenton DS. Facet joint injection and medial branch block. In: Fenton DS, Czervionke LF, editors. Image-guided spine intervention. Philadelphia: Saunders; 2003.
6. Raj PP, Lou L, Erdine S, Staats PS, Waldman SD. Chapter 14: thoracic facet joint blocks and neurotomy. In: Interventional pain management—image guided procedures. Philadelphia: Saunders Elsevier; 2008. p. 279–90.
7. Clemons RR, Benzon HT. Facet syndrome: facet joint injections and facet nerve blocks. In: Benzon HT, Raja SN, Molloy RE, Liu SS, Fishman SM, editors. Essentials of pain medicine and regional anesthesia. 2nd ed. Philadelphia: Elsevier; 2005.

8. Rathmell JP. Chapter 14: intercostal nerve block and neurolysis. In: Atlas of image-guided intervention in regional anesthesia and pain medicine. 2nd ed. Philadelphia: Lippincott Williams & Wilkins; 2012. p. 196–205.

9. Benzon HT. Facet syndrome: herpes zoster and postherpetic neuralgia. In: Benzon HT, Raja SN, Molloy RE, Liu SS, Fishman SM, editors. Essentials of pain medicine and regional anesthesia. 2nd ed. Philadelphia: Elsevier; 2005.

10. Benzon HT. Facet syndrome: truncal blocks: intercostal, paravertebral, interpleural, suprascapular, ilioinguinal, and iliohypogastric nerve blocks. In: Benzon HT, Raja SN, Molloy RE, Liu SS, Fishman SM, editors. Essentials of pain medicine and regional anesthesia. 2nd ed. Philadelphia: Elsevier; 2005.

11. Raj PP, Lou L, Erdine S, Staats PS, Waldman SD. Chapter 11: somatic blocks of the thorax. In: Interventional pain management—image guided procedures. Philadelphia: Saunders Elsevier; 2008. p. 247–54.

Lumbar Injections

41

Christopher J. Burnett and Rodney R. Lange

Abbreviations

AP	Anteroposterior
CSF	Cerebrospinal fluid
IDD	Internal Disc Disruption
LESI	Lumbar Epidural Steroid Injection
LMBB	Lumbar Medial Branch Block
LOR	Loss of resistance
RFA	Radio frequency ablation
TFESI	Lumbar Transforaminal Epidural Steroid Injection
UTI	Urinary tract infection

Introduction

Low back pain is an extremely common reason for physician visits as well as lost work time, workers' compensation claims, and disability. A comprehensive history and physical examination is important in the determination of an appropriate diagnosis and in planning treatment options. Interventions include multiple types of injections that should be part of a multimodal approach.

C.J. Burnett, M.D. (✉)
Department of Anesthesiology, Baylor Scott & White
Health/Texas A&M College of Medicine, 2401 S. 31st Street,
Temple, TX 76508, USA
e-mail: cburnett@sw.org

R.R. Lange, M.D.
Division of Pain Medicine, Department of Anesthesiology,
Baylor Scott & White Health/Texas A&M College of Medicine,
Marble Falls, TX, USA
e-mail: rlange@sw.org

Patient Positioning for Lumbar Procedures

- Patient is placed prone with 1–2 pillows underneath the mid to lower abdomen to minimize lumbar lordosis
- Additional pillows can be placed under their chest and feet for comfort

Contraindications to Lumbar Procedures

- *Absolute contraindications*
  - Patient refusal
  - Local infection at the site
  - Systemic infection (UTI, etc.)
  - Bleeding disorder
  - Full anticoagulation
  - Severe allergic reaction to injectates
  - Acute cord compression
- *Relative contraindications*
  - Pregnancy
  - Poorly controlled diabetes
  - Immunosuppression
  - Anticoagulation medications
  - Previous surgery altering the targeted anatomy
  - Congestive heart failure
  - Stenosis at the target site [1–5]

Complications of Lumbar Procedures

- *Procedural complications*
  - Headache from accidental dural puncture (most common)
  - Back pain
  - Increased radicular pain
  - Direct trauma to cauda equina or spinal nerves
  - Infection/epidural abscess
  - Hemorrhage/epidural hematoma
  - Joint damage

K.A. Sackheim, *Pain Management and Palliative Care: A Comprehensive Guide*,
DOI 10.1007/978-1-4939-2462-2_41, © Springer Science+Business Media New York 2015

- *Pharmacologic complications*
  - Allergic reaction
  - Neurotoxicity
  - Weight gain
  - Fluid retention/edema
  - Hypertension
  - Increased blood glucose
  - Changes in menstrual cycle
  - Congestive heart failure
  - Cushing's syndrome [1–9]

Lumbar Interlaminar Epidural Steroid Injection (IL-LESI)

- Most common approach to the epidural space
- The epidural space is accessed between the vertebral laminae using a posterior approach at or near midline
- A slight paramedian approach may be used in an attempt to target the more symptomatic side
- **Anatomy for interlaminar approach**
  - *Borders of the epidural space*: the laminae posteriorly, pedicles laterally and vertebral bodies anteriorly (Fig. 41.1)
  - The ligamentum flavum defines the posterior border of the epidural space and is shaped like a tent with the most midline portion being the peak of the tent's roof
  - Epidural space contains epidural fat, a venous plexus, and loose areolar tissue making it an ideal space for steroid injection [1, 2]
- **Indications**
  - Utilized for both diagnostic and therapeutic treatments
  - Nerve root inflammation/irritation resulting in *radicular symptoms* is the most common indication (this can be associated with herniated intervertebral disc, isolated neuroforaminal stenosis, ligament/facet hypertrophy, or spondylolisthesis)
  - Radiculopathy or Radiculitis

- Back/leg Pain
- Central canal stenosis (neurogenic claudication/multi-radicular levels associated)
- Neuroforaminal stenosis
- Herniated Disc
- Discogenic pain (Internal Disc Disruption IDD)
- Degenerative Disc Disease
- Postherpetic neuralgia
- Post-traumatic neuralgia
- Post-laminectomy pain
- Vertebral fractures [1–3]

- **Fluoroscopy**
  - Obtain an AP fluoroscopic image of the desired interlaminar space with slight caudal or cranial tilt to improve visualization/opening of the targeted interspace [1–3] (Fig. 41.2)

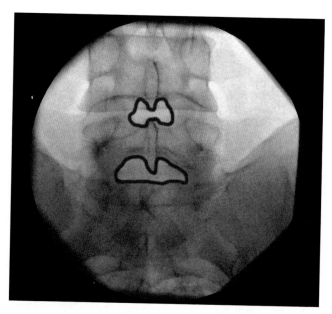

Fig. 41.1 The interlaminar space at L4–5 and L5–S1 is outlined in *blue*

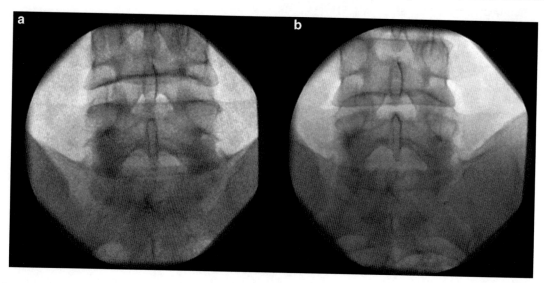

Fig. 41.2 By angling the fluoroscope in a cephalad or caudal angle the interlaminar space can be optimized for needle placement. (**a**) L5–S1 interlaminar space prior to angling the fluoroscope with a cranial tilt (**b**) Optimized fluoroscopic image of the L5–S1 interspace in the same patient

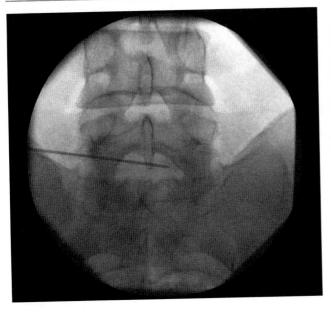
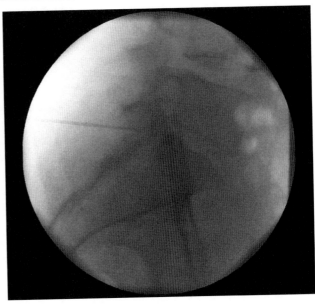

Fig. 41.3 Placing the needle onto the patient's back allows the identification of the optimal skin entry site for needle placement prior to anesthetizing the skin

Fig. 41.4 Lateral view showing depth target for LESI

- **Procedure**
  - *Entry Point*: slightly lateral to the midline of the desired open lamina
  - Anesthetize the skin over the desired space (Fig. 41.3)
  - A Tuohy needle is then inserted through the entry point
  - The needle is advanced until the ligamentum flavum is engaged. If at any time during advancement of the needle on AP view, you are not certain of your depth, check a lateral view to confirm.
  - Once ligamentum flavum is engaged change to a lateral view to assess depth (Fig. 41.4)
  - Loss of resistance (LOR) technique is initiated to locate the epidural space, while in a lateral fluoroscopic view
  - When LOR is obtained, aspirate for the presence of blood or cerebrospinal fluid (CSF)
    - *If aspiration is positive for blood*: then reposition the needle and repeat aspiration
    - *If aspiration is positive for CSF*: then reposition needle and consider access at a different level, can consider discontinuing procedure depending on circumstances. (Fig. 41.5 shows intrathecal contrast spread)
    - *If aspiration is negative*: epidural placement can be verified by injecting 1–3 mL of contrast and confirming spread in the epidural space in both the AP and lateral views, while also excluding vascular or intrathecal spread (Fig. 41.6)

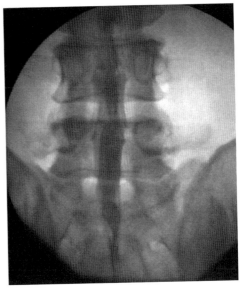

Fig. 41.5 AP fluoroscopic image of **intrathecal** contrast spread

  - Once proper needle placement is confirmed, medication mixture can be administered
- **Medications injected**
  - *Mixture of*:
    - Depomedrol 60–80 mg or equivalent steroid diluted in 1–3 mL of sterile preservative-free normal saline
    - Some clinicians choose to add 1–2 mL of 0.25 % bupivacaine
      - Use caution when injecting a high volume of anesthetic as it may cause the patient to feel

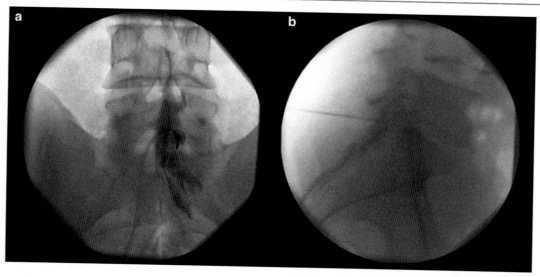

Fig. 41.6 (**a**) AP fluoroscopic image of contrast spread in the epidural space after an interlaminar L5–S1 epidural steroid injection to the right of *midline*. There is no evidence of contrast loculation, vascular run-off, or intrathecal spread. (**b**) Lateral fluoroscopic image of the same interlaminar L5–S1 epidural steroid injection showing appropriate needle depth and contrast spread into the posterior epidural space

temporary weakness and/or numbness in the lower extremities

- *Total Volume*: 5–6 mL
  - Smaller volumes may be indicated in stenotic patients or in patients with excruciating radicular pain, as increased pressure from the medications can cause a brief escalation of pain or can lead to fluid dissection of injectate into the intrathecal space [1–3]

Lumbar Transforaminal Epidural Steroid Injection

- It has been suggested that using the transforaminal approach improves outcomes by placing the injectate in closer proximity to the target nerve
- Lumbar transforaminal epidural steroid injection (TFESI) is more complicated than the interlaminar approach due to an increased risk of vascular or nerve root injury
- TFESI with local anesthetic may also be used diagnostically to determine which spinal nerve is the etiologic source of pain
- **Anatomy of the lumbar neural foramen**
  - Lateral border is formed by foramen of the lumbar vertebrae
  - Roof and floor are formed by the pedicles
  - Posterior border is formed by the superior articular process of the inferior vertebra, the inferior articular process of the superior vertebra, and the zygapophysial (facet) joint
  - Anterior border is the vertebral body and intervertebral disc
  - *Anatomical borders of the "safe" triangle*
    - Pedicules, superiorly
    - Lateral border of the vertebral body, laterally
    - Spinal nerve, inferior and medial
  - Each lumbar spinal nerve lies in the anterior–superior portion of the foramen (Fig. 41.7)
  - Vessels accompany the spinal nerves to the spinal cord
  - *The Artery of Adamkiewicz is the primary arterial supply to the anterior 2/3rds of the spinal cord. It most commonly enters the spinal cord on the left between T9 and L1, but may enter anywhere from T7 to L4. Trauma to this artery can lead to anterior spinal artery syndrome. This is a serious and devastating complication of a TFESI [4, 5].*
- **Indications**:
  - Essentially, the same as for the interlaminar approach with the potential for more selectively treating specific nerve roots
  - May also be more appropriate approach in patients who have undergone lumbar spinal surgery in order to avoid scar tissue or inadvertent dural puncture
  - Sometimes more beneficial in patients with unilateral pain

- **Fluoroscopy**
  - Start with AP view to identify the targeted level
  - Then square the superior endplate of the targeted level
    - This entails adjusting the fluoroscope in a cranial/caudal orientation until the endplates are aligned and appear as a single straight line (Fig. 41.8)
  - Once the appropriate level is identified, oblique the view 15–30° to the ipsilateral side, producing the "Scotty Dog" view (Fig. 41.9) [2, 4, 5]

- **Procedure**
  - *Entry Point*: Lateral to the desired foramen
  - Anesthetize the skin at the desired entry point
  - *Target*: On the oblique view, just below the 6 o'clock position of the pedicle or below the "chin" of the "Scotty Dog" (Fig. 41.10)
  - Insert the needle and slowly advance toward the antero/lateral aspect of the epidural space
  - The needle is advanced until the foraminal ligament is felt

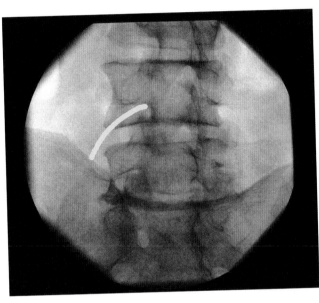

Fig. 41.7 Oblique fluoroscopic image for transforaminal approach to an epidural steroid injection at L4–L5. The L4 nerve is depicted in yellow exiting the neural foramen and descending

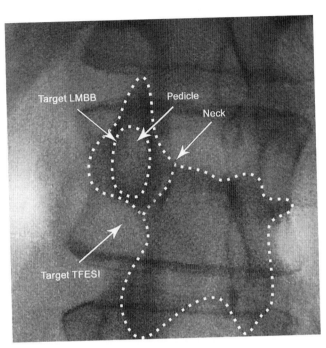

Fig. 41.9 "Scotty dog" image with targets notated for TFESI and LMBB procedures

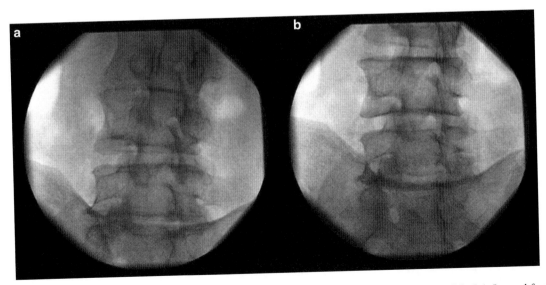

Fig. 41.8 (a) Oblique view of the L4–5 neural foramen prior to image optimization. (b) Fluoroscopic image of the L4–5 neural foramen in the same patient after slight caudal tilt of the fluoroscope to square off the inferior endplate of the L4 vertebral body

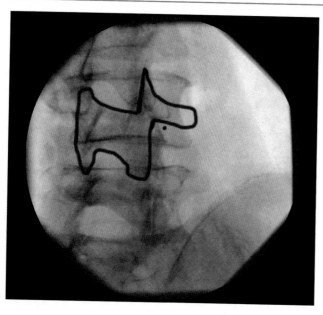

Fig. 41.10 Obliqued and optimized fluoroscopic image for a right-sided L4–L5 transforaminal epidural steroid injection. The "Scotty Dog" is outlined in *blue*. The blue dot at the six o'clock position of the pedicle depicts optimal position for needle skin entry site

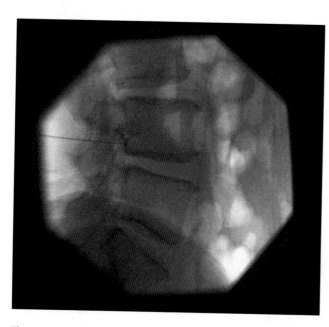

Fig. 41.11 Lateral fluoroscopic image showing the final needle position of the transformaminal epidural steroid approach. Note contrast spread in the anterior epidural space

- *Caution is maintained not to advance the needle too medial which could lead to direct contact with the nerve root*
- Once the ligament is approached, change to a lateral view to ensure appropriate depth
- The needle should be advanced beyond the posterior aspect of the neural foramen (Fig. 41.11)

- After negative aspiration, injection of contrast should show contrast spread in the anterior epidural space in the lateral view, as well as perineural and epidural spread in the AP view without vascular runoff or intrathecal spread [2, 4, 5]
  - If aspiration is positive for blood or CSF, the needle should be repositioned
- **Medications injected**
  - *Mixture of*:
    - Dexamethasone or equivalent non-particulant steroid diluted in 1–3 mL of sterile, preservative-free normal saline
      - ◆ *It is advocated to use non-particulate steroid due to the increased risk of intravascular injection and embolization with particulate steroid*
      - ◆ Some clinicians choose to add 1 mL of 0.25 % bupivacaine to the mixture for patient comfort and diagnostic value
      Use caution when injecting a high volume of anesthetic as it may cause the patient to feel temporary weakness and/or numbness of the lower extremities
  - *Total volume for each level*: 1–3 mL

Lumbar Facet Joint Injection

- **Anatomy of the lumbar facet joint**
  - Facet joints are formed from the superior articular process of the inferior vertebra and the inferior articular process of the superior vertebra (Fig. 41.12)
  - Each lumbar facet joint is innervated by two medial branch nerves
    - *First branch*: arises at the level of each joint
    - *Second branch*: originates from the level directly *above*
  - The facet joint is a true synovial joint with a limited volume that is typically <1.5 mL in the lumbar region [6–9]
- **Indications**
  - Diagnostic and therapeutic treatment of low back pain originating from the facet joints [6–9]
  - Pain from the facet joints can have a referral pattern which usually stops above the knee
- **Fluoroscopy**
  - AP view is used to identify the targeted level
  - Then oblique 25–35° to the ipsilateral side to visualize the joint space formed by the junction of the superior and inferior articular processes [6–9] (Fig. 41.13)
- **Procedure**
  - *Entry Point*: inferior one-third of the targeted facet joint
  - The skin is anesthetized at the entry point
  - A 22 gauge spinal needle is advanced in a coaxial view into the inferior aspect of the posterior joint space [6–9]

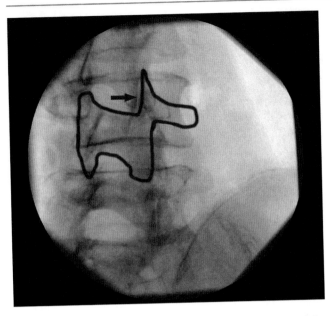

Fig. 41.12 Obliqued and optimized fluoroscopic image for a right-sided L3–4 intra-articular facet injection. The "Scotty Dog" is outlined in *blue*. The *blue arrow* depicts optimal needle skin entry site

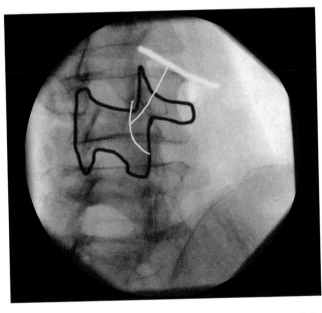

Fig. 41.13 Obliqued and optimized fluoroscopic image for a right-sided L3 medial branch block at the junction of the L4 superior articular process and transverse process. The "Scotty Dog" is outlined in *blue*. The L4 nerve root is depicted by the *thicker yellow line* with the L3 medial branch nerve descending from it illustrated by the *small yellow line*. As it descends beyond its targeted block site, it branches to give innervation to the facet joint above, as well as the facet joint below. The branching of the medial branch nerve results in the dual innervation of each facet joint from the level above and the level below

- Lateral fluoroscopy is used to confirm appropriate depth with the needle tip in the posterior aspect of the joint
- Some resistance should be felt when the needle tip enters the posterior capsule of the facet joint

- **Medications injected**
  - *Mixture of*:
    Depomedrol or equivalent steroid diluted in 0.25 % Bupivacaine. Can do diagnostic injection with anesthetic only.
  - Total Volume for Each Level: 0.5–1 mL

Lumbar Medial Branch Block

- **Anatomy of lumbar medial branch nerves**
  - Each lumbar medial branch nerve originates from the dorsal root ganglia of the spinal nerve above and descends to lie in the junction between the superior articular process and transverse process at each level
  - The medial branch nerve slopes inferomedially before branching to give innervation to the facet joint above and below (Fig. 41.13).
  - *Lumbar facet joints are innervated by the medial branch at the same level and from the level above.* Therefore, both of these nerves must be blocked in order to diagnose/treat pain emanating from a single facet joint
    - For example, the L3–L4 facet joint is innervated by the L2 and L3 medial branch nerves
  - The L5 dorsal primary ramus is blocked at the junction of the S1 superior articular process and the sacral ala [6–9]
- **Indications**: Diagnostic and therapeutic treatment of lumbar facet joint-mediated pain [6–9]
  - Most advocate starting with diagnostic blocks showing >50 % pain resolution for the duration of the local anesthetic
  - These patients are candidates for therapeutic treatment for more prolonged relief
- **Fluoroscopy**
  - Obtain an AP view to identify the appropriate level
  - Oblique the fluoroscopic view 25–35° to the ipsilateral side to optimize visualization of the "Scotty Dog"
  - Cranial or cephalad tilt can be used to square off the endplates of the targeted level
  - The target is the intersection of the transverse process and the superior articular process (the "eye" of the Scotty dog) (Fig. 41.14)
  - The one variation is the intersection of the S1 superior articular process with the sacral ala for the L5 dorsal primary ramus block [6–9] (Fig. 41.15)
- **Procedure**
  - *Entry Point*: lateral and slightly superior to the targeted pedicle
  - Anesthetize the skin at the entry point
  - Advance a 22 gauge curved spinal needle toward the target site

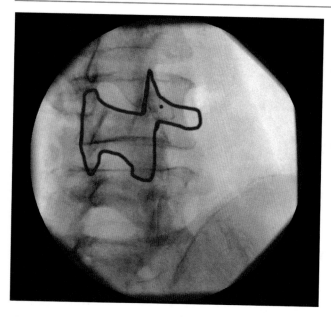

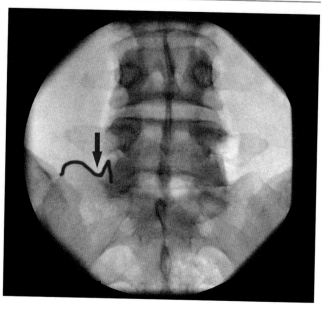

Fig. 41.14 Obliqued and optimized fluoroscopic image for a right-sided L3 medial branch nerve block at the junction of the L4 superior articular process and transverse process. The "Scotty Dog" is outlined in *blue*. The *blue dot* indicates optimal needle skin entry site

Fig. 41.15 AP fluoroscopic image optimized for blockade of the left L5 dorsal primary ramus. The left sacral ala and S1 superior articular process are outlined in *blue*. The *blue arrow* points to the groove through which the L5 dorsal primary ramus descends. Blockade should occur just below this junction

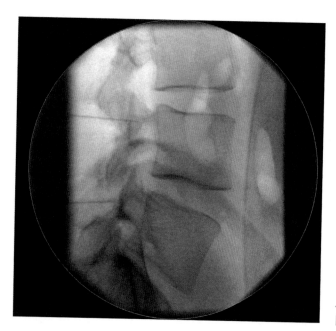

Fig. 41.16 Lateral target for LMBB

- Target is the periosteum at the junction of the superior articular process and transverse process
- Once the needle makes contact with periosteum, a lateral fluoroscopic image can be used to confirm appropriate depth (posterior to the neural foramen) (Fig. 41.16)
- Once needle position is confirmed and aspiration is negative for blood, medications are administered at each level

- **Medications injected**
  - Diagnostic block may be done with1–2 mL of local anesthetic at each level
    - A series of two injections may be performed with differing local anesthetics to monitor the amount of time that pain relief is obtained
      - Lidocaine should diminish pain for 1–2 h
      - Bupivacaine should diminish pain for 4–6 h
  - In patients who have successful diagnostic Lumbar medial branch block (LMBB), the procedure can be repeated with the addition of steroid to local anesthetic for added and prolonged therapeutic effect [6–9]
    - Depomedrol or equivalent
  - *Volume for each level*: 1–1.5 mL

Radiofrequency Ablation of Lumbar Medial Branch Nerve (RFA)

- **Anatomy**: see medial branch blocks
- **Indications**
  - Facet-mediated pain that responds well to medial branch blocks for a limited period of time
- **Contraindications**: See contraindications above
  - *Caution with pacemakers and defibrillators* [6, 9]
    Contact device manufacturer for safety recommendations before proceeding

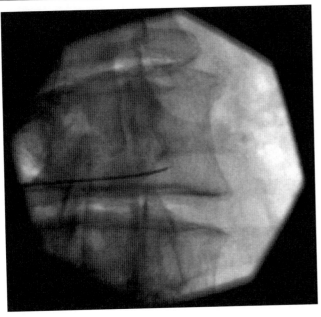

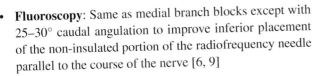

Fig. 41.17 Fluoroscopic image of needle marking appropriate skin entry site for placement of needle for radiofrequency ablation of lumbar medial branch nerve

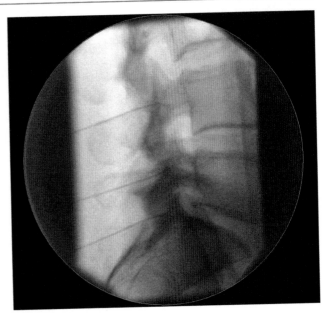

Fig. 41.18 Lateral fluoroscopic view of final needle placement for radiofrequency ablation of lumbar medial branch nerve

- **Fluoroscopy**: Same as medial branch blocks except with 25–30° caudal angulation to improve inferior placement of the non-insulated portion of the radiofrequency needle parallel to the course of the nerve [6, 9]
- **Procedure**
  - *Entry Point*: inferior to the pedicle (Fig. 41.17)
  - Anesthetize the skin at the entry point
  - A 20–22 g radiofrequency-compatible needle is inserted through the entry point with slight cephalad orientation
  - Advance until the needle lies parallel to the medial branch nerve in the groove between the transverse process and superior articular process
  - Once the needle contacts periosteum at the superior margin of the transverse process it can be walked off the superior margin and advanced 2–3 mm beyond the periosteum
  - Lateral fluoroscopy is used to verify that the needle tip does not extend into the neural foramen (Fig. 41.18)
  - *Sensory stimulation*: performed eliciting pain, pressure, or tingling in the lumbar spine
    Optimal placement should elicit stimulation at <0.5 V and 50 Hz
  - *Motor stimulation*: up to 1.5–2.0 V at 2 Hz should cause stimulation of the multifidus muscle of the back only and no motor stimulation into the lower extremity.
- Each level is then anesthetized with 1 mL of lidocaine 1 or 2 % and subsequently treated with thermocoagulation, typically at 80° Celsius for 60–90 s [6, 9].

- Patients should be counseled that there may be a delay in pain relief, as Wallerian degeneration can take up to 3 weeks to occur
- **Medications injected**
  - *Mixture of*: Depomedrol diluted with 0.25 % bupivacaine and equally distributed among treated levels
  - *Each level*: 1–2 mL
- **Complications specific to radiofrequency ablation (RFA)**
  - Exacerbation of pain
  - Dysesthesia/Neuritis
  - Injury to spinal nerve (much less common) [6, 9]
    May present as foot drop or weakness

References

1. Rathmell JP. Atlas of image-guided intervention in regional anesthesia and pain medicine. 2nd ed. Philadelphia: Lippincott Williams & Wilkins; 2012. p. 34–63. Chapter 5: Interlaminar epidural injection.
2. Stizman BT, Stizman BT. Epidural injections. In: Fenton DS, Czervionke LF, editors. Image-guided spine intervention. Philadelphia: Saunders; 2003.
3. Molloy RE, Benzon HT. Interlaminar epidural steroid injections for lumbosacral radiculopathy. In: Benzon HT, Raja SN, Molloy RE, Liu SS, Fishman SM, editors. Essentials of pain medicine and regional anesthesia. 2nd ed. Philadelphia: Elsevier; 2005.
4. Benzon HT. Selective nerve root blocks and transforaminal epidural steroid injections for back pain and sciatica. In: Benzon HT, Raja SN, Molloy RE, Liu SS, Fishman SM, editors. Essentials of

pain medicine and regional anesthesia. 2nd ed. Philadelphia: Elsevier; 2005.

5. Rathmell JP. Atlas of image-guided intervention in regional anesthesia and pain medicine. 2nd ed. Philadelphia: Lippincott Williams & Wilkins; 2012. p. 64–79. Chapter 6: Transforaminal and selective spinal nerve injection.

6. Rathmell JP. Atlas of image-guided intervention in regional anesthesia and pain medicine. 2nd ed. Philadelphia: Lippincott Williams & Wilkins; 2012. p. 80–117. Chapter 7: Facet injection: intra-articular injection, medial branch block, and radiofrequency treatment.

7. Czervionke LF, Fenton DS. Facet joint injection and medial branch block. In: Fenton DS, Czervionke LF, editors. Image-guided spine intervention. Philadelphia: Saunders; 2003.

8. Raj PP, Lou L, Erdine S, Staats PS, Waldman SD. Radiographic imaging for regional anesthesia and pain management. Philadelphia: Churchill Livingstone; 2003. p. 185–96. Chapter 30: Lumbar facet block and median branch blocks.

9. Clemons RR, Benzon HT. Facet syndrome: facet joint injections and facet nerve blocks. In: Benzon HT, Raja SN, Molloy RE, Liu SS, Fishman SM, editors. Essentials of pain medicine and regional anesthesia. 2nd ed. Philadelphia: Elsevier; 2005.

Sacral Injections

42

Christopher J. Burnett and Jared Anderson

Abbreviations

AP   Anteroposterior
CSF   Cerebrospinal fluid
ESI   Epidural steroid injection
RFA   Radiofrequency ablation
SIJ   Sacroiliac joint

Introduction

Sacral pain is very common and is categorized as a subset of back pain. A thorough history and physical examination are important in the diagnosis. Treatment should be multimodal with consideration for interventional procedures. In this chapter, interventional techniques used in the treatment of sacral pain are described.

Patient Positioning for Sacral Procedures

- Patient is placed prone with 1–2 pillows underneath the mid to lower abdomen to minimize lumbar lordosis
- Additional pillows can be placed under the chest and feet for comfort

C.J. Burnett, M.D. (✉)
Department of Anesthesiology, Baylor Scott & White Health/Texas A&M College of Medicine, 2401 S. 31st Street, Temple, TX 76508, USA
e-mail: cburnett@sw.org

J. Anderson, M.D.
Department of Anesthesiology/Pain Medicine, Baylor Scott & White Health/Texas A&M College of Medicine, College Station, TX, USA
e-mail: jeanderson@sw.org

Contraindications to Sacral Procedures

- *Absolute Contraindications*
  - Patient refusal
  - History of serious allergic reaction to injected medications
  - Proximal malignancy
  - Full anticoagulation
  - Infection at injection site
  - Allergy to injectate
- *Relative Contraindications*
  - Pregnancy
  - Proximal or systemic infection
  - Congestive heart failure
  - Coagulopathy
  - Anticoagulation medications
  - Uncontrolled diabetes mellitus

Complications of Sacral Procedures

- *Procedural complications*
  - Infection/epidural abscess
  - Hemorrhage/epidural hematoma
  - Joint damage
  - Intrathecal injection
  - Nerve ischemia/damage
  - Seizure
  - Post-procedural inflammation and pain are possible, but will typically resolve within a few weeks
- *Pharmacologic complications*
  - Allergic reaction
  - Neurotoxicity
  - Weight gain
  - Fluid retention/edema
  - Hypertension

K.A. Sackheim, *Pain Management and Palliative Care: A Comprehensive Guide*,
DOI 10.1007/978-1-4939-2462-2_42, © Springer Science+Business Media New York 2015

- Increased blood glucose
- Changes in menstrual cycle
- Congestive heart failure
- Cushing's syndrome [1–4]

Intra-Articular Sacroiliac Joint Injection

- **Anatomy**
  - Sacroiliac joint (SIJ) is the connection between the sacrum and the ilium in the pelvis on each side
  - Weight-bearing synovial joint
  - Stability of the SIJ is maintained primarily through an intricate network of ligaments
- **Indications**
  - Treatment of pain originating from the SIJ—Sacroiliitis
  - Low back or buttock pain that may radiate to the lateral thigh stopping above the knee
- **Fluoroscopy**
  - Obtain an AP view of the correct SI joint
  - To optimize fluoroscopic visualization of the SIJ, the fluoroscope is obliqued to the *contralateral side* until the inferior portion of the anterior and posterior aspects of the joint align radiographically

    This "alignment" is seen as a whitening of the joint as the joint lines overlap (Fig. 42.1)
- **Procedure**
  - *Entry Point*: Slightly medial to the inferior one-third of the joint space (Fig. 42.2)
  - Anesthetize the skin over the entry point
  - Insert a 22 g spinal needle at the desired location of the inferior joint margin
  - Approach the joint from medial to lateral (Fig. 42.3)
  - Slowly advance towards the joint
  - Lightly touch down on the bone medial to the joint

- Once you approach bone inject local anesthetic for patient comfort
- Continue to advance the needle laterally into the inferior one-third of the joint
- After negative aspiration, proper needle location can be shown with injection of contrast (0.5–1 mL) to ensure the needle tip is in the joint space (Fig. 42.4)
- **Medications Injected**
  - *Mixture of*:
    Dexamethasone or equivalent steroid
    1–3 mL of 1 % lidocaine and/or 0.25 % marcaine
  - *Total volume per side*:
    1–3 mL [1–3]

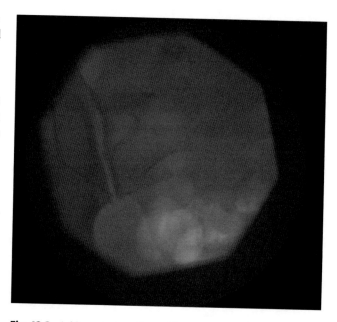

Fig. 42.2 A 22 g spinal needle marking the appropriate skin entry site for a left SIJ injection

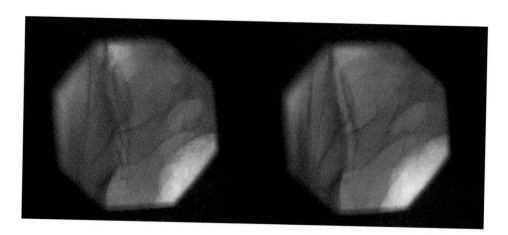

Fig. 42.1 The image on the *left* shows the SIJ before obliquing the fluoroscope to appropriately align the joint radiographically as seen in the image on the *right*

Fig. 42.3 The image to the *left* shows needle placement in the left SIJ advancing from medial to lateral. The image on the *right* shows final needle placement in the joint on the lateral fluoroscopic image

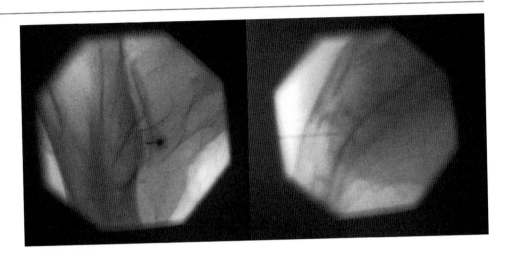

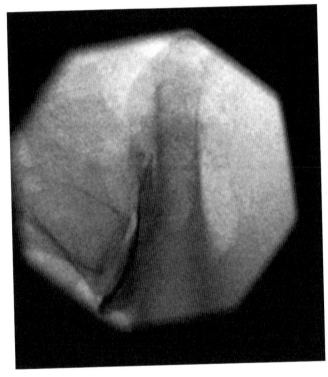

Fig. 42.4 Sacroliliac joint with contrast spread in the joint

Blockade of the Posterior Innervation of the Sacroiliac Joint (Medial and Lateral Branch Blocks)

- **Anatomy of the Posterior Sensory Innervation of the SIJ**
  - L4 medial branch nerve
  - L5 dorsal primary ramus
  - Lateral branch nerves S1–S3
    - Lateral branch nerves are located just lateral to the corresponding sacral foramen and can be blocked as they course towards the SIJ

- **Indications**
  - Blockade of the L4 medial branch nerve, the L5 dorsal primary ramus, and the lateral branch nerves S1–S3 can be utilized to treat sacroiliac-mediated pain
  - These can be done therapeutically and diagnostically to gauge potential effectiveness of radiofrequency ablation (RFA) for long-term relief
- **Fluoroscopy**
  - *L4 Medial Branch Nerve Block*
    - To optimize fluoroscopic visualization square off the superior endplate of the L5 vertebral body and oblique towards the *ipsilateral side* until the junction of the L5 superior articular process and the transverse process can be clearly seen, "scotty dog" view
  - *L5 Dorsal Primary Ramus Block*
    - AP fluoroscopic view is obtained with modest cranial/caudal or oblique angulation to optimize visualization of the junction of the ipsilateral S1 superior articular process with the sacral ala
  - *S1–S3 Lateral Branch Blocks*
    - AP fluoroscopic imaging is utilized with cranial/caudal angulation applied until each sacral foramen can be clearly visualized (Fig. 42.5)
    - This process may need to be repeated for each individual lateral branch block due to difficulty in obtaining an optimal image of all three sacral foramen in one view
- **Procedure**
  - Anesthetize the skin at the needle entry site
  - Advance needle under fluoroscopic guidance in a coaxial view
  - *Target for Each Block*
    - L4 Medial Branch Nerve Block:
      - Junction of the L5 superior articular process and transverse process (Fig. 42.6)

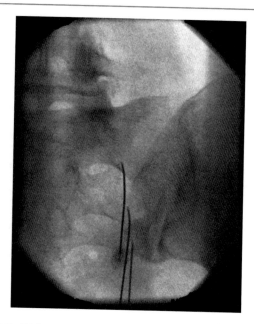

Fig. 42.5 AP fluoroscopic image of the S1–S3 foramen with needles in position for radiofrequency ablation of the lateral branch nerves

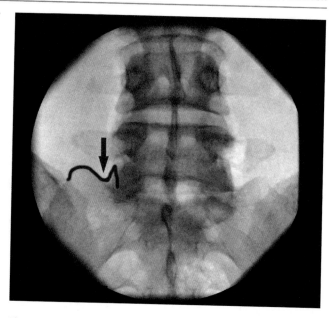

Fig. 42.7 AP fluoroscopic image optimized for blockade of the left L5 dorsal primary ramus. The left sacral ala and S1 superior articular process are outlined in *blue*. The *blue arrow* points to the groove through which the L5 dorsal primary ramus descends. Blockade should occur just below this junction

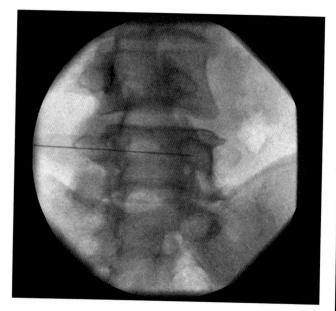

Fig. 42.6 Optimized fluoroscopic image for right L4 medial branch block. A 22-guage spinal needle is seen with the needle tip marking the approximate skin entry site for blockade of the L4 medial branch nerve at the junction of the L5 superior articular process and transverse process

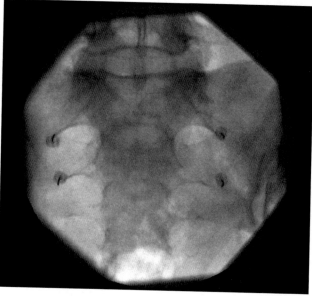

Fig. 42.8 AP fluoroscopic image showing final needle placement for bilateral S1–S2 lateral branch blocks

- L5 Dorsal Primary Ramus Block:
  - Junction of the sacral ala and the S1 superior articular process (Fig. 42.7)
- S1–S3 Lateral Branch Block:
  - Covers the lateral aspect of the respective sacral foramen to ensure adequate nerve block (Fig. 42.8)

- *Diagnostic blockade*: Injecting the L4 medial branch nerve, the L5 dorsal primary ramus, and the S1 through S3 lateral branch nerves with local anesthetic only
- *Therapeutic blocks*: Include the addition of steroid to the injected mixture in an effort to obtain prolonged pain relief [1–4]

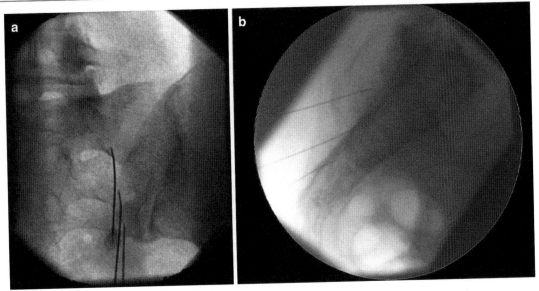

Fig. 42.9 Radiofrequency ablation of the S1–S3 lateral branch nerves. (**a**) AP fluoroscopic image with radiofrequency needles in optimal position for ablation of the right S1–S3 lateral branch nerves. (**b**) Lateral fluoroscopic image of final needle position for radiofrequency ablation of the right S1–S3 lateral branch nerves in the same patient. *Note*: The needles lie along the posterior wall of the sacrum and have not been advanced through the foramen

- **Medications Injected**
  - *Mixture of*:
    - Local anesthetic (1 % lidocaine and/or 0.25 % bupivicaine) 1–2 mL
    - Dexamethasone or equivalent steroid
  - *Total Volume at Each level*: 1–2 mL
- **Complications Specific to Medial and Lateral Branch Blocks**
  - Bowel perforation [1–4]

RFA for Sacroiliac-Mediated Pain

- **Anatomy of the Posterior Innervation of the Sacroiliac Joint**
  - See anatomy for blockade of the posterior innervation of SIJ
  - RFA treatment involves ablating the L4 medial branch nerve, the L5 dorsal primary ramus, and S1 through S3 lateral branch nerves
- **Indications**
  - Indicated after 1–2 successful diagnostic blocks or therapeutic blocks with excellent pain relief of short duration

  - RFA should only be performed on patients who received >50 % pain relief from previous diagnostic blocks [1, 4]
- **Fluoroscopy**
  - See fluoroscopic guidance for blockade of the posterior innervation of the SIJ
- **Procedure**
  - RFA Needle Positioning:
    - Needle angle with RFA should come from a more inferior approach in order to align the probe parallel to the nerve
    - *L4 Medial Branch Nerve Ablation*:
      Place the noninsulated portion of the needle parallel to the L4 medial branch nerve in the groove between the L5 transverse process and superior articular process
    - *L5 Dorsal Primary Ramus Ablation*:
      - Place the noninsulated portion of the needle parallel to the nerve at the junction of the sacral ala and S1 superior articular process
    - *Ablation of the S1–S3 Lateral Branch Nerves*:
      - Place the noninsulated portion of the radiofrequency needle parallel to the lateral edge of the sacral foramen to ensure adequate ablation of the targeted lateral branch nerve (Fig. 42.9)

- After the needle positions are confirmed radiographically on AP and lateral views, stimulation is performed at each level to ensure proximity to the nerve and as a safety measure
  - *Sensory stimulation*:
    - ◆ Goal is to elicit paresthesia of the low back and sacral region at ≤0.5 V at 50 Hz at each level
  - *Motor stimulation*:
    - ◆ Stimulation done up to 1.5 V at 2 Hz at each level to ensure no motor stimulation of the lower extremity or perineum
    - ◆ Place hand on extremity to ensure no muscle contractions
    - ◆ Contractions at the paraspinal muscles should occur
- Prior to lesioning, each level is anesthetized with 1–1.5 mL of lidocaine 1–2 %
- Thermal neurolysis is performed at 65–80 °C for 60–90 s

- **Medications Injected**
  - Pre-ablation
    - 1–1.5 mL of local anesthetic (usually 2 % lidocaine)
  - Post-ablation
    - Mixture of 0.25 % bupivacaine per level combined with Depomedrol (or equivalent steroid) can be injected at each level in an attempt to prevent post-ablation neuritis [1–4].
  - Volume Per Site Ablated: 1–2 mL [1–4]
- **Complications Specific to RFA**
  - Bowel perforation
  - Paralysis
  - Sexual dysfunction
  - Loss of bowel or bladder control
  - Post-procedure neuritis [1–4]

Sacral Transforaminal Injection

- **Anatomy of the Sacrum**
  - The sacrum is a triangular-shaped bone with a concave curvature and consists of five fused sacral vertebrae
  - There are four paired sacral foramen through which the sacral nerve roots, S1–S4, exit bilaterally
  - Sacral nerves are numbered according to the corresponding foramen through which they exit
  - Sacral formina are arranged in a linear fashion roughly 1 cm from the midline of the sacrum and are separated by approximately 1 cm
  - The S1 foramen is located about 1 cm medial to the posterior superior iliac spine and is usually the most circular in shape of the sacral foramen. The other sacral foramen are more oval in shape

- The foramen decrease in diameter from S1 to S4
- Sacral hiatus: Midline between the S4 foramen [3, 5]
- **Indications**
  - Lumbar disc herniation
  - Lumbar disc degeneration
  - Spinal stenosis
  - Sacral nerve radiculitis/neuritis
- **Fluoroscopy**
  - Obtain an AP image of the sacrum, then slightly oblique ipsilaterally, adjusting the cephalocaudal tilt until the coaxial view through the targeted foramen is attained
  - *Often, further* **cephalad tilt** *is used to place the anterior and posterior foramen out of radiographic alignment to act as a "back stop" to prevent needle passage through both foramen and potential inadvertent perforation of the bowel*
- **Procedure**
  - *Entry site*: Slightly inferior-lateral to the targeted foramen
  - Anesthetize the entry point
  - Insert a 22 g spinal needle through the entry site
  - Steer the needle superiorly and medial into the foramen
  - Many practitioners advocate lightly touching the bone surrounding the foramen to ensure proper depth
  - The needle is then advanced through the posterior foramen under fluoroscopic guidance in the coaxial view (Fig. 42.10)
  - Advance the needle until the tip is just beyond the posterior sacrum in the lateral fluoroscopic view to ensure proper depth (Fig. 42.11)

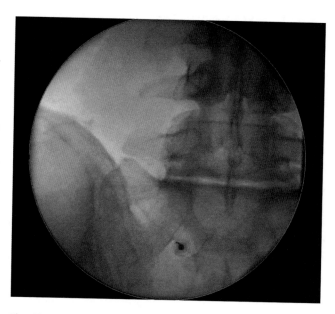

Fig. 42.10 AP fluoroscopic image of coaxial placement of a 22 g spinal needle into the left S1 foramen

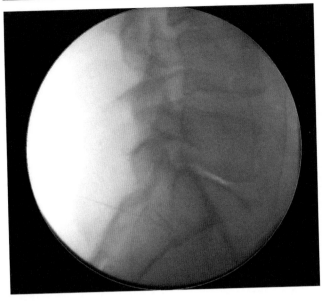

Fig. 42.11 Lateral fluoroscopic image of final needle placement for S1 transforaminal injection

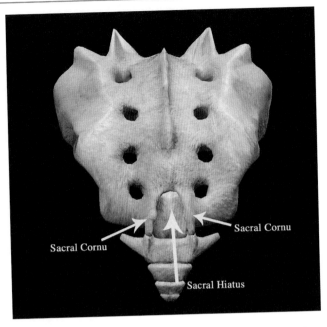

Fig. 42.13 Illustration of the posterior view of the sacral hiatus bordered laterally by the sacral cornu

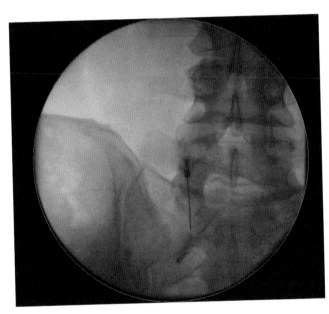

Fig. 42.12 AP fluoroscopic image of contrast spread down the left S1 nerve root

- After negative aspiration for cerebrospinal fluid (CSF) and blood, contrast should be injected to show spread down of the respective sacral nerve root without vascular runoff or uptake (Fig. 42.12)

- **Medications Injected**
  - *Mixture of*:
    0.5–1 mL of steroid (dexamethasone or equivalent nonparticulate steroid)
    1–2 mL of preservative-free normal saline

1–1.5 mL of local anesthetic
  - *Each Level*: 2.5–3.5 mL [5, 6]
- **Complications Specific to Sacral Transforaminal Injections**
  - Bowel Perforation

Caudal Epidural Steroid Injection

- **Anatomy of the Caudal Epidural Space**
  - The sacral hiatus is the most inferior aspect of the epidural space
  - The sacral hiatus is located between the two sacral cornu and is covered by the sacrococcygeal ligament (Fig. 42.13)
  - The dural sac extends to the S2 level in most adults [7]
- **Indications**
  - Lumbosacral disk herniation
  - Lumbar spinal stenosis with radicular pain (central canal stenosis, foraminal and lateral recess stenosis)
  - Compression fracture of the lumbar spine with radicular pain
  - Facet or nerve root cyst with radicular pain
  - To treat radicular pain on patients with previous surgery
- **Fluoroscopy**
  - Lateral fluoroscopy is used to visualize the sacral hiatus and confirm appropriate needle depth
  - AP view can be utilized to locate the midline of the sacral hiatus

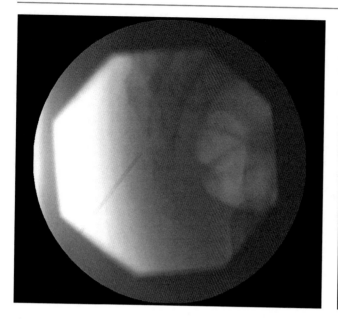

Fig. 42.14 Lateral fluoroscopic image of needle marking skin entry site for caudal epidural steroid injection. *Note*: The sacrococcygeal ligament anterior and inferior to the needle tip and the sacral hiatus just above and anterior to the needle tip

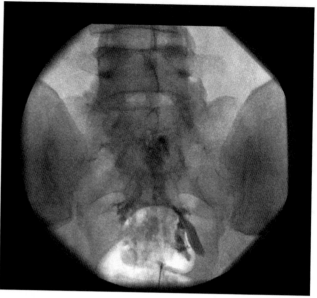

Fig. 42.15 AP fluoroscopic image of needle placement in the caudal epidural space following injection of contrast. *Note*: Nerve root runoff in the sacral distribution

- **Procedure**
  - Position the patient as above with the toes directed medially for easier access to the caudal canal
  - Identify the sacrococcygeal ligament with the sacral hiatus lying just superiorly
  - *Entry point*: Midline and inferior to the sacral hiatus
  - Anesthetize the skin overlying the entry point
  - Insert a 22 g spinal needle (or a larger specialized needle if necessary for catheter or scope placement)
  - Needle insertion is at a 45° angle between the sacral cornu directed toward the center of the hiatus
  - Lateral fluoroscopy is utilized for initial needle placement (Fig. 42.14)
  - Resistance of the sacrococcygeal ligament may be felt
  - As the needle passes through the sacrococcygeal ligament, the angle of approach should be flattened and the needle advanced an additional 1 cm
  - After negative aspiration for blood or CSF, 2–3 mL of contrast should be injected to confirm placement (Fig. 42.15)
  - Lateral and AP fluoroscopic views should be used to confirm no vascular uptake/runoff or intrathecal spread
  - Caudal epidural spread should show fatty globular pattern with sacral nerve root runoff, further confirming epidural placement
  - Once epidural placement is confirmed, the injectate is administered [7, 8]

- **Medications**
  - *Mixture of*:
    2–3 mL of local anesthetic
    Methylprednisolone, dexamethasone, or equivalent steroid
    Sterile, preservative-free normal saline comprises the remaining volume [7, 8]
  - *Total Volume*: The volume utilized should correspond to the desired height of medication spread
    10–15 mL will typically reach the level of L4 unless there is significant central stenosis
    Larger or smaller volumes may be used to reach specific levels
    Smaller volumes may be necessary in cases of spinal stenosis
- **Complications Specific to Caudal ESI**
  - Bowel perforation
  - Paralysis [7, 8]

References

1. Rathmell JP. Atlas of image-guided intervention in regional anesthesia and pain medicine. 2nd ed. Philadelphia: Lippincott Williams and Wilkins; 2012. p. 118–30.
2. Kransdorf MJ. Sacroiliac joint injection. In: Fenton DS, Czervionke LF, editors. Image-guided spine intervention. Philadelphia: Saunders; 2003.
3. Raj PP, Lou L, Erdine S, Staats PS, Waldman SD. Radiographic imaging for regional anesthesia and pain management. Philadelphia: Churchill Livingstone; 2003. p. 242–4.

4. Benzon HT. Pain originating from the buttock: sacroiliac joint dysfunction and piriformis syndrome. In: Benzon HT, Raja SN, Molloy RE, Liu SS, Fishman SM, editors. Essentials of pain medicine and regional anesthesia. 2nd ed. Philadelphia: Elsevier; 2005.

5. Raj PP, Lou L, Erdine S, Staats PS, Waldman SD. Radiographic imaging for regional anesthesia and pain management. Philadelphia: Churchill Livingstone; 2003. p. 226–30.

6. Fenton DS, Czervionke LF. Selective nerve root block. In: Fenton DS, Czervionke LF, editors. Image-guided spine intervention. Philadelphia: Saunders; 2003.

7. Rathmell JP. Atlas of image-guided intervention in regional anesthesia and pain medicine. 2nd ed. Philadelphia: Lippincott Williams and Wilkins; 2012. p. 34–63.

8. Stizman BT. Epidural injections. In: Fenton DS, Czervionke LF, editors. Image-guided spine intervention. Philadelphia: Saunders; 2003.

Sympathetic Block Injections

43

Leena Mathew and Angela Lee

Abbreviations

AP   Anteroposterior
CRPS   Complex regional pain syndrome
CSF   Cerebral spinal fluid
CT   Computed tomography

Sympathetic Blocks

Techniques of Sympatholysis

- Phentolamine infusion
- Regional anesthetic sympathetic blocks

Mechanism of Action

- Blocks/interrupts nociceptor visceral and somatic afferents with the vasomotor, sudomotor, and visceromotor fibers

Sympathetic Blocks at Different Levels

- Stellate ganglion
- Thoracic sympathetic chain blockade
- Lumbar sympathetic chain blockade
- Celiac plexus block
- Hypogastric plexus block
- Ganglion of impar

L. Mathew, M.D. (✉)
Division of Pain Medicine, Department of Anesthesiology,
New York Presbyterian Hospital, Columbia University,
New York, NY 10032, USA
e-mail: Lm370@cumc.columbia.edu; LM370@Columbia.edu

A. Lee, M.D.
Department of Anesthesiology, Columbia University Medical
Center, New York Presbyterian Hospital, New York, NY, USA
e-mail: acl9006@nyp.org

Prior to Procedures Below

- Obtain intravenous access
- Emergency vasoactive medications should be prepared
- Airway equipment should be easily accessible in the event of an emergency

Stellate Ganglion Block

- **Indications** (Table 43.1)
- **Anatomy** (Fig. 43.1)
  - *Surface landmarks*
    - C6 tubercle (Chassaignac's tubercle)
    - Medial border of the sternocleidomastoid muscle
    - Ipsilateral carotid artery
    - Surface landmarks of C7 are more difficult to palpate owing to its vestigial anterior tubercle relative to the other cervical vertebra
  - *Location and boundaries*
    - Cervical sympathetic chain is divided into the superior, middle, and inferior cervical ganglia that comprise preganglionic fibers from the upper thoracic segments of the spinal cord [1–3].
    - Stellate ganglion:
      - Formed by fusion of the inferior cervical and the first thoracic ganglia (in 80 % of population) which provides sympathetic outflow to upper extremities via the brachial plexus and to the head and neck along the carotid artery.
      - At level of the C7 and T1 interspace [4]
      - Approximately 1–3 cm in length and 3–10 mm in width
      - Bordered medially by longus colli muscle, posteriorly by head of the first rib, prevertebral fascia, and transverse process of C7, anteriorly by the vertebral artery and posterior fascia of the carotid sheath, laterally by scalene muscles, phrenic nerve, and the carotid sheath, and inferiorly by the lung pleura [5].

K.A. Sackheim, *Pain Management and Palliative Care: A Comprehensive Guide*,
DOI 10.1007/978-1-4939-2462-2_43, © Springer Science+Business Media New York 2015

Table 43.1 Indications for stellate ganglion block [1, 2]

Pain syndromes	Vascular insufficiency	Miscellaneous
Acute herpes zoster, postherpetic neuralgia	Raynaud's disease	Hyperhidrosis
Complex regional pain syndrome (CRPS) type I, II	Vasospasm	Meniere's disease
Phantom limb pain	Intractable angina pectoris	
Postradiation neuritis	Scleroderma	
Postsurgical neuropathy	Occlusive vascular disease	

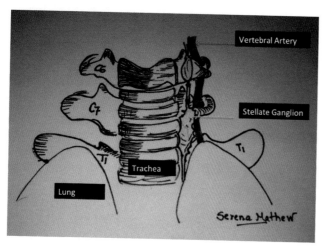

Fig. 43.1 Stellate ganglion surface anatomy

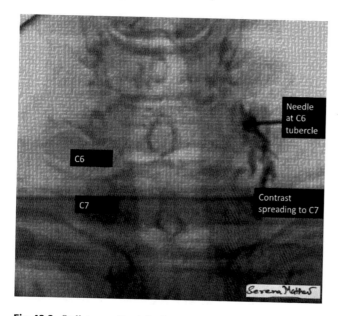

Fig. 43.2 Stellate ganglion injection with fluoroscopy

- **Fluoroscopy** (Fig. 43.2)
  - Supine position on the fluoroscopic table with a roll under the shoulder blades to provide some neck extension
  - A paratracheal approach is classic.
  - The C-arm is directed such that an anteroposterior (AP) view is obtained with the disc spaces sharply aligned between C5–C6 and C6–C7.
  - The target is the junction of the transverse process with the vertebral body.

- **Techniques**
  - C6 paratracheal approach is the most commonly used
  - Both the C6 transverse process approach and the C7 anterior paratracheal approach can be done under fluoroscopic guidance.
- Postion: patient placed supine
- **Procedure** [1, 2, 4, 6–10]
  - Neck in mild extension
  - Target point is marked after evaluating landmarks with fluoroscopy
  - The target is either the junction of the transverse process with the body at C6 or C7 level on the ipsilateral side. Local anesthesia is provided at the marked target site using 1–3 cm³ of 1 % lidocaine using a 25 G 1.5 in. needle.
  - A 25 G needle with a syringe attached via a connector is then inserted through the skin wheal.
  - Needle is advanced through the deep tissue in a gun barrel orientation until bony contact is made at the tubercle at the junction of the transverse process with the vertebral body at C6 or C7
  - At that point, withdraw the needle by a 1 mm
  - Confirm negative aspiration for blood or cerebral spinal fluid (CSF)
  - If the patient does not have a contrast allergy, inject 1–5 cm³ of radiographic contrast under real-time continuous fluoroscopy
  - Confirm the absence of intravascular uptake and appropriate localization of the needle.
  - Contrast should spread in the longus colli muscle
  - Flow of contrast extending to the head of the first rib can be observed by increasing the amount of contrast or injection of drug mixture which pushes the contrast up and down.
  - A test dose of 0.5 cm³ of 1 % lidocaine should be injected to confirm the absence of any intravascular uptake.
  - With intermittent vital sign monitoring, the medications should be injected in 1–2 cm³ increments with intermittent aspiration.
- **Medications**
  - 5–10 cm³ of a mixture of 1 % lidocaine or 0.25 % bupivacaine with or without 10–40 mg of triamcinolone or its equivalent steroid may be used for sympathetic nerve block
  - 5–10 cm³ radiographic contrast

- **Signs of effective blockade**
  - Horner's syndrome (miosis, ptosis, enophthalmos, anhidrosis)
  - Vasodilation of ipsilateral upper extremity and face
  - Ipsilateral increase in skin temperature by at least 1 °C
  - Loss of galvanic skin response
- **Side effects**
  - Recurrent laryngeal block
  - Phrenic nerve block
  - Brachial plexus block
  - Horner's syndrome
- **Complications** [2, 4, 8–10]
  - Retropharyngeal hematoma
  - Esophageal puncture, mediastinitis
  - Transverse process osteitis
  - Injury to carotid/vertebral artery causing dissection or stroke
  - Vertebral artery embolism causing stroke
  - Seizures and local anesthetic toxicity from intravascular injection
  - Total spinal from subdural or subarachnoid injection
  - Cardiac arrest
  - Pneumothorax
- **Contraindications**
  - Localized infection or sepsis
  - Coagulopathy
  - Pneumothorax
  - Contralateral hemi-diaphragmatic paralysis
  - Recent myocardial infarction
  - Glaucoma
  - Atrioventricular block

Thoracic Sympathetic Block

- **Indications**
  - Complex regional pain syndrome (CRPS)/Thoracic sympathetically mediated pain
  - Postherpetic neuralgia
  - Thoracic and upper abdominal visceral pain
  - Post-mastectomy syndrome or post-thoracotomy pain syndrome
  - Hyperhidrosis
  - Angina pectoris
- **Anatomy** (Fig. 43.3)
  - Series of ganglia, which usually correspond in number to that of the vertebrae
  - Thoracic ganglia rest against the heads of the ribs and are covered by the costal pleura
  - White and gray rami communicantes connect each ganglion with its corresponding spinal nerve
- **Patient Positioning**
  - Prone with a chest roll to maximize neck flexion and move the scapulae laterally to expose the upper thoracic ribs.
  - Scapula can be further displaced by abducting shoulders and placing forearms over the patient's head.
- **Fluoroscopy**
  - Obtain a PA view over the vertebra and costovertebral articulation of interest.
  - Using the intercostal oblique approach described by Stanton-Hicks [11], the image intensifier is rotated cephalad so axis is in the same plane as the neck of the rib.

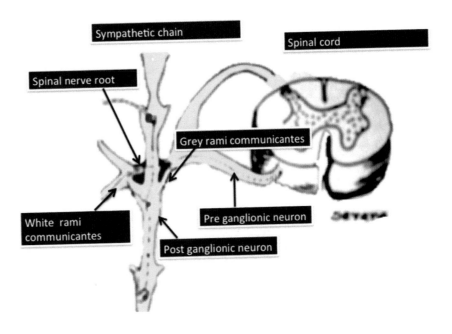

Fig. 43.3 Section of thoracic sympathetic chain anatomy

L. Mathew and A. Lee

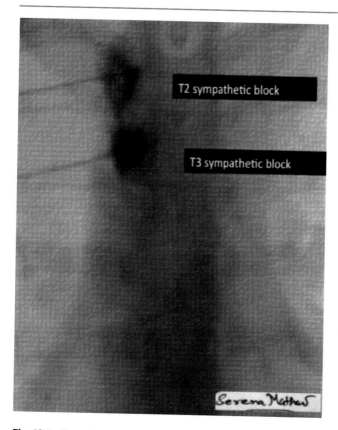

Fig. 43.4 Thoracic sympathetic block with fluoroscopy

- From this point, the C-arm is rotated to a lateral oblique position in order to superimpose the costotransverse articulation over the costovertebral articulation.
- **Procedure**
  - Sterile prep is done using betadine or chlorhexidine.
  - Local anesthesia is provided at the marked target site using 1–3 cm^3 of 1 % lidocaine using a 25 G 1.5 in. needle.
  - A 25 G needle with a syringe attached via a connector is then inserted through the skin wheal approximately 4 cm lateral to the spinous process
  - The needle is advanced under gun barrel view
  - The lateral view is checked to ensure that the needle tracks cephalad to the vertebral foramen to avoid the emerging somatic nerve.
  - The needle is advanced until the tip is immediately beside the vertebral body, anterior to the vertebral foramen, and next to the anterior aspect of the neck of the rib (Fig. 43.4)
- **Adverse effects**
  - Hypotension
  - Bradycardia
- **Complications**
  - Hematoma
  - Osteitis
  - Local anesthetic toxicity from intravascular injection

- High spinal from epidural, subdural, or subarachnoid injection
- Cardiac arrest
- Pneumothorax
- **Contraindications**
  - Localized infection or sepsis
  - Coagulopathy
  - Pneumothorax

Celiac Plexus Block

- **Indications**
  - Cancer pain in the abdomen to the level of splenic flexure of transverse colon
  - Abdominal angina
  - Hepatobiliary disorders
  - Acute or chronic pancreatitis
- **Anatomy**
  - *Surface landmarks*
    - Spinous processes of T12 and L1
    - T12 vertebral body identified by following 12th rib medially or counting up from L5
    - 5–6 cm lateral from midline for transcrural and 7–8 cm for the retrocrural approach.
    - The celiac plexus innervates most viscera in the abdominal cavity including the pancreas, liver, gallbladder, omentum, mesentery, and alimentary tract from the stomach to the transverse portion of the large colon (Fig. 43.5) [12].
    - Presynaptic sympathetic innervation of celiac plexus originates from the thoracic sympathetic trunk via the splanchnic nerves.
    - Enters abdomen through crura of diaphragm and synapses with the celiac plexus at the T12/L1 vertebral level.
    - The celiac plexus also receives parasympathetic and sensory innervation from the vagus and phrenic nerve.
    - Afferent nociceptive fibers from the abdominal viscera also travel through the celiac plexus with the sympathetic nerves and are the main target of the celiac plexus block.
    - The celiac plexus is located over the anterolateral aspect of the aorta
    - Just anterior to the diaphragmatic crus
    - Extends over origins of the celiac artery and superior mesenteric artery.
    - The plexus is composed of celiac ganglia, superior mesenteric, and the aortic renal ganglia.
    - Postganglionic fibers from the celiac plexus synapse with all the abdominal organs excluding descending colon, sigmoid colon, rectum, and the pelvic viscera.

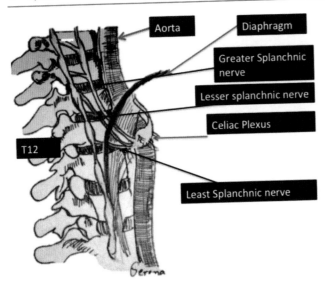

Fig. 43.5 Celiac plexus block anatomy

- **Patient Positioning**
  - Prone with a pillow underneath the abdomen to minimize lumbar lordosis

Approaches:

Transcrural Celiac Plexus Block [2, 6–9, 12]
  - In this technique, the needle penetrates the diaphragmatic crura
  - Directly blocks celiac plexus by depositing local anesthetic or neurolytic agents over anterolateral surface of aorta to surround the celiac plexus.
- **Procedure**
  - Study the abdominal CT scan carefully to identify the vertebral level corresponding to the celiac axis (may range from T12 to L2).
  - Obtain a PA view of the low thoracic and upper lumbar spine
  - L1 and T12 vertebral bodies and 12th rib should be identified with fluoroscopic imaging.
  - Needle insertion site is 5–6 cm from midline at the level of the celiac axis identified via CT scan prior to initiating the procedure.
  - Most commonly insertion is at the L1 level.
  - Rotate the image intensifier obliquely so that the tip of the L1 transverse process nearly overlies the anterolateral border of the L1 vertebral body.
  - A skin wheal is created with 1 % lidocaine over needle insertion sites on the left and right side.
  - First approach from the left side, then proceed with the right side
  - The left side is approached first so that if a complication occurs and the aorta is punctured, a single needle transaortic technique may be done instead.

- A 22-gauge styleted needle (spinal or Chiba needle 10–18 cm in length) is inserted with a gun barrel approach to the C-arm.
- Angle of insertion is 45° angle towards midline and 15° cephalad, coaxial with the image intensifier.
- The needle is advanced towards the anterolateral surface of the L1 vertebral body under intermittent imaging every 1–2 cm until bony contact is made with the vertebral body.
- At this point, redirect to walk the needle off the anterolateral edge of the L1 vertebral body.
- Once the needle is walked off the anterolateral edge of L1 vertebral body, change the C-arm view to lateral approach.
- Slowly advance the needle under lateral view so that the needle tip is 1–2 cm anterior to L1 vertebral body.
- *Correct positioning of the needle entry point is crucial*
  - Too lateral an entry point would risk injury to the renal parenchyma.
  - Cephalad approach at T11 risks puncture of the lung.
  - Too caudally towards the vertebral body of L2 risks ineffective block.
- *Caution: **Major vascular structures are being approached at this time***
  - *Left Side: **aorta***
  - *Right Side: **inferior vena cava***
- Continuous aspiration should be employed to assess for vascular puncture
- As the needle traverses the lateral surface of the L1 vertebra, a pop is often felt signifying penetration of the psoas fascia
- As the aorta is approached, transmitted vibrations can be felt through the needle.
- If the aorta is punctured, the needle should be advanced anteriorly with aspiration until there is negative aspiration.
- In the event of accidental puncture of the aorta, the block can be converted to a transaortic technique. This is why the left side is approached first. A transaortic technique then obviates the need to do the same technique on the right side as well.
- At the end point, the needle tip should be medial to the lateral border of the L1 vertebral body in the PA view.
- After confirming negative aspiration for blood, CSF, and urine, 2–5 cm³ of radiographic contrast should be injected and assess for spread over the anterior surface of the aorta.
  - Exclude intravascular and intrathecal injection. Attention for spread of contrast posteriorly towards the neuroforamina should also be noted to avoid permanent nerve injury.

- If the contrast spreads bilaterally across midline over the anterior surface of the aorta, a single puncture approach is adequate for bilateral celiac plexus block.
- If spread of contrast is unilateral, a right-sided approach is undertaken with the same technique described above.

- **Medications**
  - If a diagnostic block is to be performed prior to chemical neurolysis, a total of 10–20 cm³ of 0.25 % bupivacaine (5–10 cm³ each side) should be injected in increments with frequent interval aspiration.
  - For neurolysis, 10–20 cm³ of ethanol (30–50 % concentration) or phenol (6 % concentration) may be injected to each side.

Retrocrural Splanchnic Nerve Block [2, 6–9, 12]

- Local anesthetics or neurolytic agents are deposited posterior to the diaphragmatic crura
- Eliminates the sympathetic input to the celiac plexus

- **Fluoroscopy**
  - C-arm should is angled 20–30° cephalad to bring the inferior margin of the 12th rib cephalad to the T12 vertebral body.

- **Procedure**
  - The insertion site is approximately 5–6 cm from midline
  - A 22-gauge styleted needle (spinal or Chiba needle 10–18 cm in length) is inserted with a gun barrel approach to the C-arm
  - Repeat images should be taken intermittently and frequently every 1–2 cm of advancement
  - Make sure that the need is coaxial and contact T12 or L1 depending
  - At this point, obtain a lateral view and advance the needle until it is just medial to the lateral border of T12 or L1 vertebral body
  - 5 cm³ of radiographic contrast should be injected after ensuring negative aspiration
  - The contrast will spread in a cephalocaudal fashion over the anterolateral surface of the vertebral bodies
  - Using the same approach, position the needle on the contralateral side
  - Inevitably needs a bilateral block
  - This is distinctly different from the transcrural approach since at this angulation and level, the crura is not being breached for access.

- **Medications**
  - If a diagnostic block is performed, 10–15 cm³ of 2 % lidocaine or 0.25 % bupivacaine is injected to each side with frequent interval aspiration.
  - For neurolysis, 5–8 cm3 of either 30–50 % ethanol or 6 % phenol can be injected at each side.

- **Adverse effects**
  - Diarrhea from unopposed parasympathetic input to the GI tract
  - Orthostatic hypotension
    - Hypotension can be prevented by giving a preemptive 500–1,000 cm³ bolus of crystalloid prior to the start of the procedure
    - May last for 24–48 h

- **Complications**
  - Hematuria (usually resolves spontaneously)
  - Intravascular, intrathecal, epidural, or intradiscal injection
  - Pneumothorax
  - Renal injury
  - Retroperitoneal hematoma
  - Paresthesias due to spinal nerve injury
  - Painless paraplegia due to injury or spasm of the artery of Adamkiewicz
  - Failure of ejaculation

- **Contraindications**
  - Patients on anticoagulant therapy or those with a bleeding diathesis
  - Abdominal infection or sepsis
  - Bowel obstruction

Lumbar Sympathetic Block

- **Indications**
  - Postherpetic neuralgia in the lower extremities
  - Peripheral vascular insufficiency in the lower extremities
  - CRPS
  - Phantom pain
  - Intractable urogenital pain
  - Renal colic

- **Anatomy**
  - Lumbar sympathetic chain is located anterolateral to the lumbar vertebral bodies from L2 to L4
  - Receives preganglionic contributions from the lateral horn of the T11 to L2 spinal cord via the white communicating rami [9].
  - Postganglionic fibers exit variably:
    - Some via the gray rami communicantes traveling with the lumbar and sacral nerves
    - Smaller percentage synapse directly in the aortic plexus and the inferior and superior hypogastric plexuses [6].
  - Located in the retroperitoneal space separated spatially from the somatic nerves by the psoas muscle and fascia posteriorly.

– Abdominal aorta is anterolateral relative to the left sympathetic chain, though the position may vary with the aorta being located in the midline anterior to the vertebral body.

– Vena cava is located anterior to the right sympathetic trunk

- **Patient Positioning**
  – Prone with a pillow underneath the abdomen to minimize lumbar lordosis

- **Procedure** [2, 7–10, 13]
  – Obtain a PA view over the L2 and L3 vertebral bodies fluoroscopically (Fig. 43.6)
  – Optimal needle tip positions are in the lower 1/3 of the L2 vertebral body and in the upper 1/3 of the L3 vertebral body—because segmental lumbar vessels travel along mid-portion of the lumbar vertebral bodies.
  – Rotate the image intensifier obliquely so that the tip of the L2 transverse process overlies the anterolateral border of the L2 vertebral body.
  – Using 1 % lidocaine anesthetize the marked skin insertion site around 7 cm from midline.
  – Direct a 22 G styleted spinal needle with gun barrel approach
  – Use a 30–45° angle towards midline for a goal end-point at the inferior half of the anterolateral surface of the L2 vertebral body.
  – Advancement of the needle is done in the coaxial plane with frequent imaging every 1–2 cm and intermittent aspiration
  – The vertebral body is typically located at 7–12 cm depth
  – If bony contact is made with the vertebral body, the needle may need to be pulled and reinserted at a steeper angle in order to "walk" the needle off of the lateral margin of the L2 vertebral body.
  – At this point, obtain a lateral image (Fig. 43.7)
  – The needle should be located over the lower anterolateral aspect of the L2 vertebral body.
  – The needle is advanced until it is 1–2 cm anterior to the vertebral body on lateral view.
  – In a PA view, the needle tip should be just medial to the lateral margin of the vertebral body.
  – Remove the stylet and ensure negative aspiration of blood, urine, or CSF.
  – Inject 4–6 cm3 of radiographic contrast to visualize appropriate longitudinal spread anterior to the psoas muscle and fascia, viewed in both the PA and lateral projections.
  – Injection of the contrast will also exclude intravascular, intrathecal, or epidural puncture.

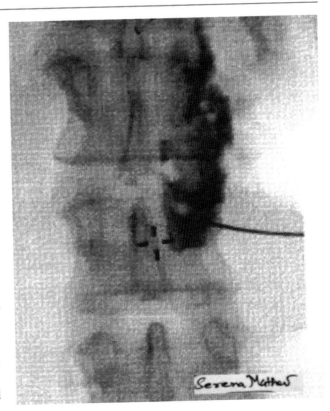

Fig. 43.6 PA fluoroscopic view for lumbar sympathetic block

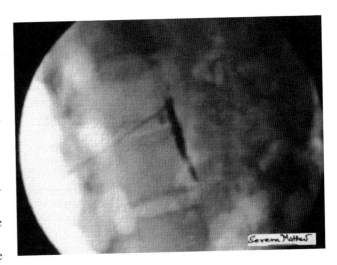

Fig. 43.7 Lateral fluoroscopic view of lumbar sympathetic block

– If the needle tip has not penetrated the psoas fascia, the contrast will outline the psoas muscle, risking ineffective sympathetic block and inadvertent block of the genitofemoral nerve.

– Once the needle is in optimal position, inject 10–20 cm3 of 0.25 % bupivacaine.

- Immediate effects of a successful sympathetic block include vasodilation and increased temperature by at least 1 ° C in the ipsilateral lower extremity.
- **Signs of effective blockade**
  - Increase in cutaneous temperature by at least 1 °C in the 15–20 min following blockade of the ipsilateral extremity
  - Absent sympatho-galvanic reflex of the blocked limb
- **Adverse effects**
  - Intravascular, intrathecal, epidural, or intradiscal injection
  - Hematuria from direct renal injury
  - Paresthesias from somatic nerve injury (genitofemoral nerve)
  - Post-sympathectomy pain following neurolysis is common in the L1 and L2 nerve root distribution
- **Contraindications**
  - Bleeding diathesis
  - Local infection
  - Anatomic anomalies which make the block exceedingly difficult or unsafe to perform

Hypogastric Plexus Block

- **Indications**
  - Pelvic pain of sympathetically mediated type
  - Visceral pain secondary to pelvic infiltration, bladder cancer, or colon cancer
- **Anatomy**
  - *Surface landmarks*
    - Dorsal midline
    - Spinous processes of L4 and L5
    - Iliac crests
    - L4–L5 interspace at the level of the superior aspect of the iliac crests
    - Mark needle entry points 5–7 cm lateral to the L4–L5 interspace
  - *Location and boundaries*
    - The superior hypogastric plexus is a retroperitoneal structure overlying the abdominal aorta below the inferior mesenteric artery and extending over its bifurcation into the right and left iliac arteries and veins.
    - Located anterior to the L5 and S1 vertebral bodies and receives input from pre- and postganglionic sympathetic fibers from the L4 and L5 sympathetic chain, the aortic plexus, and the splanchnic nerves.
    - Receives parasympathetic fibers from the S2 to S4 nerves.
    - Descends below the aortic bifurcation and splits into the right and left hypogastric nerves.

- The hypogastric nerves descend and innervate the inferior hypogastric plexuses located on either side of the rectum.
- Superior hypogastric plexus innervates the pelvic viscera including:
  - ◆ Bladder
  - ◆ Uterus
  - ◆ Vagina
  - ◆ Prostate
  - ◆ Rectum
- **Patient Positioning**
  - Prone with a pillow underneath the abdomen to minimize lumbar lordosis.
  - The inferior aspect of the pelvis pointed towards the table to angle the iliac crests posteriorly.
- **Procedure** [2, 6–9, 14, 15]
  - Sterile prep is done using betadine or chlorhexidine
  - Obtain a PA view of the L5/S1 fluoroscopically.
  - Using 1 % lidocaine anesthetize marked skin insertion sites 5–7 cm from midline at the L4–L5 interspace bilaterally.
  - A triangle is formed by the L5 transverse process superiorly, the iliac crest laterally, and the L5–S1 facet joint medially which will be the bony obstacles for needle insertion anterior to the L5–S1 junction.
  - Rotate the C-arm 25–35° obliquely over the L5/S1 junction
  - Direct the image intensifier caudally into the pelvis 25–35°
  - Advance a 22 G styleted spinal needle with a gun barrel approach at a 45° angle medial and caudad
  - Image every 1–2 cm until the needle tip is located anterolateral to L5–S1 intervertebral disc or the inferior margin of the L5 vertebral body.
  - If the iliac crest or the L5 transverse process obstructs advancement, the needle should be withdrawn and redirected.
  - If the needle tip encounters the L5 or S1 vertebral body, the needle should be withdrawn and redirected at a steeper to "walk" the needle off the vertebral body.
  - There is occasionally a loss of resistance when the needle is advanced through the psoas muscle fascia.
  - In the PA view, the needle should be at the junction of the L5 and S1 vertebral body.
  - In the lateral view, the needle should be just anterior to the vertebral body (Fig. 43.8).
  - Remove the stylet and ensure negative aspiration.
  - Inject 1–2 cm³ of radiographic contrast to visualize appropriate spread anterior to the L5–S1 intervertebral disc or the L5 vertebral body in the lateral view.
  - Position a 22-gauge styleted spinal needle on the contralateral side using the same technique.

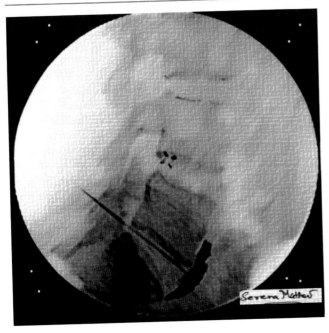

Fig. 43.8 Lateral fluoroscopic view of hypogastric plexus block

- **Medications**
  - For a diagnostic block, inject 8–10 cm³ of 0.25 % bupivacaine through each needle.
  - For neurolysis, inject 8–10 cm³ of 10 % phenol or 50 % ethanol through each needle.
- **Adverse effects**
  - Vascular puncture and intravascular injection given close proximity of iliac vessels
  - Intrathecal or epidural injection
  - Ureteral or bladder injury
  - Somatic nerve injury
- **Contraindications**
  - Bleeding diathesis
  - Local infection
- Once diagnostic sympatholysis is effective in relieving the neuropathic or visceral pain the procedure may be repeated to determine if an increasing duration of effect can be expected in any particular patient.
- Individual blocks may be all that are necessary to enable a patient to regain function by using a specific stress-loading physical therapy.
- When sympatholysis completely relieves the symptoms and facilitates exercise therapy but is limited in its duration

of effect, it is appropriate to consider a prolonged block by using one of the neurolytic techniques.

- The simplest method is that with a neurolytic agent such as phenol or by using radiofrequency lesions. Duration of effect from 3 to 6 months may be achieved, thereby allowing the progress of exercise therapy to continue.
- Continuous block of the brachial or lumbar plexus can be successfully used for periods of up to 6 weeks.
  - The main difficulties associated with these techniques are dislodgment of the catheter or infection.
  - Catheters that are implanted for a long duration should be treated as minor surgical procedures requiring the utmost sterility.

Acknowledgement Medical illustrations—Serena Christine Mathew

References

1. Rauck RL. Stellate ganglion block. Tech Reg Anesth Pain Manage. 2001;5:88–93.
2. Raj PP, Erdine S. Pain-relieving procedures the illustrated guide. Chichester: Wiley; 2012.
3. Walls WK. The anatomical approach in stellate ganglion injection. Br J Anaesth. 1955;27:616–21.
4. Carron H, Litwiller R. Stellate ganglion block. Anesth Analg. 1975;54:567–70.
5. Kastler B, Boulahdour H. Interventional radiology in pain treatment. New York: Springer; 2007.
6. Raj PP. Radiographic imaging for regional anesthesia and pain management. New York: Churchill Livingstone; 2003.
7. Rathmell JP, Neal JM, Viscomi CM. Regional anesthesia: the requisites in anesthesiology. 1st ed. St. Louis: Mosby; 2004.
8. Brown DL. Atlas of regional anesthesia. 3rd ed. Philadelphia: Elsevier Saunders; 2006.
9. Rathmell JP. Atlas of image-guided intervention in regional anesthesia and pain medicine. Philadelphia: Lippincott Williams and Wilkins; 2006.
10. Ballantyne J, Fishman S, Bonica JJ. Bonica's management of pain, vol. 1. 4th ed. Philadelphia: Lippincott, Williams & Wilkins; 2010. online resource.
11. Stanton-Hicks M. Thoracic sympathetic block: a new approach. Tech Reg Anesth Pain Manage. 2001;5:94–8.
12. Prithvi R. Celiac plexus/splanchnic nerve blocks. Tech Reg Anesth Pain Manage. 2001;5:102–15.
13. Mekhail NO. Lumbar. Sympathetic blockade. Tech Reg Anesth Pain Manage. 2001;5:99–101.
14. Plancarte R, Amescua C, Patt RB, Aldrete JA. Superior hypogastric plexus block for pelvic cancer pain. Anesthesiology. 1990;73:236–9.
15. Gundavarpu SL, Lema MJ. Superior hypogastric nerve block for pelvic pain. Tech Reg Anesth Pain Manage. 2001;5:116–9.

Injection Complications and Management

44

Sudhir Diwan, Rudy Malayil, and Staicey Mathew

Abbreviations

ASA	Aspirin
CRP	C-reactive protein
CSF	Cerebrospinal fluid
CT	Computed tomography
DSA	Digital subtraction angiography
EMLA	Lidocaine 2.5 % and prilocaine 2.5 %
ESI	Epidural spinal injections
ESR	Erythrocyte sedimentation rate
IV	Intravenous
IVIG	Intravenous immunoglobulin
MPA	Methylprednisolone acetate
MRI	Magnetic resonance imaging
NSAIDs	Nonsteroidal anti-inflammatory drugs
PDPH	Post-dural puncture headache
PO	Per os
SI	Sacroiliac
TEN	Toxic epidermal necrolysis
US	Ultrasound

S. Diwan, M.D., F.I.P.P., A.B.I.P.P. (✉)
Manhattan Spine and Pain Medicine, SUNY Downstate Medical
Center, Lenox Hill Hospital, New York, NY, USA

R. Malayil, M.D.
Beth Israel Medical Center, New York, NY, USA
e-mail: RudyMalayil@Gmail.com

S. Mathew, M.D.
Department of Orthopedics, Hospital for Joint Disease at
NYULMC, New York, NY, USA

Introduction

Generally, epidural injections, facet joint injections, and radiofrequency ablation neurectomies have rare minor adverse effects and rarer major complications. One study of 1,036 injections in 844 patients found an overall complication rate of 1.64 % [1]. Another study of 4,265 ESI showed no major complications and a low rate of minor complications (2.4 % overall) [2].

Some of these complications include:
- Vasovagal response
- Post-dural puncture headache (PDPH)
- Adverse reactions to medications
- Persistent hiccups (rare)
- Epidural lipomatosis
- Epidural hematoma
- Infections (i.e., skin, epidural abscess, osteomyelitis, and discitis)
- Aseptic meningitis
- Adhesive arachnoiditis
- Cauda equina syndrome
- Spinal cord injury and vertebrobasilar infarction

Although minor side effects are more frequently reported, including increased low back pain, numbness, paresthesia, flushing, and injection site discomfort, they raise concern for major complications. Clinicians are often faced with difficult decisions regarding the urgency of re-evaluation and the need for emergency imaging studies for prompt treatment to avoid long-term neurological deficit. Awareness of the nature and frequency of these complications may help in clinical decision-making [2].

Vasovagal Response

- *Symptoms*: Light headedness, nausea, visual changes, tinnitus, and weakness. When severe, may lead to loss of consciousness.

K.A. Sackheim, *Pain Management and Palliative Care: A Comprehensive Guide*,
DOI 10.1007/978-1-4939-2462-2_44, © Springer Science+Business Media New York 2015

- *Treatment*: Place patient in supine/Trendelenburg position, and monitor vitals (to avoid hypotension). Encourage PO fluids, or start IV fluids if severe.

Post-dural Puncture Headache

PDPH is a common complication of ESI caused by an accidental dural puncture during procedure. This may lead to persistent opening of the dura mater resulting in leakage of cerebrospinal fluid. The incidence is 0.16–1.3 % among experienced physicians [3] and can occur within hours to days following a procedure.

- *Risk Factors*
  - Female
  - Ages between 20 and 50 years old
  - Absence of fluoroscopic guidance
  - Use of a large bore needle
- *Symptoms*: Positional frontal or occipital headache that radiates to the neck or shoulders that worsens within 15 min after sitting or standing and improves within 15 min after lying down; presents with at least one symptom of neck stiffness, tinnitus, hypacusia, photophobia, or nausea; can be associated with diplopia, scalp paresthesia, upper and lower limb pain, and altered mental status
- *Diagnosis*: Based on history and symptoms. If needed, imaging can be done with CT myelogram and MRI.
- *Treatment*
  - Bed rest/supine position
  - Aggressive hydration (PO or IV if needed)
  - Medications, such as caffeine, methylxanthines, theophylline, sumatriptan, and corticosteroids, can be used
  - Fioricet for short-term symptomatic relief
  - Gold standard is epidural blood patch. In a majority of cases, the problem will resolve spontaneously. However, in some patients, the headache lasts for months or even years. Surgical closure of the dural tear is an option of last resort [4]

Adverse Effects of Medications

Adverse effects of corticosteroids may include:
- Fluid retention
- Elevated blood pressure
- Hyperglycemia
- Generalized erythema
- Facial flushing
- Hypothalamic–pituitary–adrenal axis suppression
- Cushing syndrome

- Alterations in female menstrual cycle
- Bone demineralization
- Allergic reactions

Prior Known Allergy to Contrast

If know allergy, you can use omniscan or magnevist instead of contrast, but these may be difficult to see on fluoroscopy. If you are doing a case that requires contrast, you can premedicate patient with steroids and Benadryl prior to avoid reaction to the medication. Use caution when deciding to proceed [5]

12 h Prior to Contrast Exposure
- Prednisone 20–50 mg PO
- Ranitidine 50 mg PO
- Diphenhydramine 25–50 mg PO

2 h Prior to Contrast Exposure
- Prednisone 20–50 mg PO
- Ranitidine 50 mg PO
- Diphenhydramine 25–50 mg PO

Just Prior to Injection
- Diphenhydramine 25 mg IV

Adapted and modified from Essentials of Pain Management, Benzon [5]

Allergy to Corticosteroids and Local Anesthetics

Allergic reactions to corticosteroids are extremely rare, but allergic reaction to steroid suspension has been documented. A delayed allergic reaction to triamcinolone diacetate beginning one-week post-procedure has been reported [6]. Allergic reactions to local anesthetics are also extremely rare; however, allergic reactions to ester local anesthetics and preservatives have been reported. One patient who had an anaphylactic reaction to EMLA cream was found to have a positive skin prick test [7].

- *Treatment*: Of a drug eruption depends on the specific type of reaction. Therapy for exanthematous drug eruptions is supportive in nature
  - First-generation antihistamines are used
  - Mild topical steroids (e.g., hydrocortisone, desonide) and moisturizing lotions are also used, especially during the late desquamative phase
  - Severe reactions, such as Steven Johnson Syndrome, toxic epidermal necrolysis (TEN), and hypersensitivity reactions, warrant hospital admission

- TEN is best managed in a burn unit with special attention given to electrolyte balance and signs of secondary infection
- Because adhesions can develop and result in blindness, evaluation by an ophthalmologist is mandatory
- In addition, mounting evidence indicates that intravenous immunoglobulin (IVIG) may improve outcomes for TEN patients [8].

Altered Glucose Tolerance

It is well known that glucocorticoids induce insulin resistance. Following an injection of steroids, diabetic patients generally have an increase in blood glucose levels and insulin requirements. One study by Ward et al. observed that epidural steroid injections with triamcinolone acetate resulted in an increased serum insulin level at 24 h, which normalized after one week post-procedure [9]. Patients should consult their endocrinologist prior to the procedure if they have uncontrolled diabetes mellitus.

Cushing Syndrome

Cushing Syndrome is a disorder that occurs due to exposure of high levels of endogenous cortisol or exogenous cortisol (steroid injections). Most reports state that the side effects of Cushing's begin between one and several weeks post-procedure.
- *Symptoms*: Facial swelling, buffalo hump, skin bruising, and scaly skin are symptoms of Cushing Syndrome.
- *Diagnosis*: Includes serum cortisol levels, dexamethasone suppression test, 24-h urine cortisol level, and creatinine and adrenocorticotropic hormone.
- *Treatment*: There is no specific treatment but repeat steroid use in procedures should be avoided.

Hiccup

A hiccup is an unintentional spasm of the diaphragm. This is followed by a quick closing of the vocal cords, which produces a distinctive sound. Hiccups are a known complication of thoracic and lumbar epidural steroid injections according to a paper by Abassi et al. [10] It reported that it is an under-reported side effect and could also be found after cervical epidural, lumbar facet blocks, and SI joint injections. The paper also stated that the injectate medication had no correlation with the risk for this side effect (Fig. 44.1).

Epidural Lipomatosis

Epidural lipomatosis is rare and may lead to spinal cord compression and neurologic deficits. It is usually associated with an excess of either endogenous or exogenous steroids in the body [11]. Roy-Camille et al. described the first reported case in 1991 and two cases reported by Choi et al. showed two non-obese patients without a history of steroid intake who developed epidural lipomatosis after epidural steroid injection [12].
- *Risk factors*: There are no known risk factors for the development of epidural lipomatosis.
- *Symptoms*: New neurological symptoms like increased or new back pain and/or weakness.
- *Diagnosis*: Made with radiological imaging including CT scan or MRI. Neurosurgical evaluation is needed if there are neurological symptoms and/or signs.

Epidural Hematoma

Epidural hematoma is a rare complication consisting of bleeding within the epidural space. Since the spinal canal is a nonexpendable space, bleeding is a serious complication that could lead to neurologic ischemia and potential paralysis. Incidence is between 1:150,000 and 1:220,000 [13, 14].
- *Risk factors*: Coagulopathy, thrombocytopenia, anticoagulants, and antiplatelet drugs such as clopidogrel and ticlopidine
  - NSAIDs including aspirin (ASA) have not shown to significantly increase the risk of epidural bleeding [9].
- *Symptoms*: New onset/increased back pain, headache, or neurological findings consisting of sensory/motor or bowel or bladder changes. *Symptoms may be delayed 1–2 days after injection*
- *Diagnosis*: Emergent MRI. MRI findings vary according to the age of the bleed:
  - In the first 24 h, the hematoma is usually isointense on T1- and hyperintense on T2-weighted images.
  - After 24 h, it becomes mostly hyperintense on both T1 and T2 [15]. Treatment includes neurosurgical consultation for decompression of the hematoma by surgical laminectomy.
- *Treatment*: Medical emergency can lead to spinal cord compression, surgical laminectomy, and hematoma evacuation

Infectious Complications

Most ESI-related infections could be prevented by meticulous sterile technique and attention to skin preparation. Steroid injections should not be used if there are any preexisting

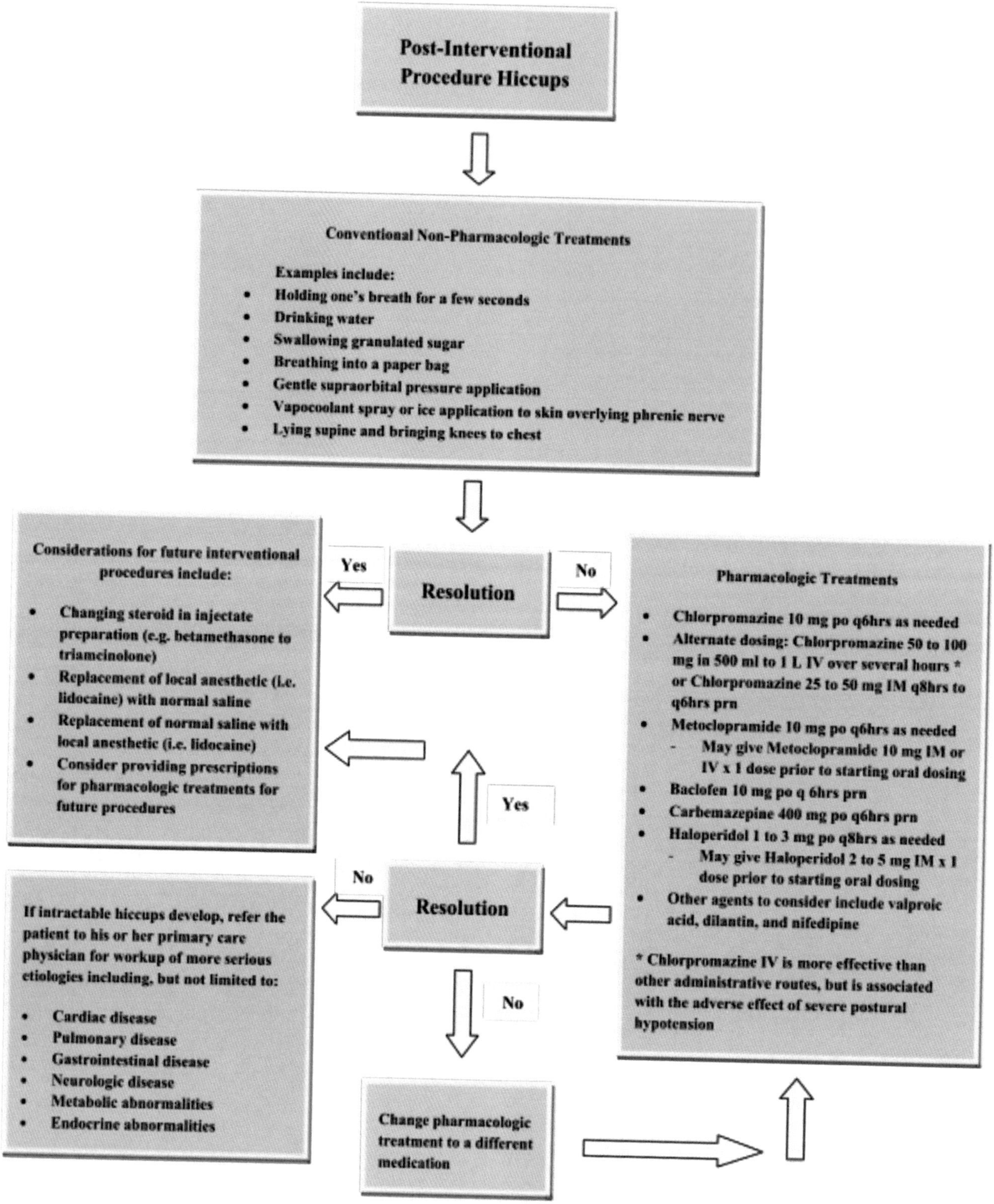

Fig. 44.1 Post-interventional procedure hiccups [1]

bacterial infections such as urinary tract infection or sinusitis. Gram-positive staph aureus is the most common causative agent. However, prophylaxic antibiotics are not recommended, even for diabetic or immunocompromised patients, as they may lead to drug-resistant strains of the pathogen. Lab tests may reveal elevated C-reactive protein (CRP), leukocytosis, and high ESR, but CT and MRI are needed to further identify the location and extent of disease [16, 17]

Superficial abscess

Collection of pus in the skin and soft tissue resulting from inflammation due to either bacteria or the injecting needle.

- *Diagnosis*: History and physical exam (heat, redness, pain, and swelling at the injection site), but bedside ultrasound (US) and computerized tomography (CT) are sometimes used to assist in the diagnosis. US is more sensitive than CT, but CT is more specific for superficial soft tissue abscesses [18]
- *Treatment*: Incision and open drainage of abscesses performed

Epidural abscess

It is a neurosurgical emergency requiring immediate action. It presents as a supperative process localized between spinal dura mater and the vertebral periosteum within the spinal epidural space.

- *Symptoms*: Back pain, fever, muscle weakness, sphincter incontinence, and sensory deficits eventually leading to paralysis.
- *Diagnosis*: MRI with contrast. Early diagnosis to avoid neurological deficits.
- *Treatment*: Early surgical decompression and abscess drainage. Laminectomy with broad antibiotic coverage. Consultation with neurosurgery or an infectious disease specialist might be necessary depending upon the clinical situation [19]

Osteomyelitis

Occurs in two adjacent vertebrae and their contiguous intervertebral disk, resulting in narrowing of the disk space. *Staphylococcus aureus* is the most common microorganism, followed by *E. coli* [20]. However, coagulase-negative staphylococci and *Propionibacterium acnes* causes exogenous osteomyelitis after spinal surgery [20]

- *Symptoms*: Focal vertebral pain that is unrelieved by lying down, with or without fever, and localized tenderness of the infected bone. Infection in the cervical region is more likely to be associated with neurological deficits, such as motor weakness or paralysis [20]
- *Diagnosis*:
  - CRP and ESR are the preferred markers of infection especially in postoperative spinal wound infections.

- If cervical osteomyelitis is suspected, MRI should be the first diagnostic step, to look for spinal epidural abscess and to rule out a herniated disk [21]
- MRI has a high accuracy (90 %) for diagnosing spinal osteomyelitis [22]. MRI without contrast is the most sensitive showing signs of bone marrow edema within a few days of onset of symptoms.
- If imaging reveals signs of disease, and blood cultures are negative, then CT-guided biopsy should be performed [21]

- *Treatment*: Surgical treatment is recommended only after IV antibiotics fail. Surgery includes spinal fusion to stabilize the affected bone [21]

Discitis

Discitis is the inflammation of the disk space between two adjacent vertebrae. May lead to osteomyelitis or epidural abscess.

- *Diagnosis*: MRI is the imaging modality of choice for discitis; a biopsy may or may not help isolate the organism [23]
- *Treatment*: Reduce mobility of the area with brace. Treat the causative organism with antibiotics [23]

Aseptic Meningitis

- *Risk factors*:
  - Polyethylene glycol
  - Benzyl Alcohol
- *Symptoms*: Burning pain in the legs, headache, meningismus, and seizures.
- *Diagnosis*: On lumbar puncture, CSF reveals pleocytosis, elevated proteins, and decrease glucose.
- *Treatment*: Symptomatic relief and reassurance [16]

Arachnoiditis

Arachnoiditis is an inflammatory condition of the arachnoid membrane and the underlying space, which undergoes fibrosis and adhesion formation within the subarachnoid space. It can be subdivided into three causes: Surgery/trauma induced, chemically induced, and infection induced. The polyethylene glycol in methylprednisolone acetate (MPA) is thought to cause chemically induced chronic adhesive arachnoiditis [24]

- *Risk factors*: Injection of MPA spreading from the epidural space into the intrathecal space.
- *Symptoms*: Gradual onset, constant burning pain in the lower legs, urinary frequency or incontinence, muscle spasm, variable sensory loss, variable motor dysfunction [9]
- *Workup*: An MRI with contrast is 99 % accurate showing "clumping" of the nerve roots suggests arachnoiditis. CT

myelogram results are variable with homogeneous contrast pattern without root shadows [24]

- *Treatment*: Surgical intervention is not recommended as it leads to further scar tissue formation.
- *Prevention*: Dilution of steroid with saline or local anesthetic before injection into the epidural space lowers the concentration of polyethylene glycol.

Cauda Equina Syndrome

Cauda equina syndrome refers to a characteristic pattern of neuromuscular and urogenital symptoms resulting from the simultaneous compression or the anesthetizing of multiple lumbosacral nerve roots below the level of the conus medullaris. Vigilance for neurologic deterioration after epidural steroid injections is important [25].

- *Risk factors*: Injectate into the intrathecal space
- *Symptoms*: Bilateral radiculopathy, saddle hypesthesia, weakness, and bowel and bladder dysfunction
- *Diagnosis*: CT or MRI scan can both confirm diagnosis.
- *Treatment*: Close monitoring of patient and vital signs and symptomatic management. Emergency surgical decompression if symptoms exist.

Spinal Cord Injury and Vertebrobasilar Infarction

Damage to the spinal cord can be caused by:

1. *Injection of medication into the spinal cord or vasculature*

   Most commonly by accidental injection of particulate material into radicular arteries lying adjacent to the targeted nerve root.

   - **Particulate steroids** (triamcinolone, betamethasone) are delivered by a carrier and are less soluble leading to their long-acting properties lasting 36–72 h but contain microcrystals.
   - **Non-particulate steroids** (dexamethasone) have been demonstrated to dissipate rapidly and therefore may have a limited duration of effect

2. *Direct needle trauma either to the spinal cord or dorsal root ganglion*

   - Needle placement into the dorsal root ganglion following transforaminal injection. The shorter length of the dorsal roots at the cervical level increases the likelihood that the injectate could enter into the spinal cord. Brainstem infarcts have also been associated with cervical transforaminal epidural steroid injections

3. *Vascular damage*

   The artery of Adamkiewicz, which is susceptible to damage, arises at T10 on left side; however, its position may vary from T7 to L4. Under fluoroscopic guidance of intra-arterial injection, the contrast dye is likely to spread within both the epidural space and intravascularly. Since the pattern of intra-arterial spread is thin, it may be overlooked [26]

   - *Symptoms*: New onset of neurological signs and symptoms including weakness, paresis, and stroke.
   - *Diagnosis*: Can be made with signs and symptoms and radiological imaging including CT or MRI. Digital subtraction fluoroscopy can enhance the visualization of intravascular dye [22]
   - *Treatment*:
     - High-dose IV corticosteroids within hours of the infarct show significant reduction in neurological injury [9]
     - To minimize potential devastating neurological injury, the use of fluoroscopic digital subtraction angiography (DSA) is suggested for all injections
     - The use of non-particulate steroids, specifically on the left side [22]

"Appendix 1" post-procedure instruction form to assist in anticipating complications.

Appendix 1

POST – PROCEDURE INSTRUCTIONS

1. After the procedure you should take it easy. You may resume your normal daily routine the next day. However, be careful to avoid strenuous activity or any activities that cause pain or discomfort.

2. Your injection included Lidocaine and/or Marcaine (numbing medication) and Celestone, Kenalog, Dexamethasone or Depo-medrol (steroid medication). The numbing medication will last for the next 3-5 hours, 24 hours at most. The steroid will begin working within 2- 7 days (for some patients it may take 2 weeks to start working)

3. Immediately following the procedure, your legs may feel shaky or weak. These sensations are temporary and will resolve.

4. Temporary typical side effects include stomach upset, flushing, headaches, increased energy level, increased appetite, rapid heart beat, abnormal menstrual cycle and irritability. Some females may experience missed menstrual cycle or increased bleeding for many days from the steroid medications.

5. *Refrain from the following for the 24-48 hours after your procedure:*
    *   Do not take a bath, swim, or sit in a hot tub. Showers are ok.
    *   Do not sit for more than 1-2 hours in any one position.
    *   Do not exercise.

6. Tenderness at the site of the injection is normal and can last for a few days. To dull the pain, use ice packs over the injection site for 15-20 minutes, only once per hour for the first 24 hours.

7. Headaches are another possible rare side effect. They only occur in less than 1% of all patients and are usually from the steroid medication. Lying down for 24-36 hours with your head no higher than one pillow and resting are the best treatments. If you experience a headache following a procedure that is extreme please call the office.

8. You are allowed to take any prescribed pain medications. You may also restart taking advil, aleve, aspirin and any other blood thinning medications you stopped prior to the procedure **unless otherwise told**.

9. Eat a well-balanced diet and try to avoid fatty and high-sugar foods.

If you have any questions regarding your procedure, please call the physician's office. If you have any emergencies and the office is closed please call 911 or go to local emergency room.

Post-procedure instructions (with permission from Danesh H, Sayanlar J. Interventional Pain Management. In: Sackheim K. Rehab Clinical Pocket Guide. Rehabilitation Medicine. Springer, New York, 2013: 427–465) [27]

References

1. Landa J, Kim Y. Outcomes of interlaminar and transforaminal spinal injections. Bull NYU Hosp Jt Dis. 2012;70(1):6–10.
2. McGrath JM, Schaefer MP, Malkamaki DM. Incidence and characteristics of complications from epidural steroid injections. Pain Med. 2011;12(5):726–31.
3. Gahleb A, et al. Post-dural puncture headache. Int J Gen Med. 2012;5:45–51.
4. Turnbulland DK, Shepherd DB. Post-dural puncture headache: pathogenesis, prevention and treatment. Br J Anaesth. 2003;91(5):718–29.
5. Benzon H, et al. Essentials of pain management. New York: Elsevier; 2011.
6. Blume JE, et al. Drug eruptions treatment & management. Medscape: http://emedicine.medscape.com/article/1049474-treatment
7. Even JL, et al. Effects of epidural steroid injection on blood glucose levels in patient with Diabetes Mellitus. Spine. 2012;37(1):E46–50.

8. Wheeless' Orthopedic textbook of Orthopaedics, 2008. http://www.wheelessonline.com/ortho/blood_supply_of_the_spinal_cord

9. Ward A, Watson J, Wood P, Dunne C, Kerr D. Glucocorticoid epidural for sciatica: metabolic and endocrine sequelae. Rheumatology (Oxford). 2002;41(1):68–71.

10. Abassi A, et al. Persistent hiccups after interventional pain procedures. PM R. 2012;4:144–51.

11. Rajput D, et al. Spinal epidural lipomatosis: an unusual cause of relapsing and remitting paraparesis. J Pediatr Neurosci. 2010;5(2):150–2.

12. Choi KC, et al. Rapid progression of spinal epidural lipomatosis. Eur Spine J. 2012;21(4):408–12.

13. Brinda Vihari SOMANCHI, Saeed MOHAMMAD. Raymond ROSS an unusual complication following caudal epidural steroid injection: a case report. Acta Orthop Belg. 2008;74:720–2.

14. Shanthanna H, Park J. Acute epidural haematoma following epidural steroid injection in a patient with spinal stenosis. Anaesthesia. 2011;66(9):837–9.

15. Simon DL, et al. Allergic or pseudoallergic reaction following epidural steroid deposition and skin testing? Reg Anesth. 1989;14:253–5.

16. Neal JM, Rathmell JP. ASRA practice advisory on neurologic complications in regional anesthesia and pain medicine. Reg Anesth Pain Med. 2007;33:404–15.

17. Kainer MA, Reagan DR, Nguyen DB, Wiese AD, Wise ME, Ward J, Park BJ, Kanago ML, Baumblatt J, Schaefer MK, Berger BE, Marder EP, Min JY, Dunn JR, Smith RM, Dreyzehner J, Jones TF, Tennessee Fungal Meningitis Investigation Team. Fungal infections associated with contaminated methylprednisolone in Tennessee. N Engl J Med. 2012;367:2194–203. doi:10.1056/NEJMoa1212972.

18. Gaspari R, Dayno M, Briones J, Blehar D. Comparison of computerized tomography and ultrasound for diagnosing soft tissue abscesses. Crit Ultrasound J. 2012;4(1):5. doi:10.1186/2036-7902-4-5.

19. Reihsaus E, Waldbaur H, Seeling W. Spinal epidural abscess: a meta-analysis of 915 patients. Neurosurg Rev. 2000;23(4):175–204.

20. Pigrau C, Almirante B, Flores X, et al. Spontaneous pyogenic vertebral osteomyelitis and endocarditis: incidence, risk factors, and outcome. Am J Med. 2005;118:1287.

21. Zimmerli W. Clinical practice. Vertebral osteomyelitis. N Engl J Med. 2010;362:1022–9.

22. Palestro CJ, Love C, Miller TT. Infection and musculoskeletal conditions: imaging of musculoskeletal infections. Best Pract Res Clin Rheumatol. 2006;20:1197–218.

23. Nasto A, Colangelo D, Rossi B, Fantoni M, Pola E. Post-operative spondylodiscitis. Eur Rev Med Pharmacol Sci. 2012;16 Suppl 2:50–7.

24. Rice I, Wee MY, Thomson K. Obstetric epidurals and chronic adhesive arachnoiditis. Br J Anaesth. 2004;92(1):109–20.

25. Morais-Almeida M, et al. Allergy to local anesthetics of the amide group with tolerance to procaine. Allergy. 2003;58:827–8.

26. Smuck M, et al. Incidence of simultaneous epidural and vascular injection during cervical transforaminal epidural injections. Spine. 2011;36:E220–3.

27. Danesh H, Sayanlar J. Interventional pain management. In: Sackheim K, editor. Rehabi clinical pocket guide, Rehabilitation medicine. New York: Springer; 2013. p. 427–65.

Neuromodulation

45

Tim Canty

Abbreviations

ADL	Activity of daily living
AP	Anteroposterior
ASC	Ambulatory surgical center
CBC	Complete blood count
CNS	Central nervous system
CPT	Current procedural terminology
CRPS	Complex regional pain syndrome
CT	Computed tomography
DRG	Dorsal root ganglia
ECG	Echocardiogram
ESR	Erythrocyte sedimentation rate
FDA	Food and Drug Administration
GABA	Gamma-aminobutyric acid
IPG	Implantable pulse generator
IV	Intravenous
MAC	Minimal anesthetic concentration
MRI	Magnetic resonance imaging
MRSA	Methicillin-resistant staphylococcus aureus
NSAID	Non-steroidal anti-inflammatory drug
PCN	Penicillin
PDPH	Postdural puncture headache
SCI	Spinal cord injury
SCS	Spinal cord stimulator
UA	Urinalysis
VAS	Visual analog scale

History and Theory

- First use of electrical stimulation for the treatment of pain was documented in 600 BC when fish capable of electrical discharge were applied to painful areas by Scribonius Largus.
- The modern resurgence in the use of stimulation was introduced by Shealy et al. in 1967 as an application of the Melzack and Wall [1] "gate control" theory of pain.
- *Mechanism*:
  - With stimulation of larger A-beta vibration/touch sensation fibers within the dorsal columns of the spinal cord, nociceptive input from the periphery transmitted by smaller C-fibers could be blocked
  - Now, it is known that other mechanisms prevail—spinothalamic inhibitory tract activation, supraspinal structure involvement, suppression of sympathetic activity, cutaneous myelinated fiber activation, activation of inhibitory neurotransmitters GABA and adenosine.
  - Multiple structures beside the dorsal horn of the spinal cord can be stimulated to provide pain relief (DRG, peripheral nerves).

Patient Selection

Carefully consider the pain mechanism when opting for SCS treatment

- *Increased Success*: [2] Neuropathic and sympathetically mediated pain tends to respond better than mechanical or inflammatory pain.

Indications

- Failed back surgery syndrome/post-laminectomy syndrome
- Complex regional pain syndrome (CRPS)
- Radiculopathy/Radiculitis

T. Canty, M.D. (✉)
Comprehensive Spine and Pain Center, State University of
New York Downstate Medical Center, New York, NY, USA
e-mail: Timcanty@NYSpinePainCenter.com

K.A. Sackheim, *Pain Management and Palliative Care: A Comprehensive Guide*,
DOI 10.1007/978-1-4939-2462-2_45, © Springer Science+Business Media New York 2015

- Spinal stenosis (nonoperative)
- Plexopathy
- Arachnoiditis
- Epidural or perineural fibrosis [2]
- Painful peripheral neuropathy, i.e., diabetic, postherpetic neuralgia, chemotherapy induced, idiopathic
- Chronic intractable pain of trunk and limbs
- Intractable low back pain and leg pain
- Postoperative chronic pain (abdominal, thoracic, pelvic, post-mastectomy, post-thoracotomy, post-nephrectomy, post-herniorrhaphy)
- Multiple sclerosis with lower extremity pain
- Motor disorders, i.e., cerebral palsy
- Ischemic pain related to severe peripheral vascular disease or refractory angina
- Occipital neuralgia
- Other peripheral neuropathic diagnoses

Contraindications

- *Not recommended for the following diagnoses*: [3]
  - Complete SCI
  - Paraplegia/quadraplegia
  - Incomplete SCI with loss of posterior column
  - Nerve root avulsion
  - Centralized pain
  - Nociceptive pain
- Coagulopathy/Anticoagulation
- Pregnancy
- Neurological deficit that may be corrected upon surgical intervention
- *Comorbidities*:
  - Systemic infection
  - Local infection at the lead insertion or generator implant site
  - Immunosuppression/Malnutrition/Chronic Illnesses/Tobacco use/Current corticosteroid use (relative contraindication—can inhibit wound healing)
- *Anatomic changes*: may prohibit lead passage [3]
  - Prior surgery causing loss of epidural space—e.g., Posterior laminectomy/scar
  - Severe thoracic spinal stenosis: *Caution should be taken if severe spinal stenosis is present*
    - Case reports of thoracic paraplegia during/after trials due to trauma in the stenotic space
    - Some have advocated thoracic MRIs prior to lead placement. Lead diameter ranges from 1.4 to 2.6 mm, adequate space must exist so that cord compression does not occur with placement
  - Severe scoliosis or spondylosis
  - Instability of spine

- Psychological [4]
  - Cognitive impairment: patient inability to care for device or properly use device
  - Uncontrolled current drug abuse
  - Other severe uncontrolled psychiatric disease/instability
- Requirement for future MRIs: an SCS would previously be contraindicated; however, as of late 2013 the FDA has approved a Medtronic system that is compatible for MRI use
- Prior to proceeding with SCS be sure there is no surgically correctable pathology: [3]
  - Order current imaging—MRI typically study of choice
  - Surgical evaluation
  - Rule out other causes of patients' pain syndrome including referred pain from: Facet pathology, sacroiliac joint, piriformis syndrome, muscular pain, and internal disc disruption

Lead Placement

- Final lead placement is critical to obtain a successful trial and implantation
- Consider any anatomical constraints that may prohibit adequate lead placement
- A single lead placed just lateral to the midline may provide unilateral coverage; however, a single lead placed in the midline may capture bilateral dermatomes.
- Most often, for bilateral symptoms, double lead placement just at the midline 1–3 mm apart is used.
- Leads can be staggered to cover more vertebral segments
- According to the literature, curved lead placements crossing over the midline have also been met with success.
- Table 45.1 shows a list of common spinal and peripheral lead contact placements used to obtain adequate coverage for specific anatomic pain locations. Variances will exist between patients and lead placement should be individualized for each patient. This table is only for reference and should be used as a loose guideline and adjusted accordingly.

SCS Trial

Documentation/Approval

- Reserved for patients who have failed standard conservative management including but not limited to: Physical therapy, Medications (NSAIDs, opiates, neuropathic agents), and Injections
- Some insurance plans require psychological evaluation prior to submitting to insurance for pre-approval (Workers' Compensation in particular)

Table 45.1 Common spinal and peripheral lead contact placements used to obtain coverage for specific anatomic pain locations

Pain location/paresthesia coverage area	Level for lead contact placement
Occipital neuralgia	C1–C2 (subcutaneous)
Face below maxilla	C2
Neck, shoulder to hand	C2–C4
Forearm to hand	C4–C7
Anterior shoulder, anginal pain	C7–T1
Intercostal neuralgia, PHN, post-thoracotomy pain	T1–T6 (far lateral gutter/dorsal root entry zone. Also subcutaneous lead placement just medial to scar, parallel to spine)
Abdomen, pelvis	T5–T7
Low back	T7–T9 (can also consider subcutaneous array in paraspinal region)
Lower extremity	T8–T11
Pelvis	L1 (conus)
Foot	T12–L1
Knee	L3 (DRG)
Foot	L5, S1 retrograde
Pelvis, rectum	S2–S4
Coccyx	Sacral hiatus
Interstitial cystitis	S3 (four contact lead placed through dorsal foramina extending out ventral)

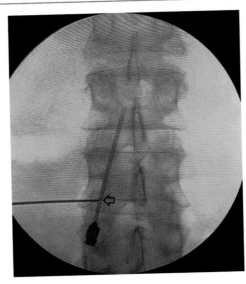

Fig. 45.1 Skin insertion site mid-pedicular (*arrow*) 1.5–2 vertebral levels below epidural entry

- Some insurance plans require a surgical evaluation to state there is no surgically treatable pathology (recommended in all patients to ensure proper patient selection)
- Patients with severe pain, VAS >5
- Patients with pain limiting the patient's activities of daily living (ADLs) and functioning
- Document all above criteria in preoperative evaluation note to facilitate insurance authorization

Equipment and Supplies
- Trial electrode kit(s) (includes epidural Tuohy needle)
- Stimulator box with connecting cables
- Loss of resistance syringe
- 25 gauge 1.5 in. needle
- 18 gauge needle
- 10 mL syringe
- 1 % lidocaine
- Skin marker
- Needle driver
- 2-0 nonabsorbable nylon or silk suture on a curved needle
- Alternate to suture—Steri-strips and benzoin/mastisol

Trial Technique Steps and Pearls: (Percutaneous Lead Placement)
- Preoperative testing as per guidelines based on age and medical history. Check CBC with diff, UA, and ESR to help identify at-risk patients [3].

- Performed at office-based fluoroscopy suite, ASC, or hospital under local anesthesia±light sedation with versed/fentanyl.
- *Pre-procedure medication*: IV antibiotics given preoperatively 30–60 min prior to incision. Ancef 1 g (2 g if >70 kg), if allergic—Clindamycin 600 mg or Vancomycin 1 g × 1 dose (if MRSA colonized) [3]
- *Lead selection*: 4, 8, 16, 32 contact leads of varying diameter with wide or narrow spacing of contacts. Up to four leads may be powered by a single generator.
- *Positioning*: prone with pillow under abdomen to reduce lumbar lordosis.
- *Sterile prep*: 2 % Chlorhexidine Gluconate/70 % Isopropyl Alcohol—*Chloraprep*. Full sterile draping.
- *Entry Level*: typically the L1/2 interspace but can also be L2/3 or L3/4. For cervical cases, it is T1–T4; however, some practitioners use lumbar insertion.

Procedure
- 14–15 gauge Tuohy needle is inserted in a paramedian approach through the anesthetized skin (1 % lidocaine) at 1.5–2 vertebral levels below the anticipated insertion level to the epidural space. This allows for about a 30° angle of entry, which facilitates the lead exiting the needle to the dorsal epidural space without lead trauma and steering of the lead cephalad.
- Needle should be advanced just medial to the pedicle until desired intralaminar epidural space is located by loss of resistance technique (see Fig. 45.1).
- If two leads are used, then needles may be inserted bilaterally paramedian with an epidural target as close to the midline as possible. May also insert both Tuohy needles on ipsilateral side of the spinous process (see Fig. 45.2).

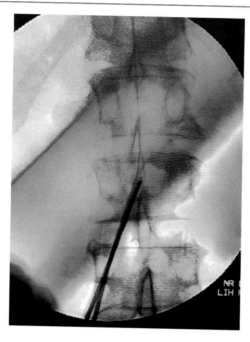

Fig. 45.2 Ipsilateral needle insertion is a technique that allows for smaller incision and facilitates single incision non-tunneled flank pocket

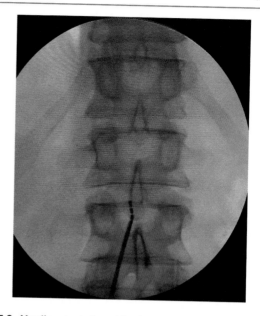

Fig. 45.3 Needle entry to the epidural space close to the midline facilitates proper lead exit to the dorsal space. If the lead moves laterally, then often it has entered the ventral epidural space

This is particularly important for permanent implant so as to limit incision size and may also be useful when a non-tunneled flank pocket/single incision technique is used.

- Lateral needle entry to the epidural space will often send the lead to the ventral epidural space. Rotating the Tuohy needle so that the opening is ventral and medial facilitates good dorsal lead placement (see Fig. 45.3). Lateral fluoroscopic views are performed initially to assure the lead is in the dorsal epidural space (see Fig. 45.4).
- *If a "wet tap" occurs*:
  - Needle can be removed and entry re-attempted on the contralateral side or at one spinal level cephalad with extreme caution
  - If concern for persistent CSF leak or other complications, procedure can be aborted and rescheduled at a later date.
- Bending a slight curve into the tip of the stylet facilitates "steering" the lead as it is inserted cephalad with AP fluoroscopic guidance. Once the lead is advanced to the proper location, the patient should be alert so that they can give feedback on where paresthesia is felt as the lead is activated.
- If a second lead is to be placed, it is beneficial to test the initial lead first to determine laterality. The physiologic midline of the spinal cord may be as much as 2 mm lateral/medial to the anatomic midline.
- The "trolling method" can be used if coverage is not obtained with lead placement in the seemingly correct

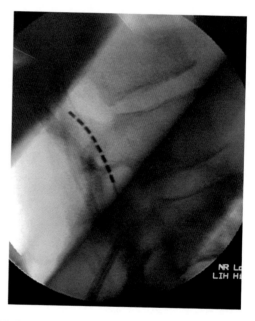

Fig. 45.4 Lateral fluoroscopic views are performed initially to assure the lead is in the dorsal epidural space

location. The lead is advanced cephalad several levels above the expected "sweet spot" and then a low level of energy is applied to the contacts so that the patient feels a slight paresthesia. The lead is then withdrawn slowly until the paresthesia is felt in the desired area(s).

- If scar or epidural adhesion is encountered with lead placement, it can often be bypassed using a non-curved stylet.
- Manufacturer representatives are usually available help program the correct combination of anodes and cathodes,

amplitude, pulse width, and stimulation frequency that provides the most complete coverage of the targeted pain area with a pleasant paresthesia sensation. Stimulation-induced paresthesia should cover at least 80 % of the distribution of pain in order to attain optimal outcomes.

- Once this is achieved, the stylet and Tuohy needle are removed cautiously with fluoroscopic guidance so as to not advance or withdraw the leads from the "sweet spot" location. A final lead placement image should be documented. The leads can then be sutured or benzoin/tegaderm fixated and dressing applied.
- Patient is then brought to recovery area, where detailed programming and patient education is performed by manufacturer representatives. Once stable patient is discharged.
- For a trial, leads are left in place for 3–5 days so that there is adequate time for the patient to determine if they are satisfied with the sensation and coverage. It may be extended to 7–10 days if the patient is uncertain; however, longer trials may increase infectious risk.
- Post-procedure antibiotics have not been shown to reduce incidence of infection [4–6]; however, many practitioners will give Keflex 500 mg PO qid for the duration of trial until leads removed. Alternative (if PCN allergic): Ciprofloxacin 500 mg PO bid.

SCS Permanent Percutaneous Implantation

SCS Implantation Documentation/Approval

Need documentation during the trial period that the patient experienced:

- >50 % pain reduction
- Increased the ability to perform ADLs (specifics)
- Increased functioning (specifics)
- Decreased pain medication intake (encouraged, not essential)
- Satisfaction with stimulation sensation

Equipment and Supplies

- Implantation kit(s)—includes lead, anchor, epidural Tuohy needle, stylettes, guidewire, tunneling needle and sheath, lead extension
- Pulse generator battery
- #10 blade scalpel
- Surgical kit for implant (forceps, needle driver, retractors, mayo scissors, etc.)
- 2-0 silk/nylon nonabsorbable on CT needle (anchors)
- 2-0 vicryl (deep fascia)
- 3-0 monocryl (subdermal)
- 4-0 monocryl (subcuticular) vs. steri-strips vs. derma-bond vs. staples
- 1 % lidocaine
- Triple antibiotic irrigation and soaking implant

Implantation Technique Pearls

- Preoperative testing as per guidelines based on age and medical history. Check CBC with diff, UA, and ESR to help identify at-risk patients [3].
- Permanent implantation is done at an ASC or hospital with local and MAC anesthesia.
- *Pre-procedure medication*: IV antibiotics given preoperatively 30–60 min prior to incision. Ancef 1 g (2 g if >70 kg), if allergic—Clindamycin 600 mg or Vancomycin 1 g × 1 dose (if MRSA colonized) [3]
- *IPG selection*: Rechargeable generator—smaller size. Needs to be charged every 1–7 days depending on the energy requirements of stimulation program. Nonrechargeable generator—typically last 3–7 years before they will need to be replaced surgically.
- *Pocket location*: chosen and skin marked preoperatively. Buttocks pocket should be placed on the dominant side to facilitate external placement of recharging device by patient. It should be lower than the beltline and not press against the ilium but cephalad enough that it will not be compressed by ischium in the seated position. Flank pocket should be inferior to the ribs but superior to the iliac crest and no more than 10 cm lateral to the midline so that lying on one's side is not uncomfortable. For cervical IPG placement, the anterior chest wall is often selected; however, flank or buttocks pockets are also used.
- Percutaneous leads can be replaced (see steps in trial section above) to the prior recorded spinal location as in the trial with intraoperative patient testing to confirm adequate coverage. Alternatively, a laminectomy can be performed surgically under general anesthesia with a paddle lead placed under direct vision. Laminectomy placed paddle leads result in less lead migration and may prolong battery life by lowering energy requirements. Some practitioners advocate paddle leads for better low back coverage however outcomes are comparable between the two techniques in studies at 3 years. Paddle leads now exist in up to five column arrays containing 20 total contacts for more precise direction of stimulation.
- Dissection of the midline or paramedian incision down to the spinous process facilitates suturing lead anchors to the deep interspinous fascia with 2-0 silk/nylon nonabsorbable suture. This will reduce lead migration. Various lead anchoring systems are also available depending on the manufacturer chosen.
- Strain relief loops placed in the lead just distal to the anchor and just proximal to the IPG may also reduce lead migration and fracture.
- After generous local anesthetic (1 % lidocaine) is applied, the tunneling needle and sheath are inserted subcutaneously from lead incision to the pocket site so that leads can be delivered and connected to the IPG.

- Pocket formation depth should be less than 1 in. below skin surface in subcutaneous fat plane. Blunt dissection with finger rather than cutting may reduce bleeding. Some advocate anesthetizing skin with plain lidocaine without epinephrine so that any small bleeders can be identified and coagulated so as to reduce hematoma and infection or seroma.
- Both midline incision and pocket are irrigated copiously with triple antibiotic irrigation prior to closure of incisions.
- Incision is closed in 2–3 layers using 2-0 vicryl for deep fascia, 3-0 monocryl for subdermal, and 4-0 monocryl for subcuticular. Alternatively, instead of 4-0 monocryl for subcuticular layer steri-strips, dermabond, or staples can be applied.
- Patient is then brought to recovery, the SCS reprogrammed and then discharged when appropriate.

Post-procedure Instructions [3]

- If medically stable, patient is discharged home same day
- Rest for 2 days post-procedure
- It is normal to feel some pain and swelling for a couple days after the procedure. Pain medications may be prescribed to help during this time.
- Avoid sudden movements, bending, twisting, lifting, reaching, pulling, and stretching for 4–6 weeks following.
- Avoid showering for 1–2 days. Then keep wound dry 10–14 days or 1–2 days after sutures/staples are removed

Complications

- Lead migration—13 %
- Lead fracture/breakage—9 %
- Infection—3–4 %—requiring hardware removal (9 % for diabetics)
- Seroma
- Hematoma
- Wound dehiscence
- Perforated viscus from tunneling
- Dural puncture leading to CSF leak, CSF hygroma
- Postdural puncture headache (PDPH)
- Pain at generator site
- Cord injury and nerve trauma may result in neurological symptoms and/or paraplegia

Complication Management/Troubleshooting

- **Wound Infection**: May present with pain, erythema, swelling, and wound discharge with possible fever and chills. Postoperative inflammation usually diminishes 5–7 days following procedure while infection swelling can begin 3–5 days following procedure. Evaluate carefully to

see if swelling is associated with increased tenderness [3]. Majority result from Staphylococcus, Streptococcus, and MRSA. Post-procedure antibiotics have not been shown to reduce incidence of infection [6]; however, many practitioners prescribe 5–7-day prophylactic postoperative antibiotics. This can lead to resistant organisms, and decisions should be made based on clinical judgment. If after this period signs of superficial incision site infection occur (erythema, tenderness), then an empiric 7–14-day course of broad-spectrum oral antibiotics could be given. Labs can be ordered including wound cultures, CBC, ESR, CRP. These labs may be nonspecific but once cultures are back change antibiotic appropriately. Ultrasound can help differentiate between seroma, hematoma, and infection [3]. If infection has reached the hardware (systemic infection), this would necessitate hardware removal and prolonged course of IV antibiotics.
- **Hematoma at IPG site**: Most small hematomas resolve within a few weeks postoperatively. While large progressing hematomas may lead to infection and/or wound dehiscence. Hematomas are more likely to lead to infection than seromas. Monitor carefully
- **Seroma**: Collection under the wound consisting of serum, lymphatic fluid, and liquefied adipose tissue. Similar presentation to hematoma. Relatively benign complication when small in size, but can develop into infection so should be followed closely [3].
  - If infection suspected—order labs CBC, ESR, CRP
  - Ultrasound can help distinguish between hematoma, seroma, and infection
  - If necessitated, aspirate fluid with large bore 14 g needle, send for culture, and sensitivity prior to antibiotic initiation (only if warranted).
    If culture is positive, initiate appropriate antibiotics.
    If culture is negative, then place a small seroma drain and have patient wear compression belt for 2–3 days.
    If seroma recurs, then incision will need to be opened and the internal capsule either dissected out completely or scored with cautery extensively to promote adequate healing. May also spray scored/resected pocket with fibrin sealant to reduce oozing when pocket is being revised for seroma.
- **Epidural Hematoma**: Symptoms include: back or leg pain, sensory or motor changes, and/or bowel or bladder changes. If patient develops neurological symptoms, emergent MRI obtained. If positive, emergent decompression/evacuation may be warranted to prevent persistent/progressive neurological compromise. Best recovery has been seen with surgical intervention within 6 h of symptom onset [4].

- *Anticoagulation*: Full explanation of managing anticoagulation is described in previous chapter dedicated to this important topic. To avoid hematomas on implantation, obtain permission from prescribing physician to stop Plavix and for 7 days and Ticlid for 14 days prior to procedure. Coumadin can be held for 4–5 days (can bridge with heparin, last heparin dose 24 h prior to procedure) and check INR on the day of or prior to procedure (should be <1.2 for epidural lead placement, <1.5 for IPG changes) [3].

- **Epidural Abscess**: presentation is similar to hematoma with delayed onset of days to weeks. Labs to order include CBC, ESR, CRP, and emergent MRI scan. Signs of severity are new neurological symptoms, persistent fever, increasing pain, and increased WBC; this requires emergent surgical evacuation, explantation, and antibiotics [3]

- **Lost or inadequate stimulation**: AP and lateral fluoroscopic images of the leads, connections, IPG to rule out lead migration, lead fracture, disconnection. If normal, then interrogate the IPG and reprogram varying amplitude, pulse width, and active electrodes. Check impedance and if two contacts are identical this indicates a short circuit. Programmer will also indicate if there is battery failure requiring replacement surgery. Leads and/or connectors may need replacement if battery is found to be intact and there are no disconnections.

- **SCS and pacemakers**: SCS can be safely utilized in conjunction with a non-demand type cardiac pacemaker and even an ICD [7]. Both devices should be programmed in bipolar mode. When placing an SCS, the cardiac device should be monitored for any sign of interference. Every time the SCS is reprogrammed continuous ECG should be monitored for signs of interference. An SCS will not damage an ICD, but if and ICD discharges, the SCS IPG may be damaged therefore after every discharge the SCS IPG should be interrogated to check the status of the device.

- **Decreased stimulation threshold**: May indicate intrathecal migration of lead abutting spinal cord. Imaging would be required.

Outcomes

- 50–70 % patients achieve >50 % pain relief with improved function (*successful trial*) [5]
- 20–40 % patients have loss of effectiveness, 2 years after implantation—indicating possible neuroplasticity within the CNS [8].
- Better SCS outcomes than reoperation for failed back surgery syndrome [9]
  - Prospective randomized crossover study
  - Outcomes: >50 % pain relief, patient satisfied
  - 9/19 SCS successful vs. 3/26 reoperation
- Improved 5-year patient satisfaction vs. medical management for CRPS-I [10]
  - 95 % patients would reimplant if given the option

References

1. Melzack R, Wall PD. Textbook of pain. Edinburgh: Churchill Livingstone; 1989.
2. Stojanovic MP. Neuromodulation techniques for the treatment of pain. In: Ballantyne JC, editor. The Massachusetts general hospital handbook of pain management. Philadelphia: Lippincott Williams & Wilkins; 2006. p. 193–203.
3. Kreis P, Fishman M. Spinal cord stimulation implantation: percutaneous implantation techniques. Oxford: Oxford University Press; 2009. p. 2, 12–14, 47, 129–130, 132–141.
4. Kebaish KM, Awad JN. Spinal epidural hematoma causing acute cauda equina syndrome. Neurosurg Focus. 2004;16:e1.
5. Kumar K, Toth C, Nath RK, Laing P. Epidural spinal cord stimulation for treatment of chronic pain—some predictors of success. A 15-year experience. Surg Neurol. 1998;50(2):110–20.
6. Wheeler AH, Burchiel KJ. Spinal Cord Stimulation. Medscape. 2013.
7. Molon G, Perrone C, Maines M, Costa A, Comisso J, Boi A, Moro E, Vergara G, Barbieri E. ICD and neuromodulation devices: is peaceful coexistence possible? Pacing Clin Electrophysiol. 2011;34(6):690–3.
8. Stojanovic MP, Abdi S. Spinal cord stimulation. Pain Physician. 2002;5(2):156–66.
9. North RB, Kidd DH, Farrokhi F, Piantadosi SA. Spinal cord stimulation versus repeated lumbosacral spine surgery for chronic pain: a randomized, controlled trial. Neurosurgery. 2005;56(1):98–106.
10. Kemler MA, de Vet HC, Barendse GA, van den Wildenberg FA, van Kleef M. Effect of spinal cord stimulation for chronic complex regional pain syndrome type I: five-year final follow-up of patients in a randomized controlled trial. J Neurosurg. 2008;108(2):292–8.

Intrathecal Drug Delivery Systems

Eli Soto

Abbreviations

ACTH	Adrenocorticotropic hormone
ASRA	American Society of Regional Anesthesia
CPT	Current Procedural Terminology
CSF	Cerebrospinal l fluid
CT	Computed tomography
DDS	Drug delivery systems
FDA	Food and Drug Administration
GB	Glycoprotein
HIV	Human immunodeficiency virus
IDDS	Intrathecal drug delivery systems
IT	Intrathecal
LMWM	Low molecular weight marker
MRI	Magnetic resonance imaging
NSAIDs	Nonsteroidal anti-inflammatory drugs
PDPH	Post-dural puncture headache

Introduction

Intrathecal drug delivery systems (IDDS) have been utilized for the past few decades for the long-term management of patients with intractable malignant [1, 2] and chronic non-malignant pain [3–5]. The deposit of medications directly into the intrathecal (IT) space in the vicinity of the dorsal horn and nerve roots is an ideal route for the administration of analgesics. In addition, the medication dosages needed are significantly lower causing a marked reduction in side effects. This chapter will briefly review the most important aspects of IDDS. It does not suffice as an only resource for practitioners involved with ITP placement or trial.

E. Soto, M.D., D.A.B.P.M., F.I.P.P. (✉)
Anesthesia Pain Care Consultants, Tamarac, FL, USA
e-mail: esoto2001@gmail.com

Indications for IDDS

- Inadequate analgesia with other oral/systemic analgesic methods
- Intolerable side effects from oral/systemic therapy

Pain Types/Conditions Treated with IDDS

- *Nociceptive*
  - Cancer pain
  - Post-laminectomy syndrome
  - Intractable angina
- *Neuropathic*
  - Complex Regional Pain Syndrome (I/II)
  - Post-herpetic neuralgia
  - Painful peripheral neuropathy
  - Post-stroke pain
  - Nerve root injury
  - Adhesive spinal arachnoiditis
  - Spinal cord injury
  - Phantom limb pain
- *Mixed*
  - HIV-related pain

Contraindications for IDDS

- *Absolute Contraindications*
  - Coagulopathy, bleeding disorders (not corrected)
  - Systemic infections
  - Local cutaneous infections near surgical sites
  - Known allergies or reactions to the implantable materials
  - Allergy to medications to be infused
  - Active intravenous drug abuse
  - Major psychiatric illness
  - Poor compliance
  - Short life expectancy (<3 months)

K.A. Sackheim, *Pain Management and Palliative Care: A Comprehensive Guide*,
DOI 10.1007/978-1-4939-2462-2_46, © Springer Science+Business Media New York 2015

- *Relative Contraindications*
  - Anticoagulation therapy (must be reversed before invasive procedures)
  - Preexisting anatomic abnormalities
  - Poor family or social support
  - Body habitus not conductive to implant
  - Metabolic disorder
  - Recovering drug addiction (patients need a thorough assessment)
  - Poor healing

Success of Neuraxial Analgesia Relies on Many Factors Including [6]

- Accurate diagnosis
- Proper patient selection
- Appropriate assessment of coexisting medical conditions as well as psychological comorbidities
- Prior therapies and results
- Spinal and anatomical technical factors
- Device-related limitations
- Socioeconomic factors

Patient Selection

- *Inclusion Criteria*
  - Identifiable pathology and/or pain generators (listed from above indication list)
  - Measurable opioids responsiveness
  - Failure of oral/systemic opioids therapy
  - Pain refractory to other less invasive therapies
  - No indication for medical or surgical therapy
  - No contraindications
  - Proper psychological screening and behavioral assessment
- *Psychological Screening*
  - Assessment of these conditions in the context of medical decision making is essential
  - Performed by a trained clinical psychologist
  - Patient and treating physician must have similar expectations
  - Even though several psychological conditions such as personality disorders, depression, substance abuse, and secondary gain could be absolute contraindications for IDDS implantation; a patient should not be included or excluded solely on the basis of a single psychological test.
  - In patients with psychological comorbidities, ongoing psychological monitoring is recommended

- For cancer patients, an initial psychological evaluation may not be necessary if the IT therapy can significantly improve their quality of life

Trialing for IDDS

The wide variety of agents available for IT analgesia either single-drug [7] or multi-drug regimen [8] (FDA-approved and off-label use), some of them with rather limited scientific evidence, have led pain physicians to focus their attention to develop practice guidelines for the use of these drugs for the long-term management of malignant [9] and nonmalignant pain [10, 11]. The trial period has been used as a measure of success in the subsequent IDDS implantation. However, the value of the trial as predictor of clinical outcome has not been supported by the literature. The trial process and device implantation techniques vary to a great extent based on the physician's skills, preferences, practice facilities, and health insurance coverage (Fig. 46.1).

Trialing

- *Goals of Trialing*
  - Physician must have an honest discussion with the patient regarding realistic expectations in terms of:
    - Pain control
    - Improvement in functional capacity
    - Reduction in systemic opioids analgesics
    - Management of adverse effects and complications
  - Objective measures for functional outcomes and patient satisfaction should be utilized
  - *"Successful trial"—commonly defined as a pain intensity reduction of >50 % in visual analog score*
- *Pretrialing Assessment*
  - *Comorbidities*:
    - Comorbidities such as diabetes, immunosuppression, sleep apnea, and bleeding disorders need special attention during the IT trial.
    - Medications for chronic conditions must be continued throughout the duration of the trial.
    - It is recommended to use prophylactic antibiotics continuously during trial of intrathecal infusions.
  - *Anticoagulation*: Discontinuation of anticoagulation therapy is required before the trial. Physicians must follow the American Society of Regional Anesthesia (ASRA) and Pain Medicine guidelines for spinal injections and catheter placement [12]. Permission must be obtained from prescribing physician before discontinuing these medications.

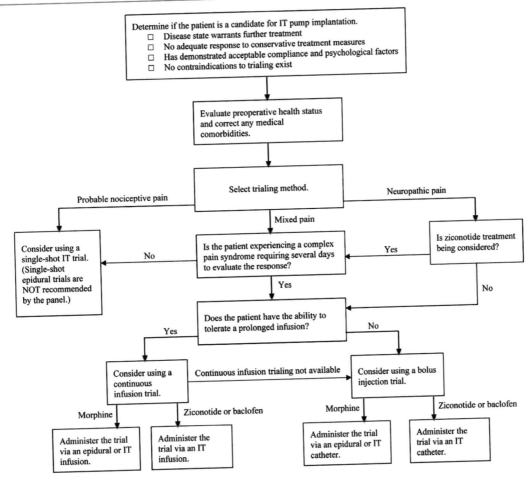

Fig. 46.1 Determination of patient's candidacy for intrathecal pump implantation

- Antiplatelet medications
  - NSAIDs: no contraindication
  - Clopidogrel: discontinue for 7 days
  - Ticlopidine: discontinue for 14 days
  - GP IIb/IIIa inhibitors: discontinue for 8–48 h
- Subcutaneous unfractioned heparin
  - Twice a day dosing or <10,000 U/day: no contra-indication; consider delaying the heparin if a technically difficult case
  - More than twice a day dosing or >10,000 U/day: safety not established
- Intravenous unfractioned heparin
  - Restart heparin 1 h after procedure
    Remove catheter 2–4 h after last heparin dose
- Low molecular weight marker (LMWM)
  - Single dose: Perform procedure 10–12 h after LMWM; next dose 4 h after needle or catheter placement
  - Twice a day dosing: restart LMWM 24 h after procedure; remove catheter at least 2 h before first dose LMWM
  - Therapeutic dose: delay procedure for 24 h

- *Pretrialing Systemic Analgesics*: In patients on chronic opioids therapy several options can be considered before the trial:
  - Complete conversion of systemic opioid therapy into epidural or intrathecal route
  - Complete weaning off medications before the trial: this could unmask an underlying opioid-induced hyperalgesia. Some patients may not require IDDS after they are completely weaned off opioids.
  - Partial weaning to minimal required dosages
  - No weaning
- *Unnecessary trials*: In several conditions, the addition of an IT trial before the implantation may be an unnecessary and counterproductive step.
  - *Cancer pain*: advanced oncologic disease with minimal control on chronic opioids therapy or unable to tolerate medication side effects. The reduction of side effects and better pain control may improve their quality of life. Intrathecal therapy in this patient population must be weighed against the risk of surgery, infection, and medication management.

- *Cerebrovascular disease*: Patient on anticoagulation after stroke with chronic pain. Stopping prophylactic anticoagulation in two separate occasions or having to bridge with heparin therapy may outweigh the benefits of the procedure.
- *Cerebral Palsy*: Patients with cerebral palsy and spasticity may benefit from IDDS with baclofen without undergoing a trial if oral baclofen therapy has been tolerated in the past.
- *Spinal instrumentation at multiple levels*: Patient with anatomic challenges may benefit from an open surgical IT catheter placement. In this scenario, a prior IT trial may be unnecessary.

Medications

Opioids: Inhibition of C-fiber transmission by binding to pre-/postsynaptic μ receptors at the dorsal horn and substantia gelatinosa

- *Morphine*:
  - Remains the "gold standard" for intrathecal opioid analgesia
  - Only opioid approved by the FDA for IDDS
- *Hydromorphone*:
  - Semisynthetic hydrogenated ketone of morphine
  - Greater lipophilic properties than morphine, thus resulting in more potency and faster onset of action
- *Fentanyl/Sufentanil*:
  - These highly lipophilic medications have the fastest onset, action peak, and clearance.
  - Fentanyl and sufentanil have potencies of 100× and 1,000× when compared to morphine, respectively.
  - Due to their rapid clearance from the intrathecal space, these medications are thought to have less rostral spread causing less supraspinal side effects.

Local anesthetics: Bind to plasma membrane of nerve cells causing modifications of the fast sodium channels preventing sodium influx which initiates the action potential

- *Bupivacaine*:
  - Most commonly used local anesthetic
  - Not been approved by the FDA to use in IDDS
  - Synergistic effect when combined with opioids

Alpha-2 adrenergic agonists: Inhibit neurotransmission and slow down the release of C-fiber transmitters including substance P by binding to pre/postsynaptic α-2 receptors in the dorsal horn

- *Clonidine*:
  - Adjuvant to opioid therapy
  - Has an effect on postsynaptic G-coupled potassium channels resulting in hyperpolarization and can also activate spinal cholinergic receptors potentiating the analgesic effect
  - Due to its lipophilic properties, results in rapid onset, peak action, and clearance from IT space.
  - Approved by the FDA for IT administration
  - Most common side effect is postural hypotension

GABA B agonists: Reduces terminal neurotransmitter release by evoking hyperpolarization of the membrane

- *Baclofen*:
  - Scientific evidence for pain conditions is limited
  - Approved by the FDA for IDDS use
  - Side effects include drowsiness, weakness, confusion, sedation, hypotension, among others
  - Overdose and withdrawal from baclofen can both be fatal. Initiation of this intrathecal medication requires extreme caution.

Calcium channel antagonists: Inhibition of substance P and glutaminergic transmission through N-type voltage-sensitive calcium channels in the substantia gelatinosa.

- *Ziconotide*:
  - Synthetic derivative of a toxin produced by the *Conus magnus*
  - Commonly used for neuropathic pain syndrome as well as chronic nonmalignant pain
  - Approved by the FDA for intrathecal use
  - Narrow therapeutic window with an extensive list of adverse effects including: changes in mental status, confusion, changes in mood or perception, postural hypotension, drowsiness, dizziness, nystagmus, visual problems, among others.

Other agents

- *Gabapentin*:
  - Reduces mechanical allodynia and thermal hyperalgesia in animal models
  - Potency of gabapentin is tenfold greater than its subcutaneous and intraperitoneal routes
  - Minimal effects on heart rate and blood pressure
- *Neostigmine*:
  - Quicker onset of sensory block and longer duration of motor and sensory block when compared with bupivacaine
- *Adenosine*:
  - Reduces the area of allodynia and hyperesthesia
- *Ketorolac*:
  - Even though prostaglandins play an important role in central sensitization, ketorolac does not reduce pain.

Medication selection for IT analgesia

- Multiple factors must be taken into consideration:
  - Pain type, lipid solubility of the drug, comorbid conditions, and concomitant medications

Table 46.1 2013 Polyanalgesic algorithm for intrathecal (IT) therapies in neuropathic pain

Line 1—Morphine/Ziconotide/Morphine + Bupivacaine

Line 2—Hydromorphone/Hydromorphone + Bupivacaine or Hydromorphone + Clonidine/Morphine + Clonidine

Line 3—Clonidine/Ziconotide + opioid/Fentanyl/Fentanyl + Bupivacaine or Fentanyl + Clonidine

Line 4—Opioid + Clonidine + Bupivacaine/Bupivacaine + Clonidine

Line 5—Baclofen

Adapted from Deer TR, Levy R, Prager J, et al. Polyanalgesic Consensus Conference—2012: Recommendations on Trialing for Intrathecal (Intraspinal) Drug Delivery: Report of an Interdisciplinary Expert Panel. Neuromodulation 2012;15:436–464 [11]

Table 46.2 Polyanalgesic algorithm for intrathecal therapies in neuropathic pain

Line 1—Morphine/Hydromorphone/Ziconotide/Fentanyl

Line 2—Morphine + Bupivacaine/Ziconotide + Opioid/Hydromorphone + Bupivacaine/Fentanyl + Bupivacaine

Line 3—Opioid (Morphine, Hydromorphone, or Fentanyl) + Clonidine/Sufentanil

Line 4—Opioid + Clonidine + Bupivacaine/Sufentanil + Bupivacaine or Clonidine

Line 5—Sufentanil + Bupivacaine + Clonidine

Adapted from Deer TR, Levy R, Prager J, et al. Polyanalgesic Consensus Conference—2012: Recommendations on Trialing for Intrathecal (Intraspinal) Drug Delivery: Report of an Interdisciplinary Expert Panel. Neuromodulation 2012;15:436–464 [11]

Table 46.3 Recommended dosages and concentrations for intrathecal medications

Drug	IT Bolus dose	Starting daily dose	Maximum daily dose	Maximum concentration
Morphine	0.2–1.0 mg	0.1–0.5 mg/day	15 mg	20 mg/mL
Hydromorphone	0.04–0.2 mg	0.02–0.5 mg/day	10 mg	15 mg/mL
Fentanyl	25–75 µg	25–75 µg/day	No upper limits	10 mg/mL
Sufentanil	5–20 µg	10–20 µg/day	No upper limits	5 mg/mL
Bupivacaine	0.5–2.5 mg	1–4 mg/day	10 mg	30 mg/mL
Clonidine	5–20 µg	40–100 µg/day	40–600 µg	1,000 µg/mL
Ziconotide	1–5 µg	0.5–2.4 µg/day	19.2 µg	100 µg/mL

Adapted from Deer TR, Levy R, Prager J, et al. Polyanalgesic Consensus Conference—2012: Recommendations on Trialing for Intrathecal (Intraspinal) Drug Delivery: Report of an Interdisciplinary Expert Panel. Neuromodulation 2012;15:436–464 [11]

– Due to the challenges that medication selection impose in the treating physician, a panel experts have created several guidelines for the utilization of IDDS. The following recommendations are based on the algorithms from the 2012 Polyanalgesic Consensus Conference [11].

- Neuropathic Pain (Table 46.1)
  - *Line 1*—Morphine alone or in combination with bupivacaine are considered first-line therapy for neuropathic pain. Ziconotide is also recommended as first-line treatment for neuropathic and nociceptive pain.
  - *Line 2*—Hydromorphone alone or in combination with bupivacaine or clonidine; morphine in combination with clonidine.
  - *Line 3*—Fentanyl alone or in combination with bupivacaine or clonidine; clonidine alone and the combination of ziconotide and an opioid.
  - *Line 4*—Bupivacaine in combination with clonidine with or without opioids.
  - *Line 5*—Baclofen monotherapy

- Nociceptive Pain (Table 46.2)
  - *Line 1*—Morphine, hydromorphone, and ziconotide monotherapy are considered first-line therapy for nociceptive pain. Fentanyl has also been incorporated as a first-line drug due to the lack of granuloma formation and lipophilic nature.
  - *Line 2*—Morphine, hydromorphone, or fentanyl in combination with bupivacaine; ziconotide in combination with an opioids.
  - *Line 3*—Morphine, hydromorphone, or fentanyl in combination with clonidine; sufentanil mono-therapy.
  - *Line 4*—Morphine, hydromorphone, or fentanyl in combination with bupivacaine and clonidine; sufentanil in combination with bupivacaine or clonidine.
  - *Line 5*—Sufentanil in combination with bupivacaine and clonidine.
- Starting dosages for IT bolus/continuous infusion and maximum concentrations (Table 46.3)
- Trialing methods: There are multiple ways of trialing neuraxial medications (i.e., epidural versus intrathecal, bolus

versus continuous infusion). Due to the lack of scientific evidence, no method can be considered superior to the others.
- Epidural versus intrathecal: The use of these routes of administration may depend on the pain sensitivity of patients. Any of the routes may be appropriate.
- Single versus multiple injection
- Bolus versus continuous: Either of these trialing methods should be performed before the permanent implant to test for possible adverse reactions and analgesic effect. However, none of them can be used as predictor of outcome.
  - *Bolus*
    Advantage: cost, convenience, and safety
    Disadvantage: limited information regarding long-term effects
  - *Continuous*:
    Advantage: More representative of pharmacokinetic and pharmacodynamic effects; provides more time for functional assessment
    Disadvantage: Higher costs due to close hospital monitoring, higher infection risk
- Trial setting: The experts from 2012 Polyanalgesic Consensus Conference recommend that patients should be monitored for at least 24 h [11]. Inpatient setting is warranted for patient with cancer-related pain (higher life expectancy) and for patients with chronic pain receiving opioids.
  - *Outpatient*
    - Advantages: Lower costs, more convenient
    - Disadvantages: Limited monitoring, slow titration
  - *Inpatient*
    - Advantages: Appropriate monitoring, rapid titration
    - Disadvantages: Higher costs, time consuming
- Initiation of IT medications after trial
  - Conservative dosing should be consider using the lower possible reasonable dose
  - Close monitoring during the postoperative period is recommended to prevent respiratory depression

Complications from Trialing

- *Post-dural puncture headache (PDPH)*
  - Treatment:
    - Supine position
    - Hydration
    - Caffeine intake
    - Intravenous dexamethasone
    - Analgesics
    - Epidural blood patch

- *Urinary retention*
  - Treatment:
    - Catheterization
    - Bethanechol
    - Opioid rotation
- *Orthostatic hypotension*
  - Treatment:
    - Hydration
- *Catheter dislodgment*
  - Treatment:
    - Place the catheter over the lower lumbar area
    - Anchor over the sacrum
    - Tunneling prevents the occurrence of dislodgment
- *Meningitis*
  - Treatment:
    - Use proper sterile techniques
    - Limit duration of trial (<3 days)
    - Tunnel the catheter
    - Maintain appropriate aseptic conditions
    - Consider the use of antibiotics through the catheter

Implantable Pump System

- *Preoperative preparation*:
  - Expectations should be discussed again including the possibility of achieving less analgesia than during the trial
  - Patient should be assessed for pulmonary function and risk of respiratory depression
  - Long-acting medications should be discontinued, as the IDDS will replace this, if a continuous infusion is used. Medications for breakthrough pain should be continued until the pain is stable.
  - *Pump size*: The treating physician should have a discussion about which pump size is appropriate for a particular patient. As a general rule, the patient should receive the largest pump that the anatomic area allows to facilitate a longer refill interval.
  - *Identify the pump pocket site*:
    - Consideration is made to belt lines, comfort positioning, wheelchair arms, physical activities, and other rehabilitation matters.
    - Pump should be positioned away from anatomic landmarks such as the rib cage, iliac crest, and current or future surgery sites.
    - Most common sites for implantation of the pump are the lower abdominal quadrants.
  - Initiate discussion about program settings and medications that will be used. Changes can always be done once the therapy has been started but the patient should

have an active role on deciding which programming modality is being chosen.

– *Intravenous hydration*: maintain adequate hydration for before procedure to prevent hypovolemic states and hypotension

– Risks and benefits of the procedure (including the risk of anesthesia) should be discussed.

• *Equipment* [13]

– Tunneled percutaneous catheters: same catheter used for continuous neuraxial analgesia but internalized/tunneled to prevent catheter dislodgement

– Implanted catheter with subcutaneous injection site: catheters can be placed in the epidural or intrathecal space; however, they have been approved for epidural infusions only. Placement requires fluoroscopy guidance and sterile conditions.

  ▪ Epidural Port-a-Cath (Smiths Medical): It can be used for patients with malignant pain with short life expectancy (<3 months). The catheter is internalized, tunneled, and connected to the reservoir. The reservoir site is usually implanted above a bony structure and anchored to the fascia to prevent movement of the port during access with a noncoring needle. The Port-a-Cath is connected to an external pump for continuous infusion.

Pump Options:

• *Fixed-rate intrathecal pump*: These pumps are set to deliver a constant volume of solution per unit of time. There is no external device to program the flow rate. They are driven by an injected pressurized gas or by an elastomeric diaphragm. The flow rate is determined by the diameter of the orifice. They can be used to infuse intrathecal pain medications and intravenous chemotherapeutic agents.

– *Advantages*:

  ▪ No programming required

  ▪ Availability of qualified physicians to manage the pump is not necessary (Easier for patients to relocate or travel)

  ▪ Smaller profile device

  ▪ Do not require periodic battery changes

– *Disadvantages*:

  ▪ Patient selection is more difficult

  ▪ More difficult to make changes in delivery doses

  ▪ More difficult to stop in the event of an emergency

– *Current options for fixed-rate pumps*

  ▪ Codman 3000 (Codman and Shurtleff, Inc., a Johnson & Johnson Co., Raynham, MA)

  ▪ IsoMed (Medtronic, Inc., Minneapolis, MN)

• *Programmable pumps*: Can be used to treat malignant and chronic pain as well as spasticity. They can also be used as hepatic or intravenous infusions. They equipment consists of an implantable pump, intrathecal catheter, and external device to program the pump.

– *Advantages*

  ▪ Adaptability—easy alteration of medication dosages

  ▪ Use of bolus dosing for breakthrough pain with option of handheld device for patient's self-administration

  ▪ Complex-continuous programming for variable but predictable pain throughout the day

– *Disadvantages*

  ▪ Programming errors

  ▪ Closer follow-up needed for safe and effective use

  ▪ Trained physicians must be available in the event of travel or relocation

– *Programmable factors*

  ▪ Patient information

  ▪ Date and time of setting changes

  ▪ Medications names, dosages (per unit of time), and concentrations

  ▪ Infusion mode
    Single bolus
    Simple continuous
    Single bolus plus simple continuous
    Periodic bolus
    Complex continuous

  ▪ Total volume of medication in the reservoir and alarm volume

  ▪ Clinician-delivered bolus doses

  ▪ Patient-delivered bolus doses

  ▪ Current options for programmable pumps
    SynchroMed EL (Medtronic, Inc., Minneapolis, MN)
    SynchroMed II (Medtronic, Inc., Minneapolis, MN)
    Prometra (Flowonix Medical, Mount Olive, NJ)

ITP Implantation Procedure

• **Positioning**

– Depends on the physician preference: the lateral decubitus position with the pocket side up versus the prone position for IT catheter placement with rotation of the patient to a supine position for creation of the pocket.

- If prone position is preferred, the use of pillows underneath the abdominal area increases the separation of the spinous processes in the lumbar spine to facilitate access to the intrathecal space. For practitioners that prefer the lateral decubitus position, the patient must be positioned with the lumbar spine slightly flexed.
- The use of pillows or pads to avoid pressure points is also encouraged.
- Position the table and drape the patient to allow fluoroscopic visualization of the anatomic landmarks were the catheter will be inserted.

- **Needle placement**
  - After the skin and subcutaneous tissues have been infiltrated with local anesthetic, the spinal needle is inserted using a shallow, paramedian oblique insertion technique (30° off the spine).
  - Entry point should be 1–2 cm lateral to the spinous processes and 1–1.5 vertebral levels below the site were the dura will be punctured (for entry point through the skin or open incision)
  - Needle tip should enter the dura at the L2–3 or L3–4 level (unless anatomic variations dictate otherwise).
  - Keeping the bevel parallel to the longitudinal fibers, the needle should be advanced until the dura is puncture.
  - The stylet should be removed at different depths to confirm correct placement until free flowing, clear CSF is observed.
  - The stylet is reinserted to prevent the unnecessary flow of CSF.

- **Implanting the catheter** (lateral decubitus position)
  - After correct placement of the needle in the intrathecal space, the bevel is oriented cephalad (to minimize shearing of the catheter) and the stylet removed and the distal tip of the catheter threaded to the desired location.
  - A slight increase in resistance could be felt when the catheter has been threaded to the tip of the needle.
  - The physician must make sure that the catheter guide wire remains in place during all the catheter manipulations.
  - Caution must be exerted when pulling the catheter back as this backward motion could cause damage to the catheter.
  - With the needle in place to protect the catheter, an incision is made at the needle site to expose the underlying fascia for anchoring of the catheter.
  - Undermining of the subcutaneous tissue is necessary to create a smooth fascial plane for anchoring of the catheter.

- With extreme caution, remove the needle from the intrathecal space, and hold the catheter near the needle tip.
- Remove the needle and guide wire at the proximal side simultaneously, holding the catheter in place to prevent migration.
- Tie nonabsorbable sutures to the fascia close to the catheter to secure the anchor and catheter in place (This step will depend on the type of anchor and catheter used).
- Tie the proximal end of the catheter to prevent further CSF leakage while tunneling and creating the pocket site.

- **Preparing the pocket**
  - An incision is made over the area previously marked for the pump placement.
  - The size of the pocket should be large enough for the pump without any pulling in the skin or subcutaneous tissue.
  - Incision should not lie over the pump or main port.
  - Recommended depth is no more than 2.5 cm underneath the skin. (Deep placement of the pump reservoir will make subsequent medication refills more difficult).

- **Tunneling the catheter**
  - Tunnel subcutaneously using the appropriate catheter passer
  - Pass the catheter through the tunneler from the spinal incision site to the pocket
  - Leave enough catheter to form several coils behind the pump
  - Untie the proximal portion of the catheter
  - If any part of the catheter is trimmed, it should measure for catheter volume calculations

- **Connecting the pump to the catheter**
  - Connect the spinal catheter tubing to the pump
  - This step will vary depending on the connector type and catheter

- **Securing the pump**
  - Use nonabsorbable sutures to secure the pump to the pocket fascia
  - Make sure the main port is facing the right way
  - Insert the pump in the pocket, verifying that the pocket is the adequate size; no skin pulling or too much room for the pump to flip

- Both incisions are then close in a standard fashion

Postoperative Care/Follow-up

- Patient must be aware of the possibility of suboptimal analgesia after the permanent implant as the postoperative pain can play an important role and confounding factor

- Titration may continue for several weeks post-implantation before reaching an optimal level
- Patients should understand the basic pump functions and maintenance (including refills)
- Educate patients about the device volume warnings and encouraged not to let the pump run dry as severe and potentially fatal withdrawal symptoms (e.g., baclofen withdrawal) may occurred.
- Physician must discuss an emergency plan if the above occurs.

Complications [14]

Surgical complications

- *CSF leakage/Post-dural puncture headache (PDPH)*: IT catheter placement can increase the risk of PDPH
  - Treatment:
    - Adequate hydration during the preoperative period
    - If prior history of PDPH, a prolonged period of bed rest and hydration may be warranted
    - Minimize trauma using a paramedian approach, low angle (30° from skin), and dural entry point at midline
    - Most dural punctures may resolve with conservative therapy including hydration, caffeine, analgesics, and bed rest
    - Treat nausea aggressively as the inability to tolerate oral hydration may worsen the headache
    - Consider admission if severe headache, new visual or neurologic symptoms, dehydration
    - Refractory cases may require an epidural blood patch. (Risk of damaging the catheter or introducing a new infection)
- *Infections, abscess formation*: Infection rate varies from 0.7 to 10.3 % per year, with the majority occurring within 60 days of implantation [15]. *Staph epidermidis* is the most common pathogen.
  - Recommendations:
    - Preoperative assessment of increased risk of infection in patients with chronic diseases such as diabetes mellitus, malignancy, HIV, among others.
    - Know prior history of local or systemic infections
    - Use preoperative antibiotics to be completed prior to the incision. (Be familiar with prior bacterial sensitivities and regional resistance patterns)
    - Chlorohexidine bathing prior to surgery in patient with high infection risk

- Postoperative antibiotics are also encouraged
- Use a new, sterile catheter (different from the trial) for the permanent implant
- Consider rapid internalization of intrathecal catheter if IDDS is considered
- A sterile operating room should be used for the implantation of the device
- The use of antibiotics wound irrigation is encouraged
- Careful attention should be paid to wound closure to prevent dehiscence and bacterial growth
  - Treatment:
    - If superficial wound infection occurs, it should be treated with antibiotics aggressively for 7–14 days and monitored closely.
    - If a deeper infection is suspected, there is no response to antibiotics or the infection recurs, the system should be removed.
- *Bleeding*: It is important to recognize and correct any factors that may contribute to intra- or postoperative bleeding. A thorough review of medications (including herbal supplements) and medical conditions such as platelet dysfunction, hepatic disease, and coagulation disorders must be performed. The ASRA guidelines for anticoagulation prior to neuraxial analgesia should be followed [12].
  - Treatment:
    - Bleeding from surgical site
      - Intraoperative bleeding occurs from inefficient hemostasis
      - Serosanguinous drainage from surgical sites in the immediate postoperative period is norma
    - Epidural hematoma
      - Depending on the severity of signs and symptoms of neurological compromise, a surgical evacuation must be warranted.
      - The appropriate imaging should be requested without delaying a surgical evaluation
- *Seroma at the implantation site*: usually noticeable after 2 weeks post-implantation. Extensive cauterization and dissection can contribute to this phenomenon.
  - Treatment:
    - Observation if no signs of infection
    - Initial treatment could include a pressure dressing with a gauze and tape; alternatively, an abdominal binder could also be used in the postoperative period as a preventive method
    - If the pocket increases in size, an abdominal X-ray may be order to rule out any mechanical complications such as disconnection at the pump site

- The fluid should not be aspirated unless an infectious process is suspected; this could potentially introduce more pathogens to the area
- If aspiration is performed, the utilization of fluoroscopy guidance is recommended to avoid any damage to pump and catheter

Device-related complications (Mechanical)

- *Catheter problems*
  - Catheter disconnection at the pump site, breakage, or displacement
    - Treatment:
      - If there is a suspicion of catheter displacement from the IT space, breakage, or disconnection at the pump site, the catheter should be investigated carefully
      - A site port access for CSF aspiration and/or contrast injection (dye study) under fluoroscopy guidance should be considered to assess the cause of catheter malfunction. (Caution: the catheter must be aspirated to remove any remaining medication before injecting contrast. Failure to do this may result in overdose if the catheter remains in the IT space). The CSF should flow freely with aspiration and the contrast should be injected without resistance.
      - A blockage on the CSF flow with aspiration of large amounts of medications suggests a mechanical obstruction
      - If there is any evidence of catheter migration, breakage or disconnection, a surgical exploration (revision) must take place for catheter replacement or reconnection.
- *Rotation of the pump*: related to the creation of a large pocket or poor anchoring technique
  - Treatment:
    - Create a pocket of the appropriate dimensions to fit the pump reservoir without pulling on the subcutaneous tissue
    - For anchoring,
      - Dacron pouch—facilitates scaring formation around the pump for anchoring
      - Nonabsorbable sutures—secure the pump to the fascia
- *Refill-related problems*
  - Pocket fill
    - Treatment:
      - Interrogate the pump before starting the process to know the amount of volume that will be aspirated

- Examine the patient palpating the area above and surrounding the pump before inserting the needle
- The use of fluoroscopy or ultrasound is encouraged if a difficult refill (due to obesity or deep pump placement) is expected
- Use a template to confirm the position of the main port while refilling the pump
- If the pump moves or it is too deep, ask a colleague to secure (hold) the pump
- Once the refill needle is inserted, the septum should be engaged and the medication aspirated. (The volume should be within 3 mL of the predicted value).
- When the new medication is injected, attention should be paid to avoid injecting air into the reservoir as it can damage the pump.
- Aspirate every 3–5 mL to confirm injection in the reservoir; if the drug cannot be aspirated a pocket fill should be suspected.
- The medication should be aspirated from the pocket immediately and the patient treated accordingly.
  - Programming errors
    - Treatment:
      - Special attention should be paid while reprogramming the pump (dosage/concentration changes, bridge bolus, etc.) as small errors can result in fatalities
      - The length of the catheter, internal/external volumes as well as the medication's doses and concentrations need to be known before administering a bridge bolus
      - When reinitiating the pump after a temporary interruption in therapy, a dose reduction should be considered

Drug-related complications

- *Adverse reactions*
  - Respiratory depression: most clinically important. It may occur due to rostral spread of medications (i.e., hydrophilic agents) or systemic absorption (i.e., lipophilic agents). Supraspinal interaction of the medication with μ-2 opioids receptors in the brainstem
    - Risk Factors
      - Opioid naïve
      - Advanced age
      - Preexisting pulmonary conditions
      - Sleep apnea
      - Minimal pain

♦ Opioid administration via different routes
- Treatment:
  ♦ Respiratory support
  ♦ Use μ receptor antagonists to reverse respiratory depression only when strictly necessary taking the appropriate precautions
- *Gastrointestinal symptoms*: Less common than with systemic therapy. Mediated by interaction of medications with the chemotherapy trigger zone
  ▪ Treatment:
    ♦ Symptomatic treatment
- *Urinary dysfunction:* Caused by reduction of detrusor muscle tone and sphincter dyssynergia. Mediated through μ and δ receptors. It is often self-limited.
  ▪ Treatment:
    ♦ Intermittent bladder catheterization
    ♦ Opioid antagonist or phenoxybenzamine
    ♦ Opioid rotation
- *Hormonal alterations*: Due to inhibition of gonadotropin and corticotropin-releasing hormones from hypothalamus, and reduction of luteinizing hormone, follicle-stimulating hormone, ACTH and β-endorphins, resulting in reduction of cortisol and testosterone.
  ▪ Treatment:
    ♦ Serum lipids, 24-h urinary cortisol, and serum androgen or estrogen levels should be monitored regularly
    ♦ Replacement with testosterone, estrogen, and corticosteroids should be initiated if the level is low
    ♦ If any concerning endocrine issue related to IDDS, the patient should be referred to a specialist
- *Peripheral edema*: Know side effects of opioid analgesia. It usually occurs early in the course of the therapy.
  ▪ Treatment:
    ♦ Assess the patient's risk factors to develop peripheral edema
    ♦ In high-risk patients such as those with cardiac, renal failure as well as venous stasis and peripheral neuropathy, the opioid should be minimized
    ♦ Leg elevation, diuretics, and compression stockings should be considered before making any changes to the medications
    ♦ Ziconotide or the addition of adjuvants with opioid-sparing effects should be consider to lower the opioid dose

- *Itching*: Common in opioids naïve patients. Morphine is the most common opioids causing pruritus.
  ▪ Treatment:
    ♦ Antihistamines
    ♦ Opioid rotation
- Recommendations:
  ▪ Be familiar with patient's history of prior drug reactions and allergies
  ▪ Be familiar with the side effects of all the intrathecal medications, especially if multiple medications are used at the same time
  ▪ If the patient experience mild adverse reactions, try reducing the dose until they disappear
  ▪ If moderate/severe adverse reactions, stop the offending agent and rotate to a different medication
- *Catheter tip granuloma*: Inflammatory mass at the tip of the catheter due to high concentration/dosage of intrathecal medications. The most common medications are morphine and hydromorphone[16].
  - Recommendations:
    ▪ Concentrations and dosages should be kept at the lowest levels that are clinical appropriate
    ▪ Rotation to ziconotide or the addition of adjuvant medications (opioid-sparing effect) should be considered if high medication dosages are reached or inadequate analgesia
    ▪ **RED FLAGS** suggesting granuloma formation:
      ♦ Worsening pain on a stable infusion rate unresponsive to dose increases
      ♦ Changes in motor, sensory, and/or proprioceptive function
    ▪ Imaging:
      ♦ Plain X-ray: to identify the position of the catheter tip
      ♦ MRI with/without gadolinium: best option to evaluate the catheter tip
      ♦ CT myelogram: for patients that cannot obtain MRI
  - Treatment: depends on symptomatology, presence of spinal cord or nerve compression
    ▪ Spine consultation
    ▪ Replacement of medication with normal saline with serial MRIs or CT myelograms
    ▪ Catheter revision, replacement or removal of the system
      ♦ Asymptomatic—discontinuation of offending agent or replacement with ziconotide or normal saline

- *Withdrawal*: Pump malfunctioning; disruption of the catheter and/or errors during refill or programming could result in withdrawal symptoms that range from mild to lethal.
  - Opioid withdrawal
    - Signs and symptoms
      - Irritability, agitation, restlessness
      - Gastrointestinal symptoms (nausea, vomiting, diarrhea, abdominal cramping)
      - Pilomotor erection
      - Excessive yawning
      - Increased lacrimation/rhinorrhea
      - Mydriasis
      - Increased pain
      - Pulmonary edema and/or cardiovascular collapse (severe acute withdrawal)
    - Treatment
      - Respiratory/Cardiovascular support
      - Restoration of the IT medication as soon as possible; if not possible start at least of the 50 % of oral equianalgesic drug dose the medication
  - Baclofen withdrawal: Can lead to life-threatening complications if left untreated
    - Signs and symptoms
      - Increased spasticity/Rigidity
      - Hyperthermia
      - Drowsiness/Obtundation
      - Respiratory depression
      - Rhabdomyolysis
      - Acute renal failure
      - Multi-system failure
      - Death
    - Treatment:
      - Early recognition of signs and symptoms
      - Respiratory/Cardiovascular support
      - Severe withdrawal—IT catheter placement with baclofen infusion may be considered. (Oral baclofen may not be sufficient to treat severe acute withdrawal)
  - Clonidine withdrawal:
    - Signs and symptoms
      - Rebound hypertension
    - Treatment:
      - Start clonidine orally or topical (patch) form
- *Opioid tolerance*: The progressive increase of medication dosages to achieve the same level of analgesia. It may be due to desensitization of opioids receptors after prolonged exposure to the medication and/or opioids receptor down regulation
  - Treatment
    - Before establishing the presence of opioids tolerance as the cause for lack of analgesia, the treating physician should rule out the possibility of catheter/pump malfunction and/or disease progression
    - Dose titration by 10–30 % of daily dose (consider an increase in concentration if the daily volume limit is reached)
    - Opioid rotation (assuming incomplete tolerance between medications)
    - Consider adding medication with opioid-sparing effect (e.g., clonidine)
    - Substitute opioids for local anesthetic to provide an opioid-free interval
- *Opioid-induced hyperalgesia*: Increase in sensitivity to a noxious stimuli and/or allodynia in patients on chronic opioids therapy. This could be another potential cause for loss of analgesia with IT infusions in the context of stable disease.

Outcomes [3]

- Moderate evidence of IDDS for chronic nonmalignant pain
- Mortality can be associated with respiratory therapy in the post-implant period after IT therapy is initiated in patients with nonmalignant pain
- Higher mortality rates have been reported for IDDS than spinal cord stimulator
- Further clinical trials are necessary to confirm these results

Billing (Table 46.4) [17]

Table 46.4 CPT codes for Intrathecal Implantables

Code	Description
Trial—Single dose, spinal injection (Percutaneous Placement)	
62310	Injection(s), of diagnostic or therapeutic substance(s) (including anesthetic, antispasmodic, opioid, steroid, other solution), not including neurolytic substances, including needle or catheter placement, includes contrast for localization when performed, epidural or subarachnoid; cervical or thoracic
62311	Injection(s), of diagnostic or therapeutic substance(s) (including anesthetic, antispasmodic, opioid, steroid, other solution), not including neurolytic substances, including needle or catheter placement, includes contrast for localization when performed, epidural or subarachnoid; lumbar or sacral
Trial—Continuous epidural catheter (Percutaneous Placement)	
62318	Injection(s), including indwelling catheter placement, continuous or intermittent bolus, of diagnostic or therapeutic substance(s) (including anesthetic, antispasmodic, opioid, steroid, other solution), not including neurolytic substances, includes contrast for localization when performed, epidural or subarachnoid; cervical or thoracic
62319	Injection(s), including indwelling catheter placement, continuous or intermittent bolus, of diagnostic or therapeutic substance(s) (including anesthetic, antispasmodic, opioid, steroid, other solution), not including neurolytic substances, includes contrast for localization when performed, epidural or subarachnoid; lumbar or sacral
Tunneled Intrathecal or Epidural Catheter	
62350	Implantation, revision or repositioning of tunneled intrathecal or epidural catheter, for long-term medication administration via an external or implantable reservoir/infusion pump; without laminectomy
62351	Implantation, revision, or repositioning of tunneled intrathecal or epidural catheter, for long-term medication administration via an external or implantable reservoir/infusion pump; with laminectomy
Permanent implantation of reservoir or pump	
62360	Implantation or replacement of device for intrathecal or epidural drug infusion; subcutaneous reservoir
62361	Implantation or replacement of device for intrathecal or epidural drug infusion; non-programmable pump
62362	Implantation or replacement of device for intrathecal or epidural drug infusion; programmable pump, including preparation of pump, with or without reprogramming
95991	Refilling and maintenance of implantable pump or reservoir for drug delivery, spinal (intrathecal, epidural) or brain (intraventricular); includes electronic analysis of pump, when performed; requiring physician's skill
Other codes	
62367	Electronic analysis of programmable, implanted pump for intrathecal or epidural drug infusion (includes evaluation of reservoir status, alarm status, drug prescription status); without reprogramming or refill
62368	Electronic analysis of programmable, implanted pump for intrathecal or epidural drug infusion (includes evaluation of reservoir status, alarm status, drug prescription status); with reprogramming
62355	Removal of previously implanted intrathecal or epidural catheter
62365	Removal of subcutaneous reservoir or pump

CPT current procedural terminology
Adapted from Manchikanti L, Falco F. Essentials of Practice Management, Billing, Coding and Compliance, Interventional Pain Management. Padduka: ASIPP Publishing; 2012 [17]

Conclusion

IDDS is an accepted therapy for the treatment of refractory malignant and nonmalignant pain that has been well established in the literature. However, there is no consensus in the many of the steps involved in this process including the trialing techniques or medication selection. Successful treatment requires careful patient selection and appropriate techniques to trial neuraxial analgesia and for the permanent implantation of the system.

References

1. Smith TJ, Staats PS, Deer T, et al. Randomized clinical trial of an implantable drug delivery system compared with comprehensive medical management for refractory cancer pain: impact on pain, drug-related toxicity, and survival. J Clin Oncol. 2002;20:4040–9.
2. Hawley P, Beddard-Huber E, Grose C, McDonald W, Lobb D, Malysh L. Intrathecal infusions for intractable cancer pain: a qualitative study of the impact on a case series of patients and caregivers. Pain Res Manag. 2009;14:371–9.
3. Patel VB, Manchikanti L, Singh V, Schultz DM, Hayek SM, Smith HS. Systematic review of intrathecal infusion systems for long-term

management of chronic Non-cancer pain. Pain Physician. 2009; 12:345–60.

4. Thimineur MA, Kravitz E, Vodapally MS. Intrathecal opioid treatment for chronic non-malignant pain: a 3-year prospective study. Pain. 2004;109:242–9.

5. Turner JA, Sears JM, Loeser JD. Programmable intrathecal opioid delivery systems for chronic noncancer pain: a systematic review of effectiveness and complications. Clin J Pain. 2007;23: 180–95.

6. Deer TR, Smith HS, Cousins M, et al. Consensus guidelines for the selection and implantation of patients with noncancer pain for intrathecal drug delivery. Pain Physician. 2010;13:E175–213.

7. Wallace MS, Rauck R, Fisher R, Charapata SG, Ellis D, Dissanayake S. Intrathecal ziconotide for severe chronic pain: safety and tolerability results of an open-label, long-term trial. Anesth Analg. 2008;106:628–37.

8. Goucke CR, Dusci LJ, Van Leeuwen S, Fairclough D, Ilett KF. Stability and tolerability of high concentrations of intrathecal bupivacaine and opioid mixtures in chronic noncancer pain: an open-label pilot study. Pain Med. 2010;11:1612–8.

9. Deer TR, Smith HS, Burton AW, et al. Comprehensive consensus based guidelines on intrathecal drug delivery systems in the treatment of pain caused by cancer pain. Pain Physician. 2011;14: E283–312.

10. Deer T, Krames ES, Hassenbusch SJ, et al. Polyanalgesic consensus conference 2007: recommendations for the management of pain by intrathecal (intraspinal) drug delivery: report of an interdisciplinary expert panel. Neuromodulation. 2007;10:300–28.

11. Deer TR, Levy R, Prager J, et al. Polyanalgesic consensus conference: 2012—recommendations on trialing for intrathecal (intraspinal) drug delivery: report of an interdisciplinary expert panel. Neuromodulation. 2012;15:436–64.

12. Horlocker TT, Wedel DJ, Rowlingson JC, et al. Regional anesthesia in the patient receiving antithrombotic or thrombolytic therapy: american society of regional anesthesia and pain medicine evidence-based guidelines (third edition). Reg Anesth Pain Med. 2010;35:64–101.

13. Peck D, Diwan S. Programmable versus fixed-rate pumps for intrathecal drug delivery. In: Deer TR, Diwan S, Buvanendran A, editors. Intrathecal drug delivery for pain and spasticity. Philadelphia: Elsevier/Saunders; 2012. p. 84–9.

14. Deer TR, Levy R, Prager J, et al. Polyanalgesic consensus conference: 2012—recommendations to reduce morbidity and mortality in intrathecal drug delivery in the treatment of chronic pain. Neuromodulation. 2012;15:467–82.

15. Naumann C, Erdine S, Koulousakis A, et al. Drug adverse events and system complications of intrathecal opioid delivery for pain: origins, detection, manifestations, and management. Neuromodulation. 1999;2(2):92–107.

16. Deer TR, Levy R, Prager J, et al. Polyanalgesic consensus conference: 2012—consensus on diagnosis, detection, and treatment of catheter-Tip granulomas (inflammatory masses). Neuromodulation. 2012;15:483–96.

17. Manchikanti L, Falco F. Essentials of practice management, billing, coding and compliance, interventional pain management. Paducah: ASIPP Publishing; 2012.

Joint, Tendon, and Nerve Injections

Karina Gritsenko, Samir Tomajian, Melinda Aquino,
and Alan David Kaye

Introduction

In this chapter, we are briefly covering some commonly used peripheral injections. It is recommended to use other resources to expand your knowledge, as there are numerous injections that may help manage your patients. Prior to proceeding with any injection full medical history, allergies, and full medication list should be overviewed prior to assure no contraindications. Proper sterile technique is recommended on all below injections. Fluoroscopy or ultrasound can aid in precise delivery of injectate in obese or complicated patients and help to avoid sensitive structures.

Knee

Knee Intra-articular Injection

- *Indications:*
  - Knee pain
  - Osteoarthritis

K. Gritsenko, M.D. (✉) • M. Aquino, M.D.
Department of Anesthesiology, Montefiore Medical Center,
Albert Einstein College of Medicine, Bronx, NY, USA

Department of Family and Social Medicine, Montefiore Medical
Center, Albert Einstein College of Medicine, Bronx, NY, USA
e-mail: karina.gritsenko@gmail.com; melindaaquino@aol.com

S. Tomajian, M.D.
Gulfport Memorial Hospital, Gulfport, MS, USA
e-mail: stomajian@gmail.com

A.D. Kaye, M.D., Ph.D.
Department of Anesthesiology, Interim LSU Hospital and Ochsner
Kenner Hospital, New Orleans, LA, USA

Department of Pharmacology, Interim LSU Hospital and Ochsner
Kenner Hospital, New Orleans, LA, USA
e-mail: alankaye44@hotmail.com

- Rheumatoid arthritis
- Gout
- *Injection technique:*
  Two different approaches: *midpatellar and anterior*
  1. **Midpatellar approach**: patient supine with knee extended on a pillow
     - *Lateral approach*: intersection of a line drawn between the lateral and proximal border of the patella (Fig. 47.1), needle inserted between the patella, and the femur at the intersection point directed at a 45° angle toward the middle of the medial side of the joint
     - *Medial approach*: needle entry point from the medial side of the knee under the middle of the patella and aiming to the opposite patellar midpole (Fig. 47.2)
  2. **Anterior approach**:
     - *Infrapatellar* (medial or lateral approach)
       - Patient positioning: seated on the exam table allowing gravity to facilitate opening of the joint space, Knees flexed 60–90°
       - Palpate the joint space opening, mark this with a marking pen or make an impression with a retractable pen
       - Clean with betadine × 3 or chlorhexidine to prep the area of insertion
       - Needle is directed through insertion site either medially or laterally to the joint space opening (Fig. 47.3)
     - *Suprapatellar*
       - Patient supine
       - Best used to drain large infusions
       - Ultrasound approach: patient supine, knee flexed at 20–30°
         High-resolution transducer parallel to the tendon quadriceps femoris, then the transducer is rotated to the axial plane.

K.A. Sackheim, *Pain Management and Palliative Care: A Comprehensive Guide,*
DOI 10.1007/978-1-4939-2462-2_47, © Springer Science+Business Media New York 2015

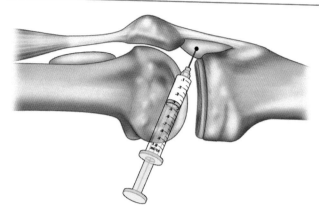

Fig. 47.1 Intra-articular knee injection. Lateral approach. Note that needle is inserted between the patella and the femur at a 45° angle

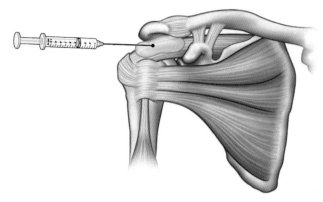

Fig. 47.3 Intra-articular shoulder injection

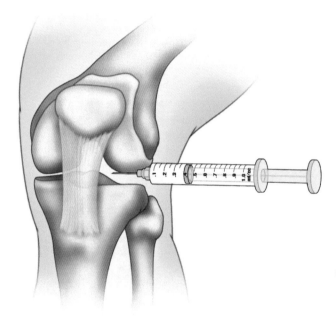

Fig. 47.2 Intra-articular knee injection. Medial approach. Note the needle enters from the medial side of the knee, under the patella, aiming to the opposite patellar mid-pole

Largest dimension of synovial recess should be identified and should be the target of the injection

Using sterile technique, a 22-gauge 3.5 in. needle is advanced into the plane of the suprapatellar recess. 2 mL of iohexol should be injected to determine intra-articular spread. Once confirmed medication should be deposited.

- *Medications:* Depomedrol or Kenalog 40–60 mg with 1–2 cm^3 of 1 % lidocaine and 1–2 cm^3 of 0.25 % bupivacaine mixture total of about 5 cm^3

Shoulder [1]

Posterior Intra-articular Shoulder Injection

- *Indications:*
  - Arthritis of the shoulder joint
  - Shoulder pain
- *Patient positioning:*
  - Supine or seated
  - Arm hanging by patient's side to allow gravity to widen the joint space
- *Injection technique:*
  - Identify the midpoint of the acromion
  - Approximately 1 in. below this midpoint is the shoulder joint space, and the intra-articular space is more lateral
  - Prep the skin overlying the posterior shoulder/subacromial region/joint space opening in sterile fashion
  - A 1½ in 25 g needle is carefully advanced through the skin and subcutaneous tissues through to the joint.
    If bone is encountered: pull back slightly and redirect with slight increased superior or medial tilt to proceed properly through the joint.
    If resistance is encountered: the needle may be in ligament or tendon, it should be advanced properly into the joint space.
- *Medications*: Depomedrol or Kenalog 40–60 mg with 1–2 cm^3 of 1 % lidocaine and 1–2 cm^3 of 0.25 % bupivacaine mixture total of about 5 cm^3

- *Complications*:
  - *Infection*: exceedingly rare with proper sterile technique
  - Transient increase in pain following injection
  - Ecchymosis and hematoma formation: decreased if pressure is placed on the injection site immediately following injection.

Elbow

Epicondyle Injections

Tennis Elbow (Lateral Epicondylitis) [1, 2, 4]

- *Patient positioning*:
  - Patient supine or seated
  - Arm placed on exam table with affected epicondyle exposed, elbow bent
  - Palmar aspect of hand resting on the table or a folded towel to relax the affected tendons.
- *Injection Technique*
  - Identify and mark the lateral epicondyle
  - Prep the skin in sterile fashion
  - Insert a 1 in. 25-gauge needle perpendicularly to the lateral epicondyle into the subcutaneous tissue overlying the affected tendon.
    If bone is encountered: pull back needle slightly before injecting medications
    If resistance is encountered: the needle may be in the tendon and should be withdrawn until the injection proceeds without significant resistance.
- *Medications*: Total mixture of 2–3 mL: 1–2 mL of local anesthetic mixed with 20–40 mg of Depomedrol or Kenalog

Golfer's Elbow (Medial Epicondylitis) [1, 6]

- *Patient positioning*:
  - Patient supine or in seated position
  - Arm fully adducted with effected epicondyle exposed, elbow fully extended
  - Dorsum of the hand resting on the exam table or a folded towel to relax the affected tendons
- *Injection technique*:
  - Identify and mark the medial epicondyle
  - Prep the skin in sterile fashion
  - Insert a 1 in. 25 g needle perpendicularly to the medial epicondyle into the subcutaneous tissue overlying the affected tendon.
    If bone is encountered: pull back needle slightly before injecting medications
    If resistance is encountered: the needle may be in the tendon and should be withdrawn until the injection proceeds without significant resistance.

- *Medications*: Total mixture of 2–3 mL: 1–2 mL of local anesthetic mixed with 20–40 mg of Depomedrol or Kenalog

Epicondyle Injection Complications

- Radial tunnel syndrome (lateral epicondyle injection)
- Ulnar nerve injury at the medial ulnar groove (medial epicondyle injection)
- Bursa injection/irritation
- Rupture/injury of the affected tendons can result from:
  - Direct injection into the tendon which increases risk of tendinitis or tendon rupture
- Infection
- Transient increase in pain following the injection in approximately 25 % of patients

Olecranon Bursitis [7–10]

- *Activities causing this pathology*
  - Direct trauma to the elbow from playing sports such as hockey or falling directly onto the olecranon process.
  - Repeated microtrauma from leaning on the elbow when arising or from working long hours at a drafting table
  - In rare cases, infection such as gout or bacterial infection
- *Patient positioning*:
  - Supine position
  - Arm fully adducted at the patient's side
  - Elbow flexed
  - Palm of the hand resting on the patient's abdomen or exam table
- *Injection technique*:
  - Identify the olecranon process and overlying bursa
  - Prep the skin overlying the posterior aspect of the joint in sterile fashion
  - Insert a 1 in. 25 g needle through the skin and subcutaneous tissues directly into the bursa
    If bone is encountered, the needle is withdrawn into the bursa
- *Medications*: Total of 5 mL: 2 mL of local anesthetic with 40 mg of methylprednisolone or equivalent steroid
- *Complications*: infection, sterile conditions will minimize this potential complication.
- *Pearl*: coexisting tendinitis may require additional treatment

Wrist

Carpal Tunnel Syndrome

- The palmaris longus tendon is bound on dorsal and lateral surfaces by the carpal bones and intercarpal joints
- The carpel tunnel is formed by the carpel bones dorsally and the transverse carpal ligament (aka flexor retinaculum)

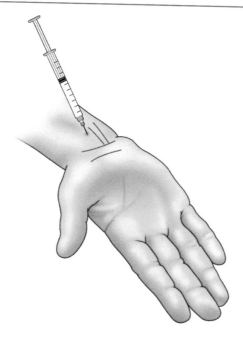

Fig. 47.4 Injection for Carpal Tunnel syndrome. Boundaries of the Carpal Tunnel. Palmaris longus tendon and flexor retinaculum are noted here

ventrally. Tendons of flexor digitorum profundus, sublimus and flexor pollicus longus, and median nerve pass through the carpal tunnel.

- *Patient positioning*: Patient is supine, arm is supinated to expose inner portion of wrist
- *Injection technique*: (Fig. 47.4) The injection is performed at a site just distal to the palmaris longus tendon and at the proximal wrist crease. The needle is inserted at a 30° angle and directed toward the ring finger.
- *Medications*: Local corticosteroid injections into the carpal tunnel may be useful for those with CTS of short duration (less than a year). A solution of 20–40 mg of corticosteroid with 1–2 cm³ of 1 % lidocaine and 1–2 cm³ of 0.25 % bupivacaine or 0.2 % ropivacaine mixture, a total of about 5 cm³, is injected along the transverse carpal ligament.
- *Complications*: Major complication: exceedingly rare if strict aseptic technique is adhered to.

Transient increase in pain following the intra-articular injection ecchymosis and hematoma formation: decreased if pressure is placed on the injection site immediately following injection.

Recommendations

- Always follow sterile technique to avoid infection.
- Instruct patients to avoid vigorous exercises following injection.
- Relative rest and ice is recommended afterwards.
- Osteoarthritis of the shoulder must be distinguished from other causes of shoulder pain including rotator cuff tear pathology to ensure proper treatment regimen.
- Coexisting bursitis and tendinitis may contribute to shoulder pain and require additional localized injection.
- Caution should be used when doing these injections to avoid tendon rupture/injury.

References

1. Waldman SD. Shoulder pain. In: Waldman SD, editor. Atlas of common pain syndromes. Philadelphia: Saunders; 2002.
2. Waldman S. Tennis elbow. In: Waldman S, editor. Pain management. Philadelphia: Saunders/Elsevier; 2007. p. 633–6.
3. Waldman SD. The tennis elbow test. In: Waldman SD, editor. Physical diagnosis of pain: an atlas of signs and symptoms. Philadelphia: Saunders; 2006.
4. Waldman SD. Tennis elbow. In: Waldman SD, editor. Atlas of pain management injection techniques. Philadelphia: Saunders; 2000.
5. Waldman SD. Golfer's elbow. In: Waldman SD, editor. Atlas of common pain syndromes. Philadelphia: Saunders; 2002.
6. Waldman S. Golfer's elbow. In: Waldman S, editor. Pain management. Philadelphia: Saunders/Elsevier; 2007. p. 637–40.
7. Waldman S. Olecranon cubital bursitis. In: Waldman S, editor. Pain management. Philadelphia: Saunders/Elsevier; 2007. p. 641–6.
8. Groff GD. Olecranon bursitis. In: Klippel JH, Dieppe PA, editors. Rheumatology. 2nd ed. London: Mosby; 1998.
9. McAfee JH, Smith DL. Olecranon and prepatellar bursitis: diagnosis and treatment. West J Med. 1988;149:607.
10. Waldman S. Olecranon cubital bursitis. In: Waldman S, editor. Atlas of common pain syndromes. Philadelphia: Saunders/Elsevier; 2007.

Regenerative Injection Therapy

48

Felix S. Linetsky, Andrea M. Trescot,
and Matthias H. Wiederholz

Abbreviations

DMN	Dorsal median nerves
DPG	Dextrose/phenol/glycerin
FDA	Food and Drug Administration
NSAIDs	Nonsteroidal anti-inflammatory drugs
PRP	Platelet-rich plasma injections
PSIS	Posterior superior iliac spine
RIT	Regenerative injection therapy
TRPV	Transient receptor potential vanilloid

Introduction

Among many interventional techniques in current use, **Regenerative Injection therapy** (RIT), also known as **prolotherapy** or **sclerotherapy**, is a viable procedure to treat chronic musculoskeletal pain of connective tissues origin. It was originally employed for the treatment of painful peripheral joint hypermobilities secondary to ligament laxity or enthesopathies but fairly quickly evolved to include the treatment of axial joints pain as well. A common feature found in patients with chronic musculoskeletal pain is tenderness on palpation at certain sites, particularly where ligaments, tendons, or aponeuroses attach to bone.

F.S. Linetsky, M.D. (✉)
Department of Osteopathic Principles and Practice,
Nova Southeastern University of Osteopathic Medicine,
Clearwater, FL, USA
e-mail: DrTrescot@gmail.com; prolopain@aol.com

A.M. Trescot, M.D.
Trescot Pain Fellowship, Pain and Headache Center,
Wasilla, AK, USA
e-mail: DrTrescot@gmail.com

M.H. Wiederholz, M.D.
Performance Spine and Sports Medicine, Lawrenceville, NJ, USA
e-mail: mwiederholz@njspineandsports.net

History

- Since fifth century BC, practitioners have been using regenerative therapy to treat medical conditions. Hippocrates practiced one of the earliest forms of regenerative therapy by cauterizing ligaments to induce thermomodulation of collagen with scar formation and joint stabilization.
  - Hypothesis is that it induced inflammation which leads to tissue self-repair [1, 2]
- 1939—J. H. Kellgren, MD injected small doses of hypertonic saline into the interspinous ligaments and mapped out the pain patterns of distal referral, mimicking radiculopathy (Fig. 48.1) [3].
- 1954—Feinstein et al. [4] repeated the study by Kellgren done 15 years earlier, again using hypertonic saline injections into the interspinous ligament
  - They confirmed the radicular referral patterns of the interspinous ligament from C1–S3 (Fig. 48.2a, b).
  - Also showed that the pattern of pain was independent of the sympathetic system and could refer to an anesthetized area.
  - Stimulation of the trunk interspinous ligament could result in visceral-like pain.
  - In addition, they were able to reproduce "numbness" and "heaviness" in the affected limb with these noxious injections.
- 1956—George Hackett, MD coined the term *Prolotherapy* at the *Fibro-Osseous Junction* [5]
- 1963—Gustav Hemwall, MD
  - Transitioned to hypertonic dextrose as the main proliferant solution [6]

Physiologic Tissue Repair

- *Ligament and tendon structure*
  - **Ligaments** (attach bone to bone) and **tendons** (attach muscles to bone)

K.A. Sackheim, *Pain Management and Palliative Care: A Comprehensive Guide*,
DOI 10.1007/978-1-4939-2462-2_48, © Springer Science+Business Media New York 2015

Fig. 48.1 Pain patterns referred from the interspinous ligament after injection of hypertonic saline in normal volunteers. *Adapted from Kellgren JH. On the distribution of pain arising from deep somatic structures with charts of segmental pain areas. Somatic Pain. 1939: 35–46)* [3, 6]

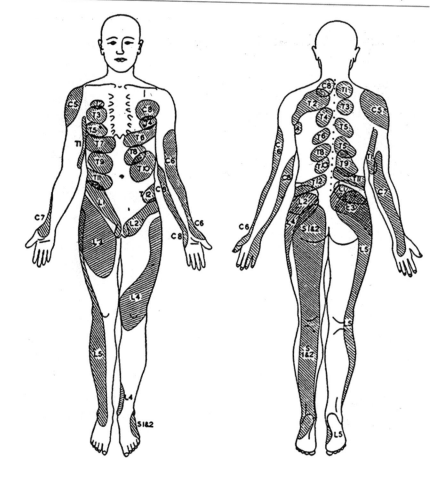

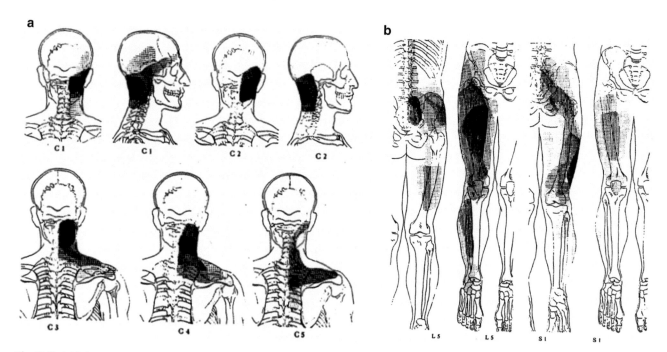

Fig. 48.2 (**a**) Pain patterns from hypertonic saline stimulation by injection of hypertonic saline into the interspinous ligaments of C1 to C5. (**b**) Pain patterns from hypertonic saline stimulation by injection of hypertonic saline into the interspinous ligaments of L5 to S1*Adapted from Feinstein B, Langton JN, Jameson RM, Schiller F. Experiments on pain referred from deep somatic tissues. J Bone Joint Surg 1954;36:981–996)* [4, 7]

- *Ligaments* are parallel bundles of fibers of primarily Type I collagen covered by a more vascular "epiligament" at the bone attachments
  - Collagen ⇒ tropocollagen ⇒ microfibrils ⇒ fascicles ⇒ endoligament ⇒ ligament ⇒ epiligament [7]
  - These fibers unfold during initial collagen loading.
  - After elongation beyond 4 % of the original length, ligaments and tendons lose their elasticity and recoil capability, becoming permanently lax, which leads to joint hypermobility with instability [8].
- *Tendons* have a similar structure but are more like woven cable
- Healing response—three phases [9]
  - *Hemorrhage with inflammation*
    - Increase in neovascularization and neoneurogenesis (Fig. 48.3)
      - Integral components of both the regenerative/reparative and degenerative processes.
      - Nerve and vascular tissue in-growth have been well documented in degenerated intervertebral discs, posterior spinal ligaments, facet joint capsules, and sacroiliac ligaments.
    - *Matrix and cellular proliferation*
      - Hypertrophic fibroblasts create a dense, disorganized collagenous connective tissue matrix
    - *Remodeling and maturation*
      - Alignment of the fibers along the long access of the structure

- Cross-linking of the fibers
- Absorption of the neovascularization
  - Deleteriously affected by
    - Denervation, inactivity, direct corticosteroid injections, NSAIDs
    - Repetitive trauma or microtrauma with insufficient time for recovery, tissue hypoxia, metabolic and hormonal abnormalities, nicotine
- *Enthesopathy*—refers to a disorder of the enthesis (attachments of ligaments and tendons to bone) [10]
  - In acute cases of sprains and torn ligaments, healing takes place by proliferation of fibrous tissue.
  - When the tissues do not heal properly, it results in ligament laxity-induced proliferation of bone and fibrous tissue strengthens the fibro-osseous junction, stabilizing the joint.

Types of Regenerative Injection Therapy

1. *Chemical injectates*
   - Utilizes an inflammatory concentration of lidocaine and dextrose (12.5–25 %)
     - Creates a fibroblastic response, increasing the tensile strength and bony attachment by 50 % (Fig. 48.4)
   - Injection is given into and around the painful area, typically the enthesis (the fibro-osseous junction)

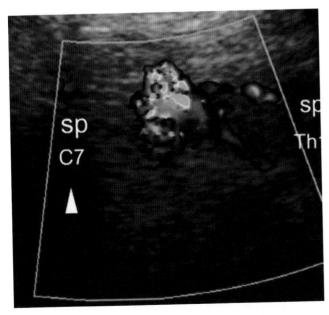

Fig. 48.3 Ultrasound image of the neovascular blood flow at the enthesopathy at C7 after a flexion-extension injury (Image courtesy of Felix Linetsky, MD)

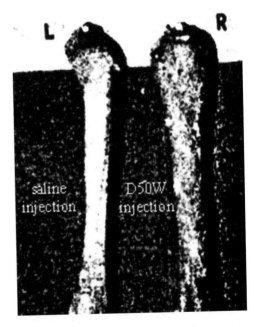

Fig. 48.4 Comparison of rabbit tendons untreated versus injected with D50W proliferant, showing 50 % increase in size, tensile strength, and bone attachment (*Modified from Hackett GS. Ligament & Tendon Relaxation (Skeletal Disability)—Treated by Prolotherapy (Fibro-osseous Proliferation). 3rd ed. Springfield, IL: Charles C. Thomas; 1958)(9) Image courtesy of Felix Linetsky, MD*

- Emphasis is on treating all painful areas and resolving joint instability by treating ligaments and other joint stabilizing structures
- Most treatments are given 4–6 weeks apart to allow for new connective tissue formation
  - Most patients require 3–6 treatments

2. *Subcutaneous neural therapy* (Neurofascial or neural therapy)
   - Involves "mini-injections" of 5 % dextrose in subcutaneous tissue at the level of the peptidergic nerves, which contain transient receptor potential vanilloid receptors (TRPV1 nerves)
     - These nerves are sensitized with trauma, injury, or constriction and represent sites of neurogenic inflammation
       - These nerves maintain the health and renewal of ligaments and tendons
     - Injections are done weekly for 5–10 visits

3. *Prolozone*
   - Utilizes ozone gas and other therapeutic substances to stimulate healing and eliminate pain in injured soft tissues and joints
     - Concentration of ozone is 1–3 %
   - Treatments are done weekly for 3–12 treatments

4. *Platelet-Rich Plasma injections* (PRP)
   - Introduced in 1987 [11] as an autologous transfusion component after an open heart operation to avoid homologous blood product transfusion
     - In the late 1990s, PRP began to be used in many fields (such as orthopedics, dentistry, wound care) to promote tissue healing [11]
   - Clinical indications—similar to RIT
   - Side effects and contraindications—similar to RIT
   - Technique
     - Consists of autologous blood collection, plasma separation (centrifuge), injection of the concentrated platelets
     - Injection releases growth factors (see below) to stimulate recovery in nonhealing soft tissues.
       - Typically given every 1–2 months for 1–6 visits

5. *Stem Cell injection*
   - Clinical indications—similar to RIT
   - Side effects and contraindications—similar to RIT with addition of pain at harvest site and possible carcinogenesis
   - Technique
     - Involves utilization of autologous adult pluripotent mesenchymal stem cells harvested from an individual's bone marrow or adipose tissue for RIT purpose.
     - Typically done for more advanced cases of joint degeneration, including osteochondral defects, or in cases where RIT with dextrose or PRP have not resolved the problem.
     - Usually combined with PRP, which is believed to enhance the healing capabilities and cellular repair.

Injection Solutions

1. *Neurolytic/chemical irritants*—Induce inflammation by altering the surface proteins of cells which causes damage, rendering them susceptible to the immune system
   - Phenol
   - Sarapin

2. *Chemotactic agents*—Directly attract immune cells to the area
   - Sodium morrhuate 5 % –30 mL sodium salts of cod liver oil (on back order for past two years)
   - Sylnasol (5 % solution of sodium salts from psyllium seed oil with 2 % benzyl alcohol) [6]—discontinued after 1962
   - Sodium tetradecyl sulfate (S.T.D. or Sotradecol®)—1 % 2 mL and 3 % 2 mL. No longer produced in multidose vials (very expensive $20 for 2 mL. vial.)
   - Polidocanol (Asclera®)—Polyethylene glycol dodecyl ether (FDA approved for vein sclerosis)

3. *Osmotic agents*—Induce inflammation by altering the surface proteins of cells, which causes damage, rendering them susceptible to the immune system
   - Local anesthetic like 1 % lidocaine diluted with 50 % dextrose provides the following the so-called proliferating concentrations and osmolarities:
     - 4:1 proportion = 10 % dextrose = 555 mOsm/L
     - 3:1 proportion = 12.5 % dextrose = 694 mOsm/L
     - 1:2 proportion = 16.5 % dextrose = 916 mOsm/L
   - Neurolytic concentrations:
     - 3:2 proportion = 20 % dextrose = 1,110 mOsm/L
     - 1:1 proportion = 25 % dextrose = 1,388 mOsm/L
     - 1 % lidocaine diluted with dextrose/phenol/glycerin (DPG):
     - 25 % dextrose, 25 % glycerin, 2.5 % phenol
   - All dilutions are neurolytic:
     - 3:1 proportion = 1,026 mOsm/L; phenol 0.62 %
     - 2:1 proportion = 1,368 mOsm/L; phenol 0.83 %
     - 3:2 proportion = 1,641 mOsm/L; phenol 1 %
     - 1:1 proportion = 2,052 mOsm/L; phenol 1.25 %
       - % dextrose solution, a 1:1 dilution is used
   - Glycerine 10–25 % solution can be used as a single agent or combined with phenol and local anesthetic; lately also used as neural therapy

4. *Particulates*—Attract macrophages that secrete growth factors for tissue healing
   - Medical-grade pumice suspension
   - Talcum

5. *Biologic agents*
   - Platelet-rich plasma
     - Autologous blood
   - Stem cells
     - Requires harvesting of the stem cells
       - Bone marrow derived—iliac crest aspiration
       - Adipose tissue derived—liposuction

Relevant Anatomy

- Arthur Steindler and J.V. Luck [12] published a fundamental work describing the clinical anatomy related to the diagnosis of low back pain based on procaine injections.
    - Posterior divisions of the spinal nerves (the dorsal median nerves or DMN) provide the sensory supply to multiple structures:
        - Ligamentous structures such as supraspinous, interspinous, iliolumbar, sacroiliac, sacrotuberous, and sacrospinous ligaments.
        - Tendon attachments
        - Origins and insertions of the aponeuroses of the tensor fascia lata, gluteal muscles, and thoracolumbar fascia.
    - Steindler and Luck also pointed out that these structures are interrelated anatomically and functionally.
        - They stated that *based on the clinical presentations alone, no definite diagnosis can be made*
            - Five postulated criteria have to be met to prove that causal relationship exists between the structure and pain symptoms:

            Contact with the needle must aggravate the local pain

            Contact with the needle must aggravate or elicit the radiation of pain

            Procaine infiltration must suppress local tenderness

            Procaine infiltration must suppress radiation of pain

            Positive leg signs must disappear

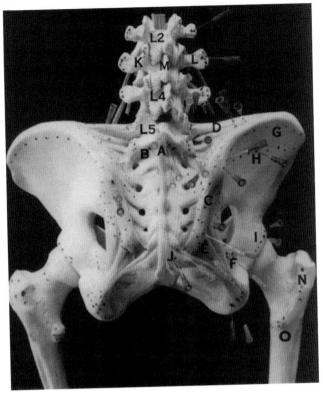

Fig. 48.5 Injection sites for low back pain. Black dots represent injection sites. *A* supraspinatus ligament, *B* interspinous ligament; *C* sacroiliac ligament; *D* iliolumbar ligament; *E* sacrotuberous ligament; *F* sacrospinous ligament; *G* insertion of gluteus maximus; *H* insertion of gluteus medius; *I* acetabular attachments of hip joint capsule; *J* sacrococcygeal ligament; *K* facet joint capsule; *L* thoracolumbar fascia attachment on to transverse process L2 to L5; *M* apex of spinous process attachments of supraspinous ligament and dorsal layer of thoracolumbar fascia; *N* trochanteric attachment of gluteal tendons; *O* lesser trochanter (Image courtesy of Felix Linetsky, MD)

Technique

- It is recommended that physicians interested in RIT train with an RIT expert.
    - Preceptorships are available through the American
    - Academy of Regenerative Orthopedic Medicine (www.aarom.org)
    - Textbooks on the subject are also available (see Suggested Reading).
- Example: Low back pain (Fig. 48.5)
    - Identify the areas of tenderness by palpation; if not comfortable with palpatory approach further confirm areas of injection with ultrasound or fluoroscopy (Fig. 48.6)

    Spinous processes

    PSIS

    Iliolumbar ligament

    Facets

    Sacrotuberous ligament (proximal and distal)

    - Injection at the fibro-osseous junction

    Needle *must* touch bone

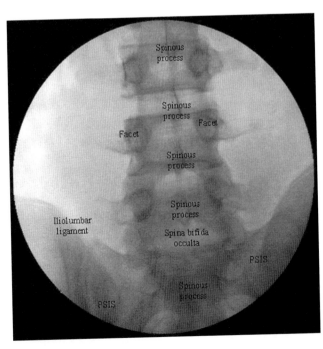

Fig. 48.6 Fluoroscopic landmarks for injections (image courtesy of Andrea Trescot, MD)

Fig. 48.7 General injection sites. Schematic drawing demonstrating sites of tendon origins and insertions, (enthesis) of the paravertebral musculature in the cervical, thoracic, lumbar, and pelvic regions with parts of the upper and lower extremities. Clinically significant enthesopathies with small fiber neuropathies and neuralgias are common at the locations identified by dots. Dots also represent most common locations of needle insertion and RIT injections. (Note: not all of the locations are treated in each patient). *Modified from Sinelnikov Atlas of Anatomy, Volume 1, Meditsina, Moskow, 1972 by Tracey James. All rights reserved. No part of this picture may be reproduced or transmitted in any form or by any means without written permission from Felix Linetsky MD*

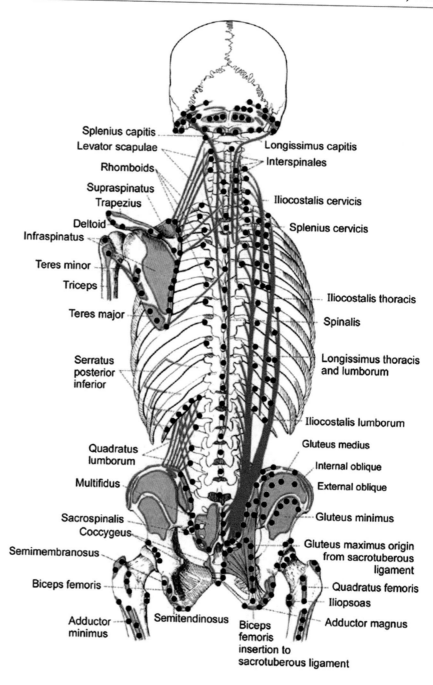

- Inject small amounts (usually 0.5–1 mL at each needle insertion or reinsertion) of the injectate; total volume depends on the number of sites injected, but total volume should be under 20 cm³ to limit local anesthetic toxicity
- Advances of diagnostic ultrasound allow precise placements of injectates at the sites of soft tissue pathology specifically fibromuscular interface, into the ligaments or tendons, large or small joints or their components
- The technique is applicable "from the head to the toes" (Fig. 48.7)

Clinical Indications

- Osteoarthritis, spondylolysis and spondylolisthesis
- Painful enthesopathies, tendinosis, or ligamentosis secondary to sprains or strains from overuse, occupational and postural conditions known as Repetitive Motion Disorders
- Painful hypermobility, instability, and subluxations of the axial joints secondary to ligament laxity accompanied by restricted range of motion at reciprocal segment(s) that improve temporarily with manipulation

- Posterior column sources of nociception refractory to steroid injections, nonsteroidal anti-inflammatory therapy (NSAID), and radiofrequency procedures
- Postsurgical cervical, thoracic, and low back pain (with or without instrumentation)
- Recurrent painful rib subluxations at the costotransverse, costovertebral, and sternochondral articulations
- Vertebral compression fractures with a wedge deformity that exert additional stress on the posterior ligamento-tendinous complex

Side Effects and Contraindications

- Main side effects are due to needle trauma and inadvertent needle placement
  - Pain
  - Stiffness
  - Bleeding
  - Bruising
  - Soreness
  - Swelling
- Serious risks are very rare but may include:
  - Nerve, ligament, tendon injury
  - Spinal headache
  - Pneumothorax
  - Nerve damage
  - Spinal cord injury
  - Disc injury
  - Infection
- Allergic or anaphylactic reactions to the proliferants may also occur
  - For instance, sodium morrhuate is a fish oil product and should be avoided in persons with a fish allergy
- Regenerative injection therapy to the spine carries similar risk as any spinal injection
  - Spinal cord injury
  - Death
  - *No injections should be done by untrained practitioners*

Billing

- There is no code for PRP or stem cell injections
- Because of misinterpreted studies, regenerative injection therapy is considered "experimental" and therefore not covered by insurance

References

1. Dorman TA. Diagnosis and injection techniques in orthopedic medicine. Baltimore: Williams and Wilkins; 1991.
2. Gedney EH. Special technic hypermobile joint: a preliminary report. Osteopath Profession. 1937;9:30–1.
3. Kellgren JH. On the distribution of pain arising from deep somatic structures with charts of segmental pain areas. Clin Sci. 1939;4:35–46.
4. Feinstein B, Langton JN, Jameson RM, Schiller F. Experiments on pain referred from deep somatic tissues. J Bone Joint Surg. 1954;36:981–96.
5. Hackett GS. Joint ligament relaxation treated by fibro-osseous proliferation. 1st ed. Springfield: Charles C. Thomas; 1956.
6. Kayfetz DO, Blumenthal LS, Hackett GS, Hemwall GA, Neff FE. Whiplash injury and other ligamentous headache–its management with prolotherapy. Headache. 1963;3:21–8.
7. Ravin TH. Tensegrity to tendonitis. Prolotherapy lecture series. Denver: American Academy of Musculoskeletal Medicine; 2012.
8. Frank CB. Ligament structure, physiology and function. J Musculoskelet Neuronal Interact. 2004;4(2):199–201.
9. Hackett GS. Ligament & tendon relaxation (skeletal disability)—treated by prolotherapy (fibro-osseous proliferation). 3rd ed. Springfield: Charles C. Thomas; 1958.
10. Weaver A, Keystone E, Mease PJ, Ritchlin CT. New applications for TNF inhibition 2000 [31/1/13]. Available from: http://www.medscape.org/viewarticle/418418_2.
11. Ferrari M, Zia S, Valbonesi M, Henriquet F, Venere G, Spagnolo S, et al. A new technique for hemodilution, preparation of autologous platelet-rich plasma and intraoperative blood salvage in cardiac surgery. Int J Artif Organs. 1987;10(1):47–50.
12. Steindler A, Luck JV. Differential diagnosis of pain low in the back; allocation of the source of pain by the procaine hydrochloride method. JAMA. 1938;110:106–13.

Suggested Reading

Ravin TH, Cantieri MS, Pasquarello GJ. Review of principles of prolotherapy. Denver: American Academy of Musculoskeletal Medicine; 2008.
Hauser R, Maddela HS, Alderman D, et al. International medical editorial board consensus statement on the use of prolotherapy for musculoskeletal pain. J Prolother. 2011;3(4):745–64.
Gordin K. Comprehensive scientific overview on the use of platelet rich plasma prolotherapy (PRPP). J Prolother. 2011;3(4):813–25.
Alderman DD, Alexander RW, Harris GR, Astourian PC. Stem cell prolotherapy in regenerative medicine: background, theory and protocols. J Prolother. 2011;3(3):689–708.
The following are available at www.AAROM.org
Linetsky F, Botwin K, Gorfine L, Miguel R, Ray A, Trescot A, et al. Position paper of the Florida academy of pain medicine on regenerative injection therapy: effectiveness and appropriate usage. Pain Clin. 2002;4(3):38–45.
Linetsky F, Derby R, Parris W, et al. Regenerative injection therapy (chapter 35). In: Manchikanti L, Slipman CW, Fellows B, editors. Low back pain: an interventional approach to diagnosis and treatment. Paducah: ASIPP Publishing; 2002.
Linetsky F, Miguel R, Torres F. Treatment of cervicothoracic pain and cervicogenic headaches with regenerative injection therapy. Curr Pain Headache Rep. 2004;8(1):41–8.
Linetsky F, Trescot A, Manchikanti L. Regenerative injection therapy (chapter 9). In: Manchikanti L, Singh V, editors. Interventional techniques in chronic non-spinal pain. Paducah: ASIPP Publishing; 2009. p. 87–98.
Linetsky F, Alfredson H, Crane D, Centeno C. (2013) Treatment of chronic painful musculoskeletal injuries and disease with regenerative injection therapy (RIT): Regenerative injection therapy, principles and practice (Chapter 81). In: Deer TR (ed.) Comprehensive treatment of chronic pain by medical intervention, and integrative approaches. pp.889–912

Index

K.A. Sackheim, *Pain Management and Palliative Care: A Comprehensive Guide*,
DOI 10.1007/978-1-4939-2462-2, © Springer Science+Business Media New York 2015

Made in the USA
Charleston, SC
12 July 2016